Kostoris Library Christie
R02683X4988

D1765136

Stem Cell Transplantation for Hematologic Malignancies

Contemporary Hematology

Gary J. Schiller, MD, Series Editor

Stem Cell Transplantation for Hematologic Malignancies, edited by *Robert J. Soiffer,* 2004

Chronic Lymphocytic Leukemia: *Molecular Genetics, Biology, Diagnosis, and Management,* by *Guy B. Faguet,* 2004

Biologic Therapy of Leukemia, edited by *Matt Kalaycio,* 2003

Modern Hematology: *Biology and Clinical Management,* by *Reinhold Munker, Erhard Hiller, and Ronald Paquette,* 2000

Red Cell Transfusion: *A Practical Guide,* edited by *Marion E. Reid and Sandra J. Nance,* 1998

Stem Cell Transplantation for Hematologic Malignancies

Edited by

Robert J. Soiffer, MD

Dana-Farber Cancer Institute
Harvard Medical School, Boston, MA

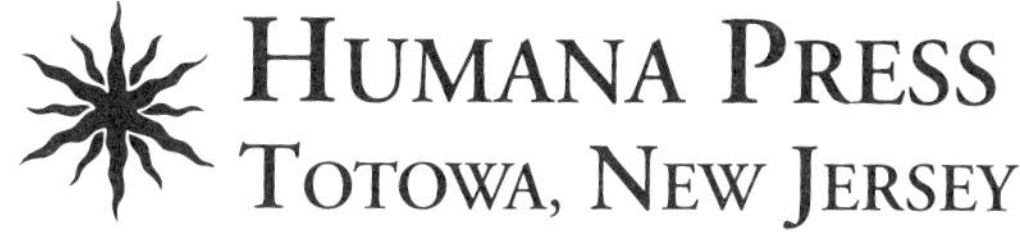

Humana Press
Totowa, New Jersey

999 Riverview Drive, Suite 208
Totowa, New Jersey 07512

humanapress.com

For additional copies, pricing for bulk purchases, and/or information about other Humana titles, contact Humana at the above address or at any of the following numbers: Tel: 973-256-1699; Fax: 973-256-8341; E-mail: humana@humanapr.com; website at humanapress.com

All articles, comments, opinions, conclusions, or recommendations are those of the author(s), and do not necessarily reflect the views of the publisher.

Due diligence has been taken by the publishers, editors, and authors of this book to ensure the accuracy of the information published and to describe generally accepted practices. The contributors herein have carefully checked to ensure that the drug selections and dosages set forth in this text are accurate in accord with the standards accepted at the time of publication. Notwithstanding, as new research, changes in government regulations, and knowledge from clinical experience relating to drug therapy and drug reactions constantly occurs, the reader is advised to check the product information provided by the manufacturer of each drug for any change in dosages or for additional warnings and contraindications. This is of utmost importance when the recommended drug herein is a new or infrequently used drug. It is the responsibility of the health care provider to ascertain the Food and Drug Administration status of each drug or device used in their clinical practice. The publisher, editors, and authors are not responsible for errors or omissions or for any consequences from the application of the information presented in this book and make no warranty, express or implied, with respect to the contents in this publication.

This publication is printed on acid-free paper. ◯
ANSI Z39.48-1984 (American National Standards Institute)
Permanence of Paper for Printed Library Materials.

Production Editor: Robin B. Weisberg.

Cover Illustration: From Fig. 1A and B in Chapter 13, "Hepatic Veno-Occlusive Disease," by Paul G. Richardson.

Cover design by Patricia F. Cleary.

Printed in the United States of America. 10 9 8 7 6 5 4 3 2 1

1-59259-733-5 (e-book)

Library of Congress Cataloging-in-Publication Data

Stem cell transplantation for hematologic malignancies / edited by Robert J. Soiffer.
p. ; cm. -- (Contemporary hematology)
Includes bibliographical references and index.
ISBN 1-58829-180-4 (alk. paper)
1. Hematopoietic stem cells--Transplantation. 2. Lymphomas --Treatment. 3. Multiple myeloma--Treatment. 4. Leukemia --Treatment. I. Soiffer, Robert J. II. Series.
[DNLM: 1. Leukemia--therapy. 2. Hematopoietic Stem Cell Transplantation. 3. Lymphoma--therapy. WH 250 S824 2004]
RC271.H45S74 2004
617.4'4--dc21

2003013960

Preface

Transplantation of human hematopoietic progenitor cells in the treatment of malignant disease has been under clinical investigation since the 1980s. During this time, indications for transplantation have been expanded considerably, and clinical outcomes have steadily improved. Yet, formidable obstacles remain. Identification of the ideal donor, prevention of transplant-related complications (e.g., organ damage, infection, graft-vs-host disease [GVHD]), and permanent eradication of the underlying malignancy are critical for success, and sadly remain elusive in many circumstances.

Fundamental notions about transplantation have changed over the past several years. No longer are patients who seek transplantation limited by the availability of a human leukocyte antigen-identical sibling. Advances in immune suppression and T-cell depletion have permitted transplantation of stem cells from haploidentical relatives or from unrelated donors. As well, it is now clear that not all allogeneic transplant recipients need to receive high doses of chemo/radiotherapy for disease control or for prevention of graft rejection. Transplantation utilizing nonmyeloablative doses of conditioning, so-called "mini-transplants," takes advantage of the recognized capacity of graft-vs-leukemia reactions to eliminate disease. Even the term bone marrow transplant is becoming increasingly outdated as mobilized peripheral blood or umbilical cord blood, rather than bone marrow, is used frequently as a stem cell source.

Stem Cell Transplantation for Hematologic Malignancies should provide students, physicians, and other health care professionals with a clear vision of the current state-of-the-art in hematopoietic stem cell transplantation for malignant disease. The first part of the book focuses on indications and results of transplantation for acute leukemias, chronic myelogenous leukemia, lymphoma, multiple myeloma, and breast cancer, providing insight into the relative merits of transplant and nontransplant approaches to these disorders. Part II examines transplant-related complications including the pathophysiology and clinical consequences of acute and chronic GVHD, delayed immune reconstitution leading to infectious complications, and organ damage to the lung and liver. Transplant-related complications do not always lead to death and their impact on survivors' quality of life is also presented.

Part III concentrates on the graft itself. Stem cell and donor source is addressed in chapters on peripheral blood stem cell transplants, unrelated and haploidentical donor transplants, and umbilical cord transplants. The effects of graft manipulation to eliminate residual contaminating tumors cells in autologous transplantation or to reduce the number of T lymphocytes causing GVHD in allogeneic transplantation is then discussed. Finally, the role of donor lymphocyte infusions in the treatment and prevention of relapse after stem cell transplantation and its influence on the development of nonmyeloablative transplantation are addressed in the final two chapters. It is our hope that *Stem Cell Transplantation for Hematologic Malignancies* will not only serve as a comprehensive review of past and current experience surrounding transplantation for malignant disease, but also provide a vision into the advances anticipated over the next several years.

Acknowledgments

I would like to thank my family for their unselfish support for all my academic endeavors. I would also like to thank Gail Delaney for her technical assistance in preparing this book.

Robert J. Soiffer, MD

Contents

PART III. SOURCES OF DONOR STEM CELLS

PART IV. GRAFT ENGINEERING

PART V. GRAFT-VS-TUMOR EFFECT

Contributors

Edwin P. Alyea III, MD • *Division of Hematologic Malignancies, Dana-Farber Cancer Institute, Harvard Medical School, Boston, MA*
Kenneth C. Anderson, MD • *Division of Hematologic Neoplasia, Dana-Farber Cancer Institute, Harvard Medical School, Boston, MA*
Joseph H. Antin, MD • *Division of Hematologic Malignancies, Dana-Farber Cancer Institute, Harvard Medical School, Boston, MA*
Lindsey Baden, MD • *Division of Infectious Diseases, Brigham and Women's Hospital, Harvard Medical School, Boston, MA*
Humberto Caldera, MD • *Department of Medicine, University of Texas M.D. Anderson Cancer Center, Houston, TX*
Nelson J. Chao, MD • *Department of Medicine, Duke University Medical Center, Durham, NC*
Sandra Cohen, MD • *Division of Hematology and Bone Marrow Transplantation, City of Hope Comprehensive Cancer Center, Duarte, CA*
Kenneth R. Cooke, MD • *Division of Hematology/Oncology, Department of Pediatrics, Comprehensive Cancer Center, University of Michigan, Ann Arbor, MI*
Corey Cutler, MD, MPH, FRCPC • *Division of Hematologic Malignancies, Dana-Farber Cancer Institute, Harvard Medical School, Boston, MA*
Faith E. Davies, MD • *Division of Hematologic Neoplasia, Dana-Farber Cancer Institute, Harvard Medical School, Boston, MA*
H. Joachim Deeg, MD • *Division of Clinical Research, Fred Hutchinson Cancer Research Center, University of Washington School of Medicine, Seattle, WA*
Lyle C. Feinstein, MD • *Transplantation Biology Program, Clinical Research Division, Fred Hutchinson Cancer Research Center, University of Washington School of Medicine, Seattle, WA*
James L. M. Ferrara, MD • *Departments of Internal Medicine and Pediatrics, Comprehensive Cancer Center, University of Michigan, Ann Arbor, MI*
Stephen J. Forman, MD • *Hematologic Neoplasia Program, City of Hope Comprehensive Cancer Center, Duarte, CA*
Sergio Giralt, MD • *Department of Medicine, University of Texas M.D. Anderson Cancer Center, Houston, TX*
Timothy F. Goggins, MD • *Department of Medicine, Duke University Medical Center, Durham, NC*
Stephen Gottschalk, MD • *Department of Pediatrics, Center for Cell and Gene Therapy, Texas Children's Cancer Center, Baylor College of Medicine, Houston, TX*
John G. Gribben, MD, DSc • *Division of Hematologic Neoplasia, Dana-Farber Cancer Institute, Harvard Medical School, Boston, MA*
P. Jean Henslee-Downey, MD • *Division of Blood Diseases and Resources, National Heart, Lung and Blood Institute, National Institutes of Health, Bethesda, MD; and South Carolina Cancer Center, University of South Carolina, Columbia, SC*
Helen E. Heslop, MD • *Departments of Medicine and Pediatrics, Center for Cell and Gene Therapy, Baylor College of Medicine, Houston, TX*

VINCENT HO, MD • *Division of Hematologic Malignancies, Dana-Farber Cancer Institute, Harvard Medical School, Boston, MA*

CAROLYN A. KEEVER-TAYLOR, PhD • *Department of Medicine, Division of Neoplastic Diseases and Related Disorders, Blood and Bone Marrow Transplantation Program, Medical College of Wisconsin, Milwaukee, WI*

THOMAS J. KENNEY, MD • *Division of Medical Oncology, University of Colorado Health Sciences Center, Denver, CO*

STEPHANIE J. LEE, MD, MPH • *Division of Population Science, Dana-Farber Cancer Institute, Harvard Medical School, Boston, MA*

COLLEEN H. MCDONOUGH, MD • *The Sidney Kimmel Comprehensive Cancer Center, Johns Hopkins University, Baltimore, MD*

YAGO NIETO, MD • *Bone Marrow Transplant Program, University of Colorado Health Sciences Center, Denver, CO*

UWE PLATZBECKER, MD • *Division of Clinical Research, Fred Hutchinson Cancer Research Center, University of Washington School of Medicine, Seattle, WA*

PAUL G. RICHARDSON, MD • *Division of Hematologic Malignancies, Dana-Farber Cancer Institute, Harvard Medical School, Boston, MA*

CLIONA M. ROONEY, PhD • *Departments of Molecular Urology and Microbiology and Pediatrics, Center for Cell and Gene Therapy, Baylor College of Medicine, Houston, TX*

ROBERT H. RUBIN, MD, FACP, FCCP • *Division of Infectious Diseases, Brigham and Women's Hospital, Harvard Medical School, Boston, MA*

BRENDA M. SANDMAIER, MD • *Transplantation Biology Program, Division of Clinical Research, Fred Hutchinson Cancer Research Center, University of Washington School of Medicine, Seattle, WA*

ELIZABETH J. SHPALL, MD • *Department of Blood and Marrow Transplantation, University of Texas M.D. Anderson Cancer Center, Houston, TX*

ROBERT J. SOIFFER, MD • *Division of Hematologic Malignancies, Dana-Farber Cancer Institute, Harvard Medical School, Boston, MA*

JOHN W. SWEETENHAM, MD • *Division of Medical Oncology, University of Colorado Health Sciences Center, Denver, CO*

TAKANORI TESHIMA, MD, PhD • *Department of Internal Medicine, Comprehensive Cancer Center, University of Michigan, Ann Arbor, MI*

GEORGIA B. VOGELSANG, MD • *The Sidney Kimmel Comprehensive Cancer Center, Johns Hopkins University, Baltimore, MD*

DANIEL WEISDORF, MD • *Division of Hematology, Oncology, and Transplantation, University of Minnesota, Minneapolis, MN*

Part I

Transplant for Malignant Disease

1 Allogeneic and Autologous Stem Cell Transplantation for Acute Leukemia and Myelodysplasia in the Adult

Sandra Cohen, MD *and Stephen J. Forman,* MD

Contents

1. ALLOGENEIC TRANSPLANTATION FOR ACUTE LYMPHOBLASTIC LEUKEMIA

1.1. Introduction

Acute lymphoblastic leukemia (ALL) is characterized by clonal proliferation, accumulation, and tissue infiltration of immature lymphoid cells of the bone marrow. Although ALL accounts for approx 80% of childhood leukemias in the United States, a second peak occurs around age 50 and there is an increase in incidence with increasing age. Age greater than 60 yr, leukocyte count greater than 30,000, non-T-cell phenotype, lack of mediastinal adenopathy, poor performance status at diagnosis, Philadelphia chromosome (Ph)+ at cytogenetic analysis, as well as the finding of other chromosomal translocations such as t(4;11), t(1;19), or t(8;14) all predict for a poor outcome even with aggressive chemotherapy. Those patients requiring more than 4 wk of induction therapy to achieve remission also have a poorer prognosis *(1–4)*.

1.2. Cytogenetics in ALL

Cytogenetic abnormalities found in patients with ALL can be powerful predictors of treatment outcome. In many instances, results of cytogenetic studies can help to direct treatment, highlighting where more aggressive treatment, such as allogeneic transplantation, should be

From: *Stem Cell Transplantation for Hematologic Malignancies*
Edited by: R. J. Soiffer © Humana Press Inc., Totowa, NJ

strongly considered. Chromosomal changes are found in 60–85% of all cases of ALL *(5,6)*. Numerical chromosome abnormalities, either alone or in association with structural changes, are found in about half of ALL cases. Although more than 30 distinct nonrandomly occurring rearrangements are presently known in ALL, a few particular cytogenetic anomalies are significantly more common than others and determine the prognosis for the patient. The Third International Workshop on Chromosomes in Leukemia (TIWCL) identified several significant differences between groups of patients, based on results of cytogenetic studies. Translocations t(8;14), t(4;11), and 14q+ correlate with a higher risk of central nervous system (CNS) involvement, whereas t(4;11) and t(9;22) were associated with higher leukocyte and blast counts and risk for relapse.

The most common cytogenetic abnormality in adult ALL is the Ph chromosome. Occurring most commonly in chronic myelogenous leukemia (CML), the Ph chromosome brings into juxtaposition the tyrosine kinase *c-abl* on chromosome 9 with the major breakpoint cluster region (m-bcr) on chromosome 22. The Ph+ chromosome appears in about 95% of patients with CML, in about 1–2% of patients with acute myelogenous leukemia (AML), as well as in up to 5% of children and 15–30% of adults with ALL *(7)*. In contrast to CML, in which patients with the bcr-abl hybrid protein almost always measures 210 kd (the p210 protein), about half of patients with ALL and the Ph+ chromosome have a 190-kd protein (p195) (see below).

Currently, the overall disease-free survival for adult patients with ALL is 35%, with those patients with T-cell ALL having the better treatment outcomes compared to all other subtypes of ALL in the adult *(8–12)*.

As with any other hematologic malignancy, the decision of whether and when to proceed to allogeneic transplant is often dictated by prognostic features identified at diagnosis. Initial treatment of adult patients with ALL has evolved over the past few decades, with a dramatic increase in intensity of treatment and with the addition of consolidation and maintenance arms of treatment. Overall, complete remission (CR) rates have risen to as high as 80–90% of those patients under the age of 60 *(13)*. However, the higher-dose regimens do select for disease that is more chemotherapy resistant when relapses do occur. Second remissions occur with lower frequency than in previous years and, when achieved, tend to be shorter lasting.

1.3. Allogeneic Transplantation in First Complete Remission

Allogeneic transplantation in first complete remission (CR1) is generally reserved for those patients who present with poor risk features, such as those described earlier. In several Phase II studies, patients with high-risk disease treated with allogeneic transplantation had a disease-free survival (DSF) longer than would have been predicted. Depending on the risk factors present at diagnosis in an individual patient, continued remissions range from less than 10% to more than 50%. Studies that have been conducted indicate that bone marrow transplantation (BMT) offers some groups of such patients long-term disease survival rates of between 40% and 60% *(13)*. At the City of Hope and Stanford, a series of 149 patients with high-risk features were transplanted in CR1. Selection criteria included white blood cells (WBC) higher than 25,000, chromosomal translocations t(9;22), t(4;11), and t(8;14), age older than 30, extramedullary disease at the time of diagnosis, and/or requiring more than 4 wk to achieve a CR. Two-thirds of the patients had at least one risk factor and the remaining patients had two or more high-risk features at presentation. The majority of these patients underwent hematopoietic cell transplantation (HCT) in the first 4 mo after achieving a CR. HCT during first remission led

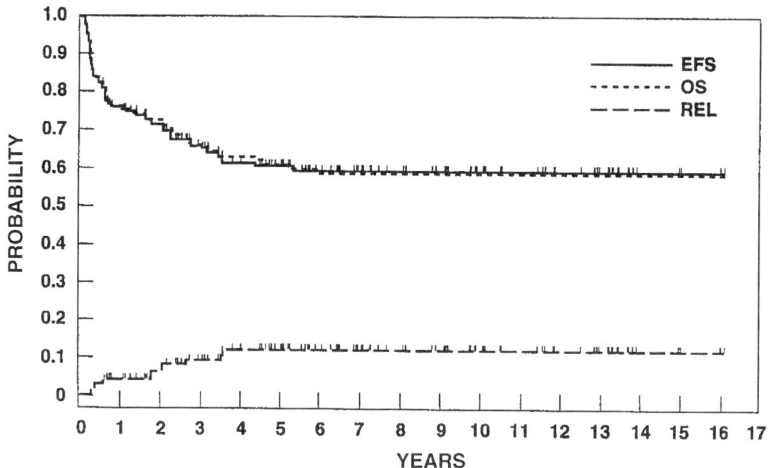

Fig. 1. Probability of event-free survival (EFS), overall survival (OS), and relapse for 149 adult patients with high-risk ALL. (Updated from ref. *15* with permission.)

to prolonged DFS in this patient population who would otherwise have been expected to fare poorly. At a median follow-up of greater than 5 yr, the actual DFS was 61%, with a relapse rate of 10% *(14,15)* (*see* Fig. 1).

The French Group on Therapy for Adult ALL conducted a retrospective study comparing chemotherapy to autologous stem cell transplantation (autoSCT) and allogeneic BMT (alloBMT). Although the overall results of treatment did not show a treatment advantage for the alloBMT group, subgroup analysis revealed that those patients with high-risk disease had a higher 5-yr survival of 44% as opposed to 20% in the other two groups.

1.4. Philadelphia Chromosome-Positive ALL

Because of the poor prognosis associated with Ph+ ALL, allogeneic transplant is generally pursued during CR1, as long as there are no absolute medical contraindications to BMT. A recent report updated this experience on 23 patients with Ph+ ALL transplanted from human leukocyte antigen (HLA)-identical siblings while in CR1 between 1984 and 1997. All but one patient were conditioned with fractionated-dose total-body irradiation (FTBI) (1320 cGy) and high-dose etoposide. The 3-yr probability of DFS and relapse were 65% and 12%, respectively. The subset of patients transplanted after 1992 had a DFS of 81% with a relapse rate of 11%, and it is speculated that these patients may have benefited from improvements in supportive care *(16)*.

Volunteer matched unrelated donors (MUD) are used when no suitable sibling donors can be found. A report from Seattle reported results for MUD BMT for 18 patients with Ph+ ALL who underwent transplantation at that center and who lacked a suitable family donor. The median patient age was 25 yr. Seven patients were in CR1, one was in second remission, three were in first relapse, and the remaining seven had more advanced or chemotherapy refractory leukemia at transplant. All patients were conditioned with cyclophosphamide and total-body irradiation followed by marrow transplants from closely HLA-matched, unrelated volunteers. Graft failure was not observed. Five patients had recurrent ALL after transplantation and another four died from causes other than leukemia. Six patients transplanted in CR1, two in first relapse, and one in second remission remain alive and leukemia-free at a median follow-up of 17 mo (range: 9–73 mo). The probability of leukemia-free survival at 2 yr is 49% *(17)*.

Of additional interest are the follow-up of patients with Ph+ ALL and the impact of the detection of minimal residual disease (MRD) after allogeneic transplant. Radich et al. reviewed the transplants of 36 patients with Ph+ ALL. Seventeen were transplanted in relapse and 19 were transplanted in remission. Twenty-three patients had at least one positive bcr-abl polymerase chain reaction (PCR) assay after BMT either before a relapse or without subsequent relapse. Ten of these 23 relapsed after a positive assay at a median time from the first positive PCR assay of 94 d (range: 28–416 d). By comparison, only 2 relapses occurred in the 13 patients with no prior positive PCR assays. The unadjusted relative risk (RR) of relapse associated with a positive PCR assay compared with a negative assay was 5.7.

The data from Radich et al. also suggest that the type of bcr-abl chimeric mRNA detected posttransplant was associated with the risk of relapse: 7 of 10 patients expressing the p190 bcr-abl relapsed, compared with 1 of 8 who expressed only the p210 bcr-abl mRNA. The RR of p190 bcr-abl positivity compared to PCR-negative patients was 11.2, whereas a positive test for p210 bcr-abl was apparently not associated with an increased relative risk. The finding that the expression of p190 bcr-abl may portend an especially high risk of relapse suggests a different clinical and biologic behavior between p190 and p210 bcr-abl *(18)*.

1.5. Relapsed or Refractory ALL

Acute lymphoblastic leukemia (ALL) is refractory to primary chemotherapy in approx 10–15% of patients. Of all those patients who do achieve a CR1 to primary therapy (65–85%), approx 60–70% will relapse. Relapsed ALL in an adult is rarely curable, but remissions are sometimes achieved with reinduction with either a standard vincristine, prednisone, and anthracycline or a cytarabine-based regimen, particularly high-dose Ara-C (HDAC) combined with an anthracycline *(19–23)*. Available data from the Interantional Bone Marrow Transplant Registry (IBMTR) shows that patients transplanted from an HLA-identical sibling for ALL in second CR (CR2) have approx a 35–40% chance of long-term DFS, whereas those transplanted with disease not in remission have a leukemia-free survival (LFS) of only 10–20%.

1.6. Unrelated BMT for ALL

Historically, the outcome after transplantation from unrelated donors has been inferior to that observed after matched-sibling transplantation because of increased rates of graft rejection and graft-vs-host disease (GVHD) resulting from increased alloreactivity in this setting. The IBMTR reports a DFS of 44% for patients receiving unrelated donor transplantations for ALL in CR1 and 33% in CR2. The National Marrow Donor Program (NMDP) reports 5-yr DFS of 35% in CR1 in adults and 46% in children, decreasing to 25% and 40%, respectively, in CR2. Over the past few years, improved results have been reported from several single-center studies, particularly in pediatric patients, reflecting improvements in donor/recipient matching, GVHD prophylaxis, and supportive care *(24–27)*. In addition, an NMDP study showed that younger donor and recipient age were associated with significantly improved outcome *(28)*.

1.7. Impact of GVL on Recurrence of ALL

Unlike patients with CML, or even AML, studies of patients with ALL who have relapsed after alloBMT have demonstrated a limited response to discontinuation of immunosuppression or to donor leukocyte infusions *(29)*. This has led some to question the existence of a therapeu-

Table 1
Relapse After Transplantation for ALL in CR1

Group	*Relapse probability at 3 yr (%)*
Allogeneic, non-T-cell-depleted	
No GVHD	44 ± 17
Acute only	17 ± 9
Chronic only	20 ± 19
Both	15 ± 10
Syngeneic	41 ± 32
Allogeneic, T-cell-depleted	34 ± 13

tic graft-vs-leukemia (GVL) effect in ALL. A comparative review of patients who underwent alloBMT for ALL suggests that patients with ALL who have had GVHD have a lower relapse rate than do patients who lack the effect (Table 1).

2. AUTOLOGOUS HEMATOPOIETIC CELL TRANSPLANTATION FOR ADULT ALL

There is much less experience with autologous transplantation for ALL and studies have been focused primarily on those patients in either first or second remission who lacked a sibling or allogeneic donor. Some studies have utilized the same criteria for autologous transplantation as has been utilized for allogeneic transplantation based on the idea that the preparative regimen does contribute to the cure of ALL because the allogeneic effect is less potent than in myeloid malignancy. Several groups have reported outcomes for large series of adults with ALL undergoing autologous hematopoietic transplantation in CR1 *(30–36)*. One study from France reported on 233 such patients with long-term DFS at 41% *(37)*. The most important prognostic factor was the interval between achieving a CR and proceeding to transplant, with those patients being transplanted later having the better DFS. This effect may represent the dropout of high-risk patients who relapse before transplantation or possibly the effect of consolidation therapy in reducing tumor burden administered prior to HCT. The European Cooperative Group report on more than 1000 patients indicated an LFS of 36%, whereas the IBMTR reported a similar plateau at 40% *(30)*.

One randomized trial showed a comparison between outcome of adults with ALL in first remission treated with chemotherapy vs autologous transplantation. The French LALA 87 trial allocated patients under 40 with HLA-matched siblings to transplantation and the remaining patients received consolidation treatment with modest-dose chemotherapy or an autologous transplant *(31)*. There was a significant dropout rate in the autologous arm because of early relapse, and the long-term follow-up showed no significant difference in overall survival between the two groups: 34% for autologous BMT and 29% for chemotherapy. This difference applied to both the standard-risk or high-risk group. This trial has been very influential, as it represents the only randomized trial of the use of autologous transplantation in ALL. A larger trial involving collaboration between the Eastern Cooperative Oncology Group and the Medical Resarch Council (MRC) is ongoing comparing allogeneic transplant, autologous transplant or chemotherapy in all adult patients with ALL who go into remission *(38)*. In addition, a collaboration between the CALGB and the Southwest Oncology Group will determine whether the utilization of STI-571 (Gleevec) consolidation therapy for patients with Ph+ ALL who lack a sibling or unrelated donor will achieve a PCR-negative state that would facilitate the collection of autologous stem cells that are relatively free of leukemia cells and then could be used for support of an autologous transplant. In general, the results for autologous transplantation for Ph+ positive ALL have been quite poor and this trial will help determine whether STI-571, in addition to its contribution to improving the response rate of patients with CML, can also benefit patients with ALL.

3. ALLOGENEIC TRANSPLANTATION FOR AML

The use of BMT for AML has expanded in the past three decades and has moved from an experimental treatment used only for patients with refractory disease to a first line of treatment for patients with AML in their first remission, depending on biological characteristics and response to initial therapy, as described in this section *(39–43)*. The following discussion summarizes the data on the results of allogeneic transplantation for AML, interpreted within the context of the evolving understanding of the molecular biology and cytogenetics of AML and the implications of these disease-related factors in the treatment and long-term survival in patients with this disease.

Historically, the classification of treatment of AML has been based completely on morphologic and clinical observations; however, the identification of the molecular events involved in the pathogenesis of human tumors have refined their classification and understanding, including the acute leukemias *(44)*. In AML, even more than ALL, a large number of leukemia-specific cytogenetic abnormalities have been identified and the involved genes cloned. These studies have helped elucidate the molecular pathways that may be involved in cellular transformation, provide methods for monitoring of patients after chemotherapy, and help evaluate the response to therapy correlated with various clinical and phenotypic characteristics *(45)*. Although the leukemia cells in many patients do not have detectable structural chromosome abnormalities at diagnosis, some may show molecular changes at diagnosis, such as involvement of the mixed lineage leukemia (MLL) gene *(46)*. Taken together, these observations have led to the concept that AML is a heterogeneous disease with its variants best defined by molecular defects and cytogenetic changes, some of which are more common in different age groups. In previous treatment trials with either standard therapy or allogeneic or autologous transplantation, patients were often treated as a homogeneous group. As described in the following subsections, recent studies have refined the way patients are allocated to various treatments, as well as in the analysis of the data, and provide the basis for now making a biologically based and response-based treatment decision, rather than a global one, for patients with AML.

3.1. Cytogenetic Characterization of AML

Cytogenetic risk groups form the backbone of a decision tree for postremission consolidation at the present time *(47–49)*. Other disease-related factors that influence the risk of relapse after induction chemotherapy include high leukocyte count at diagnosis or extramedullary disease and residual leukemia in marrow exams 7–10 d after completion of induction therapy. The availability of a sibling or unrelated donor also affects the risk assessment for consolidation treatment. HLA typing is now part of the National Comprehensive Cancer Network

(NCCN) guideline recommendations for initial evaluation of patients with newly diagnosed AML who do not have comorbid medical conditions that would be a contraindication to transplantation.

3.1.1. Stem Cell Transplantation for Acute Promyelocytic Leukemia

Patients with acute promyelocytic leukemia (APL) enjoy an excellent DFS (80–90%) with current conventional-dose chemotherapy combined with all-transretinoic acid (ATRA) in induction and maintenance *(50,51)*. Remission status can be monitored by following the level of the fusion protein (PML/RAR) produced by the t(15;17) translocation using PCR techniques *(51)*. Patients who either fail to achieve molecular remission by completion of consolidation or who show re-emergence and a rising level of the fusion protein are likely to relapse. Transplantation, using either an allogeneic donor or a molecular negative autologous stem cell product, is reserved for patients with APL who show evidence of relapse.

3.1.2. Good-Risk Cytogenetics

Patients with good-risk cytogenetics [t(8;21), inv(16), t(16;16)] may achieve long-term remission with multiple cycles of high-dose Ara-C in 40–60% of patients with relapse as the major cause of treatment failure *(52)*. Autologous transplant following one or more dose-intensive chemotherapy consolidations have shown a somewhat better DFS of 70–85% in cooperative groups and single-institution studies *(53)*. Although molecular probes exist for these translocations, their use in monitoring minimal residual disease is not as clinically useful as the probes for CML or APL *(54,55)*. Many patients with t(8;21) in clinical remission remain PCR positive for 10–20 yr without relapse. Thus, the treatment approach for consolidation therapy of this subgroup of consolidation therapy would include (1) multiple cycles of high-dose Ara-C, with allogeneic transplant reserved for treatment of relapse in patients having a sibling donor, (2) one or two cycles of HDAC followed by autologous peripheral blood stem cell transplantation (PBSCT) in CR, or (3) multiple cycles of HDAC with autologous stem cells collected in remission and reserved for salvage in patients without a sibling donor.

3.1.3. Intermediate-Risk Cytogenetics

The majority of adults with *de novo* AML are in the intermediate-risk group. Unfortunately, the DFS for this group declines to 30–35% when HDAC alone is used for consolidation. In this group of patients, both autologous and allogeneic (sibling) transplant in CR offer an improved DFS of 50–60% *(56–58)*. Factors that might influence the type of transplant are patient age, tumor burden at diagnosis, and infectious complications during induction. In younger patients (< 30 yr) in whom the risk of GVHD is relatively low, allogeneic transplantation may be more attractive because of a low (15–20%) relapse rate. In an older patient (50–60 yr), the higher treatment-related mortality (20–40%) and long-term morbidity associated with allogeneic marrow transplant suggests that autologous PBSCT offers at least an equivalent chance of relapse-free survival (RFS) with less long-term toxicity. Recent studies using peripheral blood stem cells (PBSCs) rather than marrow in the allogeneic setting have shown a significant decrease in the toxicity profile of a dose-intensive regimen that may make these treatments safer in older patients but longer follow-up is needed *(59)*. In addition, the development of nonmyeloablative allogeneic transplant approaches may allow for the use of alloBMT in older patients with AML.

3.1.4. Poor-Risk Cytogenetics

Patients with loss of chromosome 5 or 7 or complex karyotypic abnormalities as well as those patients with antecedent myelodysplasia or therapy-related leukemia have a very poor outcome when treated with conventional HDAC (10–12% 5-yr DFS). Autologous transplants have failed to improve on these results in most series. Allogeneic transplants can cure approx 40% of patients in this group *(60,61)*. In patients with any of these poor-risk features who lack a sibling donor, an unrelated donor search should be initiated early while the patient is still undergoing induction.

3.2. Transplant Strategy for Adult Patients With AML

Anthracycline-containing primary induction therapy for newly diagnosed AML will lead to CR in 65–80% of patients treated *(44)*. The likelihood of remaining in CR is, however, highly dependent on prognostic factors found at the time of diagnosis, including cytogenetic analysis as well as response to treatment. Patients who require more than one cycle of chemotherapy to achieve remission have a poor prognosis regardless of cytogenetic subgroup *(62)*. Subsequent treatment options for patients who successfully enter CR1 after primary induction therapy include repeated courses of intensive consolidation chemotherapy, autoBMT, or alloBMT.

Currently, the decision on which of the three options to choose should take into account the predicted benefit in terms of DFS and quality of life vs risk of morbidity and mortality. An important component of this decision depends on identification of an available matched sibling donor. In most series, allogeneic transplantation results in a lower rate of relapse for patients undergoing BMT for AML in first remission *(39)*. These results, however, do not always factor in the new information on the biology of AML and the impact of various treatment modalities on the outcome.

Compared to autologous transplantation or consolidation chemotherapy, alloBMT carries with it a higher potential for complications, with particular difficulty arising from regimen-related toxicity, infection, and GVHD, but it offers the therapeutic potential of the GVL effect. Decision-making should also take into account the knowledge that AML treated by allogeneic transplantation at the time of relapse is less likely to induce a lasting remission than transplantation at the time of first remission because the disease may become treatment resistant, accompanied by the development of additional somatic mutations and drug resistance. Patients who relapse and who are then treated with chemotherapy may develop organ dysfunction as a result of chemotherapy, fungal, or bacterial infections and become less able to withstand subsequent chemotherapy or a BMT-preparative regimen.

The decision to proceed to allogeneic transplantation thus becomes less controversial as patients move from lesser to greater risk of relapse (and risk of death from leukemia) (i.e., beyond CR1 and toward first relapse, CR2, or for primary refractory disease, etc.) Therefore, much research has centered on the determination of which patients are most likely to benefit from alloBMT early in their treatment course.

3.3. When to Begin Consideration for BMT

Because AML carries with it a high risk of relapse after achievement of remission, patients under the age of 60 who have no obvious contraindications for alloBMT should be evaluated regarding the number, health, and availability of siblings or other close relations who are potential candidates for bone marrow donation. HLA typing can be performed at any time, but it should be performed early so that all treatment options can be defined, particularly if the

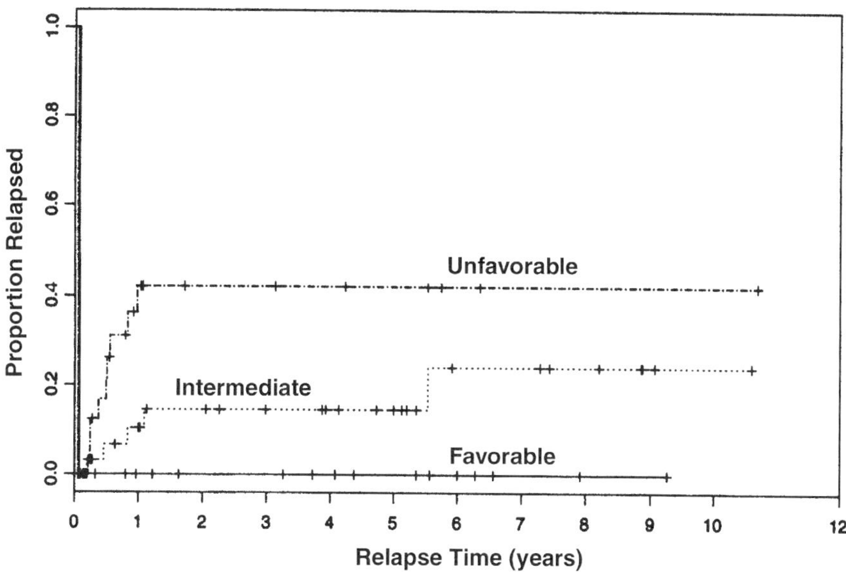

Fig. 2. Actuarial relapse rate for patients undergoing allogeneic transplantation for AML in first remission with a regimen of fractionated total body irradiation and VP-16. Based on pretransplant cytogenetics, those patients with poor-risk cytogenetics showed a higher rate of relapse compared to those with more favorable cytogenetic findings.

patient does not achieve a remission. This applies particularly to patients with poor-risk cytogenetics or other poor prognostic features who are at very high risk for early relapse. This approach provides for minimal delay for transplantation in the possible event of primary refractory disease, early disease relapse after primary therapy, or persistent cytogenetic abnormalities in the marrow after CR is attained. In addition, there is currently no evidence that consolidation therapy used before proceeding to allogeneic transplant has any benefit in reducing relapse after allogeneic transplant *(63)*. Thus, for patients in a first morphologic and cytogenetic remission who are candidates for alloBMT, consolidation therapy is not necessary and may lead to complications that either delay or increase the risk of transplantation.

3.4. Outcome After BMT for AML

Studies demonstrate a 5-yr DFS of 46–62% for patients treated with alloBMT in CR1 *(64–68)*. Cytogenetic analysis also has an impact on the outcome of transplant. In one series, relapse was 0% in patients with good-risk cytogenetics and approached 40% in those patients with poor-risk cytogenetics *(69)* (*see* Fig. 2). Additional studies from multiple institutions support a DFS ranging from 46% to 62% after 5 yr of observation *(70–75)*.

In order to reduce the limitations of GVHD on survival, Papadopoulos and colleagues at Memorial Sloan-Kettering Cancer Center studied the use of T-cell-depleted allografts in 31 patients with AML in CR1 or CR2. Patients treated in CR1 attained a DFS of 77% at 56 mo, whereas those treated in CR2 had a DFS of 50% at 48 mo. All patients were treated with a conditioning regimen of total-body irradiation (TBI), Thiotepa, and cyclophosphoride. Probability of relapse in patients treated in CR1 was 3.2%. Nonleukemic mortality in this group was 19.4%. There were no cases of grade II–IV acute GVHD *(44)*.

3.5. Effect of Conditioning Regimen on Survival or Relapse Rate

Several studies have been published comparing outcomes after different conditioning regimens. Although the use of higher doses of TBI results in a lower rate of relapse, patients suffered a higher incidence of GVHD and transplant-related mortality *(76)*. Other studies have found no significant differences between conditioning regimens using cyclophosphamide (Cy)/single-dose TBI vs Cy/fractionated-dose TBI (FTBI), CT/TBI vs Melphalan/TBI *(77)*. There are conflicting data as to whether busulfan (BU)/Cy results in a higher relapse rate than Cy/TBI, but recent data suggest that optimal use of busulfan (intravenous or targeted therapy) may have an impact on both toxicity and relapse *(78)*. Recent studies utilizing radioimmunotherapy designed to target hematopoietic tissue have shown promising results with a low relapse rate and no increase in transplant-related toxicity *(79)*. Presently, there are no data to determine whether one regimen is more or less effective for each of the cytogenetic subtypes of AML.

3.6. AlloBMT for AML in First Relapse or CR2

For patients in relapse after failure of standard therapy for AML, allogeneic transplantation offers the only chance for cure for those patients who lack a sibling donor. For those patients who are able to achieve a second remission, particularly after a long first remission and lack a sibling donor, an autologous transplant is a potentially curative therapy *(80,81)*. A common dilemma is the question of whether to proceed directly to allogeneic transplantation at the time of relapse (if a suitable donor has been identified) or whether to proceed to reinduction chemotherapy first in an attempt to reach a CR2 (required for autoBMT). Although no randomized data are available, one study demonstrates statistically nonsignificant survival rates differences of 29% in patients transplanted in untreated first relapse (R1) vs 22% in second remission (R2) and in 10% with refractory relapse *(39,82,83)*. Another study retrospectively evaluated outcomes in patients transplanted at various stages of disease. DFS was significantly better in patients transplanted in R1, but no statistical difference was found between the various groups transplanted beyond CR1. Thus, the decision concerning reinduction is often based on the age, condition, duration of R1 and cytogenetic category of the patient with relapsed AML *(39)*. Figure 3 shows an approach to the timing and use of BMT based on prognostic features found at diagnosis and in response to treatment *(39)*.

3.7. Approach to the Patient With Primary Refractory AML

The survival of patients with AML who do not achieve a remission with primary therapy is very poor and, in general, is independent of all other cellular characteristics. The lack of achievement of remission is the clearest demonstration of the resistance of the disease to chemotherapy. Some studies have been performed that indicate that the use of allogeneic transplantation in patients who have not achieved a remission may result in long-term DFS in approx 5–30% of patients *(84–86)*. A recent analysis of 71 patients with primary refractory AML who underwent a transplant from a sibling donor was performed to determine whether there are pretransplant features of this unique patient population that predict treatment outcome *(87)*. Unfavorable cytogenetics before stem cell transplantation (SCT) was significantly associated with decreased DFS and a TBI-based regimen appeared to convey a better outcome. The actuarial probability of DFS and relapse at 3 yr was 44% and 38% for patients with intermediate cytogenetics and 18% and 68% for those patients with unfavorable cytogenetics. Figure 4

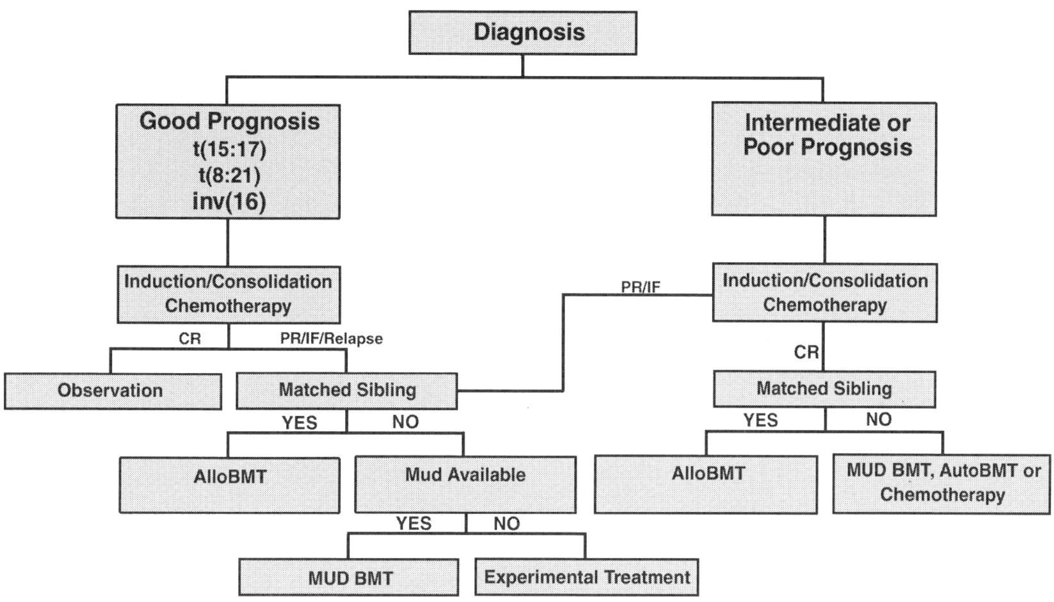

Fig. 3. Algorithm for the treatment of patients with AML. (Reprinted with permission from ref. *39*.)

shows the DFS for a group of patients who failed to achieve a remission and were then treated with an alloBMT from a sibling donor.

The data suggest that allogeneic transplantation can cure some patients with primary refractory AML and that cytogenetic analysis before SCT correlates with transplant outcome as well as relapse. Thus, for patients who do not achieve remission with either one or two cycles of induction therapy, particularly with a HDAC-based regimen, proceeding to allogeneic transplantation when a sibling donor is identified appears to be the optimal strategy rather than utilizing repeated courses of chemotherapy, which are unlikely to result in remission. Patients who require more than one cycle of chemotherapy to achieve a remission should also be considered at high risk for relapse and should be considered for early BMT *(88)*.

4. AUTOLOGOUS SCT FOR AML IN CR1

Many studies have been published utilizing unpurged marrow or purged marrow for treatment of patients with AML in R1, usually after consolidation therapy (89–94). DFS for patients in CR1 have varied between 34% and 80%. Although each trial demonstrates the potential efficacy of the approach, many of these studies have been criticized for including patients who had received widely varying induction therapies, types and numbers of consolidation cycles before autologous HCT, duration of CR before transplant, and relatively short follow-up times. In addition, there are differences in the stem cell product manipulation and preparative regimens. In many of these studies, similar to many reports of allogeneic transplant for AML in R1, a number of patients who otherwise would have been candidates for autoSCT suffered a relapse prior to transplant and were not part of the subsequent analysis.

The Medical Research Council Leukemia Working Parties (MRC10) conducted a clinical trial to determine whether the addition of autoBMT to intensive consolidation chemotherapy improved RFS for patients with AML in R1 *(90)*. After three courses of intensive consolidation

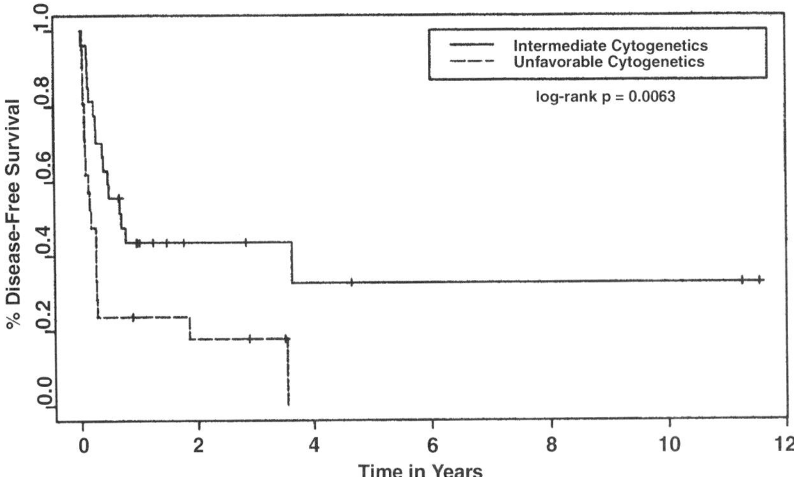

Fig. 4. Disease-free survival for a group of patients with AML undergoing allogeneic transplantation after having failed to achieve a remission with either Ara-C, idarubicin, or HDAC and an anthracycline. Patients with intermediate cytogenetics had a better DFS than those with unfavorable cytogenetics. Overall, the actual probability of DFS at 3 yr was 44% for patients with intermediate cytogenetics and 18% for those with unfavorable cytogenetics.

therapy, bone marrow was harvested from patients who lacked a donor. These patients were then randomized to receive, after one additional course of chemotherapy, either no further treatment or an autoBMT or preparation with cyclophosphamide and total-body irradiation. On an intent to treat analysis, the number of relapses was substantially lower in the group assigned to transplant (37% vs 58%, $p = 0.007$), which resulted in superior DFS at 7 yr (53% vs 40%, $p = 0.04$). This benefit for transplant was seen in all cytogenetic risk groups (*see* Fig. 5).

In a North American study, patients in R1 with a histocompatible sibling donor were assigned to allogeneic transplantation and the remainder were randomized between autoHCT utilizing 4-HC-purged marrow or one course of 3 g/m^2 HDAC every 12 h for 6 d. The preparative regimen for both the allogeneic and autologous transplant was busulfan and cyclophosphamide. The 4-yr DFS for chemotherapy, autologous transplant, and allogeneic transplant was 35%, 37%, and 42%, respectively; however, as noted earlier, the impact of any of these therapies needs to take into account the pretreatment characteristics of the disease in order to assess the efficacy of the postremission therapy *(95)*. In the above-noted trial, patients were categorized into favorable, intermediate, unfavorable, and unknown cytogenetic risk groups based on pretreatment karyotypes that had, as described earlier, an impact on achievement of remission; however, among postremission patients, survival from CR varied significantly among the favorable, intermediate, and unfavorable groups, with significant evidence of interaction between the effects of treatment and cytogenetic risk status on survival. In this trial, patients with favorable cytogenetics did significantly better following autologous transplantation and alloBMT than with chemotherapy alone, whereas patients with unfavorable cytogenetics did better with an allogeneic transplant. These data, combined with that obtained from the CALGB concerning the dose–response curve of Ara-C in postremission therapy, indicate, again, the importance of cytogenetic analysis on the outcome of any particular postremission induction therapy.

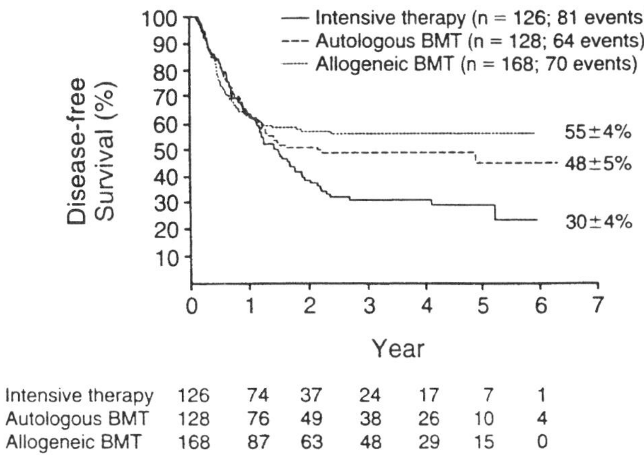

Intensive therapy	126	74	37	24	17	7	1
Autologous BMT	128	76	49	38	26	10	4
Allogeneic BMT	168	87	63	48	29	15	0

Fig. 5. Disease-free survival of patients randomized between autologous transplantation and intensive chemotherapy in the MRC10 trial. (Reprinted with permission from ref. *56*.)

5. POST-AUTOLOGOUS-TRANSPLANT IMMUNOTHERAPY

Several groups have attempted to determine whether the addition of an immunotherapeutic strategy after achievement of minimal residual disease and autologous transplant might improve DFS for patients *(96–99)*. Interleukin-2 (IL-2) is a cytokine that has a broad range of antitumor effects and has been used in some patients undergoing autologous transplant for a variety of malignancies. A Phase II study from the City of Hope utilizing high-dose IL-2 following HDAC/idarubicin-mobilized autoSCT was conducted with 70 patients *(100)*. The treatment strategy consisted of consolidation postinduction with high-dose cytosine arabinoside and idarubicin followed by granulocyte colony-stimulating factor and autologous PBSC collection and then autoSCT utilizing TBI (12 Gy), VP-16 (60 mg/kg), and cyclophosphamide (75 mg/kg). IL-2 was administered upon hematologic recovery at a schedule of 9×10^6 IU/m^2 for 24 h on d 1–4 and 1.6×10^6 IU/m^2 IL-2 on d 9–18. Seventy patients with a median age of 44 were treated in the study. Of these patients, 29% had good-risk cytogenetics, 38% had intermediate-risk cytogenetics, and 36% had either unfavorable-risk or unknown cytogenetics. Of 70 patients, 60 were able to undergo autoSCT following consolidation. With a median follow-up of 33 mo, the 2-yr probability of DFS for the whole group of patients on an intention to treat analysis is 66% and 73% for the 39 patients who actually made it to autoSCT (*see* Fig. 6). Whether IL-2 or any other post-BMT immunotherapeutic approach mimicking an allogeneic GVL has an impact on overall DFS will require a randomized trial stratified by cytogenetic risk groups.

Taken together, these results indicate that autologous transplant in CR1 after one or more courses of consolidation therapy can improve DFS in selected groups of patients. There still remain questions about the number and type of courses of consolidation chemotherapy, the type of regimen used for BMT, and the treatment of MRD after transplant.

6. MYELODYSPLASTIC SYNDROMES

The myelodysplastic syndromes (MDSs) encompass a spectrum of marrow disorders with variable degrees of ineffective hematopoiesis and predisposition to leukemic transformation

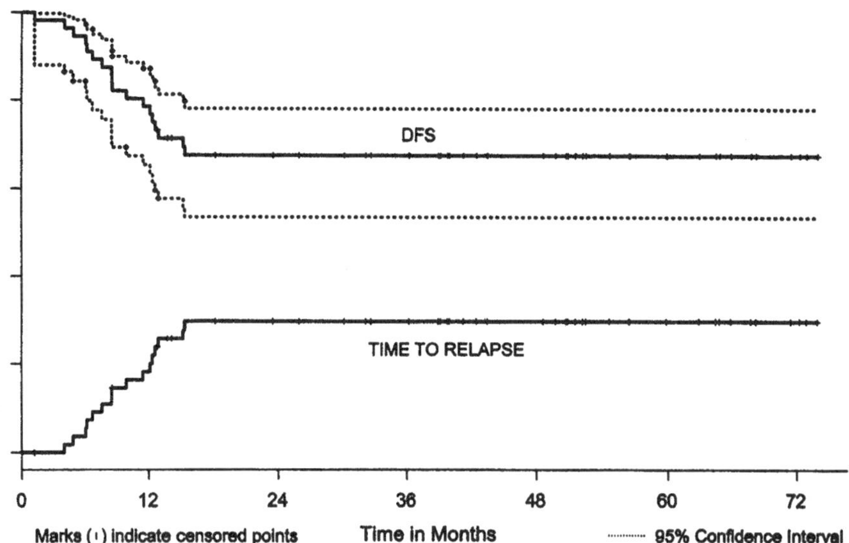

Fig. 6. Disease-free survival and time to relapse for patients with AML undergoing autologous transplant in R1 followed by posttransplant IL-2.

with survival ranging from months to decades after diagnosis *(101)*. Factors influencing outcome are the number of significant cytopenias and cytogenetic abnormalities and the presence of increasing marrow blasts, which have recently been codified into a prognostic index that reflects both survival and leukemic transformation, as described later in this chapter *(102)*. Whereas the majority of patients with MDS are above 60 yr of age and, therefore, above the usual age for transplant, there are an increasing number of younger patients developing MDS as a sequelae of chemotherapy or radiation for lymphomas, germ cell tumors, and breast cancer *(103,104)*. These secondary MDS patients tend to be at high risk for early transformation to AML and often have poor-risk cytogenetics.

Decisions to utilize transplantation to replace the defective stem cells are influenced by the patient's age, prognostic index score, and comorbid conditions. Patients with low-risk disease are usually not recommended for transplant until they progress, unless they have treatment-related MDS. For patients with intermediate-risk disease, full-dose allogeneic transplant from a sibling or volunteer unrelated donor should be considered as primary therapy for patients under 55 yr of age; such procedures successfully restore normal hematopoiesis in 40–50% of patients *(105)*. For patients with high-risk disease (with >15% blasts in the marrow) or secondary AML, there is controversy as to whether induction chemotherapy to reduce the "leukemic" burden is beneficial. Whereas the relapse rate is less in patients who respond to induction treatment, there are also many who fail to respond and who become too debilitated to receive a transplant. In patients who do not have a sibling donor, induction chemotherapy may be necessary as a temporizing measure while a donor is sought.

6.1. IPSS Classification of MDS

The first clinically useful staging system, the French–American–British (FAB) classification, as proposed by Bennett and colleagues, categorized MDS on the basis of the proportion of myeloblasts in the marrow (and blood) into refractory anemia (RA), RA with ringed

Table 2
Classification of MDS Acccording to FAB

Classification	*% Marrow blasts*	*% Peripheral blood blasts*	*Ringed sideroblasts >15% of bone marrow*	*Monocytes >1000/μL*
RA	<5	<1	–	–
RARS	<5	<1	+	–
RAEB	5–20	<5	±	–
RAEB-T	21–30	>5	±	±
CMML[a]	<5	<5	±	+

Note: +, always present; –, always absent; ±, variable.

[a]Recently reclassified as an MPD.

sideroblasts (RARS), RA with excess blasts (RAEB), and RAEB in transformation (RAEB-T) (*see* Table 2) *(101)*. An additional subcategory, chronic myelomonocytic leukemia (CMML), has recently been reclassified as a myeloproliferative disorder. Several additional classification alternatives followed by the FAB proposal, and, recently, Greenberg and colleagues presented the IPSS, which, in addition to the proportion of blasts, considers the number of peripheral blood cytopenias and clonal chromosomal abnormalities *(102)*. Normal cytogenetics, -y, 5q-, and 20q-, are considered good risk, chromosome 7 abnormalities and complex karyotypes are considered poor risk, and all other findings are considered intermediate risk (*see* Table 3). Combining blast counts, cytopenias, and cytogenetics, the International Prognostic Scoring System (IPSS) divides MDS into four risk groups: low risk, intermediate-1, intermediate-2, and high risk. With conventional management, the median life expectancies for these four groups were 5.7, 3.5, 1.2, and 0.4 yr, respectively. Disease progression was faster in older patients than in younger patients.

6.2. Clinical Results of Allogeneic Transplant for MDS

A rapidly growing number of patients with MDS have undergone allogeneic HSCT, and results show that stage by FAB or IPSS classification at the time of transplantation significantly impacts the posttransplant outcome. As expected from the natural history of the different risk categories, patients with RA/RARS and with low IPSS scores, especially with low-risk cytogenetics, generally do better after HSCT, predominantly because of a lower relapse rate *(106)*. Disease recurrence and nonrelapse mortality (NRM) have been the major causes of treatment failure in patients with "advanced" or "high-risk" MDS treated with allogeneic transplantation. The European Bone Marrow Transplant (EBMT) group has reported 5-yr RFSs with myeloablative HSCT of 46%, 35%, 27%, and 0% for patients with RA/RARS, RAEB, RAEB-T, and secondary acute myeloid leukemia, respectively *(107)*. Dependent on the interval from diagnosis to transplant, patient age, the source of stem cells, and conditioning regimen used, nonrelapse mortality (NRM) in the range of 25–65% has been observed *(100)*.

Efforts to improve outcomes in patients with primary and secondary MDS have focused on attempts to reduce NRM and relapse. One approach has been to carefully adjust the dose of BU according to plasma levels in order to minimize the risk of excessive dosing leading to toxicity and inadequate dosing leading to an increased risk of relapse. Deeg et al. *(108)* evaluated 109

Table 3
IPSS: Parameters, Scores, and Risk Groups

	Score value				
Prognostic variable	0	0.5	1.0	1.5	2.0
Marrow blasts (%)	<5	5–10	—	11–20	21–30
Karyotype[a]	Good	Intermediate	Poor		
Cytopenias	0/1	2/3			

[a]Good = normal, -y, del(5q), del(20q); poor = complex (3 abnormalities) or chromosome 7 anomalies; intermediate = all other abnormalities.

patients with MDS aged 6–66 yr (median: 46 yr) who were treated with tBUCY (BU targeted to plasma concentrations of 800–900 ng/mL plus CY, 2 × 60 mg/kg) and HSCT from related (*n*=45) or unrelated donors (*n*=64). At the time of transplant, 40 patients had less than 5% myeloblasts in the marrow, and 69 had less advanced disease. NRM at 100 d (3 yr) was 12% (28%) for related and 13% (30%) for unrelated recipients. Kaplan–Meier estimates of 3-yr RFS were 56% for related and 59% for unrelated recipients. The only factor significant for RFS was the etiology of MDS (*de novo* > treatment related). The cumulative incidences of relapse were 16% for related and 11% for unrelated recipients. Factors significantly correlated with relapse were advanced FAB classification and IPSS score, poor-risk cytogenetics, and treatment-related etiology. None of the factors examined was statistically significant for NRM. RFS tended to be superior in patients transplanted with peripheral blood rather than marrow stem cells. Patient age and donor type had no significant impact on outcome.

6.3. Induction Therapy for Advanced MDS Prior to Transplant

The question arises whether pre-transplant induction (debulking) chemotherapy would improve results in patients with advanced/high-risk disease by reducing the incidence of posttransplant relapse. Anderson et al. from the Fred Hutchinson Cancer Research Center (FHCRC) reported a retrospective analysis *(109)* of 46 patients (median age: 42 yr) with secondary AML (17 therapy related, 29 myelodysplasia related) who had not received remission induction chemotherapy and underwent allogeneic (*n*=43) or syngeneic (*n*=3) HSCT. The 5-yr actuarial RFS was 24.4%, and the cumulative incidences of NRM and relapse were 44.3% and 31.3%, respectively. A shorter time from AML diagnosis to transplant was associated with a lower risk of NRM and improved RFS, whereas a lower peripheral blood blast count was associated with a lower risk of relapse. Results in these 46 previously untreated patients were compared to 20 patients (median age: 36 yr; 12 therapy related, 8 myelodysplasia related) transplanted with chemotherapy-sensitive disease after induction chemotherapy (CR1 [*n*=6], CR2 [*n*=3], first untreated relapse [*n*=11]). The 5-yr actuarial RFS was 15% (3/20), and the cumulative incidences of NRM and relapse were 60% (12/20) and 25% (5/20), respectively. Difference in outcome between the two groups of patients were not significant and suggested that induction therapy before myeloablative HSCT did not provide an advantage for survival in this study.

A different study by Yakoub-Agha et al. included 70 patients with t-MDS (*n*=31) or therapy-related AML (*n*=39) who underwent myeloablative allogeneic HSCT *(110)*. Thirty-three patients had received induction chemotherapy before HSCT. At the time of transplantation, 24 patients were in CR and 46 had active disease. With a median follow-up of 7.9 yr (range: 1.1–

18.8 yr) years after HSCT, 16 patients were alive, 34 died of NRM, 19 died of relapse, and one died of relapse of the primary disease. Patients in CR at HSCT died less often of relapse (8%) than did patients not in CR (44%), whereas the NRM was not significantly different (46% vs 51%). The RFS for patients who achieved a CR after induction therapy prior to HSCT was 45%. In contrast, the RFS for patients who had active AML or MDS at the time of HSCT was 26% and 15%, respectively (p=0.052). In multivariate analysis, the absence of CR at HSCT was one of the factors associated with poor outcome. Thus, this study would suggest that HSCT was effective treatment for patients with t-MDS or t-AML who had responsive disease and were in remission at the time of HSCT.

REFERENCES

1. Copelan EA, McGuire EA. The biology and treatment of acute lymphoblastic leukemia in adults. *Blood* 1995;85:1151–1168.
2. Hoelzer D, Ludwig WD, Thiel D, et al. Improved outcome in adult B-cell acute lymphoblastic leukemia. *Blood* 1996;87:495–508.
3. Hoelzer D, Thiel E, Loffler T, et al. Prognostic factors in a multricentric study for treatment of acute lymphoblastic leukemia in adults. *Blood* 1988;71:123–131.
4. Laport GF, Larson RA. Treatment of adult acute lymphoblastic leukemia. *Semin Oncol* 1997;24:70–82.
5. Sutton L, Chastang C, Ribaud P, et al. Factors influencing outcome in de novo myelodysplastic syndromes treated by allogeneic bone marrow transplantation: a long-term study of 71 patients Societe Francaise de Greffe de Moelle. *Blood* 1996;88:358–365.
6. Third International Workshop on Chromosomes in Leukemia. Chromosomal abnormalities and their clinical significance in acutee lymphoblastic leukemia. *Cancer Res* 1983;43:868.
7. Faderl S, Kantarjian M, Talpaz M, et al. Clinical significance of cytogenetic abnormalities in adult acute lymphoblastic leukemia. *Blood* 1998;91:3996–4019.
8. Linker CA, Leavitt LJ, O'Donnell M, et al. Treatment of adult acute lymphoblastic leukemia with intensive cyclical chemotherapy: a follow-up report. *Blood* 1991;78(11):2814–2822.
9. Larson RA, Dodge RK, Burns PC, et al. A five-drug remission induction regimen with intensive consolidation for adults with acute lymphoblastic leukemia: Cancer and Leukemia Group B study 8811. *Blood* 1995;85(8):2025–2037.
10. Hoelzer D, Thiel H, Loffler H, et al. Prognostic factors in a multicenter study for treatment of acute lymhoblastic leukemia in adults. *Blood* 1988;71(1):123–131.
11. Kantarjian HM, O'Brien S, Smith TL, et al. Results of treatment with hyper-CVAD, a dose-intensive regimen, in adult acute lymphoblastic leukemia. *J Clin Oncol* 2000;18(3):547–561.
12. Boucheix C, David B, Sebban C, et al. Immunophenotype of adult acute lymphoblastic leukemia, clinical parameters, and outcome: an analysis of a prospective trial including 562 tested patients (LALA87). *Blood* 1994;84(5):1603–1612.
13. Linker CA, Levitt LJ, O'Donnell M, et al. Treatment of adult acute lymphoblastic leukemia with intensive cyclical chemotherapy: a followup report. *Blood* 1991;78:2814–2822.
14. Forman SJ. The role of allogeneic bone marrow transplantation in the treatment of high-risk acute lymphocytic leukemia in adults. *Leukemia* 1997;11(suppl 4):S18–S19.
15. Chao NJ, Forman SJ, Schmidt GM, et al. Allogeneic bone marrow transplantation for high-risk acute lymphoblastic leukemia during first complete remission. *Blood* 1991;78:1923–1927.
16. Snyder D. Allogeneic bone marrow transplantation for Philadelphia chromosome-positive acute lymphoblastic leukemia in first complete remission: long term followup. *Biol Blood Marrow Transplant* 2000; 6:537–603.
17. Sierra J, Radich J, Hansen JA, et al. Marrow transplants from unrelated donors for treatment of Philadelphia chromosome-positive acute lymphoblastic leukemia. *Blood* 1997;90:1410–1414.
18. Radich J, Gehly G, Lee A, et al. Detection of bcr-abl transcripts in Philadelphia chromosome-positive acute lymphoblastic leukemia after marrow transplantation. *Blood* 1997;89:2602–2609.
19. Giona F, Testi A, Amadori G, et al. Idarubicin and high-dose cytarabine in the treatment of refractory and relapsed acute lymphoblastic leukemia. *Ann Oncol* 1990;1:51–55.

20. Hiddemann W, Kreutzman H, Straif K, et al. High-dose cytosine arabinoside in combination with mitoxantrone for the treatment of refractory acute myeloid leukemia and lymphoblastic leukemia. *Semin Oncol* 1987;14:73–77.
21. Kantarjian HM, Walters RL, Keating MJ, et al. Mitoxantrone and high-dose cytosine arabinoside for the treatment of refractory acute lymphoblastic leukemia. *Cancer* 1990;65:5–8.
22. Toze CL,l Shepherd JD, Nantel SH, et al. Allogeneic bone marrow transplantation for low grade lymphoma and chronic lymphocytic leukemia. *Blood* 1999;90(suppl):4513.
23. Weiss MA. Treatment of adult patients with relapsed or refractory acute lymphoblastic leukemia (ALL). *Leukemia* 1997;11(suppl 4):S28–S30.
24. Hongeng S, Krance RA, Bowman LC, et al. Outcomes of transplantation with matched-sibling and unrelated-donor bone marrow in children with leukemia. *Lancet* 1997;350:767–770.
25. Oakhill A, Pamphilon DH, Potter MN, et al. Unrelated donor bone marrow transplantation for children with relapsed acute lymphoblastic leukemia in second complete remission. *Br J Haematol* 1996;94:574–578.
26. Balduzzi A, Gooley T, Anasetti C, et al. Unrelated donor marrow transplantation in children. *Blood* 1995;86:3247–3256.
27. Saarinen-Pihkala UM, Gustafsson G, Ringden O, et al. No disadvantage in outcome of using matched unrelated donors as compared with matched sibling donors for bone marrow transplantation in children with acute lymphoblastic leukemia in second remission. *J Clin Oncol* 2001;19:3406–3414.
28. Kollman C, Howe CW, Anasetti C, et al. Donor characteristics as risk factors in recipients after transplantation of bone marrow from unrelated donors: the effect of donor age. *Blood* 2001;98:2043–2051.
29. Kanamori H, Sasaki S, Yamazaki E, et al. Eradication of minimal residual disease during graft-versus-host reaction induced by abrupt discontinuation of immunosuppression following bone marrow transplantation in a patient with Ph1-ALL. *Transpl Int* 1997;10:328–330.
30. Gorin NC. Autologous stem cell transplantation in acute lymphocytic leukemia. *Stem Cells* 2002;20:3–10.
31. Fiere D, Lepage E, Sebban C, et al. Adult acute lymphoblastic leukemia: a multicentric randomized trial testing bone marrow transplantation as postremission therapy. *J Clin Oncol* 1993;11(10):1990–2001.
32. Attal M, Blaise D, Marit G, et al. Consolidation treatment of adult acute lymphoblastic leukemia: a prospective, randomized trial comparing allogeneic versus autologous bone marrow transplantation and testing the impact of recombinant interleukin-2 after autologous bone marrow transplantation. *Blood* 1995;86(4):1619–1628.
33. Powles R, Sirohi B, Singhal S, et al. The role of maintenance therapy after autotransplantation in adult acute lymphoblastic leukemia. *Blood* 1998;(suppl 1):689a.
34. Hunault M, Harousseau JL, Delain M, et al. Improved outcome of high risk acute lymphoblastic leukemia (ALL) with late high dose therapy. A GOELAMS's trial. *Blood* 1998;(suppl 1):803a.
35. Linker C, Damon L, Navarro W, et al. Autologous stem cell transplantation for high-risk adult acute lymphoblastic leukemia (ALL). *Blood* 1998;(suppl 1):689a.
36. Martin H, Fauth F, Atta J, et al. Singe versus double autologous BMT/PBSCT in patients with BCR-ABL-positive acute lymphoblastic leukemia. *Blood* 1994;(suppl 1):580a.
37. Gorin N, Aegerter P, Auvert B. Autologous bone marrow transplantation (ABMT) for acute leukemia in remission: an analysis on 1322 cases. *Bone Marrow Transplant* 1990;4:35.
38. Rowe JM, Richards SM, Burnett AK, et al. Favorable results of allogeneic bone marrow transplantation (BMT) for adults with philadelphia (Ph)-chromosome-negative acute lymphoblastic leukemia (ALL) in first complete remission (CR): results from the international ALL trial (MRC UKALL XII/ECOG E2993). *Blood* 1998;(suppl 1):481a.
39. Stockerl-Goldstein KE, Blume KG. Allogeneic hematopoietic cell transplantation for adult patients with acute myeloid leukemia. In: Thomas ED, Blume KG, Forman SJ, eds. *Hematopoietic Cell Transplantation*, 2nd ed. London: Blackwell Science, 1999:823–834.
40. Forman SJ, Krance RA, O'Donnell MR, et al. Bone marrow transplantation for acute nonlymphoblastic leukemia during first complete remission. An analysis of prognostic factors. *Transplantation* 1987;43:650–653.
41. Mehta J, Powles R, Treleaven J, et al. Long-term follow-up of patients undergoing allogeneic bone marrow transplantation for acute myeloid leukemia in first complete remission after cyclophosphamide-total body irradiation and cyclosporine. *Bone Marrow Transplant* 1996;18:741–746.
42. Snyder DS, Chao NJ, Amylon MD, et al. Fractionated total body irradiation high-dose etoposide as a preparatory regimen for bone marrow transplantation for 99 patients with acute leukemia in first complete remission. *Blood* 1993;82:2920–2928.

43. Keating S, Suciu S, de Witte T, et al. Prognostic factors of patients with acute myeloid leukemia (AML) allografted in first complete remission: an analysis of the EORTC-GIMEMA AML 8A trial. The European Organization for Research and Treatment of Cancer (EORTC) and the Gruppo Italiano Malattie Ematologiche Maligne dell' Adulto (GIMEMA) Leukemia Cooperative Groups. *Bone Marrow Transplant* 1996;17:993–1001.
44. Löwenberg B, Downing J, Burnett A. Acute myeloid leukemia. *N Engl J Med* 1999;341:1051–1062.
45. Golub TR, Slonim DK, Tamayo P, et al. Molecular classification of cancer: class discovery and class pr gene expression monitoring. *Science* 1999;286:531–537.
46. Caligiuri MA, Strout MP, Lawrence D, et al. Rearrangement of ALL1 (MLL) in acute myeloid leukemia with normal cytogenetics. *Cancer Res* 1998;58:55–59.
47. Yunis JJ, Brunning RD, Howe RB, et al. High-resolution chromosomes as an independent prognostic indicator in adult acute nonlymphocytic leukemia. *N Engl J Med* 1984;311:812–818.
48. Keating MJ, Smith TL, Kantarjian H, et al. Cytogenetic pattern in acute myelogenous leukemia: a major reproducible determinant of outcome. *Leukemia* 1988;2:403–412.
49. Mrozek K, Heinonen K, de la Chapelle A, et al. Clinical significance of cytogenetics in acute myeloid leukemia. *Semin Oncol* 1997;24:17–31.
50. Fenaux P, Chastang C, Chevret S, et al. A randomized comparison of all-transretinoic acid (ATRA) followed by chemotherapy and ATRA plus chemotherapy and the role of maintenance therapy in newly diagnosed acute promyelocytic leukemia. *Blood* 1999;94:1192–1200.
51. Niu C, Yam H, Yu T, et al. Studies on treatment of acute promyelocytic leukemia with arsenic trioxide: remission induction, follow-up, and molecular monitoring in 11 newly diagnosed and 47 relapsed acute promyelocytic leukemia patients. *Blood* 1999;94:3315–3324.
52. Bloomfield CD, Lawrence D, Byrd JC, et al. Frequency of prolonged remission duration after high-dose cytarabine intensification in acute myeloid leukemia varies by cytogenetic subtype. *Cancer Res* 1998;58:4173–4179.
53. Stein AS, Slovak ML, Sniecinski I, et al. Immunotherapy with IL-2 after autologous stem cell transplant for acute myelogenous leukemia in first remission. Proceedings of the Ninth International Symposium on Autologous Blood and Marrow Transplantation 1999;1:46–53.
54. Saunders MJ, Tobal K, Liu Yin JA. Detection of t(8;21) by reverse transcriptase polymerase chain reaction in patients in remission of acute myeloid leukaemia type M2 after chemotherapy or bone marrow transplantation. *Leukemia Res* 1994;18:891–895.
55. Nucifora G, Larson RA, Rowley RD. Persistence of the 8;21 translocation in patients with acute myeloid leukemia type M2 in long term remission. *Blood* 1993;82:712–715.
56. Burnett AK, Goldstone AH, Stevens RMF, et al. Randomised comparison of addition of autologous bone-marrow transplantation to intensive chemotherapy for acute myeloid leukemia in first remission. Results of MRC AML 10 trial. *Lancet* 1998;351:700–708.
57. Zittoun RA, Mandelli F, Willemze R, et al. Autologous or allogeneic bone marrow transplantation compared with intensive chemotherapy in acute myelogenous leukemia. *N Engl J Med* 1995;332:217–223.
58. Cassileth PA, Harrington DP, Appelbaum FR, et al. Chemotherapy compared with autologous or allogeneic bone marrow transplantation in the management of acute myeloid leukemia in first remission. *N Engl J Med* 1998;339:1649–1656.
59. Bensinger W, Martin P, Storer B, et al. Transplantation of bone marrow as compared with peripheral blood cells from HLA-identical relatives in patients with hematologic malignancies. *N Engl J Med* 2001;344:175–181.
60. Thomas ED, Buckner CD, Banaji M, et al. One hundred patients with acute leukemia treated by chemotherapy, total body irradiation, and allogeneic marrow transplantation. *Blood* 1977;49:511–533.
61. Slovak ML, Kopecky KJ, Cassileth PA, et al. Karyotypic analysis predicts outcome of preremission and postremission therapy in adult acute myeloid leukemia: a Southwest Oncology Group/Eastern Cooperative Oncology Group study. *Blood* 2000;96:4075–4083.
62. Estey EH, Shen Y, Thall PF. Effect of time to complete remission on subsequent survival and disease-free survival time in AML, RAEB-t, and RAEB. *Blood* 2000;95:72–77.
63. Tallman MS, Rowlings PA, Milone G, et al. Effect of postremission chemotherapy before human leukocyte antigen-identical sibling transplantation for acute myelogenous leukemia in first complete remission. *Blood* 2000;96:1254–1258.
64. Blaise D, Maraninchi D, Archimbaud E, et al. Allogeneic bone marrow transplantation for acute myeloid leukemia in first remission: a randomized trial of a busulfan–cytoxan versus cytoxan–total body irradia-

tion as preparative regimen: a report from the Group d'Etudes de la Greffe de Moelle Osseuse. *Blood* 1992;79:2578–2582.
65. Soiffer RJ, Fairclough D, Robertson M, et al. CD6-depleted allogeneic bone marrow transplantation for acute leukemia in first complete remission. *Blood* 1997;89:3039–3047.
66. Thomas ED, Buckner CD, Clift RA, et al. Marrow transplantation for acute nonlymphoblastic leukemia in first remission. *N Engl J Med* 1979;301:597–599.
67. Appelbaum FR, Dahlberg S, Thomas ED, et al. Bone marrow transplantation or chemotherapy after remission induction for adults with acute nonlymphoblastic leukemia: a prospective comparison. *Ann Intern Med* 1984;101:581–588.
68. Champlin RE, Ho WG, Gale RP, et al. Treatment of acute myelogenous leukemia: a prospective controlled trial of bone marrow transplantation versus consolidation chemotherapy. *Ann Intern Med* 1985;102:285–291.
69. Fung H, Jamieson C, Snyder D, et al. Allogeneic bone marrow transplantation (BMT) for AML in first remission (1CR) utilizing fractionated total body irradiation (FTBI) and allogeneic bone marrow transplantation for bcr-abl positive acute lymphoblastic leukemia. VP-16: analysis of risk factors for relapse and disease-free survival. *Blood* 1999;94:167a.
70. Bostrom B, Brunning RD, McGlave P, et al. Bone marrow transplantation for acute nonlymphoblastic leukemia in first remission: analysis of prognostic factors. *Blood* 1985;65:1191–1196.
71. Clift RA, Buckner CD, Thomas ED, et al. The treatment of acute nonlymphoblastic leukemia by allogeneic transplantation. *Bone Marrow Transplant* 1987;2:243–258.
72. Forman SJ, Spruce WE, Farbstein MJ, et al. Bone marrow ablation followed by allogeneic marrow grafting during first complete remission of acute nonlymphocytic leukemia. *Blood* 1983;61:439–442.
73. Helenglass G, Powles RL, McElwain, TJ, et al. Melphalan and total body irradiation (TBI) versus cyclophosphamide and TBI as conditioning for allogeneic matched sibling bone marrow transplants for acute myeloblastic leukemia in first remission. *Bone Marrow Transplant* 1988;3:21–29.
74. Kim TH, McGlave PB, Ramsay N, et al. Comparison of two total body irradiation regimens in allogeneic bone marrow transplantation for acute nonlymphoblastic leukemia in first remission. *Int J Radiat Oncol Biol Phys* 1990;19:889–897.
75. McGlave PB, Haake RJ, Bostrom BC, et al. Allogeneic bone marrow transplantation for acute nonlymphocytic leukemia in first remission. *Blood* 1988;72:1512–1517.
76. Mehta J, Powles R, Singhal S, et al. Clinical and hematologic response of chronic lymphocytic and prolymphocytic leukemia persisting after allogeneic bone marrow transplantation with the onset of acute graft-versus-host disease: possible role of graft-versus-leukemia effect. *Bone Marrow Transplant* 1996;18:371–375.
77. Popplewell L, Forman SJ. Allogeneic hematopoietic stem cell transplantation for acute leukemia, chronic leukemia, and myelodysplasia. *Hematol/Oncol Clin North Am* 1999;13:987–1015.
78. Andersson BS, Gajewski J, Donato M, et al. Allogeneic stem cell transplantation (BMT) for AML and MDS following IV busulfan and cyclophosphamide (i.v. BuCy). *Bone Marrow Transplant* 2000;25:S35–S38.
79. Appelbaum FR. Radioimmunotherapy and hematopoietic cell transplantation. In: Thomas ED, Blume KG, Forman SJ, eds. *Hematopoietic Cell Transplantation*, 2nd ed. London: Blackwell Science, 1999:168–175.
80. Stein AS, Forman SJ. Autologous hematopoietic cell transplantation for acute myeloid leukemia. In: Thomas ED, Blume KG, Forman SJ, eds. *Hematopoietic Cell Transplantation*, 2nd ed. London: Blackwell Science, 1999:287–295.
81. Miller CB, Rowlings PA, Zhang MJ, et al. The effect of graft purging with 4-hydroperoxycyclophosphamide in autologous bone marrow transplantation for acute myelogenous leukemia. *Exp Hematol* 2001;29:1336–1346.
82. Appelbaum FR, Clift RA, Buckner CD, et al. Allogeneic marrow transplantation for acute nonlymphoblastic leukemia after first complete relapse. *Blood* 1983;61:949–953.
83. Buckner CD, Clift RA, Thomas ED, et al. Allogeneic marrow transplantation for patients with acute nonlymphoblastic leukemia in second remission. *Leukemia Res* 1982;6:395–399.
84. Forman SJ, Schmidt GM, Nademanee AP, et al. Allogeneic bone marrow transplantation as therapy for primary induction failure for patients with acute leukemia. *J Clin Oncol* 1991;9:1570–1574.
85. Mehta J, Powles R, Horton C, et al. Bone marrow transplantation for primary refractory acute leukemia. *Bone Marrow Transplant* 1994;14:415–418.
86. Biggs JC, Horowitz MM, Gale RP, et al. Bone marrow transplants may cure patients with acute leukemia never achieving remission with chemotherapy. *Blood* 1992;80:1090–1093.

87. Fung HC, O'Donnell M, Popplewell L, et al. Allogeneic stem cell transplantation (SCT) for patients with primary refractory acute myelogenous leukemia (AML): impact of cytogenetic risk group on the transplant outcome, in press.
88. Tallman MS, Kopecky KJ, Amos D, et al. Analysis of prognostic factors for the outcome of marrow transplantation or further chemotherapy for patients with acute nonlymphocytic leukemia in first remission. *J Clin Oncol* 1989;7:326–337.
89. Stein AS, Forman SJ. Autologous hematopoietic cell transplantation for acute myeloid leukemia. In: Forman SJ, Blume KG, Thomas ED, eds. *Hematopoietic Cell Transplantation*, 2nd ed. London: Blackwell Science, 1999:963–977.
90. Burnett AK, Goldstone AH, Stevens RMF, et al. Randomised comparison of addition of autologous bone-marrow transplantation to intensive chemotherapy for acute myeloid leukemia in first remission. Results of MRC AML 10 trial. *Lancet* 1998;351:700–708.
91. Zittoun RA, Mandelli F, Willemze R, et al. Autologous or allogeneic bone marrow transplantation compared with intensive chemotherapy in acute myelogenous leukemia. *N Engl J Med* 1995;332:217–223.
92. Ball ED, Mills LE, Cornwell GG 3rd, et al. Autologous bone marrow transplantation for acute myeloid leukemia using monoclonal antibody-purged bone marrow. *Blood* 1990;75:1199–1206.
93. Cassileth PA, Andersen J, Lazarus HM, et al. Autologous bone marrow transplant in acute myeloid leukemia in first remission. *J Clin Oncol* 1993;11:314–319.
94. Löwenberg B, Verdonck LJ, Dekker AW, et al. Autologous bone marrow transplantation in acute myeloid leukemia in first remission: results of a dutch prospective study. *J Clin Oncol* 1990;8:287–294.
95. Cassileth PA, Harrington DP, Appelbaum FR, et al. Chemotherapy compared with autologous or allogeneic bone marrow transplantation in the management of acute myeloid leukemia in first remission. *N Engl J Med* 1998;339:1649–1656.
96. Fefer A. Graft-versus-tumor responses. In: Forman SJ, Blume KG, Thomas ED, eds. *Hematopoietic Cell Transplantation* 2nd ed, London: Blackwell Science, 1999:316–326.
97. Weisdorf DJ, Anderson PM, Kersey JH, et al. Interleukin-2 therapy immediately after autologous marrow transplantation: toxicity, T cell activation and engraftment. *Blood* 1991;78:226.
98. Klingemann HG, Eaves CJ, Barnett MJ, et al. Transplantation of patients with high risk acute myeloid leukemia in first remission with autologous marrow cultured in interleukin-2 followed by interleukin-2 administration. *Bone Marrow Transplant* 1994;14:389–396.
99. Robinson N, Benyunes MC, Thompson JA, et al. Interleukin-2 after autologous stem cell transplantation for hematologic malignancy: a phase I/II study. *Bone Marrow Transplant* 1997;19:435–442.
100. Stein AS, Slovak ML, Sniecinski I, et al. Immunotherapy with IL-2 after autologous stem cell transplant for acute myelogenous leukemia in first remission. Proceedings of the Ninth International Symposium on Autologous Blood and Marrow Transplantation 1999;1:46–53.
101. Bennett JM, Catovsky D, Daniel MT, et al. Proposals for the classification of the myelodysplastic syndromes. *Br J Haematol* 1982;51:189–199.
102. Greenberg PL. Myelodysplastic syndrome. In: Hoffman R, Benz Jr. EJ, Shattil SJ, Furie B, Cohen HJ, Silberstein LE, McGlave P, eds. *Hematology. Basic Principles and Practice*, 3rd ed. New York: Churchill Livingstone, 2000:1106–1129.
103. Krishnan, A., Bhatia, S., Slovak, M., et al. Predictors of therapy-related leukemia and myelodysplasia following autologous transplantation for lymphoma: an assessment of risk factors. *Blood* 2000;96:1588–1593.
104. Tucker MA, Coleman CN, Cox RS, et al. Risk of second cancers after treatment for Hodgkin's disease. *N Engl J Med* 1988;318:76–81.
105. Deeg HJ, Appelbaum FR. Hemopoietic stem cell transplantation for myelodysplastic syndrome. *Curr Opin Oncol* 2000;12:116–120.
106. Witherspoon RP, Deeg HJ, Storer B, et al. Hematopoietic stem-cell transplantation for treatment-related leukemia or myelodysplasia. *J Clin Oncol* 2001;19:2134–2141.
107. de Witte T. Stem cell transplantation in myelodysplastic syndromes. *Forum* 1999;9:75–81.
108. Deeg HJ, Storer B, Slattery JT, et al. Conditioning with targeted busulfan and cyclophosphamide for hemopoietic stem cell transplantation from related and unrelated donors in patients with myelodysplastic syndrome. *Blood* 2002, in press.
109. Anderson JE, Gooley TA, Schoch G, et al. Stem cell transplantation for secondary acute myeloid leukemia: evaluation of transplantation as initial therapy or following induction chemotherapy. *Blood* 1997;89:2578–2585.

110. Yakoub-Agha I, de La Salmoniere P, Ribaud P, et al. Allogeneic bone marrow transplantation for therapy-relatedd myelodysplastic syndrome and acute myeloid leukemia: a long-term study of 70 patients—report of the French society of bone marrow transplantation. *J Clin Oncol* 2000;18:963–971.

2 Hematopoietic Stem Cell Transplantation for Chronic Myelogenous Leukemia

Humberto Caldera, MD *and Sergio Giralt,* MD

CONTENTS

1. INTRODUCTION AND HISTORICAL PERSPECTIVE

Chronic myelogenous leukemia (CML) is a myeloproliferative disorder characterized by specific hematologic and cytogenetic abnormalities. It was the first malignant disease to be linked to a consistent chromosomal abnormality: the Philadelphia (Ph) chromosome, which was first described in 1960 by Nowell and Hungerford *(1–3)*.

The natural course of CML is very well characterized and usually follows a triphasic process through chronic, accelerated, and blastic phases *(4)*; the median survival of patients with CML treated with hydroxyurea is 4–5 yr. Over the last two decades, the goals of treatment for CML have changed from palliative measures that could result in symptom control to curative therapies aimed at achieving complete disappearance of the disease as measured by cytogenetic and molecular markers. High-dose chemotherapy followed by allogeneic hematopoietic stem cell transplantation (HSCT) was the first curative therapy described for CML and remains the curative treatment with the longest established track record in this disease *(5)*.

Fefer et al. reported the first syngeneic bone marrow transplantations (BMT) for the treatment of CML in 1979 *(5)*. The leukemic clone was successfully eliminated in four patients with chronic-phase CML who were treated with a combination of cyclophosphamide, dimethylbusulfan, and 920 cGy of total-body irradiation (TBI) followed by an infusion of syngeneic bone mar-

From: *Stem Cell Transplantation for Hematologic Malignancies*
Edited by: R. J. Soiffer © Humana Press Inc., Totowa, NJ

row. In this initial series as well as the updated series from the same institution, more than half of the patients remained alive and free of disease *(6)*. These results demonstrated that permanent eradication of the leukemic clone as defined by the absence of cells containing the Ph chromosome on standard cytogenetic evaluations was possible and that high-dose chemoradiotherapy could result in long-term disease control without evidence of disease transformation.

The results from syngeneic transplants were the basis for the development of allogeneic BMT from human leukocyte antigen (HLA)-matched siblings for the treatment of chronic-phase CML. Goldman et al. *(7)* reported in 1982 the first series of 14 patients undergoing HLA-identical sibling BMT using high-dose cyclophosphamide (Cy) and TBI (Cy/TBI). Twelve of those patients survived and had normalization of blood counts and no evidence of Ph-positive cells in the bone marrow or in the peripheral blood.

The allograft experience demonstrated that complete cytogenetic remission (as defined by the absence of the Ph+ chromosome using conventional cytogenetic techniques) could be used as a surrogate marker for long-term disease control and probable cure. The importance of cytogenetic remissions as a surrogate marker for disease control has also been demonstrated for nontransplant therapies such as interferon and the novel tyrosine kinase inhibitor imatinib mesilate (STI-571) *(8–13)*.

2. PATHOGENETIC MECHANISMS OF CHRONIC MYELOGENOUS LEUKEMIA: IMPLICATIONS FOR PROGENITOR STEM CELL TRANSPLANTATION

In 1973, Rowley (3) recognized that the Ph chromosome resulted from a balanced translocation between chromosomes 9 and 22 (9;22). The translocation involves a reciprocal transfer of the Abelson proto-oncogene (c-abl) sequence in the long arm of chromosome 9 to variable locations in the breakpoint cluster region (bcr-1) in the short arm of chromosome 22 *(3,14)*. The fusion gene resulting from the translocation (9;22) can direct the synthesis of one of the following chimeric proteins with tyrosine kinase activity: p210 (bcr-abl) or p190 (bcr-abl) *(15)*. Irradiated mice treated with a retrovirus encoding the protein p210 sequence will develop a disease with the characteristics of chronic-phase human CML *(16)*, providing definite evidence that the bcr-abl translocation is essential in the pathogenesis of the disease. Thus, cure of CML will, by definition, imply elimination of all clonogenic cells containing the Ph chromosome. One of the hallmarks of CML progenitor cells is their genetic instability, which leads to additional chromosomal abnormalities, which, in turn, will eventually lead to the loss of normal differentiation and the accumulation of immature forms, characteristic of the transformed phases of the disease *(17,18)*.

Chronic myelogenous leukemia progenitor cells that give rise to the transformed phenotype of the disease are more resistant to conventional as well as high-dose chemoradiotherapy regimens and, generally, are also resistant to immune therapeutic maneuvers such as allografting and interferon *(19–22)*. This resistance explains why patients with transformed-phase disease have poorer outcomes and it has been the primary motivation to promote the use of allografting early in the course of the disease, despite the morbidity and mortality associated with this therapeutic modality *(23–25)*. Thus, optimal application of curative therapies (i.e., allogeneic transplantation) require that these therapies be applied early in the course of the disease (before disease transformation occurs) and preferably before the emergence of a large number of resistant clones.

3. RESULTS OF HEMATOPOIETIC STEM CELL TRANSPLANTATION

3.1. Syngeneic Transplantation

Results of syngeneic transplantation are informative because they provide the clinical evidence that high-dose chemoradiotherapy can eradicate CML, that purging may be beneficial, and that there is an important graft-vs-leukemia (GVL) effect operating in the allograft setting. Results from single institution and registry analysis demonstrate that high-dose chemoradiotherapy with syngeneic transplants can achieve a 59% leukemia-free survival (LFS) at 3 yr in patients with CML. Nonrelapse mortality rates (NRM) are low (<10%), and the 3-yr relapse rate is around 40% for patients in the chronic phase *(6,26)*. These results confirm the efficacy of dose-intensive therapy in promoting long-term disease control in CML. Results for patients with transformed phase are significantly inferior, particularly in the setting of blast crisis, primarily the result of an increased incidence of relapse posttransplant.

3.2. HLA-Identical Sibling Transplantation

For many years, allogeneic transplantation from an HLA-identical sibling was considered the only curative treatment option for patients with CML *(27)*. Despite a 30% NRM, the 50–60% cure rate justified the recommendation of using allogeneic transplantation as front-line therapy for CML *(27–29)*. The most popular conditioning regimens used have been chemoradiotherapy (Cy/TBI) and combination chemotherapy with busulfan (BU) and cyclophosphamide (BU-Cy) *(29–35)*. In 1994, Clift et al. *(31)* from the Seattle group reported the results of a randomized trial comparing BU-Cy (16 mg/kg BU over 4 d, followed by 60 mg/kg/d Cy for 2 d) vs Cy-TBI (60 mg/kg/d Cy for 2 d, followed by six fractions of TBI at 2 Gy/d) as conditioning regimens prior to allogeneic BMT (alloBMT) from HLA-identical siblings in patients with chronic-phase CML. Seventy-three patients received BU-Cy and 69 received Cy/TBI. There were no differences in overall survival (80% in both groups) and relapse rate (13% in both groups) at 3 yr. The Cy/TBI regimen was clearly more toxic: There were more cases of acute graft-vs-host disease (GVHD), more fever days, positive blood cultures, more prolonged hospitalizations, and increases in the creatinine level. The incidence of veno-occlusive liver disease was similar, as was the speed of engraftment.

Those results were updated in 1999 *(32)* after a median follow-up of 7.7 yr. The Kaplan–Meier probabilities of survival at 9 yr are 73% for patients treated with the BU-Cy regimen and 65% for the CyTBI regimen (*p* nonsignificant). The cumulative incidence of relapse was 19% for the BU-Cy regimen and 22% for the Cy/TBI regimen (*p* nonsignificant); the event-free survival (EFS) probabilities were 55% for the BU-Cy group and 48% for the Cy/TBI group, respectively. In a recent meta-analysis of the largest published randomized trials, the projected 10-yr survival estimates were 65% and 63% with BU-Cy vs Cy/TBI, respectively. The disease-free survival (DFS) estimates at 10 yr were 52% for the BU-Cy group and 46% for the Cy/TBI group. The 5-yr incidence of chronic extensive GVHD was not different: 37% in the BU-Cy group and 39% in the Cy/TBI group *(33–35)*.

In summary, for patients with CML in chronic phase undergoing allogeneic stem cell transplantation (alloSCT) from HLA-identical sibling donors, no optimal regimen has been identified. Both Cy/TBI and BU-Cy regimens provide similar efficacy and long-term results, but the BU-Cy regimen is better tolerated and is, at the moment, the most commonly used regimen for this indication.

In the classic BU-Cy regimen, the busulfan is given orally; because of the large number of pills that the patients need to take to achieve an appropriate dosage and the significant incidence of gastrointestinal problems in the allogeneic transplant setting, the absorption of the drug becomes very unpredictable and, therefore, oral bioavailability can vary as much as sixfold from patient to patient *(36)*. The interpatient and intrapatient variability in oral busulfan absorption results in significant disparities in measured busulfan levels among patients. Busulfan plasma levels have correlated with engraftment, disease control, and toxicity. Slattery et al. *(37,38)* reported that patients with CML whose busulfan-steady state plasma concentration was less than 917 ng/mL had a higher rejection rate and relapse rate than patients with area under curve (AUC) greater than 917 ng/mL. Likewise levels below 200 ng/mL were associated with high rejection rates and autologous reconstitution. In the pediatric population, high busulfan plasma concentrations have been associated with a higher incidence of veno-occlusive disease *(39)*.

To overcome the variability of busulfan dosing, two strategies have been proposed. Pharmacologic monitoring requires measuring plasma levels of busulfan and adjusting busulfan administration to obtain a target dose. The Seattle group reported their experience with this approach and have demonstrated that dose adjustment is feasible and results in more than 70% of patients achieving long-term remissions *(38,40)*. The second strategy has involved the use of an intravenous formulation of busulfan. Intravenous busulfan results in more predictable dosing and better patient tolerability; pharmacokinetic studies have demonstrated that adequate blood levels can be achieved when the drug is given intravenously every 6 h for 16 doses *(41)*. Long-term results with intravenous busulfan as well as comparative trials of intravenous busulfan vs pharmacologic monitoring with oral busulfan are not available. For now, both strategies seem to represent the standard of care for allogeneic transplantation for CML in chronic phase.

The results of allogeneic transplantation for the treatment of patients with CML in the accelerated or blastic phase are not as encouraging as those obtained in the chronic phase of the disease. There is an increased risk of transplant-related complications, increased relapse rate and decreased survival, ranging from 0% to 25% in patients in blastic phase and from 15% to 40% in patients in the accelerated phase *(27,30,42)*. It has been suggested that younger age and cytogenetic abnormalities additional to the Ph+ chromosome as sole manifestations of accelerated disease are independent factors for better survival in this group *(43)*. More intensive regimens may be beneficial for patients in the accelerated phase but not in the blastic phase *(44)*.

Although many patients with CML undergoing BMT are cured, the consequences and side effects of allogeneic transplants can still be felt many years afterward. Socié et al. from the Late Effects Working Committee of the International Bone Marrow Transplant Registry (IBMTR) reviewed 2146 patients with CML that were disease-free 2 yr after transplantation; the relative mortality rate at 5 yr after BMT was 11.2 and it was 19.1 after 10 yr. The most common causes for mortality were relapsed disease (*n*=47) and chronic GVHD (*n*=36). Thus, although many patients are cured with transplant, the mortality rate remains higher than that expected for the general population for many years *(45)*.

3.3. Alternative Donor Transplantation

When an HLA-identical sibling is not available, an alternative donor must be found. These alternative donors include phenotypically HLA-matched or near-matched family members, phenotypically matched unrelated volunteers, and phenotypically matched or mismatched cord blood stem cells. Up to 10% of patients will be able to find a suitably matched donor within an extended family search (phenotypic match or one-antigen-mismatched donor). The probability of identifying a compatible donor within the unrelated donor registries will depend on the ethnic background of the patient and the degree to which his or her ethnic group is represented in the different volunteer donor registries that are searched *(46)*.

The comparative outcomes of 974 patients receiving progenitor SCT for CML from different donor sources were reported to the IBMTR and published in 1997 *(47)*. Five hundred twenty-seven patients received a transplant from an HLA-identical sibling donor, 92 had a one-HLA-antigen-mismatched relative donor, 44 had a two-HLA-antigen-mismatched relative donor, 251 had an HLA-matched unrelated donor (MUD), and 60 patients had a one-HLA-antigen-mismatched unrelated donor. Recipients of alternative-donor transplants were, in general, "sicker" than those that received HLA-identical related transplants; they tended to have a worse performance status, more advanced disease, and higher white cell count. The interval time between diagnosis and transplant was shortest for HLA-identical sibling transplants, longer for alternative-related-donor transplants, and longest for unrelated donors. The conditioning regimen was more intensive for the alternative-donor transplants, who received more TBI, and other chemotherapies in addition to cyclophosphamide. Thirty-nine percent of unrelated-donor transplants and 49% of the related HLA-mismatched donors received T-cell-depleted grafts. Transplant-related mortality (TRM) was greater than 50% in all of the alternative-donor groups. The incidence of graft failure, acute and chronic GVHD, and relapse rate were all significantly higher in the alternative-donor transplants. NRM was similar in MUD and one-HLA-antigen-mismatched related donors, with risks 1–2.5 times higher than HLA-identical sibling transplants. NRM rates with two-HLA-antigen-mismatched relative donor and one-HLA-antigen-mismatched unrelated donor were similar and three times higher than HLA-identical sibling transplants.

In 1998, the Seattle team reported the outcome of 196 patients with CML who received unrelated transplants at that institution *(48)*. After a median follow-up of 5 yr, survival was estimated at 57%, with a relapse rate of 10%. The survival was negatively affected by an interval from diagnosis to treatment of more than 1 yr, an HLA-DRB1 mismatch, high body-weight index, and age older than 50 yr. Prophylactic use of antibiotics (ganciclovir and fluconazole) was associated with an improved survival. Five-year survival was 74% for patients younger than 50 yr who received a transplant from an HLA-matched donor within 1 yr of diagnosis.

Most recently, the National Marrow Donor Program reported the outcome of 916 matched unrelated donor transplantations for chronic-phase CML facilitated through them *(49)*. Eighty-six percent of the patients were conditioned with Cy/TBI, and 81% of the transplants were perfectly matched. Five-year overall survival (OS) was 47% for patients older than 35 yr and 67% for those 20–35 yr old. The overall DFS was 43%. The most recent survival data comes from the IBMTR *(50)*: One thousand three hundred patients with CML received transplants from matched unrelated donors between 1991 and 1997. The 3-yr probability of survival was 50% for those transplanted in the first year after the diagnosis (n=403) and 40% for those transplanted later in their disease (n=897). Results of representative studies for allografts in CML are summarized in Table 1.

The worse outcome observed in alternative-donor transplant when compared to HLA-identical sibling donors may be in part related to an underestimation of HLA mismatching by standard serologic techniques *(51)*; more sensitive DNA-based techniques were not available during the last decade. With improved molecular and DNA-based HLA typing techniques, it

Table 1
Results of Representative Series of Allogeneic Transplants for CML in Chronic Phase According to Donor Type

n donor type	*Regimen*[a]	*OS*[a]	*DFS*[a]	*NRM*[a]	*RR*[a]	*Ref.*
142/HLA-identical sibling	Cy/TBI (n=69) BU-Cy (n=73)	65% at 9 yr 73% at 9 yr	48% at 9 yr 55% at 9 yr	25% 20%	22% 19%	33
120/HLA-identical sibling	Cy/TBI (n=55) BU-Cy (n=65)	66% at 5 yr 61% at 5 yr	51% at 5 yr 59% at 5 yr	NR[a]	4% 4%	35
916/MUD (19% one AgMM)	Cy/TBI (86%) BU-Cy (14%)	47% at 5 yr (>35 yr old) 67% at 5 yr (20–35 yr old)	43% at 5 yr	NR	6%	49
196/MUD	Cy/TBI	57% at 5 yr	NR	39%	10%	48

[a]Abbreviations: OS, overall survival; DFS, disease-free survival; NRM, nonrelapse mortality; RR, relapse rate; Cy, cyclophosphamide; BU, busulfan; TBI, total body irradiation; MUD, matched unrelated donor; AgMM, antigen mismatch; NR, not reported.

will be possible to identify better matched donors, which, in turn, will likely improve the outcome of these transplants in the near future. Furthermore, improved GVHD prophylaxis and therapy and more aggressive management of bacterial, viral, and fungal infections, including the use of prophylactic agents, will also have a positive effect in the outcome of matched unrelated donor BMT.

3.4. Umbilical Cord Blood Transplantation

Umbilical cord blood transplantation (UCBT) is an alternative source of stem cells for those patients lacking a suitable donor. Since the first successful transplantation was performed in 1989 *(52)*, this treatment became popular over the last decade. Initial experiences with HLA-identical and HLA-1-mismatched sibling grafts proved that engraftment was possible in children with hematologic and metabolic disorders. The incidence of acute and chronic GVHD was very low, and the survival after 19 mo was 72% *(53)*. It was later demonstrated that this therapy was effective even when using HLA-mismatched grafts from unrelated donors *(54)*.

The experience of cord blood transplantation in adults is more limited, and to the present there are no large series reporting the outcome of this strategy in adult CML patients. The largest two series *(55,56)* reported 90 adult patients with hematologic and congenital metabolic disorders, including 27 patients with CML. Results in both series were similar, with a high transplant-related mortality (more than 40%). Most patients developed grade II acute skin GVHD. Chronic GVHD, mostly limited, developed in about 40% of the surviving patients. DFS was 53% at 1 yr in one study *(55)* and 26% at 40 mo in the other *(56)*, and it was not influenced by the diagnosis (CML vs others).

The current available data indicate that unrelated cord blood transplant may induce durable engraftment in the majority of the adult patients with hematologic malignancies. Better outcomes are seen in younger patients who receive the transplant in earlier stages of their disease. With the limited available data, it is clear that this approach should be reserved for patients in whom matched unrelated donors are not available. Newer strategies, including graft manipulation (i.e., expansion, multiple cord transplants) and nonmyeloablative conditioning regimens, are under investigation and may contribute to improve the outcome of cord blood transplantation in the near future.

3.5. Autologous Transplantation

Autologous BMT for CML has been investigated as an alternative strategy for patients lacking a suitable allogeneic donor. In the last decade, several studies have shown that benign Ph-negative stem cells may coexist in the bone marrow with the Ph-positive clone, particularly in the earlier stages of the disease *(17,18,57)*. Furthermore, treatment with interferon or intensive chemotherapy plus or minus hematopoietic growth factors can induce or reestablish Ph-negative hematopoiesis *(8,9,57)*.

High-dose chemotherapy with autologous bone marrow or peripheral blood stem cell transplantation has been explored extensively in CML. When performed in patients with advanced disease, the results are poor, with few, if any, patients achieving long-term disease control, despite the use of purging, chronic-phase marrow, and posttransplant interferon *(58)*.

Several studies evaluating high-dose chemotherapy followed by autologous bone marrow or peripheral stem transplantation for patients with chronic-phase CML have been conducted in Europe and North America *(56–67)*. Outcomes are significantly better in patients with a lower percentage of Ph+ cells in the infused product, transplanted earlier in the course of their disease, and who received posttransplant interferon *(66,67)*. The Genoa Group reported minimal graft failure and zero transplant-related mortality in a small cohort of patients (n=30) transplanted in the early chronic phase followed by posttransplant immunotherapy with interferon and interleukin-2. The actuarial survival rate after 3.5 yr of follow-up was 87% *(60)*.

Autologous transplant in CML should still be considered an investigational strategy. Autografting will need to be re-explored in the context of imatinib mesylate-induced remissions. Stem cell collections and transplants with in vivo imatinib-purged marrows have been performed in a small number of patients with rapid engraftment and good outcomes (S. Giralt, unpublished data).

3.6. Novel Transplantation Techniques

The results of high-dose chemotherapy and autologous transplant demonstrate that in most patients the high-dose chemoradiotherapy may not eradicate the malignant clone. The therapeutic benefit of allogeneic HSCT in CML is largely related to the immunologically mediated GVL effect. This observation is best supported by the fact that up to 70% of patients with relapsed CML after an allogeneic BMT (alloBMT) can achieve cytogenetic and molecular remission after donor lymphocyte infusions *(68–73)*.

High-dose chemotherapy followed by "standard" allogeneic transplantation carries a significant risk of morbidity and mortality depending on disease status, histocompatibility, and patient's age and overall medical condition; therefore, allogeneic transplants are generally reserved for younger patients (less than 50–55 yr old) without comorbid conditions *(30–35,74–77)*.

Because some malignancies, including CML, can be cured by a GVL effect induced by donor lymphocyte infusion (DLI), alternative therapeutic strategies consisting of a less toxic, nonmyeloablative conditioning regimen followed by allogeneic transplantation have been developed. These regimens would potentially decrease the risk of complications, expanding the indications for alloBMT to older and medically debilitated patients *(77–82)*. Combinations of purine analogs and alkylating agents, as well as low-dose TBI have been used as nonablative conditioning regimens by several investigators *(79–82)*.

Chronic myelogenous leukemia would intuitively be the disease in which nonablative transplant should be most effective because of the strong GVL effect that is operative in this entity. Notwithstanding the experience with nonablative transplantation in this disease, it is still limited, primarily as a result of the availability of other nontransplant options. Table 2 summarizes the most important series reported to date *(83–88)*.

The following conclusions can be derived from the current experience:

1. Nonablative transplantation is feasible in older patients with CML.
2. Graft failure is a cause of treatment failure and occurs more commonly in the patients who did not receive fludarabine.
3. Graft-vs-host disease still occurs, but NRM seems to be lower than that seen after conventional preparative regimens.
4. Disease-free survival is comparable to younger patients in the chronic phase; however, patients with advanced disease may have better disease control with reduced intensity conditioning over true nonablative therapies.
5. The role of imatinib in this setting has not been formally explored and may be important for outcomes.

Table 2
Results of Nonablative Transplantation for CML

n	*Age (yr)*	*No. of Patients CP1*[a]	*Regimen*[a]	*Graft failure*	*aGVHD*	*NRM*	*DFS*	*Ref.*
10	59 (42–72)	5	FAI	2/10	10%	10%	3/5 CP, 0/5 advanced	82
21	39 (3–57)	NS	FB	0/17	70%	12%	81% at 1 yr	83
12	56 (40–71)	8	TBI F-TBI	4/12	50%	16%	8/12 at 1 yr	84
13	34 (15–67)	8	FC	4/13	50%	0%	3/8 CP1, 1/5 advanced	85
45	NS	20	FB (80%)	15/45	48%	28%	33% at 1 yr	86
46	50 (29–62)	23	FM (67%)	7/39	24%	35%	80% CP1, 45% advanced	87

[a]Abbreviations: CP1, chronic phase 1; FAI, fludarabine; Ara-C, idarubicine; FB, fludarabine busulfan; TBI, total-body irradiation; FC, fludarabine cyclophosphamide; FM, fludarabine melphalan; aGVHD, acute graft-vs-host disease; NRM, nonrelapse mortality; DFS, disease-free survival.

6. The current indications for nonablative transplantation for the treatment of CML are not clear and this approach remains investigational; controlled trials comparing this approach vs standard myeloablative allogeneic transplantation are needed. These regimens can presently be recommended only for older or infirm patients with relatively stable CML.
7. The optimal posttransplant immunosuppressive therapy is not clear; a variety of regimens, including tacrolimus, methotrexate, or the combination of cyclosporine and mycophenolate mofetil have been used.

4. PROGNOSTIC FACTORS FOR TRANSPLANT OUTCOMES IN CML

The most important and well-established prognostic factor for transplant outcome in CML is the stage of the disease at the time of transplant. Other well-established prognostic factors include age, histocompatibility, and cytomegalovirus (CMV) status. In contrast to prior busulfan therapy, which has been demonstrated to affect transplant outcome in a negative fashion, pretreatment with interferon does not alter the outcome of patients with CML undergoing allogeneic transplantation. The IBMTR *(89)* reported the outcome of 209 patients treated with interferon-α (with or without concurrent hydroxyurea) for a median duration of 2 mo (range: 1–39 mo) compared to 664 patients who received only hydroxyurea prior to the transplantation. All patients received transplantations from HLA-identical sibling donors. The incidence of GVHD, NRM, survival, and DFS were similar and not affected by a short course of interferon prior to alloBMT *(89)*. These results have been confirmed by other groups *(90,91)*. A summary of prognostic factors is stated in Table 3.

T-Cell depletion has been shown to reduce the incidence of acute and chronic GVHD, but at the expense of increases in relapse and graft failure, therefore providing no definite benefit in survival (92–95). T-Cell depletion with pre-emptive donor lymphocyte infusions (DLIs) using molecular monitoring of bcr-abl may compensate for the increase relapse risk seen after T-cell-depleted allografts without increasing the risk of GVHD *(96)*.

5. TREATMENT OF RELAPSE POSTALLOGENEIC TRANSPLANTATION

5.1. Defining Relapse

Despite significant improvement in the outcome after allogeneic bone marrow transplantation in the last decade, CML relapse after allografting is an important cause of treatment failure *(97)*. Defining relapse is important not only to allow for comparisons among different treatment strategies, but also to determine who may need further therapy. Three types of relapses have been defined in CML *(97)*:

1. Hematologic relapses: recurrence of signs and symptoms of the disease
2. Cytogenetic relapses: recurrence of Philadelphia chromosome-positive-containing cells as determined by conventional cytogenetic techniques
3. Molecular relapses: as determined by the presence of the bcr/abl gene using polymerase chain reaction (PCR) technology

When clinical and/or hematologic relapse is evident, those patients will invariably progress to the accelerated and blastic phase if left untreated. Patients relapsing or progressing to transformed CML after transplant have an extremely poor outcome with a median survival of less than 2 yr. Patients with cytogenetic relapse may have a spontaneous cytogenetic remission up to 20% of the times if they had T-cell-repleted grafts, T-cell-depleted transplants will rarely

Table 3
Prognostic Factors for Outcome After Allogeneic Transplantation for CML

	Factor	*Favorable*	*Unfavorable*	*Comment*
Established	Age	Younger	Older	May be ameliorated by tailoring therapy (i.e., T-cell depletion or reduced intensity conditioning for older patients).
	Disease status	Chronic phase	Other	Advanced-phase disease should be considered for novel therapies (i.e., imatinib maintenance, prophylactic DLI, novel regimens, etc.).
	Histocompatibility	Matched sibling	Other	Modern typing techniques can identify unrelated donors who are 10/10 matched by molecular techniques. Results of transplants from these donors have been similar to those of fully matched donors.
	Time To Transplant	Less than 2 yr from diagnosis	Greater than 2 yr	Confounded by disease transformation
	Prior interferon therapy	None/Yes	Yes/none	Confounding results. Most series report no effect on outcome. Potential reduce risk of relapse versus increase risk of GVHD.
	T-Cell depletion	None	Yes	May change with PCR monitoring and pre-emptive DLI therapy.
	Stem cell source	Peripheral blood	Bone marrow	Benefit for peripheral blood may be seen only in patients with advanced disease and may actually be deleterious for patients in the chronic phase.

show transient cytogenetic relapses and will generally have rapid hematologic progression. Interferon therapy can delay hematologic progression after cytogenetic relapse, but may have only a minimal effect on long-term survival *(98,99)*.

The significance of having a positive PCR test is controversial and does not always predict cytogenetic or hematologic relapse, although a single positive PCR test is associated with a significant risk of relapse *(100)*. The detection of bcr-abl at 6–12 mo after BMT was associated with a 42% risk of relapse at a median of 200 d, compared to 3% risk of relapse in the PCR-negative patients. The detection of bcr-abl later in the posttransplant period may have a different significance. Two groups have reported a high incidence of bcr-abl positivity of 25% and 56% at a median of 36 mo after BMT *(100,101)*. The relapse rate was just 8–10%, indicating that this finding may not confer a high risk for "late" relapse.

In order to assess the risk of relapse in patients who test positive for the bcr-abl translocation by PCR, Radich et al. *(102)* evaluated 379 patients who were alive at 18 mo or longer after alloBMT for CML. Ninety patients (24%) had at least one positive PCR test, and 13 of them relapsed (14%). Quantification assays were performed on the bcr-abl-positive samples. It was found that the median bcr-abl level at relapse was 40,443 bcr-abl copies per microgram of RNA. Sixty-nine percent of the bcr-abl-positive patients who did not relapse had only one positive test at a median of 24 copies of bcr-abl per microgram of RNA. This observation may have a prognostic implication and may prompt an earlier therapeutic intervention.

5.2. Treating Relapse

Treatment of patients that relapse after an alloBMT for CML has changed dramatically over the last 10 yr. Initially, only a second BMT was the only potential curative intervention, although few patients achieved durable remissions because of the high rates of morbidity and mortality *(103,104)*. Interferon therapy was shown to reinduce remissions, in a proportion of patients who relapsed after allograft; although delays in disease progression were documented as well as achievement of complete cytogenetic remissions, the impact on survival was marginal at best *(98,99)*.

Lymphocyte infusion from the original donor (DLI) has become the most effective treatment for patients with CML that relapse after an alloBMT. A direct GVL reaction can be induced by the administration of these immunocompetent cells, and complete remissions with acceptable toxicity and without additional therapy can be achieved. The probability of maintaining a remission after 2–3 yr is between 70% and 90% in patients with chronic-phase relapse *(68–70,105–109)*. Responses in patients with accelerated- or blastic-phase relapses are significantly inferior and less durable. Chronic-phase relapse, time between BMT and DLI shorter than 2 yr, pre-DLI chronic GVHD, and development of acute or chronic GVHD post-DLI predict better outcomes for DLI therapy *(68–70)*.

The most common complications of DLI are infections, acute and chronic GVHD, and pancytopenia *(68–70)*. Up to 60% of the patients will develop acute GVHD, about half of them grade III or IV. More than 50% of the patients will also develop extensive chronic GVHD *(68–70)*. Patients with hematologic relapse tend to develop more myelosuppression than those with only cytogenetic relapse. Pancytopenia is less likely to occur if the hematopoiesis is still driven by donor cells; hence, DLI given early in the course of the relapse will likely minimize the incidence and severity of bone marrow aplasia *(105)*.

Two strategies have been used to reduce the risk of GVHD after DLI. The M.D. Anderson group reported on the use of CD8-depleted DLI and demonstrated a low incidence of acute

Table 4
Results of Imatinib Mesylate as Treatment for CML Relapse After Allogeneic Transplantation

n	*Stage*[a]	*% Response CHR/CMR*[a]	*Toxicity*[a]	*Ref.*
13	CP=6/>CP=7	100/60%	WBC, edema	110
28	CP=5/>CP=23	75/52%	GVHD	111
15	NS	80/50%	WBC	112
13	>CP=13	60/40%	WBC	113
12	CP=5/>CP=12	50/30%	LFTs, WBC	114
17	CP=10/>CP=7	100/70%	GI, WBC	115

[a]Abbreviations: CP, chronic phase; CHR, complete hematologic response; CMR, complete molecular response; WBC, white blood cell; GVHD, graft-vs-host disease; LFT, liver function tests; GI, gastrointestinal.

GVHD (10%) with a high durable response rate (80%) in patients with chronic-phase CML relapsing after an allograft *(106)*. These results have been confirmed by Alyea et al. and expanded to other diseases such as myeloma *(107)*. Dose-escalated DLI has also been effective in reducing the risk of GVHD without affecting the efficacy of DLIs for the treatment of CML relapsing after an allograft. Dazzi et al. *(108)* compared, in a nonrandomized fashion, the administration of DLI as a single-dose (1.0×10^8 cells/kg) vs a sequential, escalating dose regimen (starting at 1×10^7). Patients in the escalating group received a total dose of 1.9×10^8 lymphocytes/kg. The probability of achieving a cytogenetic remission was not different between the two groups, but the incidence of GVHD was much lower in the second group (10% vs 44%, respectively; p=0.011). These findings suggest that administering the same doses of lymphocytes over several infusions may decrease the incidence of GVHD.

Imatinib mesylate has also been used in patients relapsing after an allograft, including those who have failed to respond to donor lymphocyte infusions *(110–115)*. The reported experience to date is summarized in Table 4. These results show that imatinib can be an effective treatment for patients with CML relapsing after an allogeneic transplantation. However, long-term follow-up is unavailable, and the experience is still limited; thus, imatinib therapy should not replace DLIs in this setting unless it is in the context of a clinical trial or in the event that donor lymphocytes are not available.

6. ROLE OF HIGH-DOSE CHEMOTHERAPY AND ALLOGENEIC HSCT IN THE IMATINIB ERA

Based on the best available data, the American Society of Hematology published in 1999 the following recommendations for the treatment of CML with high-dose chemotherapy and allogeneic HSCT *(24)*:

1. Bone marrow transplantation should preferably be offered to patients within the first 2 yr after the diagnosis.

2. Early BMT over a trial of interferon should be offered to those patients with high-risk disease.
3. Younger patients are most likely to benefit from the treatment and there is virtually no experience in patients older than 65 yr; however, an upper age limit for BMT has not been fully defined and varies from center to center.
4. Bone marrow transplantation is most successful if the donor is an HLA-matched sibling (according to observational studies); results at most centers are inferior when a matched unrelated donor is used.
5. Patients who received busulfan therapy prior to BMT may do worse; there is no evidence of benefit in receiving prior hydroxyurea therapy, and the prior use of interferon does not seem to alter the outcome in related transplants. However, in at least one study, there appears to be deleterious result in transplants from matched unrelated donors.

These recommendations will probably change with our current therapeutic options for CML. The first change that has occurred is that allogeneic transplantation is not seen by many patients or investigators as the only curative option for CML. This view has been successfully challenged by the long-term results of patients who achieved a complete cytogenetic remission with interferon therapy. Results from the European Registry *(116)* demonstrated that for CML patients who achieved a complete remission to interferon, the OS at 5 yr was 86% and, more importantly, the progression-free survival was 58%. These results underscore the fact that long-term disease control can be achieved without allografting as long as complete cytogenetic remissions are obtained. Moreover, although some of these patients may be PCR negative, the relevance of PCR negativity in this setting is unknown, and changes in quantitative levels of disease as measured by PCR will probably be more relevant in predicting outcomes.

With the current age limitation of transplantation and the relatively low complete remission rate to interferon-based therapy, the development of the tyrosine kinase inhibitor imatinib mesylate has become the single most important therapeutic advance in CML. This agent has demonstrated an outstanding efficacy and safety profile. For patients with chronic-phase CML, the major and complete cytogenetic remission rates are 60% and 40%, respectively *(10–13)*. The median duration of remission in these patients has not been reached, and although follow-up is short, based on the experience with interferon-resistant and interferon-intolerant patients, recurrence is not a universal phenomenon. The response rate in patients with accelerated-phase and blast crisis are significantly lower and the duration of remission is shorter, with few, if any, patients achieving long-term disease control. As with interferon, the risk of fatal and serious life-threatening toxicities is extremely small.

The development of imatinib has obligated the CML community to rethink the standard approach for newly diagnosed patients. Prior to imatinib, the standard algorithm for patients with CML would include early transplantation for young patients with an HLA-identical sibling donor; the threshold for young was defined by each institution according to local results. Patients who were considered at higher risk for transplant complications either because of age or comorbidities or patients without an HLA-compatible donor would get a therapeutic trial of interferon. In the event of achieving major or complete cytogenetic remissions, transplantation would be deferred until signs of disease progression were evident; in the event of failure to respond to interferon, patients could undergo allografts if deemed eligible and if an alternative donor was available.

Despite the body of evidence supporting the early use of alloSCT for the treatment of CML, the current results with imatinib make it difficult not to recommend a therapeutic trial of imatinib for all patients—first to achieve hematologic remissions and then cytogenetic re-

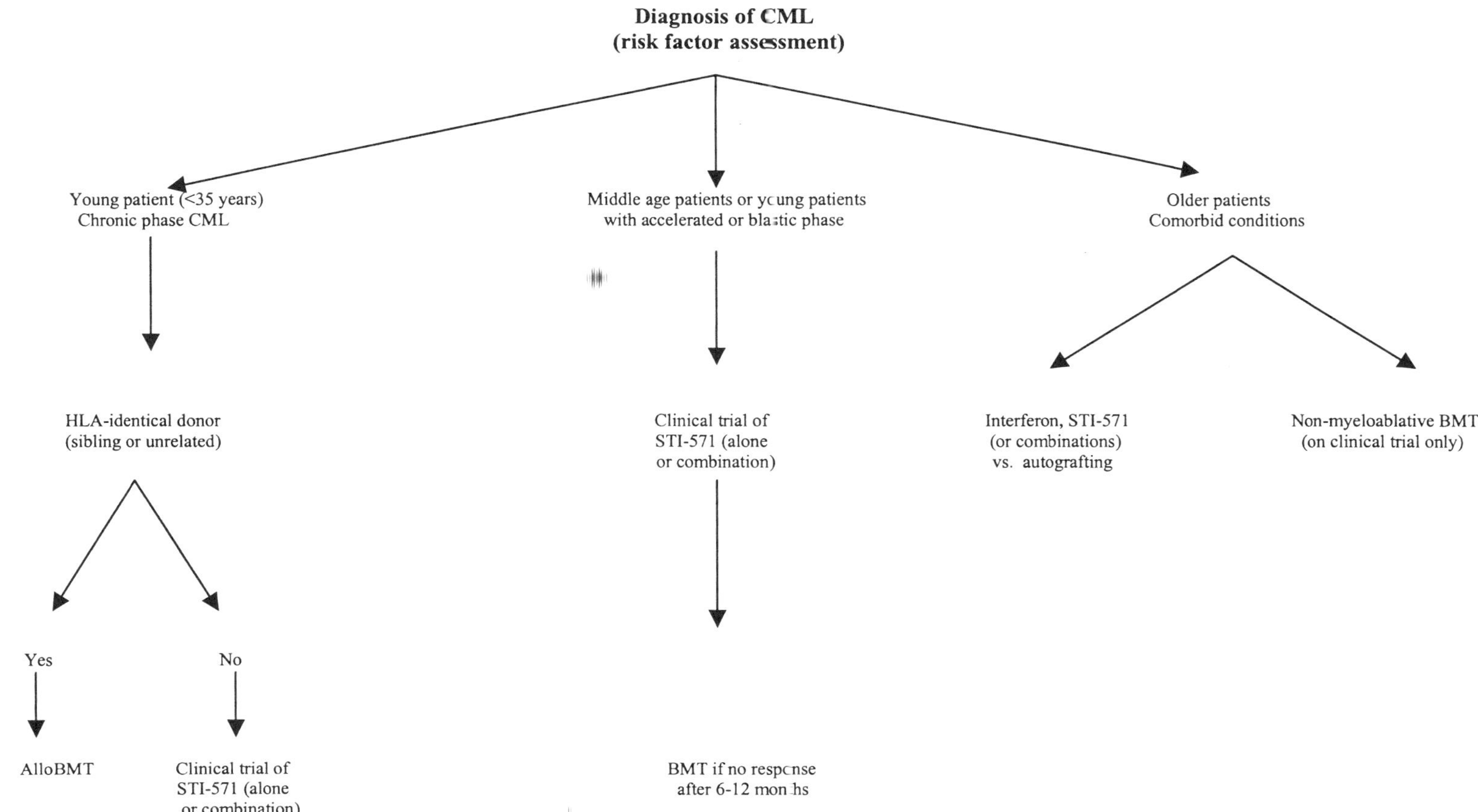

Fig. 1. Propsed algorithm for the teatment o patients with newly diagnosed CML.

sponses. This response would identify those patients in whom an early allograft would be considered appropriate (i.e., failure to achieve cytogenetic response within 6–12 mo of imatinib therapy) versus those in whom a more conservative strategy of continued imatinib therapy would be warranted. Notwithstanding, very young patients (i.e., less than 30 yr of age) could be considered for up-front transplantation if a donor is available because the morbidity and mortality of allografts in this patient population is relatively low and continues to improve. Thus, we and others have proposed the algorithm that is summarized in Fig. 1.

Imatinib will positively impact the field of transplantation in other ways beyond reducing the number of patients who will eventually need allografts for control of their disease. These include the following:

1. Imatinib therapy for relapse prevention postallograft in the high-risk setting (i.e., T-cell depletion or allografts in advanced-phase disease)
2. Imatinib purging (in vivo and in vitro) for collection of Ph-negative autologous stem cells
3. Imatinib maintenance after autografting

In conclusion, the field of transplantation for CML has undergone profound evolution, from the use of PCR monitoring for minimal residual disease to the risk stratification of patients according to their response to imatinib therapy. These advances will hopefully allow for the achievement of complete cytogenetic and molecular remission for most patients with CML and improve the natural history for all patients with this disease.

REFERENCES

1. Nowell PC, Hungerford DA. Chromosomes studies on normal and leukemic human leukocytes. *J Natl Cancer Inst* 1960;25:85–109.
2. Nowell PC, Hungerford DA. A minute chromosome in human granulocytic leukemia. *Science* 1960;132:1497.
3. Rowley JD. A new consistent chromosomal abnormality in chronic myelogenous leukemia identified by quinacrine and giemsa staining. *Nature* 1973;243:290–293.
4. Sokal JE, Baccarani M, Russo D, et al. Staging and prognosis in chronic myelogenous leukemia. *Semin Hematol* 1988;25(1):49–61.
5. Fefer A, Cheever MA, Thomas ED, et al. Disappearance of Ph(1)-positive cells in four patients with chronic granulocytic leukemia after chemotherapy, irradiation and marrow transplantation from an identical twin. *N Engl J Med* 1979;300(7):333–337.
6. Fefer A, Cheever MA, Greenberg PD, et al. Treatment of chronic granulocytic leukemia with chemoradiotherapy and transplantation of marrow from identical twins. *N Engl J Med* 1982;306(2):63–68.
7. Goldman JM, Baughan ASJ, McCarthy DM, et al. Marrow transplantation for patients in the chronic phase of chronic granulocytic leukaemia. *Lancet* 1982;2(8299):623–625.
8. Kantarjian HM, Smith TL, O'Brien S, et al. Prolonged survival in chronic myelogenous leukemia after cytogenetic response to interferon-α therapy. *Ann Intern Med* 1995;122(4):254–261.
9. Kantarjian HM, O'Brien S, Anderlini P, et al. Treatment of chronic myelogenous leukemia: current status and investigational options. *Blood* 1996;87(8):3069–3081.
10. Kantarjian HM, Sawyers CL, Hochhaus A, et al. Hematologic and cytogenetic responses to imatinib mesylate in chronic myelogenous leukemia. *N Engl J Med* 2002;346:645–652.
11. Druker BJ, Talpaz M, Resta DJ, et al. Efficacy and safety of a specific inhibitor of the BCR-ABL tyrosine kinase in chronic myeloid leukemia. *N Engl J Med* 2001;344(14):1031–1037.
12. Druker BJ, Sawyers CL, Kantarjian HM, et al. Activity of a specific inhibitor of the BCR-ABL tyrosine kinase in the blast crisis of chronic myeloid leukemia and acute lymphoblastic leukemia with the Philadelphia chromosome. *N Engl J Med* 2001;344(14):1038–1042.
13. Druker BJ for the International Randomized Interferon vs. STI-571 Study Group. STI571 versus interferon + cytarabine as initial therapy for patients with CML: results of a randomized study. *Proc Am Soc Clin Oncol* 2002;21:1a.

14. Kawasaki ES, Clark SS, Coyne MY, et al. Diagnosis of chronic myelogenous and acute lymphocytic leukemias by detection of leukemia-specific mRNA sequences amplified in vitro. *Proc Natl Acad Sci USA* 1988;85(15):5698–5702.
15. Knopka JB, Kriz R. An alteration of the human c-abl protein in K562 leukemia cells unmasks associated tyrosine kinase activity. *Cell* 1984;37:1035–1042.
16. Daley GQ, Van Etten RA, Baltimore D. Induction of chronic myelogenous leukemia in mice by the P210 bcr-abl gene of the Philadelphia chromosome. *Science* 1990;247(4944):824–830.
17. Kurzrock R, Gutterman JU, Talpaz M. The molecular genetics of Philadelphia chromosome-positive leukemias. *N Engl J Med* 1988;319(15):990–998.
18. Kurzrock R, Talpaz M. The molecular pathology of chronic myelogenous leukemia. *Br J Haematol* 1991;79(suppl 1):34–37.
19. Alimena G, Dallapiccola B, Gastaldi R, et al. Chromosomal, morphological, and clinical correlations in blastic crisis of chronic myelogenous leukaemia: a study of 69 cases. *Scand J Haematol* 1982;28(2):103–117.
20. Cervantes, F, Ballesta F, Mila M, et al. Cytogenetic studies in blast crisis of Ph-positive chronic granulocytic leukemia: results and prognostic evaluation in 52 patients. *Cancer Genet Cytogenet* 1986;21(3):239–246.
21. Swolin B, Weinfeld A, Westin J, et al. Karyotypic evolution in Ph-positive chronic myeloid leukemia in relation to management and disease progression. *Cancer Genet Cytogenet* 1985;18(1):65–79.
22. Singh S, Wass J, Vincent PC, et al. Significance of secondary cytogenetic changes in patients with Ph-positive chronic granulocytic leukemia in the acute phase. *Cancer Genet Cytogenet* 1986;21(3):209–220.
23. Sawyers CL. Chronic myeloid leukemia. *N Engl J Med* 1999;340:1330–1340.
24. Silver RT, Woolf SH, Hehlmann R, et al. An evidence-based analysis of the effect of busulfan, hydroxyurea, interferon, and allogeneic bone marrow transplantation in treating the chronic phase of chronic myeloid leukemia: developed by the American Society of Hematology. *Blood* 1999;94(5):1517–1536.
25. Lee SJ, Anasetti C, Horowitz MM et al. Initial therapy for chronic myelogenous leukemia: playing the odds. *J Clin Oncol* 1998;16(9):2897–2903.
26. Gale RP, Horowitz MM, Ash RC, et al. Identical-twin bone marrow transplants for leukemia. *Ann Intern Med* 1994;120(8):646–652.
27. Thomas ED, Clift RA, Fefer A, et al. Marrow transplantation for the treatment of chronic myelogenous leukemia. *Ann Intern Med* 1986;104(2):153–163.
28. Goldman JM, Szydlo RM, Horowitz MM, et al. Choice of pretransplant treatment and timing of transplants for chronic myelogenous leukemia in chronic phase. *Blood* 1993;82(7):2235–2238.
29. Giralt S, Kantarjian H, Talpaz M. The natural history of chronic myelogenous leukemia in the interferon era. *Semin Hematol* 1995;32(2):152–158.
30. Biggs JC, Szer J, Crilley P, et al. Treatment of chronic myeloid leukemia with allogeneic bone marrow transplantation after preparation with BuCy2. *Blood* 1992;80(5):1352–1357.
31. Clift RA, Buckner CD, Thomas ED, et al. Marrow transplantation for chronic myeloid leukemia: a randomized study comparing cyclophosphamide and total body irradiation with busulfan and cyclophosphamide. *Blood* 1994;84(6):2036–2043.
32. Clift RA, Radich J, Applebaum FR, et al. Long-term follow up of a randomized study comparing cyclophosphamide and total body irradiation with busulfan and cyclophosphamide for patients receiving allogeneic marrow transplants during chronic phase of chronic myeloid leukemia. *Blood* 1999;94(11):3960–3962.
33. Socié G, Clift RA, Blaise D, et al. Busulfan plus cyclophosphamide compared with total-body irradiation plus cyclophosphamide before marrow transplantation for myeloid leukemia: long-term follow-up of four randomized studies. *Blood* 2001;98(13):3569–3574.
34. Ringden O, Ruutu T, Remberger M, et al. A randomized trial comparing busulfan with total body irradiation as conditioning in allogeneic marrow transplant recipients with leukaemia-A report from the Nordic Bone Marrow Transplantation Group. *Blood* 1994;83(9):2723–2730.
35. Devergie A, Blaise D, Attal M, et al. Allogeneic bone marrow transplantation for chronic myeloid leukemia in first chronic phase: a randomized trial of busulfan–cytoxan versus cytoxan–total body irradiation as preparative regimen: a report from the French Society of Bone Marrow Graft (SFGM). *Blood* 1995;85(8):2263–2268.
36. Hassan M, Ljungman P, Bolme P, et al. Busulfan bioavailability. *Blood* 1994;84(7):2144–2150.
37. Slattery JT, Sanders JE, Buckner CD, et al. Graft-rejection and toxicity following bone marrow transplantation in relation to busulfan pharmacokinetics. *Bone Marrow Transplant* 1995;16(1):31–45.

38. Slattery JT, Clift RA, Buckner CD et al. Marrow transplantation for chronic myeloid leukemia: the influence of plasma busulfan levels on the outcome of transplantation. *Blood* 1997;89(8):3055–3060.
39. Grochow LB, Jones RJ, Brundrett RB, et al. Pharmacokinetics of busulfan: correlation with veno-occlusive disease in patients undergoing bone marrow transplantation. *Cancer Chemother Pharmacol* 1989;25(1):55–61.
40. Deeg HJ, Shulman HM, Anderson JE, et al. Allogeneic and syngeneic marrow transplantation for myelodysplastic syndrome in patients 55 to 66 years of age. *Blood* 2000;95(4):1188–1194.
41. Anderson BS, Kashyap A, Gian V, et al. Conditioning therapy with intravenous busulfan and cyclophosphamide (IV BuCy2) for hematologic malignancies prior to allogeneic stem cell transplantation: a phase II study. *Biol Blood Marrow Transplant* 2002;8:145–154.
42. Martin PJ, Clift RA, Fisher LD, et al. HLA-identical marrow transplantation during accelerated phase chronic myelogenous leukemia: analysis of survival and remission duration. *Blood* 1988;72(6):1978.
43. Clift RA, Buckner CD, Thomas ED, et al. Marrow transplantation for patients in accelerated phase of chronic myeloid leukemia. *Blood* 1994;84(12):4368–4373.
44. Przepiorka D, Khouri I, Thall P, et al. Thiotepa, busulfan and cyclophosphamide as a preparative regimen for allogeneic transplantation for advanced chronic myelogenous leukemia. *Bone Marrow Transplant* 1999;23(10):977–981.
45. Socié G, Stone JV, Wingard JR, et al. Long-term survival and late deaths after allogeneic bone marrow transplantation. *N Engl J Med* 1999;341(1):14–21.
46. Beatty PG, Dahlberg S, Mickelson EM, et al. Probability of finding HLA-matched unrelated marrow donors. *Transplantation* 1988;45(4):714–718.
47. Szydlo R, Goldman JM, Klein JP, et al. results of allogeneic bone marrow transplants for leukemia using donors other than HLA-identical siblings. *J Clin Oncol* 1997;15(5):1767–1777.
48. Hansen JA, Gooley TA, Martin PJ, et al. Bone marrow transplants from unrelated donors for patients with chronic myeloid leukemia. *N Engl J Med* 1998;338(14):962–968.
49. McGlave PB, Shu XU, Wen W, et al. Unrelated donor marrow transplantation for chronic myelogenous leukemia: 9 years experience of the National Marrow Donor program. *Blood* 2000;95(7):2219–2225.
50. International Bone Marrow Transplant Registry website.
51. Petersdorf EW, Smith AG, Mickelson, et al. Ten HLA-DR4 alleles defined by sequence polymorphisms within the DRB1 first domain. *Immunogenetics* 1991;33(4):267–275.
52. Gluckman E, Broxmeyer HE, Auerbach AD, et al. Hematopoietic reconstitution in a patient with Fanconi's anemia by means of umbilical-cord blood from an HLA-identical sibling. *N Engl J Med* 1989;321:1174–1178.
53. Wagner JE, Kernan NA, Steinbuch M, et al. Allogeneic sibling umbilical-cord-blood transplantation in children with malignant and non-malignant disease. *Lancet* 1995;346:214–219.
54. Kurtzberg J, Laughlin M, Graham ML, et al. Placental blood as a source of hematopoietic stem cells for transplantation into unrelated recipients. *N Engl J Med* 1996;335(3):157–166.
55. Sanz GF, Saavedra S, Planelles D, et al. Standardized, unrelated donor cord blood transplantation in adults with hematologic malignancies. *Blood* 2001;98(8):2332–2338.
56. Laughlin MJ, Barker J, Bambach B, et al. Hematopoietic engraftment and survival in adults recipients of umbilical-cord blood from unrelated donors. *N Engl J Med* 2001;344(24):1815–1822.
57. Verfaillie CM, Bhatia R, Steinbuch M, et al. Comparative analysis of autografting in chronic myelogenous leukemia: effects of priming regimen and marrow or blood origin of stem cells. *Blood* 1998;92(5):1820–1831.
58. Mcglave PB, De Fabritis P, Deisseroth A, et al. Autologous transplants for chronic myelogenous leukaemia: Results from eight transplant groups. *Lancet* 1994;343:1486–1488.
59. Pigneaux A, Faberes C, Boiron JM, et al. Autologous stem cell transplantation in chronic myeloid leukemia: a single center experience. *Bone Marrow Transplant* 1999;24(3):265–270.
60. Carella AM, Lerma E, Corsetti MT, et al. Autografting with Philadelphia chromosome-negative mobilized hematopoietic progenitor cells in chronic myelogenous leukemia. *Blood* 1999;93(5):1534–1539.
61. Boiron JM, Cahn JY, Meloni G, et al. Chronic myeloid leukemia in first chronic phase not responding to alpha-interferon: outcome and prognostic factors after autologous transplantation. EBMT Working Party on Chronic Leukemias. *Bone Marrow Transplant* 1999;24(3):259–264.
62. Carella AM, Chimirri F, Podesta M, et al. High-dose chemo-radiotherapy followed by autologous Philadelphia chromosome-negative blood progenitor cell transplantation in patients with chronic myelogenous leukemia. *Bone Marrow Transplant* 1996;17:201–205.

63. Barnett MJ, Eaves CJ, Phillips GL, et al. Autografting with cultured marrow in chronic myeloid leukemia: results of a pilot study. *Blood* 1994;84(3):724–732.
64. Khouri IF, Kantarjian HM, Talpaz M, et al. Results of high-dose chemotherapy and unpurged autologous stem cell transplantation in 73 patients with chronic myelogenous leukemia: the MD Anderson experience. *Bone Marrow Transplant* 1996;17:775–779.
65. Corsetti MT, Lerma E, Dejana A, et al. Cytogenetic response to autografting in chronic myelogenous leukemia correlates with the amount of BCR-ABL positive cells in the graft. *Exp Hematol* 2000;28(1):104–111.
66. Podesta M, Piaggio G, Sessarego M, et al. Autografting with Ph-negative progenitors in patients at diagnosis of chronic myeloid leukemia induces a prolonged prevalence of Ph-negative hemopoiesis. *Exp Hematol* 2000;28(2):210–215.
67. Talpaz M, Kantarjian H, Liang J, et al. Percentage of Philadelphia-chromosome (Ph)-negative and Ph-positive cells found after autologous transplantation for CML depends on percentage of diploid cells induced by conventional-dose chemotherapy before collection of autologous cells. *Blood* 1995;85:3257–3265.
68. Kolb HJ, Schattenberg A, Goldman JM, et al. Graft-versus-leukemia effect of donor lymphocyte transfusions in marrow grafted patients. *Blood* 1995;86(5):2041–2050.
69. Collins RH, Shpilberg O, Drobyski WR, et al. Donor leukocyte infusions in 140 patients with relapsed malignancy after allogeneic bone marrow transplantation. *J Clin Oncol* 19997;15(2):433–444.
70. Porter DL, Collins RH, Hardy C, et al. Treatment of relapsed leukemia after unrelated donor marrow transplantation with unrelated donor leukocyte infusions. *Blood* 2000;95(4):1214–1221.
71. Helg C, Starobinski M, Jeannet M, et al. Donor lymphocyte infusion for the treatment of relapse after allogeneic hematopoietic stem cell transplantation. *Leuk Lymphoma* 1998;29(3–4):301–313.
72. Drobyski WR, Keever CA, Roth MS, et al. Salvage immunotherapy using donor lymphocyte infusions as treatment for relapsed chronic myelogenous leukemia after allogeneic bone marrow transplantation: efficacy and toxicity of a defined T-cell dose. *Blood* 1993;82(8):2310–2318.
73. Porter DL, Roth MS, McGarigle C, et al. Induction of graft-versus-host disease as immunotherapy for relapsed chronic myeloid leukemia. *N Engl J Med* 1994;330(2):100–106.
74. Goldman JM, Szydlo RM, Horowitz MM, et al. Choice of pretransplant treatment and timing of transplants for chronic myelogenous leukemia in chronic phase. *Blood* 1993;82(7):2235–2238.
75. Van Rhee F, Szydlo RM, Hermans J, et al. Long-term results after allogeneic bone marrow transplantation for chronic myelogenous leukemia in chronic phase: a report from the Chronic Leukemia Working Party of the European Group for Blood and Marrow Transplantation. *Bone Marrow Transplant* 1997;20:553–560.
76. Goldman J, Gale R, Horowitz M, et al. Bone marrow transplantation for chronic myelogenous leukemia in chronic phase. *Ann Intern Med* 1988;108(6):806–814.
77. Giralt S, Estey E, Albitar M, et al. Engraftment of allogeneic hematopoietic progenitor cells with purine analog-containing chemotherapy: harnessing graft-versus-leukemia without myeloablative therapy. *Blood* 1997;89:4531–4536.
78. Champlin R, Khouri I, Avichai S, et al. Harnessing graft-versus-malignancy: non-myeloablative preparative regimens for allogeneic hematopoietic transplantation, an evolving strategy for adoptive immunotherapy. *Br J Haematol* 2000;111:18–29.
79. Storb R, Yu C, Sandmaier B, et al. Mixed hematopoietic chimerism after hematopoietic stem cell allografts. *Transplant Proc* 1999;31(1–2):677–678.
80. Slavin S. Nonmyeloablative stem cell transplantation and cell therapy as an alternative to conventional bone marrow transplantation with lethal cytoreduction for the treatment of malignant and nonmalignant hematologic diseases. *Blood* 1998;91:756–763.
81. Giralt S, Thall PF, Khoury I, et al. Melphalan and purine analog-containing preparative regimens: reduced-intensity conditioning for patients with hematologic malignancies undergoing allogeneic progenitor cell transplantation. *Blood* 2001;97(3):631–637.
82. Champlin R, Shimoni A, Cohen A, et al. FLAG–IDA, a non ablative preparative regimen with allogeneic PBSC transplantation for CML. *Blood* 2000;96:410a[Abstract 1764].
83. Slavin S, Nagler A, Shapira M, et al. Non-myeloablative allogeneic stem cell transplantation for the treatment of patients with chronic myeloid leukemia. *Blood* 2000;96:203a[Abstract 867].
84. Sandmaier B, Niederwieser D, McSweeney P, et al. Induction of molecular remissions in chronic myelogenous leukemia (CML) with nonmyeloablative HLA identical sibling allografts. *Blood* 2000;96:201a[Abstract 861].

85. Sloan E, Childs R, Greene A, et al. Non-myeloablative peripheral blood stem cell transplantation for chronic myelogenous leukemia. *Blood* 2000;96:783a[Abstract 3387].
86. Ehringer G, Kiehl M, Siegert W, et al. Dose reduced conditioning for allografting in 48 patients with CML: a retrospective analysis. *Blood* 2000;96:783a[Abstract 3385].
87. Lalancette M, Rezvani K, Szydlo R, et al. Favorable outcome of non-myeloablative stem cell transplant (NMSCT) for chronic myeloid leukemia (CML) in first chronic phase: a retrospective study of the European Group for Blood and Marrow Transplantation (EBMT). *Blood* 2000;96:545a.
88. Giralt S, Khouri I, Braunschweig I, et al. Melphalan and purine analog containing preparative regimens. Less intensive conditioning for patients with hematologic malignancies undergoing allogeneic progenitor cell transplantation. *Blood* 1999;94(10):564a[Abstract 2518].
89. Giralt S, Szydlo R, Goldman JM, et al. Effect of short-term interferon therapy on the outcome of subsequent HLA-identical sibling bone marrow transplantation for chronic myelogenous leukemia: an analysis from the International Bone Marrow Transplant Registry. *Blood* 2000;95(2):410–415.
90. Pigneux A, Tanguy ML, Michallet M, et al. Prior treatment with alpha interferon does not adversely affect the outcome of allogeneic transplantation for chronic myeloid leukemia. *Br J Haematol* 2002;116(1):193–201.
91. Hehlmann R, Hochhaus A, Kolb HJ, et al. Interferon-α before allogeneic bone marrow transplantation in chronic myelogenous leukemia does not affect the outcome adversely, provided it is discontinued at least 90 days befor the procedure. *Blood* 1999;94(11):3668–3677.
92. Horowitz M, Gale R, Sondel P, et al. Graft-versus-leukemia reactions after bone marrow transplantation. *Blood* 1990;75:555–562.
93. Apperley J, Mauro F, Goldman J, et al. Bone marrow transplantation for chronic myeloid leukaemia in first chronic phase: importance of graft-versus-leukaemia effect. *Br J Haematol* 1988;69(2):239–245.
94. Marmont A, Horowitz M, Gale R, et al. T-Cell depletion of HLA-identical transplants in leukemia. *Blood* 1991;78(8):2120–2130.
95. Porter DL, Antin JH. Infusion of donor peripheral blood mononuclear cells to treat relapse after transplantation for chronic myelogenous leukemia. *Hematol Oncol Clin North Am* 1998;12(1):123–150.
96. Mackinnon S, Papadopoulus EB, Carabasi MH, et al. Adoptive immunotherapy evaluating escalating doses of donor leukocytes for relapse of chronic myeloid leukemia after bone marrow transplantation: separation of graft-versus-leukemia responses from graft-versus-host disease. *Blood* 1995;86(4):1261–1268.
97. Giralt SA, Goldman J, Anasetti C, et al. Recommendations for assessment and definitions of response and relapse in chronic myelogenous leukemia. A report from the chronic Leukemia Working Committee of the International Bone Marrow Transplant Registry. In press.
98. Arcese W, Goldman JM, D'Arcangelo E, et al. Outcome for patients who relapse after allogeneic bone marrow transplantation for chronic myeloid leukemia. Chronic Leukemia Working Party. European Bone Marrow Transplantation Group. *Blood* 1993;82(10):3211–3219.
99. Giralt SA, Champlin RE. Leukemia relapse after allogeneic bone marrow transplantation: a review. *Blood* 1994;84(11):3603–3612.
100. Radich JP, Gehly G, Gooley T, et al. PCR detection of the bcr-abl fusion transcript after allogeneic marrow transplantation for chronic myeloid leukemia: results and implications in 346 patients. *Blood* 1995;85(9):2632–2638.
101. Costello RT, Kirk J, Gabert J. Value of PCR analysis for long term survivors after allogeneic bone marrow transplant for chronic myelogenous leukemia: a comparative study. *Leuk Lymphoma* 1996;20(3–4):239–243.
102. Radich JP, Gooley T, Bryant E, et al. The significance of bcr-abl molecular detection in chronic myeloid leukemia patients "late," 18 months or more after transplantation. *Blood* 2001;98(6):1701–1707.
103. Mrsic M, Horowitz M, Atkinson K, et al. Second HLA-identical sibling transplants for leukemia recurrence. *Bone Marrow Transplant* 1992;9(4):269–275.
104. Radich J, Sanders J, Buckner C, et al. Second allogeneic marrow transplantation for patients with recurrent leukemia after initial transplant with total-body irradiation-containing regimens. *J Clin Oncol* 1993;11(2):304–313.
105. Van Rhee F, Lin F, Cullis J, et al. Relapse of chronic myeloid leukemia after allogeneic bone marrow transplant: the case for giving donor leukocyte transfusions before the onset of hematologic relapse. *Blood* 1994;83;3377.
106. Shimoni A, Anderlini P, Andersson B, et al. CD8-depleted donor lymphocytes for the treatment of CML relapse after allogeneic transplant: long term follow up and factors predicting outcome. *Blood* 1999;94(suppl 1):160a.

107. Alyea EP, Soiffer RJ, Canning C, et al. Toxicity and efficacy of defined doses of CD4(+) donorlymphocytes for treatment of relapse after allogeneic bone marrow transplant. *Blood* 1998;91:3671–3680.
108. Dazzi F, Szydlo RM, Craddock C, et al. Comparison of single-dose and escalating-dose regimens of donor lymphocyte infusion for relapse after allografting for chronic myeloid leukemia. *Blood* 2000;95(1):67–71.
109. Guglielmi C, Arcese W, Hrmans J, et al. Risk assessment in patients with Ph+ chronic myelogenous leukemia at first relapse after allogeneic stem cell transplant: an EBMT retrospective analysis. *Blood* 2000;95:3328–3334.
110. Moreira VA, Setubal DC, Albuquerque DG, et al. Gleevec (STI-571) as therapy for relapse after bone marrow transplantation. *Blood* 2001;98(11)[Abstract 4788].
111. Kantarjian HM, O'Brien S, Cortes J, et al. Results of imatinib mesylate (STI-571) therapy in patients with chronic myelogenous leukemia in relapse after allogeneic stem cell transplantation. *Blood* 2001;98(11):137a[Abstract 575].
112. Chambon-Pautas C, Cony-Makhoul P, Giraudier S, et al. Glivec (STI-571) treatment for chronic myelogenous leukemia in relapse after allogeneic stem cell transplantation: a report of the French experience (on behalf of the SFGM and FILMC). *Blood* 2001;98(11):140a[Abstract 587].
113. Wassmann B, Pfeifer H, Scheuring U, et al. Glivec (STI-571) in the treatment of patients with chronic myeloid leukemia relapsing in accelerated or blastic phase after allogeneic stem cell transplantation. *Blood* 2001;98(11):140a[Abstract 588].
114. Soiffer RJ, Galinsky I, DeAngelo D, et al. Imatinib mesylate (Gleevec) for disease relapse following allogeneic bone marrow transplantation. *Blood* 2001;98(11):400a[Abstract 1682].
115. Ullmann AJ, Beck J, Kolbe K, et al. Clinical and laboratory evaluation of patients treated with STI-571 (Gleevec) after allogeneic and syngeneic stem cell transplantation with relapsed Philadelphia chromosome-positive leukemia. *Blood* 2001;98(11):401a[Abstract 1685].
116. Bonifazi F, de Vivo A, Rosti G, et al. Chronic myeloid leukemia and interferon-α: a study of complete cytogenetic responders. *Blood* 2001;98(10):3074–3081.

3 Stem Cell Transplantation for Hodgkin's and Non-Hodgkin's Lymphomas

Thomas J. Kenney, MD
and John W. Sweetenham, MD

Contents

The role of high-dose therapy (HDT) and stem cell transplantation (SCT) in the treatment non-Hodgkin's lymphoma (NHL) and Hodgkin's disease (HD) continues to evolve. There is considerably more experience with autologous SCT (autoSCT) than allogeneic SCT (alloSCT). AutoSCT has an established role in relapsed/refractory intermediate-grade NHL and relapsed/ refractory HD. Uncertainty still exists about the benefit of autoSCT as front-line therapy for high-risk NHL and HD and in indolent NHL. AlloSCT does not have a well-established role in NHL or HD, whereas reduced intensity alloSCT is under active investigation. Many questions remain to be answered regarding the optimal timing of SCT, ideal preparative regimen, best source of stem cells, role of stem-cell-purging procedures, and importance of pre-SCT cytoreduction.

1. AUTOLOGOUS STEM CELL TRANSPLANTATION

1.1. Hodgkin's Disease

Hodgkin's disease afflicts roughly 8000 people each year in the United States. Current conventional chemotherapy and radiotherapy regimens cure 70–80% of patients with early-stage disease and 60–70% of patients with advanced disease. Currently, the use of HDT and autoSCT is widely accepted in relapsed and refractory HD. The role of HDT and autoSCT in the primary treatment of high-risk patients is less defined.

From: *Stem Cell Transplantation for Hematologic Malignancies*
Edited by: R. J. Soiffer © Humana Press Inc., Totowa, NJ

1.1.1. Relapsed Disease

Up to 30–40% of HD patients will relapse after first-line treatment. The likelihood of long-term survival is generally low with standard salvage chemotherapy. In an extended follow-up of HD patients treated at the National Cancer Institute, the estimated 20-yr overall survival (OS) for patients who relapsed after mechlorethamine, vincristine, procarbazine, and prednisone (MOPP) chemotherapy was only 17% *(1)*. The single strongest predictor of outcome in this series was initial remission duration. Long-term survival was 24% for those with an initial remission longer than 1 yr and 11% for those with an initial remission less than 1 yr. Despite an estimated 20-yr disease-free survival (DFS) of 45%, OS was compromised by secondary leukemia and other treatment-related complications. Similar results were reported by the Milan group *(2)*. In their series, the 8-yr OS for relapsed HD patients treated with salvage chemotherapy was 54%, 28%, and 8% for patients with relapse after 1 yr, within 1 yr, and with induction failure, respectively.

The poor results with standard salvage chemotherapy have led to the investigation of HDT and autoSCT for relapsed HD. Modern supportive care and growing experience with HDT have made HDT and autoSCT a more attractive option in recent years. The transplant-related mortality (TRM) is now under 5% at experienced centers *(3,4)*. Multiple studies have been reported *(3–31)*, including four large publications from transplant registries *(13–15,23)* that demonstrate a DFS of around 50% in relapsed HD treated with HDT and autoSCT (*see* Table 1). The patient populations in these studies were diverse regarding disease status at transplant, time to relapse, and degree of previous treatment. The results seen in the SCT studies compare favorably with those previously reported for standard salvage chemotherapy in relapsed HD *(1,2)*. A recent study from Stanford University specifically compared outcomes of 60 relapsed or refractory HD patients who received HDT and autoSCT with 103 historically matched controls who had received conventional salvage therapy *(5)*. Freedom from progression (FFP) at 4 yr was significantly improved in the SCT group (62% vs 32%; $p< 0.01$) while OS was not significantly different (54% vs 47%, $p= 0.25$).

The excellent results with HDT and autoSCT in HD have made it difficult to accrue adequate numbers of patients for randomized trials comparing SCT to standard salvage chemotherapy. Two randomized trials have been completed, however. In the larger of the two trials, 161 patients with relapsed HD were randomized between two cycles of Dexa-BEAM (dexamethasone, carmustine (BCNU) etoposide, cytaribine, melphalan) followed either by two further cycles of Dexa-BEAM or HDT and autoSCT. Patients continued on the protocol only if they had chemosensitive disease (i.e., achieved a partial remission [PR] or complete remission [CR] with the initial two cycles of Dexa-BEAM). Freedom from treatment failure at 3 yr for the chemosensitive patients was significantly improved in the SCT arm (55% vs 34%; $p= 0.019$) (*see* Fig. 1), whereas OS did not differ significantly between treatment arms (71% vs 65%; $p= 0.331$) *(21)*. A smaller trial of 40 patients by Linch et al. also demonstrated improved 3-yr event-free survival (EFS) without improved OS for the SCT group *(22)*. The lack of OS advantage in these trials may be related in part to successful salvage with SCT in the standard chemotherapy arms.

It is conceivable that certain groups of "high-risk" relapsed HD patients may benefit the most from SCT. The definition of a "high-risk" patient varies among studies, and there is no accepted set of prognostic factors that are used to stratify relapsed HD patients. Some prognostic factors that have been identified include B symptoms at relapse *(5,16,20)*, chemoresponsiveness at time of relapse *(5,9,10,15,20,23,24)*, performance status *(3,7,15,29)*, disease status at the

Table 1
HDT and AutoSCT for Relapsed/Refractory Hodgkin's Disease

Author	*n*	*Preparative regimen*	*TRM*	*PFS*[a]	*OS*	*Years follow-up*
Horning et al. *(4)*	119	TBI or CCNU or BCNU + VP-16/Cy	5%	48% (EFS)	52%	4
Nademanee et al. *(12)*	85	TBI or BNCU +VP16/Cy	13%	58% (DFS)	75%	2
Reece et al. *(7)*	56	CBV	21%	47% (EFS)	53%	5
Chopra et al. *(9)*	155	BCNU/VP-16/AraC/Melph	10%	50%	55%	5
Bierman et al. *(3)*	128	CBV	4%	25%	77%	4
Wheeler et al. *(24)*	102	CBV	12%	42%	65%	3
Arranz et al. *(28)*	47	CBV	9%	34%	52%	7
Sureda et al. *(14)* (Registry)	494	CBV, BEAM, BEAC TBI-containing (10%)	9%	45% (TTF)	55%	5
Lazarus et al. *(15)* (Registry)	414	CBV, other	7%	NR	63%	3
Sweetenham et al. *(13)* (Registry)	139	BEAM, CBV, other	7%	45%	49%	5
Brice et al. *(23)* (Registry)	280	BEAM, BEAC/CBV, other	6%	60%	66%	3

[a]Abbreviations: TRM, treatment-related mortality, PFS, progression-free survival; OS, overall survival; TBI, total body irradiation; VP16/Cy, VP16/cyclophosphamide; CBV, cyclophosphamide, BCNU, VP16; Melph, Melphalan; BEAM, BCNU, VP16, Ara-C, Melphalan; BEAC, BCNU, VP16, Ara-C, cyclophosphamide. EFS, event-free survival; DFS, disease-free survival; TTF, time to treatment failure.

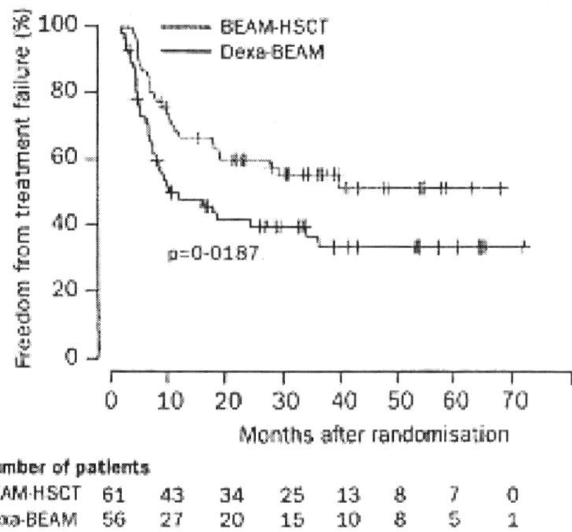

Fig. 1. Freedom from treatment failure for patients with relapsed chemosensitive Hodgkin's disease. (From ref. *21*.)

time of transplant *(4,23,26,28,30)*, remission duration *(16,26,31)*, tumor bulk at relapse *(9,11,19,26,30)*, and extranodal relapse *(4,12,16,23,24,26)*. Disease status at the time of transplant has been the most consistently identified factor across multiple studies, whereas remission duration has been the most controversial. Reece et al. reported a study of relapsed HD patients treated with SCT in which progression-free survival (PFS) was superior in patients with a remission duration of more than12 mo vs less than 12 mo (85% vs 48%) *(26)*. Conversely, other studies have shown no difference in PFS or OS in relapsed HD patients *(5,27)*.

Several groups have published prognostic indices for relapsed and refractory HD patients undergoing SCT *(4,24,25,31)*. In a series from Stanford University, disseminated disease, B symptoms, and greater than minimal disease at the time of SCT were identified as "high-risk" factors *(4)*. Patients with no, one, two, or three risk factors had a 3-yr FFP of 85%, 57%, 41%, and <20%, respectively (*see* Fig. 2). In another series, more than one extranodal site of relapse, poor performance status, and progressive disease at the time of HDT correlated with outcome *(24)*. Patients with no, one, two, or more factors had a 3-yr OS of 82%, 56%, and 19%, respectively, after HDT and autoSCT.

Based on the available data, HDT and autoSCT is indicated for most relapsed HD patients. Patients with chemorefractory disease at relapse or who are not in CR at the time of SCT will do worse but still should receive HDT and autoSCT. Some patients in late relapse may do as well with conventional salvage chemotherapy, but this remains controversial.

1.1.2. Primary Refractory Disease

Primary refractory patients are those who do not achieve a CR or progress during primary combination chemotherapy. These patients do poorly with conventional salvage chemotherapy *(1,2)*. Multiple investigators have reported on HDT and autoSCT in patients with primary refractory disease *(9,20,28,32–36)*. Most series report a DFS of 30–40% with HDT and autoSCT in early follow-up (*see* Table 2). The exact definition of primary refractory disease has become clouded by increasingly sensitive imaging technology and was not uniform among series.

No randomized studies have been reported comparing HDT and autoSCT with standard salvage chemotherapy for primary refractory disease. However, several investigators have

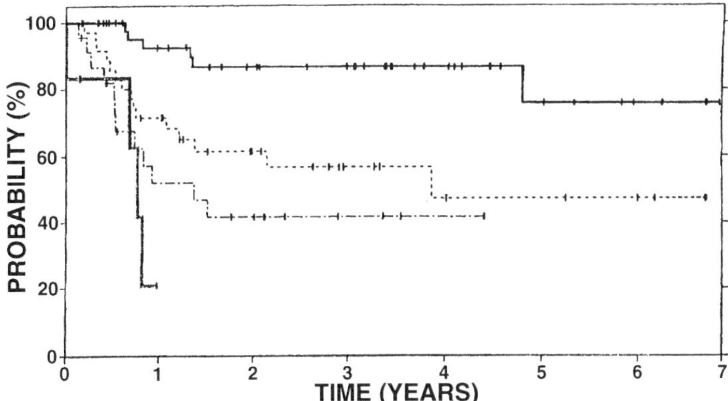

Fig. 2. Freedom from progression in 119 patients with recurrent or refractory Hodgkin's disease treated with high-dose therapy and autografting according to number of prognostic factors.

compared SCT data to matched controls that received conventional chemotherapy. André et al. reported a trend toward improved OS with HDT and autoSCT compared to matched controls *(32)*. In a retrospective analysis of 67 HD patients with primary progressive disease by Josting et al., the 25 patients undergoing HDT and SCT had significantly improved 5-yr OS compared to those receiving conventional chemotherapy (53% vs 0%) *(36)*. These data are confounded by the fact that the healthiest patients were likely selected for SCT. Despite the lack of randomized data, autoSCT appears to be the best option for patients with primary refractory disease.

1.1.3. HDT and AutoSCT as Primary Therapy

Aggressive combination chemotherapy ± radiation therapy cures 60–70% of patients with advanced HD *(37)*. Groups from Stanford and Germany have obtained even more impressive early results in single-arm studies using high-intensity regimens *(38,39)*.Whether these newer regimens are superior to doxorubicin, bleomycin, vinblastine, and dacarbazine (ABVD) awaits results of ongoing clinical trials. The success of conventional combination chemotherapy in curing HD and the favorable salvage rates has precluded as much interest in HDT and autoSCT as primary therapy.

Despite the excellent results seen with first-line conventional chemotherapy, there are some patients at high risk for relapse *(40,41)* who might benefit from more intensive treatment such as HDT and autoSCT. Recently, the International Prognostic Factors Project on Advanced Hodgkin's Disease identified a widely accepted set of prognostic factors has that included serum albumin less than 4q/dL, hemoglobin less than 10.5 g/dL, male sex, stage IV disease, age 45 years or older, white cell count greater than or equal to 15,000/mm^3, and lymphocyte count less than 600/mm^3 or less than 8% of the white-cell count *(42)*. Risk of relapse increased predictably with increasing numbers of factors, and patients with four or more risk factors had only a 42% 5-yr FFP. The consistent incorporation of these factors into the study design may ultimately help to identify patients who would benefit from first-line HDT and autoSCT.

Several groups have published series of up-front HDT and autoSCT for high-risk HD patients with DFS and OS rates of 80–100% and improved outcome relative to historical controls in some cases *(43–48)*. Three randomized studies have now also been published or reported in abstract form that compared HDT and autoSCT to either standard front-line chemotherapy or high-intensity front-line chemotherapy *(49–51)*. Proctor et al. identified 178 "poor-risk" patients based on their own Scotland and Newcastle Lymphoma Group (SNLG) index *(41)*, of

Table 2
HDT and AutoSCT for Primary Refractory HD

Author	*n*	*Preparative regimen*	*PFS*	*OS*	*Years follow-up*
Sweetenham et al. *(33)* (Registry)	175	BEAM, CBV, other	32%	36%	5
Lazarus et al. *(35)* (Registry)	122	CBV and other	38%	50%	3
André et al. *(32)*	86	BEAM, CBV	25% (EFS)	35%	5
Reece et al. *(34)*	30	CBV ± P	42% (EFS)	60%	5
Arranz et al. *(28)*	47	CBV	34% (DFS)	52%	7

Note. *See* Table 1 for definitions.

whom 126 were entered into their study *(49)*. One hundred twenty patients were treated with three cycles of an intensive chemotherapy regimen, prednisolone, vinblastine, doxorubicin, chlorambucil, etoposide, bleomycin, vincristine, and procarbazine (PVACE-BOP). Of these patients, 93% responded. Only 65 of 107 patients accepted randomization between HDT and autoSCT and two further cycles of PVACE-BOP. The 5-yr time to treatment failure was similar in the SCT and chemotherapy groups (79% vs 85%; $p= 0.35$). Federico et al. reported initial results on a study that enrolled HD patients with two or more of the following risk factors: high serum LDH levels, large mediastinal mass, more than one extranodal involved site, low hematocrit, or inguinal involvement. One hundred sixty HD patients were randomized to four cycles of ABVD followed by either HDT and autoSCT or four more cycles of ABVD. Patients were required to have a CR or PR after the first four cycles of ABVD in order to continue with the study. The 5-yr FFS in the SCT and chemotherapy arms were not significantly different (85% vs 83%; $p= 0.61$) and OS was similar. The GOELAMS group also recently presented an abstract that showed no difference in OS or FFP in high-risk HD patients with a median follow-up of 42 mo randomized to intensive chemotherapy or HDT and autoSCT *(51)*.

No trial reported to date has shown superior outcome for HDT and autoSCT as part of front-line therapy for newly diagnosed high-risk HD patients. Additionally, most studies were started before the introduction of the International Prognostic Factor scoring system, making the comparison of patient populations among studies difficult. HDT and autoSCT remains experimental for first-line therapy of HD.

1.1.4. Role of Involved-Field Radiotherapy

Hodgkin's disease relapses after SCT often occur at previous sites of disease. Involved-field radiotherapy (IFRT) has been incorporated into HDT regimens both before and after SCT with the goal of decreasing the rate of relapse at previous sites of disease and improving survival. Although IFRT clearly decreases local relapse rates and may improve PFS, it is has not been shown to improve survival *(52–55)*. Poen et al. retrospectively reported on 100 relapsed and refractory HD undergoing HDT and autoSCT, of whom 24 received IFRT. Improved PFS was seen only in stage I–III patients getting IFRT *(52)*. Mundt et al. reviewed 54 HD patients who underwent HDT and autoSCT, of whom 20 received IFRT *(53)*. IFRT significantly reduced the rate of relapse at previous sites of disease and improved PFS in patients with persistent disease after SCT. Patient selection based on lack of prior radiotherapy or the presence of bulk disease make these studies difficult to interpret. In addition, IFRT along with SCT may increase the risk of pulmonary toxicity and secondary malignancy *(56–58)*. Although IFRT may have some benefit, its role in HDT and autoSCT for HD is still not well defined.

1.1.5. High-Dose Preparative Regimens in HD

The most common preparative regimens used with SCT in HD are cyclophosphamide, BCNU, and VP-16 (CBV) and BCNU, VP-16, cytaribine, and melphalan (BEAM). Total-body irradiation (TBI) has also been incorporated; however, its use is limited by the fact that many patients have already received radiotherapy as part of their initial HD treatment. No randomized trials exist that compare preparative regimens. Historical comparisons have shown some difference in toxicity but no difference in outcome among different preparative regimens *(12,59–61)*. Randomized trials are required to determine if one preparative regimen is truly superior to others regarding efficacy and long-term toxicity.

1.2. Non-Hodgkin's Lymphoma

1.2.1. Diffuse Large B-Cell Lymphoma

Diffuse large B-cell lymphoma (DLBCL) is the most common aggressive NHL *(62)*. With conventional combination chemotherapy, patients with DLBCL can expect a 40–50% chance of long-term survival *(63)*. The remaining patients relapse or have primary refractory disease. The outlook for this group of patients is generally poor with conventional chemotherapy. The most widely accepted set of prognostic factors for predicting the outcome in DLBCL patients treated with primary doxorubicin-containing regimens is the International Prognostic Index (IPI) *(64)*. Risk factors identified included age greater than 60 yr, elevated lactate dehydrogenase (LDH) level, poor performance status, Ann Arbor stage III/IV, and more than one site of extranodal disease. Patients were divided into low risk (no to one risk factors), low-intermediate risk (two risk factors), high-intermediate risk (three risk factors), and high risk (four to five risk factors). An age-adjusted IPI was applied to patients under the age of 60.

1.2.1.1. Relapsed or Refractory Disease

The poor outcomes seen with conventional salvage chemotherapy regimens have led to the investigation of HDT and autoSCT. The largest randomized study of HDT and autoSCT in relapsed or refractory intermediate- and high-grade NHL (most with DLBCL) was reported by the Parma group in 1995 *(65)*. In this study, 109 relapsed patients with a response to two cycles of salvage dexamethasone, cytaribine, and cisplatin (DHAP) were randomized to four further cycles of DHAP or high-dose carmustine, etoposide, cytaribine, and cyclophosphamide (BEAC) and autoSCT. The trial excluded patients with bone marrow or central nervous system (CNS) involvement and those over the age of 60 yr. The 5-yr EFS (46% vs 12%, $p= 0.0001$) and OS (53% vs 32%, $p= 0.038$) were both significantly improved in the SCT arm (*see* Fig. 3). Based primarily on these results, HDT and autoSCT is the treatment of choice for patients with chemotherapy-sensitive relapsed DLBCL.

Several factors predict the outcome in relapsed DLBCL patients undergoing HDT and autoSCT. The most important of these is chemosensitivity. In a series by Philip et al. of 100 patients with relapsed or refractory aggressive NHL undergoing HDT and autoSCT, patients with chemotherapy-sensitive disease at relapse had a DFS of 36% in contrast to 14% in those with chemotherapy-resistant disease *(66)*. Patients who failed to achieve a CR with primary chemotherapy had no long-term DFS. Other predictors of poor outcome after HDT and autoSCT include a short relapse-free interval after primary therapy (<12 mo), bulky disease, and higher age-adjusted IPI score *(67–69)*. The 5-yr OS for patients in the PARMA study with low-risk,

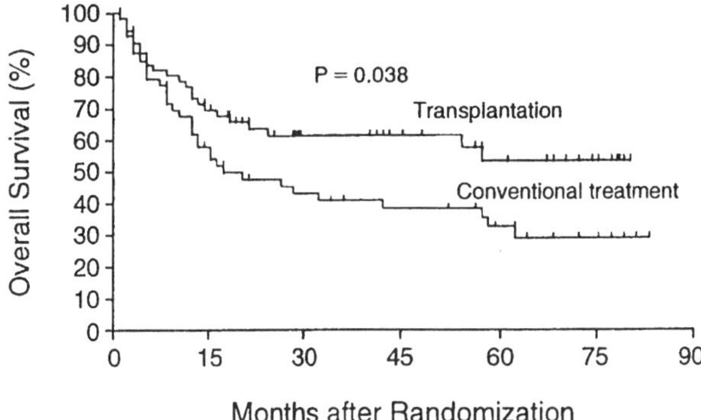

Fig. 3. Overall survival after high-dose therapy and autologous stem cell transplantation vs conventional therapy in patients with relapsed aggressive non-Hodgkin's lymphoma.

low-intermediate-risk, high-intermediate-risk, and high-risk IPI score were 83%, 69%, 46%, and 32%, respectively *(69)*. Notably, SCT patients in the PARMA study still had a better outcome relative to DHAP patients regardless of IPI score or time to relapse *(68,69)*.

1.2.1.2. Primary Therapy

The 50–60% relapse rate seen with first-line combination chemotherapy has led investigators to examine the role of HDT and autoSCT as initial treatment in high-risk DLBCL patients. Multiple trials of HDT and autoSCT as front-line therapy have been reported using variable inclusion criteria and chemotherapy regimens (*see* Table 3) *(70–77)*. Most trials published to date did not prospectively stratify patients by their IPI score, although some have looked retrospectively at IPI subgroups.

The LNH-87 trial recruited 916 high-risk patients under the age of 55 for induction chemotherapy *(70)*. High-risk patients were defined as those with at least one of the following factors: Eastern Cooperative Oncology Group (ECOG) performance status of 2–4, two or more extranodal sites, tumor burden of at least 10 cm in largest dimension, bone marrow or CNS involvement, and Burkitt or lymphoblastic subtypes. The 464 patients who achieved CR were randomized to consolidative sequential chemotherapy or HDT and autoSCT. Preliminary results showed a 3-yr DFS of 52% and OS of 71% in the sequential chemotherapy arm vs 59% and 69%, respectively, in the SCT arm. These differences were not statistically significant. The same group recently published a retrospective analysis based the IPI score *(71)*. For high- and high-intermediate risk patients, the 8-yr DFS and OS for the SCT arm was 55% and 64% vs 39% and 49%, respectively, for the sequential chemotherapy arm. In this case, the results were statistically significant. The Italian NHL Cooperative Study Group published a randomized trial of etoposide, doxorubicin, cyclophosphamide, vincristine, and bleomycin (VACOP-B) with DHAP for salvage versus VACOP-B followed by HDT and autoSCT *(72)*. In this study of 124 patients under the age of 60 with intermediate-grade NHL, there was no significant difference in 6-yr DFS or OS. In the SCT arm, 29% of patients did not actually undergo SCT. A retrospective analysis of high-risk and high-intermediate-risk patients by the IPI demonstrated a significant improvement in DFS in the SCT arm over the chemotherapy arm (87% vs 48%, $p = 0.008$).

Table 3
HDT and AutoSCT as Initial Treatment of DLBCL

Author	*n*	*Randomization*	*DFS chemo/SCT*	*OS chemo/SCT*	*Years follow-up*
Haioun et al. *(70)*	464	Sequential chemo vs HDT and auto-SCT in those who had CR with induction chemo	52% / 59% (p=0.46)	71%/69% (p=0.60)	3
Santini et al.*(72)*	124	VACOP-B alone with DHAP salvage as needed vs VACOP-B followed by HDT and auto-SCT	60%/80% (p=0.1)	65%/65% (p=0.5)	6
Kluin-Nelemans et al. *(73)*	194	CHVmP/BV (same as induction) vs HDT and auto-SCT in patients who achieved PR/CR with induction chemo	56%/61% (p=0.712) (TTP)	77%/68% (p=0.336)	5
Gianni et al. *(75)*	98	MACOP-B vs high-dose sequential chemo followed by HDT nd auto-SCT	49%/76% (p=0.004) (EFS)	55%/81% (p=0.09)	7
Gisselbrecht et al. *(76)*	370	ACVBP followed by sequential consolidation chemo vs shortened escalating-dose chemo followd by HDT and auto-SCT	76%/58% (p=0.004)	60%/46% (p=0.007)	5

The European Organization for Research and Treatment of Cancer (EORTC) recently published a trial of 194 patients with aggressive NHL under the age of 65 that randomized patients achieving a CR or PR with three cycles of combination chemotherapy to either HDT and autoSCT or further chemotherapy *(73)*. The 5-yr OS among the 194 randomized patients was 68% for the SCT arm and 77% for the chemotherapy arm and was not statistically significant. Notably, 70% of the patients in this study were low or low-intermediate risk by the IPI. A subset analysis based on IPI groups also did not show any difference among treatment arms. Gianni et al. randomized 98 patients with poor-risk features (defined as stage I/II with a mass greater than10cm or stage III/IV) to methotrexate, leucovorin, doxorubicin, cyclophosphamide, vincristine, bleomycin, and prednisone (MACOP-B) vs high-dose sequential chemotherapy followed by HDT and autoSCT *(75)*. Most of the patients in this trial were high or high-intermediate risk by the IPI. The 7-yr FFP in the SCT arm was significantly improved over the chemotherapy arm (84% vs 49%, $p< 0.001$). A trend toward improved OS for the SCT arm was also seen.

The LNH93-3 trial was conducted with 370 NHL patients under 60 yr old who were either high or intermediate-high risk by the age-adjusted IPI *(76)*. Patients were randomized to doxorubicin, cyclophosphamide, vindesine, bleomycin, and prednisone (ACVBP) or a shortened standard-dose regimen followed by HDT and autoSCT. The 5-yr OS and EFS for the ACVBP and SCT arms were 60% vs 46% ($p= 0.007$) and 52% vs 39% ($p= 0.01$) in contrast to results from previous studies of SCT in DLBCL. Vitolo et al. have reported preliminary results in a study of 131 DLBCL patients under age 60 with high-intermediate or high risk by age-adjusted IPI or bone marrow involvement *(77)*. Patients were randomized to conventional chemotherapy followed by HDT and autoSCT or to dose-intensive conventional chemotherapy. With a median follow-up of 36 mo, no differences were noted in OS or DFS between groups.

Thus, the benefit of HDT and autoSCT in patients with high-risk DLBCL remains controversial. Trials to date have suffered in particular from variable definitions of what constitutes a high-risk patient and from the use of nonstandard chemotherapy in control arms. Ongoing randomized trials may identify a subset of patients that will benefit from HDT and autoSCT.

1.2.1.3. Slow Responders

The issue of whether HDT and autoSCT is beneficial for patients with a slow response to chemotherapy has been addressed in several trials *(78–80)*. A retrospective analysis by Vose et al. examined the outcome of 184 Autologous Blood and Bone Marrow Transplant Registry (ABMT) patients with diffuse aggressive lymphoma who failed to achieve a CR with front-line chemotherapy and went on to HDT and autoSCT *(78)*. The 5-yr PFS and OS were 31% and 37%, respectively, for the group. Poor performance status, chemotherapy resistance, age greater than 55 yr, multiple chemotherapy regimens, and lack of pretransplant or posttransplant involved-field radiation correlated with poor outcome in multivariate analysis. Verdonck et al. reported a randomized study of slowly responding NHL patients in 1995 *(79)*. In this study, 69 of 106 previously untreated intermediate- or high-grade NHL patients who achieved a slow response (defined as 25–90% decrease in total tumor volume) after three cycles of cyclophosphamide, doxorubicin, vincristine, and prednisone (CHOP) were randomized to five further cycles of CHOP or HDT and autoSCT. No difference in 4-yr OS or DFS was observed between the two groups and the 4-yr DFS in both groups was comparable to that of the fast-responding patients. In another study by Martelli et al., patients achieving only a PR (defined as 50–80%

reduction in total tumor volume) two-thirds of the way through front-line chemotherapy were randomized to DHAP or HDT and autoSCT *(80)*. Again, there was no statistically significant difference in OS or PFS between treatment arms. Despite the fact that the Verdonck and Martelli trials suffered from small patient numbers, no data to date support the use of HDT and autoSCT in slowly responding DLBCL patients.

1.2.2. Follicular Lymphoma

A portion of patients with early-stage follicular lymphoma (FL) can achieve long-term survival with local radiation therapy *(81)*. However, the majority of patients with follicular NHL have disseminated disease at diagnosis. This group has a median survival of 8–10 yr, a number that has not changed with the introduction of multiagent chemotherapy *(82)*. HDT and autoSCT has recently been applied to this disease with hopes of improving long-term OS and DFS. Conversely, there has also been reluctance to use aggressive and potentially toxic therapy like HDT and autoSCT in FL based on the long natural history of the disease. In addition, the high incidence of bone marrow involvement complicates the transplant process. Studies have been published on HDT and autoSCT for relapsing/refractory patients and for those in first remission. These series differed in the use of purging, disease status at transplant, and degree of inclusion of other histologies.

1.2.2.1. Relapsed and Refractory Disease

Patients with relapsed and refractory disease can still respond to chemotherapy after multiple relapses. However, response rates are lower and remission duration shorter with each subsequent cycle of chemotherapy *(83)*. The continuing chemoresponsiveness of FL makes HDT and autoSCT an attractive strategy for prolonging remission and ideally survival.

Several centers have published series of HDT and autoSCT in relapsed/refractory FL patients containing heterogeneous patient populations (*see* Table 4) *(84–95)*. In a series from the Dana Farber Cancer Institute, 153 relapsed/refractory patients received HDT and anti-B-cell monoclonal antibody (MAb)-purged autoSCT *(84)*. The 8-yr DFS and OS were 42% and 66%, respectively (*see* Fig. 4). In a similar series from St. Bartholomew Hospital, 99 relapsed FL patients underwent HDT with purged autoSCT with a 5-yr freedom from recurrence (FFR) and OS of 63% and 69%, respectively *(85)*. The University of Nebraska treated 100 relapsed/ refractory FL patients without bone marrow involvement with HDT and unpurged autoSCT *(86)*. The 4-yr failure-free survival (FFS) and OS were 44% and 65%, respectively.

The St. Bartholomew group compared results of HDT and autoSCT with a matched historical control group *(87)*. The SCT group had a significantly better PFS but not OS. One small randomized trial has been completed. The Chemotherapy Unpurged Purged (CUP) trial randomized relapsed chemosensitive FL patients to chemotherapy, HDT, and purged autoSCT, or HDT, and unpurged autoSCT *(88)*. At a median follow-up of 26 mo, there was a significant improvement in the progression/relapse rate seen for HDT and autoSCT over chemotherapy (66% for chemotherapy, 39% for unpurged SCT, 37% for purged SCT, $p = 0.002$).

The results of studies of HDT and autoSCT for FL are encouraging. Caution, however, is indicated in interpreting these results, as study participants were highly selected. Moreover, no randomized data exist that actually shows improved OS. Evidence for actual cure or plateau in survival curves with HDT and autoSCT in relapsed/refractory FL is also lacking.

Table 4
HDT and AutoSCT in Relapsed/Refractory FL

Author	*n*	*Preparative regimen*	*Purging*	*DFS*	*OS*	*Years follow-up*
Freedman et al. *(84)*	153	Cy/TBI	Yes	42%	66%	8
Apostolides et al. *(85)*	99	Cy/TBI	Yes	63% (FFR)	69%	5
Bierman et al. *(86)*	100	Cy/TBI	No	44% (FFS)	65%	4
Brice et al. *(89)*	83[a]	TBI or BEAM	Yes	42% (FFP)	58%	5
Molina et al. *(90)*	58[b]	Cy/TBI±VP-16 or BCNU	No	42%	67%	5
Cao et al. *(91)*	49	Cy/VP-16 ± BCNU or TBI	Yes	44%	60%	4
Voso et al. *(95)*	41	Cy/TBI	Yes	43% (RFS)	72%	3.7
Weaver et al. *(93)*	49	BU/Cy or BEAC	No	35% (EFS)	55%	3.6
Colombat et al. *(94)*	42	Cy/TBI or BEAM	Yes (40%)	58% (EFS)	83%	3.6

[a]29% transformed FL.

[b]18% transformed FL.

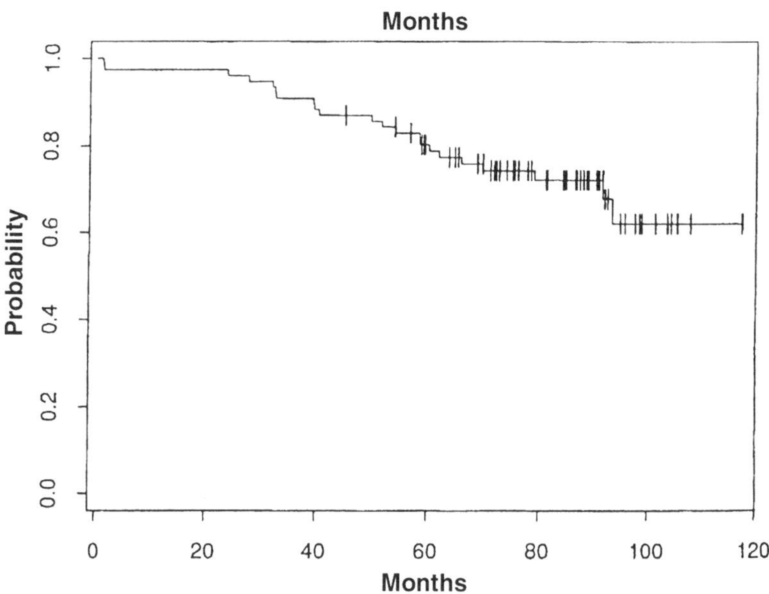

Fig. 4. Overall survival after high-dose therapy and autologous stem cell transplantation in patients with relapsed follicular non-Hodgkin's lymphoma.

1.2.2.2. First-Line Therapy

Several groups have reported series of patients receiving HDT and autoSCT in first remission (*see* Table 5) *(96–103)*. As with relapsed/refractory disease, results in these nonrandomized studies have been superior to what one would expect with standard chemotherapy. The most impressive results are from the Stanford University group, which recently published an update of their first-line treatment series *(97)*. They enrolled 37 previously untreated patients 50 yr or younger with stage III or IV FL who achieved a minimal disease state with a standard conventional chemotherapy regimen. With a median follow-up of 6.5 yr, the estimated 10-yr OS and disease-specific survival of the 37 patients after HDT and autoSCT were 86% and 97%, respectively. The Dana Farber Cancer Institute group transplanted 77 previously untreated FL patients who achieved a minimal residual disease state using slightly less stringent criteria *(98)*. The 3-yr DFS and OS in this series were 66% and 89%, respectively.

More recently, the GITMO reported results in untreated FL patients using intensive chemotherapy to achieve a minimal disease state before HDT and unpurged autoSCT *(103)*. As opposed to the previously discussed studies, patients were selected before it was known what their response to initial chemotherapy would be. Eighty-seven percent of patients enrolled obtained a CR with initial intensive chemotherapy and 47% had polymerase chain reaction (PCR)-negative peripheral blood stem cell (PBSC) grafts at the time of SCT without purging. DFS and OS at 4 yr was 67% and 84%, respectively. Early results of the first 150 randomized patients in the GOELAMNS 064 trial have been reported in abstract form *(104)*. In this trial, newly diagnosed FL patients with high tumor burdens and under the age of 60 were randomized to HDT and SCT or conventional chemotherapy with interferon. At a median follow-up of 31 mo, the estimated 4-yr EFS was significantly better in the SCT group (61% vs 27%, $p < 0.027$).

Table 5
HDT and AutoSCT as First-Line Therapy in FL

Author	*n*	*Preparative regimen*	*Purging*	*DFS*	*OS*	*Years follow-up*
Horning et al. *(97)*	37	Cy/TBI/VP-16	Yes	86%	97%	10
Freedman et al. *(98)*	77	Cy/TBI	Yes	66%	89%	3
Ladetto et al. *(103)*	92	MTX/Cy/VP-16	No	67%	84%	4
Tarella et al. *(99)*	29	MTX and L-PAM	Yes	59% (EFS)	79%	9
Colombat et al. *(100)*	27	Cy/TBI	Yes	55% (EFS)	64%	6
Seyfarth et al. *(96)*	33	Cy/TBI or BEAM	No	76% (EFS)	92%	4
Voso et al. *(95)*	70	Cy/TBI	Yes	78% (RFS)	86%	3.7

Table 6
HDT and AutoSCT in Transformed FL

Author	*n*	*Preparative regimen*	*DFS*	*OS*	*Years follow-up*
Williams et al. *(112)* (Registry)	50	Cy/TBI, BEAM, or other	30% (PFS)	51%	5
Friedberg et al. *(114)*	27	Cy/TBI	46%	58%	5
Chen et al. *(113)*	35	TBI/VP-16/Melphalan	36% (PFS)	37%	5
Foran et al. *(111)*	27	Cy/TBI	52%		2.4
Cao et al. *(91)*	17	Cy/VP-16±BCNU or TBI	49%	50%	4

Accumulating data suggest that younger patients with FL can achieve significant PFS with HDT and autoSCT when used as first-line treatment. Whether this actually translates into improved long-term survival or cure is still unclear.

1.2.2.3. Transformed Disease

Transformation occurs in 30–70% of cases of FL *(105–107)*. Transformed FL is associated with a median survival of under 1 yr with standard chemotherapy, although a subgroup of patients with limited disease and no previous exposure to chemotherapy may do better *(108,109)*. HDT and autoSCT has also been applied to transformed follicular NHL in hopes of improving the outcome. Results from nonrandomized series have demonstrated 5-yr OS in the range of 50% (*see* Table 6) *(110–114)*. This compares favorably to trials of conventional chemotherapy and needs to be confirmed in a randomized clinical trial.

1.2.2.4. Role of Purging

The role of purging stem cell grafts in FL remains controversial. Although contamination of bone marrow and stem cell collections may contribute to relapse after SCT, FL most often recurs at previous sites of disease. The Dana Farber Cancer Institute data have suggested that ex vivo purging of bone marrow with monoclonal antibodies improves outcome *(84,115,116)*. In their series, 113/153 patients had bone marrow harvests PCR positive for the bcl-2/JH rearrangement *(84)*. After purging, 42% of these patients became PCR negative. Patients with PCR-negative bone marrow harvests after purging had a significantly longer FFR than those with positive harvests. Patients who remained PCR-negative during follow-up also did better. The PCR status of the bone marrow harvest did not correlate with outcome in the St. Bartholomew's series, however *(85)*. Several other studies have argued against a benefit in PFS with purging as well *(117,118)*. No difference in outcome was observed in early follow-up between purged and unpurged stem cells in the CUP trial *(88)*.

The use of PBSCs and/or in vivo purging with rituximab may eliminate the need for complicated ex vivo purging procedures. The use of intensive chemotherapy and unpurged PBSC collection resulted in a 47% rate of PCR-negative harvests in the GITMO study *(103)*. Magni et al. achieved a 93% PCR-negative PBSC harvest in 15 FL and mantle cell lymphoma patients with bone marrow involvement using a combination of rituximab and intensive chemotherapy *(119)*. Other centers have shown comparable results in small early studies *(120–123)*. Rituximab may also be able to convert FL patients with minimal residual disease (MRD) after autoSCT to a MRD-negative state *(124)*.

The benefits of purging remain unclear. There has been a more consistent association between PCR negativity at follow-up than PCR-negative harvest with improved DFS. Randomized trials are required to resolve the issue. The use of rituximab as in vivo purging appears promising in early studies.

1.2.2.5. Prognostic Factors

Several prognostic factors have been shown to affect DFS and/or OS in patients with FL undergoing HDT and autoSCT, although no widely accepted index has been established. These include older age *(86)*, increased LDH, presence of B symptoms *(84)*, number of previous chemotherapy regimens *(86,87,92)*, disease chemosensitivity *(87,92,95)*, presence of histologic transformation *(91,111,113,114)*, and PCR positivity of the bone marrow at follow-up *(84,85)*.

1.2.3. Mantle Cell Lymphoma

Mantle cell lymphoma (MCL) comprises approx 6% of all NHL *(62)*. Most patients present with advanced disease. The reported median survival in most published series is 3–4 yr with no evidence of cure. There is no widely accepted standard first-line therapy for MCL. Anthracycline-containing regimens such as CHOP are often used, as well as fludaribine-containing combinations and dose-intensive third-generation NHL regimens *(125–132)*. The use of MAbs alone or in combination with chemotherapy has been reported recently and studies of radiolabeled MAbs are in progress *(133,134)*.

1.2.3.1. AutoSCT Results

High-dose therapy and autoSCT has been used a salvage therapy and as a component of first-line therapy for patients with MCL (*see* Tables 7 and 8) *(135–148)*. Multiple series reported a worse outcome for patients receiving SCT after relapse, particularly in patients who have received multiple prior chemotherapy regimens. In the study from the University of Nebraska Medical Center, the 2-yr EFS for patients who had received less than three prior therapies was 45% compared to 0% for those receiving more than three prior therapies *(143)*. In another recent study from Stanford and the City of Hope, the 3-yr EFS was 88% for patients undergoing autoSCT in first CR compared with 41% for those in subsequent CR *(144)*.

Favorable results from the M.D. Anderson Cancer Center (MDACC) were seen in 45 patients undergoing hyper-CVAD and high-dose methotrexate and cytaribine induction followed by SCT (autoSCT and alloSCT) *(145)*. The 3-yr EFS and OS rates of 72% and 92%, respectively, for previously untreated patients compared with 17% and 25%, respectively, for patients who had received prior therapy. Comparison of these patients with 25 historical controls who had received CHOP-like chemotherapy without proceeding to SCT showed a markedly superior EFS and OS in the SCT group. Whether these data are a result of patient selection, the intensive induction regimen, or the incorporation of SCT is not clear. Very early results from another MDACC study incorporating rituximab into the hyper-CVAD/high-dose cytaribine/high-dose methotrexate without SCT have shown equivalent outcome to patients who underwent SCT as well *(146)*. Early data from the first randomized study of autoSCT in MCL were recently presented *(149)*. The 102 of 143 patients with newly diagnosed MCL who achieved a CR or PR with initial CHOP-like chemotherapy were assigned to HDT and autoSCT or interferon-α maintenance. After a maximum of 4 yr follow-up, the EFS was significantly better in the SCT group (53% vs 17%, $p = 0.011$).

The role of autoSCT in MCL is still not well defined. Lack of randomized studies, lack of a standard chemotherapy regimen to which to compare results, and heterogeneous patient

Table 7
HDT and AutoSCT for Previously Treated MCL

Author	*n*	*Transplant regimen*	*EFS*	*OS*	*Years follow-up*
Ketterer et al. *(138)*	16	TBI-based	24%	24%	3
Vandenberghe et al. *(131)* (Registry)	150	Various	30%	48%	2
Malone et al. *(144)*	29	Cy/TBI/VP-16	38%	61%	3
Freedman et al. *(142)*	28	Cy/TBI	31% (DFS)	62%	4
Vose et al. *(143)*	40	Various	36%	65%	2
Milpied et al. *(141)*	18	TBI-based or BEAM	48% (DFS)	80%	4
Blay et al. *(140)*	18	Various	75% (PFS)	91%	2
Khouri et al. *(145)*	20	Hyper-CVAD, Ara-C/MTX then Cy/TBI	17%	25%	

Table 8
HDT and AutoSCT in MCL Patients in First CR

Author	*n*	*Transplant regimen*	*EFS*	*OS*	*Years follow-up*
Stewart et al. *(135)*	14	CAP/BOP then various HDT	8% (FFS)	23%	5
Malone et al. *(144)*	16	Cy/VP-16/TBI or CBV	87%	94%	3
Khouri et al. *(145)*	25	Hyper-CVAD, Ara-C/MTX then Cy/TBI	72%	92%	3

populations complicate interpretation of any SCT study in this disease. Patients who have received multiple prior chemotherapy regimens appear to do poorly, whereas patients treated earlier may do better. Long-term follow-up of ongoing randomized trials is needed to determine if HDT and autoSCT leads to improved OS.

1.2.3.2. Stem Cell Purging

Both peripheral blood (PB) and bone marrow involvement are frequent in MCL. Thus, several groups have investigated the role of ex vivo purging. Jacquy et al. demonstrated that the use of chemotherapy/granulocyte colony-stimulating factor protocols in MCL actually increased the number of t(11;14) cells in the PB of 10 of 12 patients, suggesting a rationale for ex vivo purging *(150)*. However, Anderson et al. were only able to eradicate PCR-detectable MCL in 2/19 patients undergoing autoSCT for MCL *(151)*. MCL cells may therefore be relatively resistant to purging. Several encouraging small studies of in vivo purging using rituximab have been reported that include MCL patients *(119,123,152)*. No study to date includes sufficient patient numbers to be able to identify an OS or EFS difference according to whether or not purging was performed. The ideal purging strategy is also unclear.

1.2.3.3. Role of Radioimmunoconjugates

The use of radioimmunoconjugates as part of the SCT preparative regimen have shown promise in relapsed MCL *(153–155)*. In a recent series of 16 patients with relapsed MCL, treatment with tositumomab (anti-CD20 antibody conjugated with I-131) along with high-dose etoposide and cyclophosphamide resulted in a 3-yr OS and PFS or 93% and 61%, respectively *(154)*. Further studies are needed to confirm these results.

1.2.4. Lymphoblastic Lymphoma

Lymphoblastic lymphoma accounts for approx 2% of all cases of NHL *(62)*. It is a neoplasm of precursor B or T lymphocytes with an aggressive clinical course. Intensive chemotherapy/radiotherapy regimens produce CR rates of 70–80% with 40–60% of patients achieving long-term survival *(156–158)*. Both autoSCT and alloSCT have been used to consolidate first remissions in this disease in attempts to improve long-term survival. Retrospective series from single centers and registries have reported 50–80% long-term survival with SCT *(159–164)*. More recently, a study by Sweetenham et al. randomized patients who achieved a CR or PR after standard remission-induction therapy to HDT and autoSCT or a conventional consolidation/maintenance protocol *(165)*. Only 65 of 119 patients started on induction chemotherapy were eligible for randomization, because of patient refusal, early disease progression, excessive toxicity with induction therapy, or elective alloSCT. A trend toward improved relapse-free survival (RFS) was noted without any improvement in overall OS. The lack of difference between arms may be explained in part by low numbers and the application of SCT in relapsing patients. The exact role of HDT and autoSCT has yet to be determined in lymphoblastic lymphoma.

1.2.5. Burkitt's Lymphoma

Burkitt's lymphoma is a rare subset of NHL with an aggressive clinical course. The disease is characterized by an 8;14 chromosomal translocation. Burkitt-like lymphoma is a less well-defined subtype. The largest series on HDT and autoSCT was reported by Sweetenham et al. and retrospectively analyzed 117 cases reported to the European Group for Blood and Marrow Transplantation (EBMT) *(166)*. The 3-yr OS was 72% for patients in first CR, 37% for patients in chemosensitive relapse, and only 7% for chemoresistant patients. Although results for autoSCT in patients with chemosensitive relapse compared favorably to conventional salvage chemotherapy, newer intensive conventional chemotherapy regimens have shown outcomes as good or superior to those reported by Sweetenham et al. for first-line patients *(167–174)*. Magrath et al. reported a 2-yr EFS of 100% in adults treated with an alternating non-cross-resistant regimen of cyclophosphamide, vincristine, doxorubicin, high-dose methotrexate (CODOX-M) and Ifosfamide, etoposide, high-dose cytaribine (IVAC) in 20 adult patients with small noncleaved NHL *(167)*. Mead et al. more recently applied this regimen to 40 high-risk patients (any patient with an ECOG performance status greater than 1, elevated LDH, mass greater than 10 cm, or greater than stage II) with documented Burkitt's lymphoma and achieved a 2-yr EFS and OS of 60% and 70%, respectively *(168)*.

The excellent results with modern conventional chemotherapy regimens even in high-risk patients appear to limit the role of HDT and autoSCT as first-line therapy in Burkitt's lymphoma. Further comparative studies are needed to determine if any subset of patients would benefit from HDT and autoSCT in first remission. HDT and autoSCT may have some benefit in selected relapsed chemosensitive patients and should be considered in this setting. There is little role for HDT and autoSCT in relapsed chemorefractory patients.

1.2.6. Peripheral T-Cell Lymphomas

Peripheral T-cell lymphomas (PTCL) are a heterogeneous group of neoplasms that comprise the majority of T-cell NHL and roughly 10% of all cases of NHL *(175)*. Although two small series found no difference in outcome between PTCL and corresponding B-cell phenotypes *(176,177)*, several large series suggested that PTCL is associated with a worse prognosis *(178,179)*. Melnyk et al. retrospectively analyzed the outcome of 560 NHL cases treated at the MDACC *(179)*. They found that the 5-yr failure-free survival (FFS) and OS for was significantly worse for PTCL patients relative to DLBCL patients (FFS 38% vs 58%, $p< 0.0001$ and OS 39% and 62%, $p< 0.001$).

Although a small number of cases of PTCL were included series examining autoSCT in DLBCL *(70,72,79,80)*, few large studies have been published on autoSCT in PTCL alone. Vose et al. reported on results of HDT and autoSCT in a group of 41 recurrent NHL intermediate or high-grade NHL patients *(180)*. Seventeen patients had a T-cell phenotype, whereas 24 had a B-cell phenotype. There was no significant difference in 2-yr OS or DFS between the two groups. Blystad et al. performed HDT and autoSCT in 41 chemosensitive PTCL patients, 17 of whom were in first CR or PR *(181)*. The 3-yr OS and EFS were 58% and 48%, respectively. In a series from the MDACC, 36 relapsed or refractory PTCL patients underwent SCT, with 7 receiving allogeneic SCT *(182)*. The 3-yr OS and PFS were 36% and 28%, respectively. Recently, the Spanish Lymphoma Cooperative Group reported an abstract on 77 PTCL patients receiving HDT and autoSCT in first remission or after relapse *(183)*. At 23 mo median follow-up, the actuarial 5-yr OS was 49% and the DFS was 44%. The 5-yr OS for patients transplanted in first CR was 80%.

Anaplastic large-cell lymphoma (ALCL) may be a more favorable subtype of PTCL. One-third or more ALCLs actually express B-cell antigens. Several groups have reported on HDT and autoSCT in relapse or as part of first-line therapy in PTCL *(184–187)*. Fanin et al. treated 16 ALCL patients with HDT and SCT as part of first-line therapy *(184)*. Patients first received 5-flurouracil, methotrexate, cytaribine, cyclophosphamide, doxorubicin, vincristine, prednisone (F-MACHOP) followed by IFRT in patients with residual mediastinal masses. All patients received HDT and autoSCT regardless of remission status after primary chemotherapy. At a median of 33.5 mo follow-up, DFS was 100%.

The diverse patient populations, significant heterogeneity of PTCL itself, and paucity of studies make it difficult to draw conclusions about the role of HDT and autoSCT in this group of lymphomas. As more becomes known about specific PTCL subtypes, further studies may help elucidate which subtypes respond most favorably to HDT and autoSCT. The impressive results of HDT and autoSCT for ALCL needed to be confirmed in a randomized trial vs conventional chemotherapy.

1.2.7. High-Dose Preparative Regimens in NHL

As opposed to HD, TBI-containing regimens are more commonly used for NHL. Some of the most frequently used regimens include cyclophosphamide/TBI (Cy/TBI), cyclophosphamide/etoposide/TBI (Cy/VP-16/TBI), BEAM, Carmustine etoposide, cytaribine, cyclophosphamide (BEAC), and CBV. No randomized trials have compared different regimens. A retrospective analysis from Stanford University found no difference in outcome among NHL patients receiving preparative regimens with chemotherapy and radiation vs radiation alone *(188)*. Radioimmunoconjugates such as tositumomab may be promising additions to preparative regimens by delivering high doses of radiation directly to tumors while sparing normal tissue. Press et al. reported a phase I/II study combining tositumomab with high-dose cyclophosphamide and etoposide as a preparative regimen for relapsed NHL patients undergoing autoSCT *(153)*. The 2-yr OS and PFS (83% and 68%, respectively) compared favorably to that of a nonrandomized control group that received high-dose cyclophosphamide and etoposide along with TBI (OS=53% and PFS=36%). Long-term efficacy and toxicity of radioimmunoconjugates are not known.

1.3. Stem Cell Source in AutoSCT

Peripheral blood stem cells have become the preferred source of donor cells in autoSCT in both HD and NHL. Several randomized and matched-pair studies have shown that patients receiving PBSCs have reduced time to hematopoietic recovery and reduced duration in hospital stay *(189–195)*. One study also showed a significant cost savings with the use of PBSCs *(192)*. No difference in OS or PFS after SCT has been demonstrated in any of these studies. Using chemotherapy and growth factors together appears to improve mobilization and decrease time needed for collection of PBSCs but has not been shown to improve outcome *(195)*.

1.4. Toxicity From AutoSCT

Early treatment-related mortality (TRM) has decreased over time with accumulating experience in autoSCT in HD and NHL and improvements in supportive care. Experienced centers now report TRM under 5–10%. Long-term non-relapse-related toxicity is still a significant problem, however. Of particular concern is the high incidence of secondary acute myelogenous leukemia (AML) and myelodysplasia (MDS). Incidences ranging from 5% to 20% have been reported after HDT and autoSCT for HD and NHL *(56–58,196–205)*.

The median time to onset is 2–4 yr after completing therapy. Both initial chemoradiotherapy and HDT before SCT likely contribute to the incidence of secondary AML and MDS. In addition, patients with clonal cytogenetic abnormalities before SCT are likely at higher risk of developing secondary AML or MDS than those with normal cytogenetics *(200)*. Age greater than or equal to 40 and previous TBI have been identified in some series as risk factors

(186,196,201). Nonhematologic malignancies are also a significant issue in long-term survivors of HDT and autoSCT *(202–204)*. The additive impact of HDT and autoSCT to this risk has not been established.

2. ALLOGENEIC STEM CELL TRANSPLANTATION

Although autoSCT has been widely applied in HD and NHL, experience with alloSCT is far more limited. In addition, few direct comparisons between alloSCT and autoSCT exist. There are several advantages to alloSCT over autoSCT. First, there may be a graft-vs-lymphoma (GVL) effect with alloSCT *(206)*. Evidence for this phenomenon includes the apparent effectiveness of modulation of immunosuppressive therapy *(207)*, correlation of relapse rate with chronic graft-vs-host disease (GVHD) *(208)*, clinical responses to donor lymphocyte infusions (DLIs) *(209,210)*, and the effectiveness of nonmyeloablative conditioning regimens with alloSCT *(211)*. The GVL effect is, however, still controversial *(212)*. Second, by using another donor's stem cells, one avoids the potential for lymphomatous contamination of graft. Third, alloSCT may be associated with a lower risk of secondary AML and MDS. Disadvantages of alloSCT include a higher TRM, acute and chronic GVHD, the need for prolonged immunosuppression, paucity of suitable donors, and age restriction to younger patients. A common finding across HD and NHL studies comparing autoSCT to alloSCT is a lower relapse rate for alloSCT at the expense of higher TRM relative to autoSCT.

2.1. Hodgkin's Disease

Experience with HDT and alloSCT in HD is limited in part because of the success of autoSCT. Therefore, the role of alloSCT in HD has not been defined. Several series have been published to date *(213–218)*. The patient populations were heterogeneous among these series regarding the degree of previous treatment, performance status, and disease status at SCT.

The Seattle group reported on outcomes of 127 patients with relapsed or refractory HD who underwent SCT at their center over a 21-yr period *(213)*. Fifty-three patients underwent alloSCT from human leukocyte antigen (HLA)-identical siblings, 68 patients underwent autoSCT, and six patients underwent syngeneic transplant. The alloSCT group had a significantly lower relapse rate than the autoSCT group (45% vs 76%, $p = 0.05$). However, there was no significant difference in OS, EFS, or nonrelapse mortality. Although not statistically significant, the higher nonrelapse mortality in the alloSCT group likely contributed to the lack of survival difference. The EBMT compared registry results of 45 relapsed or refractory HD patients treated with alloSCT to matched patients receiving autoSCT *(214)*. The relapse rate in this series was no different between alloSCT and autoSCT (61% vs 61%). There were also no significant differences seen between alloSCT and autoSCT in 4-yr OS or PFS. However, the 4-yr toxic death rate for alloSCT was significantly worse (48% vs 27%, $p = 0.04$). For patients with chemosensitive disease, the 4-yr OS favored autoSCT (64% vs 30%, $p = 0.007$).

Gajewski et al. published an analysis of 100 consecutive patients with HD who received HLA-matched sibling alloSCT from the International Bone Marrow Transplant Registry (IBMTR) *(215)*. The majority of the patients were not in remission at the time of transplant and half had a Karnofsky score of less than 50%. The 3-yr DFS, OS, and relapse rate of the group was 15%, 21%, and 65%, respectively. Johns Hopkins recently published a series of 157 relapsed or refractory HD patients, 53 of whom received alloSCT *(216)*. The estimated 10-yr OS for autoSCT and alloSCT patients was 37% and 30%, respectively ($p = 0.2$). Patients with resistant disease at relapse who were treated with alloSCT had a significantly higher total nonrelapse mortality than those treated with autoSCT (53% vs 28%, $p= 0.04$). There was a trend toward a lower relapse rate with alloSCT in patients with sensitive disease. The estimated 10-yr survival for patients with sensitive disease was 63% of alloSCT and 44% for autoSCT ($p= 0.83$).

Several subsets of HD patients may stand to benefit the most from alloSCT. These would include relapsed HD patients in whom adequate autologous stem cells cannot be mobilized and relapsed HD patients with significant bone marrow involvement. With the limited current available data, alloSCT for HD has not been shown to be superior to autoSCT for relapsed or refractory HD. AlloSCT appears to be associated with a lower relapse rate but higher TRM, which may negate any survival benefit. More investigation is needed to resolve this issue.

2.2. Non-Hodgkin's Lymphoma

2.2.1. Follicular Lymphoma

The survival curves for FL after HDT and autoSCT have not shown any evidence of a plateau with lengthy follow-up. Moreover, autoSCT may not be very effective in patients with refractory disease or significant bone marrow involvement. Other heavily pretreated patients may not be able to mobilize adequate numbers of stem cells for autoSCT. The significant incidence of secondary MDS/AML after HDT and autoSCT is also a concern for patients whose disease may have a long natural history. All of these factors have provided impetus for investigation of alloSCT in follicular and other low-grade lymphomas.

The largest series of HDT and alloSCT in low-grade lymphoma (majority of patients with FL) was reported from the IBMTR *(219)*. The 113 patients on which the series reported had a median age of 38 yr, generally had advanced disease, and had received a median of two previous chemotherapy regimens. The 3-yr recurrence rate, TRM, OS, and DFS were 15%, 40%, 49%, and 49%, respectively. Age less than 40, chemosensitive disease, good performance status, and TBI-containing regimen correlated with improved survival. Verdonck et al. compared results of alloSCT and autoSCT in a heavily pretreated group of low-grade NHL patients *(220)*. Eighteen patients received autoSCT, whereas 10 patients received alloSCT. Notably, all autoSCT patients had chemosensitive disease at transplant, as opposed to only 7 out 10 in the alloSCT patients. Although three of seven alloSCT died of TRM, their 2-yr PFS was significantly better than the autoSCT group (68% vs 22%, $p= 0.049$). Several other series have been reported as well, mainly in heavily pretreated and often refractory patients *(221–225)*. Common among series was a high TRM, low relapse rate, and DFS rates of 50–80% in early follow-up.

Allogeneic SCT in FL and other low-grade lymphomas appears to be feasible in younger patients, even with refractory disease. There is also a suggestion that it may cure some patients relative to autoSCT, perhaps because of GVL effect. This, however, comes at the price of higher TRM. Large prospective studies with longer follow-up are needed to see if the advantages if alloSCT can translate into improved long-term survival over autoSCT.

2.2.2. DLBCL and High-Grade NHL

Few large studies have specifically examined the role of alloSCT in intermediate- and high-grade NHL and none have addressed alloSCT in specific intermediate/high-grade NHL subtypes only *(208,226–229)*. A study by Chopra et al. compared the outcomes of 101 alloSCT patients reported to the EBMTG lymphoma registry with those of 101 matched autoSCT patients *(208)*. Half of the patients had lymphoblastic lymphoma and the other half were listed as intermediate/high-grade NHL. At a median follow-up of 48 mo the PFSs were similar in both groups (49% for alloSCT vs 46% for autoSCT). Among lymphoblastic lymphoma patients, there was a significantly lower relapse rate in the alloSCT group compared to the autoSCT group. This, however, did not translate into improved OS because of a higher TRM in the alloSCT group. Notably, there was a significantly lower relapse rate among alloSCT patients who developed chronic GVHD, suggesting a GVL effect. Most of these patients had lymphoblastic lymphoma. Ratanatharathorn et al. reported a series of 66 consecutive patients with either relapsed/refractory intermediate/high-grade NHL or transformed low-grade NHL who received either alloSCT or autoSCT *(228)*. Patients under the age of 55 and with HLA-matched siblings were given allogeneic bone marrow transplant (allo-BMT). The mean age of the alloSCT group was 40 and the autoSCT group was 47. At a median follow-up of 14 mo, there was a significantly higher probability of disease progression in the autoSCT group and a nonsignificant improvement in PFS in the alloSCT group.

2.2.3. Mantle Cell Lymphoma

As with FL, curability has been elusive using HDT and autoSCT in MCL. Several small series of alloSCTs have been published to date *(131,230–232)*. Most studies have shown comparable rates of OS and DFS to autoSCT. The European Bone Marrow Transplant group reported registry data on 22 MCL patients who underwent alloSCT *(131)*. The OS and EFS at 2 yr was 62% and 52%, respectively. Khouri et al. have reported a study of 16 patients with MCL undergoing alloSCT, including 5 previously untreated patients receiving hyper-CVAD/cytaribine/methotrexate induction and 11 previously untreated patients *(230)*. With a median follow-up of 24 mo, OS and FFS were 55% with 5 of 11 patients dying of transplant-related complications. For those patients with chemosensitive disease at the time of transplantation, the corresponding figures were both 90%, results similar to those reported by the same group using autoSCT after hyper-CVAD. A GVL effect was suggested by the fact that five of seven patients positive by PCR at the time of transplant for the bcl-1 or Ig gene rearrangement became negative within 7 mo after transplant. Several other smaller reports also suggest a GVL effect based on response to donor lymphocyte infusion or “slow” responses observed after the onset of GVHD *(231,232)*. As with other types of NHL, the role of alloSCT is unclear and remains experimental.

2.2.4. Conclusion

As with HD, the role of alloSCT in NHL has not been well established. The small numbers of studies and heterogeneity of NHL makes it difficult to draw firm conclusions. The available data on alloSCT for NHL suggest that alloSCT may induce a GVL effect that contributes to a lower rate of relapse relative to autoSCT. On the other hand, there is no conclusive evidence that the lower relapse rate leads to improved long-term survival. Moreover, the patients in alloSCT studies were highly selected. It is possible that some of the outcomes seen with alloSCT were related to favorable patient characteristics, including younger age. The high TRM with alloSCT may ultimately limit its usefulness to small as of yet unidentified subsets of NHL patients.

3. REDUCED-INTENSITY ALLOGENEIC STEM CELL TRANSPLANTATION

Reduced-intensity transplant (RIT) or nonmyeloablative alloSCT for lymphoma is currently an active area of research. The technique involves using smaller doses of chemotherapy and/or TBI than traditional alloSCT preparative regimens. Rather than relying on the high-dose chemotherapy and/or TBI to eradicate the lymphoma, reduced-intensity alloSCT relies on the GVL effect. The goal of RIT is to reduce TRM associated with the preparative regimen and thus improve long-term survival.

A number of small studies and one large study have been published on RIT that include HD and NHL patients *(211,233–251)*. Most studies have included heavily pretreated heterogeneous groups of patients with very early follow-up and have demonstrated variable results. Fludaribine-based conditioning regimens were used in most studies that ideally allowed for recovery of autologous hematopoiesis in the setting of graft failure. More intensive BEAM-based regimens have also been used. Some centers have incorporated CAMPATH-1H *(234–236)* as in vivo T-cell depletion in an attempt to decrease the incidence of GVHD and promote engraftment, whereas others have used rituximab *(237)* to help prevent relapse before the GVL effect sets in. There have also been reports of successful autografting followed by RIT in refractory heavily pretreated NHL and HD patients *(238)*.

The EBMT recently published the largest series to date on RIT *(239)*. The study reports on 188 lymphoma patients (52 HD, 52 low-grade NHL, 52 high-grade NHL including DLBCL, 22 MCL) with a median age of 40 yr and median number of three prior therapies (including previous autoSCT in 48%), most of whom were treated with a fludaribine-based preparative regimen. Notably, 71% of patients had chemosensitive disease at the time of SCT. With a median follow-up of 283 d the estimated 2-yr OS and PFS for the entire group was 50% and 30%, respectively. Patients with chemoresistant disease, high-grade NHL, and MCL had a significantly worse PFS. TRM was 34% at 2 yr and significantly worse in older patients. Multiple patients responded to DLI.

The most impressive single-institution results have been reported by the MDACC *(240)*. Forty-nine patients with indolent NHL (FL or small lymphocytic lymphoma), DLBCL, and MCL and a median age of 55 yr underwent RIT. Patients had received a median of four prior chemotherapy regimens. Seventy-one percent had chemosensitive disease at the time of SCT. At 19 mo median follow-up, the 2-yr OS and DFS for indolent NHL were both 85%, and for DLBCL, they were 71% and 61%, respectively. The 1-yr OS and DFS for MCL patients was 100% and 92%, respectively. One hundred-day mortality was only 4%. Spitzer et al. reported on RIT in 20 refractory DLBCL patients *(241)*. At a follow-up of 13-52 mo, five patients were alive and free of disease. Bertz et al. recently published a series of 25 heavily pretreated NHL and HD patients *(242)*. Twelve patients received RIT, whereas 13 underwent standard alloSCT. Nonrelapse mortality was significantly worse in the standard alloSCT group (54% vs 17%, $p=$ 0.03), as was the 1-yr OS (23% vs 67%, $p = < 0.02$). Several studies have specifically addressed RIT in patients who had relapsed after autoSCT *(236,243)*. Branson et al. published a series of 38 patients with NHL, HD, and multiple myeloma who had failed after autoSCT *(236)*. The OS and PFS at 14 mo follow-up were 53% and 50%, respectively. TRM within the first 14 mo was 20% and 3 of 15 patients responded to DLI.

Reduced-intensity transplant and alloSCT shows promise in early studies for the treatment of relapsed and refractory NHL and HD patients. As with autoSCT, early data suggest that patients with chemorefractory disease at the time of SCT do poorly. The short-term OS and PFS rates in heavily pretreated patients including those who have relapsed after autoSCT are notable. These patients normally have a very poor prognosis with standard salvage therapy. Although there are no randomized data, it appears that RIT and alloSCT are associated with a lower TRM than standard alloSCT. Whether the lower TRM and the GVL effect will result in improved long-term survival remains to be seen. Many questions still need to be answered about RIT, including the ideal type of conditioning regimen, role and timing of DLI and monoclonal antibodies administration, and appropriate posttransplant immunosuppressive regimen. Moreover, patient subsets who will benefit the most from RIT need to be identified.

REFERENCES

1. Longo DL, Duffey PL, Young RC, et al. Conventional-dose salvage combination chemotherapy in patients relapsing with Hodgkin's disease after combination chemotherapy: the low probability of cure. *J Clin Oncol* 1992;10:210.
2. Bonfante V, Santoro A, Vivani S, et al. Outcome of patients with Hodgkin's disease failing after primary MOPP-ABVD. *J Clin Oncol* 1997;15:528.
3. Bierman PJ, Bagin RG, Jagganath S, et al. High dose chemotherapy followed by autologous hematopoietic rescue in Hodgkin's disease: long-term follow-up in 128 patients. *Ann Oncol* 1993;4:767.
4. Horning SJ, Chao NJ, Negrin RS, et al. High-dose therapy and autologous hematopoietic progenitor cell transplantation for recurrent or refractory Hodgkin's disease: analysis of the Stanford University results and prognostic indices. *Blood* 1997;89:801.
5. Yuen AR, Rosenberg SA, Hoppe RT, et al. Comparison between conventional salvage therapy and high-dose therapy with autografting for recurrent or refractory Hodgkin's disease. *Blood* 1997;89:814.
6. Carella AM, Congui AM, Gaozza E, et al. High-dose chemotherapy with autologous bone marrow transplantation in 50 advanced resistant Hodgkin's disease patients: an Italian study. *J Clin Oncol* 1988;6:1411.
7. Reece D, Barnett M, Connors J, et al. Intensive chemotherapy with cyclophosphamide carmustine, and etoposide with autologous bone marrow for relapsed Hodgkin's disease. *J Clin Oncol* 1991;9:1871.
8. Armitage J, Bierman P, Vose J, et al. Autologous bone marrow transplantation for patients with relapsed Hodgkin's disease. *Am J Med* 1991;91:605.
9. Chopra R, McMillan A, Linch D, et al. The place of high-dose BEAM therapy and autologous bone marrow transplantation in poor-risk Hodgkin's disease: a single-center eight-year study of 155 patients. *Blood* 1993;81:1137.
10. Yahalom J, Gulati S, Toia M, et al. Accelerated hyperfractionated total-lymphoid irradiation, high-dose chemotherapy, and autologous bone marrow transplantation for refractory and relapsing patients with Hodgkin's disease. *J Clin Oncol* 1993;11:1062.
11. Rapoport A, Rowe J, Kouides P, et al. One hundred autotransplants for relapsed or refractory Hodgkin's disease and lymphoma: value of pretransplant disease status for predicting outcome. *J Clin Oncol* 1993;11:2351.
12. Nademanee A, O'Donnell MR, Snyder DS, et al. High-dose chemotherapy with or without total body irradiation followed by autologous bone marrow and/or peripheral blood stem cell transplantation for patients with relapsed and refractory Hodgkin's disease: results in 85 patients with analysis of prognostic factors. *Blood* 1995;85:1381.
13. Sweetenham JW, Taghipour G, Milligan D, et al. High-dose therapy and autologous stem cell rescue for patients with Hodgkin's disease in first relapse after chemotherapy: results from the EBMT Lymphoma Working Party of the European Group for Blood and Bone Marrow Transplantation. *Bone Marrow Transplant* 1997;20:745.
14. Sureda A, Arranz R, Iriondo E, et al. Autologous stem-cell transplantation for Hodgkin's disease: results and prognostic factors in 494 patients from the Grupo Español de Linfomas/Transplante Atológo de Médula Ósea Spanish Cooperative Group. *J Clin Oncol* 2001;19:1395.
15. Lazarus HM, Loberiza FR, Zhang M-J, et al. Autotransplants for Hodgkin's disease in first relapse or second remission: a report from the autologous blood and marrow transplant registry (ABMTR). *Bone Marrow Transplant* 2001;27:387.
16. Moskowitz CH, Nimer SD, Zelenetz AD, et al. A 2-step comprehensive high-dose chemoradiotherapy second-line program for relapsed and refractory Hodgkin disease: analysis by intent to treat and development of a prognostic model. *Blood* 2001;97:616.
17. Argiris A, Seropian S, Cooper DL, et al. High-dose BEAM chemotherapy with autologous peripheral blood progenitor-cell transplantation for unselected patients with primary refractory or relapsed Hodgkin's disease. *Ann Oncol* 2000;11:665.

18. Josting A, Katay I, Rueffer U, et al. Favorable outcome with relapsed or refractory Hodgkin's disease treated with high-dose chemotherapy and stem cell rescue at the time of maximal response to conventional salvage chemotherapy (Dexa-BEAM). *Ann Oncol* 1998;9:289.
19. Stewart DA, Guo D, Gluck S, et al. Double high-dose therapy for Hodgkin's disease with dose-intensive cyclophosphamide, etoposide, and cisplatin (DICEP) prior to high-dose melphalan and autologous stem cell transplantation. *Bone Marrow Transplant* 2000;26:383.
20. Fermé C, Mounier N, Divine M, et al. Intensive salvage therapy with high-dose chemotherapy for patients with advanced Hodgkin's disease in relapse or failure after initial chemotherapy: results of the Groupe d'Études des Lymphomes de l'Adulte H89 Trial. *J Clin Oncol* 2002;20:467.
21. Schmitz N, Pfistner B, Sextro M, et al. Aggressive conventional chemotherapy compared with high-dose chemotherapy with autologous haemopoietic stem-cell transplantation for relapsed chemosensitive Hodgkin's disease: a randomized trial. *Lancet* 2002;359:2065.
22. Linch DC, Winfield D, Goldstone AH, et al. Dose intensification with autologous bone-marrow transplantation in relapsed and resistant Hodgkin's disease: results of a BNLI randomized trial. *Lancet* 1993;341:1051.
23. Brice P, Bouabdallah R, Moreau P, et al. Prognostic factors for survival after high-dose therapy and autologous stem cell transplantation for patients with relapsing Hodgkin's disease: analysis of 280 patients from the French registry. Société Francaise de Greffe de Moëlle. *Bone Marrow Transplant* 1997;20:21.
24. Wheeler C, Eickhoff C, Elias A, et al. High-dose cyclophosphamide, carmustine, and etoposide with autologous transplantation in Hodgkin's disease: a prognostic model for treatment outcomes. *Biol Blood Marrow Transplant* 1997;3:98.
25. O'Brien ME, Milan S, Cunningham D, et al. High-dose chemotherapy and autologous bone marrow transplant in relapsed Hodgkin's disease: a pragmatic prognostic index. *Br J Cancer* 1996;73:1272.
26. Reece DE, Connors JM, Spinelli JJ, et al. Intensive therapy with cyclophosphamide, carmustine, etoposide +/– cisplatin, and autologous bone marrow transplantation for Hodgkin's disease in first relapse after combination chemotherapy. *Blood* 1994;83:1193.
27. Fung H, Nademanee A, Kashyap, et al. Evaluation of prognostic factors in patients with Hodgkin's disease in first relapse treated by autologous stem cell transplantation: duration of first remission does not predict the transplant outcome. *Blood* 1997;90:594a[Abstract].
28. Arranz R, Tomas JF, Gil-Fernandez JJ, et al. Autologous stem cell transplantation (ASCT) for poor prognostic Hodgkin's disease (HD): comparative results with two CBV regimens and importance of disease status at transplant. *Bone Marrow Transplant* 1998;21:779.
29. Jagganath S, Armitage JO, Dicke KA, et al. Prognostic factors for response and survival after high-dose cyclophosphamide, carmustine, and etoposide with autologous bone marrow transplantation for relapsed Hodgkin's disease. *J Clin Oncol* 1989;7:179.
30. Crump M, Smith AM, Brandwein J, et al. High-dose etoposide and melphalan, and autologous transplantation in Hodgkin's disease: importance of disease status at transplant. *J Clin Oncol* 1993;11:704.
31. Josting A, Franklin J, May M, et al. New prognostic score based on treatment outcome of patients with relapsed Hodgkin's lymphoma registered in the database of the German Hodgkin's Lymphoma Study Group. *J Clin Oncol* 2002;20:221.
32. André M, Henry-Amar M, Pico JL, et al. Comparison of high-dose therapy and autologous stem-cell transplantation with conventional therapy for Hodgkin's disease induction failure: a case-control study. Société Francaise de Greffe de Moëlle. *J Clin Oncol* 1999;17:222.
33. Sweetenham JW, Carella AM, Taghipour G, et al. High-dose therapy and autologous stem-cell transplantation for adult patients with Hodgkin's disease who do not enter a remission after induction chemotherapy: results in 175 patients reported to the European Group for Blood and Bone Marrow Transplantation. Lymphoma Working Party. *J Clin Oncol* 1999;17:3101.
34. Reece DE, Barnett MJ, Shepard JD, et al. High-dose cyclophosphamide, carmustine (BCNU), and etoposide (VP-16) with or without cisplatin (CBV +/– P) and autologous transplantation for patients with Hodgkin's disease who fail to enter a complete remission after combination chemotherapy. *Blood* 1995;86:451.
35. Lazarus H, Rowlings P, Zhang M, et al. Autotransplants for Hodgkin's disease in patients never achieving remission: a report from the Autologous Blood and Marrow Transplant Registry. *J Clin Oncol* 1999;17:534.
36. Josting A, Reiser M, Rueffer U, et al. Treatment of primary progressive Hodgkin's and aggressive non-Hodgkin's lymphoma: is there a chance for cure? *J Clin Oncol* 2000;18:332.

37. Canellos GP, Anderson JR, Propert KJ, et al. Chemotherapy of advanced Hodgkin's disease with MOPP, ABVD, or MOPP alternating with ABVD. *N Engl J Med* 1992;327:1478.
38. Horning SJ, Hoppe RT, Breslin S, et al. Stanford V and radiotherapy for locally extensive and advanced Hodgkin's disease: mature results of a prospective clinical trial. *J Clin Oncol* 2002;20:630.
39. Diehl V, Franklin J, Sieber M, et al. Dose escalated BEACOPP chemotherapy improves failure free survival in advanced-stage Hodgkin's disease: updated results of the German Hodgkin's Lymphoma Study Group. *Blood* 2000;96:2474a[Abstract].
40. Straus DJ, Gaynor JJ, Myers J, et al. Prognostic factors among 185 adults with newly diagnosed advanced Hodgkin's disease treated with alternating potentially non-cross-resistant chemotherapy and intermediate-dose radiation therapy. *J Clin Oncol* 1990;8:1173.
41. Proctor SJ, Taylor P, Donan P, et al. A numerical prognostic index for clinical use in identification of poor-risk patients with Hodgkin's disease at diagnosis. Scotland and Newcastle Lymphoma Group (SNLG) Therapy Working Party. *Eur J Cancer* 1991;27:624.
42. Hasenclever D, Diehl V. A prognostic score for advanced Hodgkin's disease. *N Engl J Med* 1998;339:1506.
43. Carella AM, Carlier P, Congui A, et al. Autologous bone marrow transplantation as adjuvant treatment for high-risk Hodgkin's disease in first complete remission after MOPP/ABVD protocol. *Bone Marrow Transplant* 1991;8:99.
44. Fleury J, Legros M, Colombat P, et al. High-dose therapy and autologous bone marrow transplantation in first complete or partial remission for poor prognosis Hodgkin's disease. *Leuk Lymphoma* 1996;20:259.
45. Sureda A, Mataix R, Hernandez-Navarro F, et al. Autologous stem cell transplantation for poor prognosis Hodgkin's disease in first complete remission: a retrospective study from the Spanish GEL-TAMO Cooperative Group. *Bone Marrow Transplant* 1997;20:283.
46. Schmitz M, Hasenclever D, Brosteanu O, et al. Early high-dose therapy to consolidate patients with high-risk Hodgkin's disease in first complete remission? Results of an EBMT/GHSG matched-pair analysis. *Blood* 1995;86:439a[Abstract].
47. Carella AM, Prencipe E, Pungolino E, et al. Twelve years' experience with high-dose therapy and autologous stem cell transplantation for high-risk Hodgkin's disease patients in first remission after MOPP/ABVD chemotherapy. *Leuk Lymphoma* 1996;21:63.
48. Nademanee A, Molina A, Fung H, et al. High-dose chemo/radiotherapy and autologous bone marrow or stem cell transplantation for poor-risk advanced stage Hodgkin's disease during first complete or partial remission. *Biol Blood Marrow Transplant* 1999;5:292.
49. Proctor SJ, Mackie M, Dawson A, et al. A population-based study of intensive multi-agent chemotherapy with or without autotransplant for the highest risk Hodgkin's disease patients identified by the Scotland and Newcastle Lymphoma Group (SNLG) prognostic index. A Scotland and Newcastle Lymphoma Group study (SNLG HD III). *Eur J Cancer* 2002;38:795.
50. Federico M, Carella A, Brice P, et al. High-dose therapy (HDT) and autologous stem cell transplantation (ASCT) versus conventional therapy for patients with advanced Hodgkin's disease (HD) responding to initial therapy. *Proc Am Soc Clin Oncol* 2002;21:263a [Abstract].
51. Saghatchian M, Djeridane M, Escoffre-Barbe M, et al. Very high risk Hodgkin's disease (HD): ABVd (4 cycles) plus BEAM followed by autologous stem cell transplantation (ASCT) and radiotherapy (RT) versus intensive chemotherapy (3 cycles) (INT-CT) and RT. Four-year results of the GOELAMS H97-GM multicentric randomized trial. *Proc Am Soc Clin Oncol* 2002;21:263a [Abstract].
52. Poen JC, Hoppe RT, Horning SJ. High-dose therapy and autologous bone marrow transplantation for relapsed/refractory Hodgkin's disease: the impact of involved field radiotherapy on patterns of failure and survival. *Int J Radiat Oncol Biol Phys* 1996;36:3.
53. Mundt AJ, Sibley G, Williams S, Hallahan D, et al. Patterns of failure following high-dose chemotherapy and autologous bone marrow transplantation with involved field radiotherapy for relapsed/refractory Hodgkin's disease. *Int J Radiat Oncol Biol Phys* 1995;33:261.
54. Lancet JE, Rapoport AP, Brasacchio R, et al. Autotransplantation for relapsed or refractory Hodgkin's disease: long-term follow-up and analysis of prognostic factors. *Bone Marrow Transplant* 1998;22:265.
55. Tsang RW, Gospodarowicz MK, Sutcliffe SB, et al. Thoracic radiation therapy before autologous bone marrow transplantation in relapsed or refractory Hodgkin's disease. PMH Lymphoma Group, and Toronto Autologous BMT Group. *Eur J Cancer* 1999;35:73.

56. Krishnan A, Bhatita S, Slovak ML, et al. Predictors of therapy-related leukemia and myelodysplasia following autologous transplantation: an assessment of risk factors. *Blood* 2000;95:1588.
57. Stone RM, Neuberg D, Soiffer R, et al. Myelodysplastic syndrome as a late complication following autologous bone marrow transplantation for non-Hodgkin's lymphoma. *J Clin Oncol* 1994;12:2535.
58. Guitierrez-Delgado F, Maloney DG, Press OW, et al. Autologous stem cell transplantation for non-Hodgkin's lymphoma: comparison of radiation-based and chemotherapy-only preparative regimens. *Bone Marrow Transplant* 2001;28:455.
59. Wheeler C, Antin JH, Churchill WH, et al. Cyclophosphamide, carmustine, and etoposide with autologous bone marrow transplantation in refractory Hodgkin's disease and non-Hodgkin's lymphoma: a dose-finding study. *J Clin Oncol* 1990;8:648.
60. Weaver C, Appelbaum F, Peterson F, et al. High-dose cyclophosphamide, carmustine, and etoposide followed by autologous bone marrow transplantation in patients with lymphoid malignancies who have received dose-limiting radiotherapy. *J Clin Oncol* 1993;11:1329.
61. Reece DE, Nevill TJ, Sayegh A, et al. Regimen-related toxicity and non-relapse mortality with high-dose cyclophosphamide, carmustine (BCNU), and etoposide (VP-16-213) (CBV) and CBV plus cisplatin (CBVP) followed by autologous stem cell transplantation in patients with Hodgkin's disease. *Bone Marrow Transplant* 1999; 23:1131.
62. The non-Hodgkin's Lymphoma Classification Project: a clinical evaluation of the International Lymphoma Study Group classification of non-Hodgkin's lymphomas. *Blood* 1997;89:3909.
63. Fisher R, Gaynor E, Dahlberg S, et al. Comparison of a standard regimen (CHOP) with three intensive chemotherapy regimens for advanced non-Hodgkin's lymphoma. *N Engl J Med* 1993;328:1002.
64. The International Non-Hodgkin's Lymphoma Prognostic Factors Project: a predictive model for aggressive non-Hodgkin's lymphoma. *N Engl J Med* 1993;329:987.
65. Philip T, Guglielmi C, Hagenbeek A, et al. Autologous bone marrow transplantation as compared to salvage therapy in relapses of chemotherapy-sensitive non-Hodgkin's lymphoma. *N Engl J Med* 1995;333:1540.
66. Philip T, Armitage JO, Spitzer G, et al. High-dose therapy and autologous bone marrow transplantation after failure of conventional chemotherapy in adults with intermediate-grade or high-grade non-Hodgkin's lymphoma. *N Engl J Med* 1987;316:1493.
67. Rapoport AP, Lifton R, Constine LS, et al. Autotransplantation for relapsed or refractory non-Hodgkin's lymphoma: long-term follow-up and analysis of prognostic factors. *Bone Marrow Transplant* 1997;19:883.
68. Guglielmi C, Gomez F, Philip T, et al. Time to relapse has prognostic value in patients with aggressive lymphoma enrolled onto the PARMA trial. *J Clin Oncol* 1998;16:3264.
69. Blay J, Gomez F, Sebban C, et al. The international prognostic index correlates to survival in patients with aggressive lymphoma in relapse: analysis of the PARMA trial. *Blood* 1998;92:3562.
70. Haioun C, Lepage E, Gisselbrecht C, et al. Comparison of autologous bone marrow transplantation with sequential chemotherapy for intermediate-grade non-Hodgkin's lymphoma in first complete remission. *J Clin Oncol* 1994;12:2543.
71. Haioun C, Lepage E, Gisselbrecht C, et al. Survival benefit of high-dose therapy in poor-risk aggressive non-Hodgkin's lymphoma: final analysis of the prospective LNH87-2 protocol—a groupe d'Étude des lymphomas de l'Adulte study. *J Clin Oncol* 2000;18:3025.
72. Santini G, Salvagno L, Leoni P, et al. VACOP-B versus VACOP-B plus autologous bone marrow transplantation for advanced diffuse non-Hodgkin's lymphoma: results of a prospective randomized trial by the Non-Hodgkin's Lymphoma Cooperative Study Group. *J Clin Oncol* 1998;16:2796.
73. Kluin-Nelemans HC, Zagonel V, Anastasopoulou A, et al. Standard chemotherapy with or without high-dose chemotherapy for aggressive non-Hodgkin's lymphoma: randomized phase III EORTC study. *J Natl Cancer Inst* 2001;93:22.
74. Kaiser U, Uebelacker I, Havemann K, et al. High dose chemotherapy with autologous stem cell transplantation in high grade NHL: first analysis of a randomized multicenter study. *Bone Marrow Transplant* 1998;21:S177.
75. Gianni A, Bregni M, Salvatore S, et al. High-dose chemotherapy and autologous bone marrow transplantation compared with MACOP-B in aggressive B-cell lymphoma. *N Engl J Med* 1997;336:1290.
76. Gisselbrecht C, Lepage E, Molina T, et al. Shortened first-line high-dose chemotherapy for patients with poor-prognosis aggressive lymphoma. *J Clin Oncol* 2002;20:2472.

77. Vitolo U, Liberati AM, Deliliers GL, et al. A multicenter randomized trial by the Italian Lymphoma Intergroup (ILI) comparing high dose chemotherapy (HDS) with autologous stem cell transplantation (ASCT) vs. intensified chemotherapy MegaCEOP in high risk diffuse large B-cell lymphoma (DLBCL): no difference in outcome and toxicity. *Blood* 2001;98:252b.
78. Vose JM, Zhang M-J, Philip A, et al. Autologous transplantation for diffuse aggressive non-Hodgkin's lymphoma in patients never achieving remission: a report from the Autologous Blood and Bone Marrow Transplant Registry. *J Clin Oncol* 2001;19:406.
79. Verdonck LF, van Putten WL, Hagenbeek A, et al. Comparison of CHOP chemotherapy with autologous bone marrow transplantation for slowly responding patients with aggressive non-Hodgkin's lymphoma. *N Engl J Med* 1995;332:1045.
80. Martelli M, Vignetti M, Zinzani P, et al. High-dose chemotherapy followed by autologous bone marrow transplantation versus dexamethasone, cisplatin, and cytaribine in aggressive non-Hodgkin's lymphoma with partial response to front-line chemotherapy: a prospective randomize Italian multicenter study. *J Clin Oncol* 1996;14:534.
81. MacManus MP, Hoppe RT. Is radiotherapy curative for stage I and II low-grade follicular lymphoma? Results of a long-term follow-up study of patients treated at Stanford University. *J Clin Oncol* 1996;14:1282.
82. Horning SJ. Follicular lymphoma: have we made ant progress? *Ann Oncol* 2000;11:23.
83. Johnson PW, Rohatiner AZ, Whelan JS, et al. Patterns of survival in patients with recurrent follicular lymphoma: a 20-year study from a single center. *J Clin Oncol* 1995;13:140.
84. Freedman AS, Neuberg D, Mauch P, et al. Long-term follow-up of autologous bone marrow transplantation in patients with relapsed follicular lymphoma. *Blood* 1999;94:3325.
85. Apostolidis J, Gupta RK, Grenzelias D, et al. High-dose therapy with autologous bone marrow support as consolidation of remission in follicular lymphoma: long-term clinical and molecular follow-up. *J Clin Oncol* 2000;18:527.
86. Bierman PJ, Vose JM, Anderson JR, et al. High-dose therapy with autologous hematopoietic rescue for follicular low-grade non-Hodgkin's lymphoma. *J Clin Oncol* 1997;15:445.
87. Rohatiner A, Johnson P, Price C, et al. Myeloablative therapy with autologous bone marrow transplantation as consolidation therapy for recurrent follicular lymphoma. *J Clin Oncol* 1994;12:1177.
88. Schouten HC, Kvaloy S, Sydes M, et al. The CUP trial: a randomized study analyzing the efficacy of high dose therapy and purging in low-grade non-Hodgkin's lymphoma (NHL). *Ann Oncol* 2000;11(suppl 1):91.
89. Brice P, Simon D, Bouabdallah R, et al. High-dose therapy with autologous stem-cell transplantation (ASCT) after first progression prolonged survival of follicular lymphoma patients included in the prospective GELF 86 protocol. *Ann Oncol* 2000;11:1585.
90. Molina A, Nadenamee A, O'Donnel M, et al. Long-term follow-up and analysis of prognostic factors after high-dose therapy and peripheral blood stem cell autografting in 58 patients with a history of low grade follicular lymphoma. *Blood* 1999;94:171a.
91. Cao TM, Horning SJ, Negrin RS, et al. High-dose therapy and autologous hematopoietic-cell transplantation for follicular lymphoma beyond first remission: the Stanford University experience. *Biol Blood Marrow Transplant* 2001;7:294.
92. Bastion Y, Brice P, Haioun A, et al. Intensive therapy with peripheral blood progenitor cell transplantation in 60 patients with poor-prognosis follicular lymphoma. *Blood* 1995;86:3257.
93. Weaver CH, Schwartzberg L, Rhinehart S, et al. High-dose chemotherapy with BUCY or BEAC and unpurged peripheral blood stem cell infusion in patients with low-grade non-Hodgkin's lymphoma. *Bone Marrow Transplant* 1998;21:383.
94. Colombat P, Donadio D, Foillard L, et al. Value of autologous bone marrow transplantation in follicular lymphoma: a France Autogreffe retrospective study of 42 patients. *Bone Marrow Transplant* 1994;13:157.
95. Voso MT, Martin S, Hohaus S, et al. Prognostic factors for the clinical outcome of patients with follicular lymphoma following high-dose therapy and peripheral blood stem cell transplantation (PBSCT). *Bone Marrow Transplant* 2000;25:957.
96. Seyfarth B, Kuse R, Sonnen R, et al. Autologous stem cell transplantation for follicular lymphoma: no benefit for early transplant? *Ann Hematol* 2001;80:398.
97. Horning SJ, Negrin RS, Hoppe RT, et al. High-dose therapy and autologous bone marrow transplantation for follicular lymphoma in first complete or partial remission: results of a phase II clinical trial. *Blood* 2001;97:404.

98. Freedman AS, Gribben JG, Neuberg D, et al. High-dose therapy and autologous bone marrow transplantation in patients with follicular lymphoma during first remission. *Blood* 1996;88:2780.
99. Tarella C, Caracciolo D, Corrandini P, et al. Long-term follow-up of advanced-stage low-grade lymphoma patients treated up front with high-dose sequential chemotherapy and autograft. *Leukemia* 2000;14:740.
100. Colombat P, Cornillet P, Deconick E, et al. Value of autologous stem cell transplantation with purged bone marrow as first-line therapy for follicular lymphoma with high tumor burden: a GOELAMS phase II study. *Bone Marrow Transplant* 2000;26:971.
101. Morel P, Laporte J, Noel MP, et al. Autologous bone marrow transplantation as consolidation therapy may prolong remission in newly diagnosed high-risk follicular lymphoma: a pilot study of 34 cases. *Leukemia* 1995;9:576.
102. Bociek R, Bierman P, Vose J, et al. High dose therapy with autologous hematopoietic stem cell transplantation for patients with low-grade follicular non-Hodgkin's lymphoma in first complete or partial remission. *Blood* 1999;94:170a.
103. Ladetto M, Corrandini P, Vallet S, et al. High rate of clinical and molecular remissions in follicular lymphoma patients receiving high-dose sequential chemotherapy and autografting at diagnosis: a multicenter, prospective study by the Gruppo Italiano Trapianto Midollo Osseo (GITMO). *Blood* 2002;100:1559.
104. Colombat P, Foussard C, Bertrand P, et al. Value of autologous stem cell transplantation in first line therapy of follicular lymphoma with high tumor burden: first results of the randomized GOELAMNS 064 trial. *Blood* 2001;98:861a.
105. Acker B, Hoppe RT, Colby TV, et al. Histologic conversion in non-Hodgkin's lymphomas. *J Clin Oncol* 1983;1:11.
106. Cullen MH, Lister TA, Bearly RI, et al. Histological transformation of non-Hodgkin's lymphoma. *Cancer* 1979;44:645.
107. Bastion Y, Sebban C, Berger P, et al. Incidence, predictive factors, and outcome of lymphoma transformation in follicular lymphoma patients. *J Clin Oncol* 1997;15:1587.
108. Gallagher CJ, Gregory WM, Jones AE, et al. Follicular lymphoma: prognostic factors for response and survival. *J Clin Oncol* 1986;4:1470.
109. Yuen AR, Kamel OW, Halpern J, et al. Long-term survival after histologic transformation of low-grade follicular lymphoma. *J Clin Oncol* 1995;13:1726.
110. Schoeten HC, Bierman PJ, Vaughan WP, et al. Autologous bone marrow transplantation in follicular non-Hodgkin's lymphoma before and after histologic transformation. *Blood* 1989;74:2579.
111. Foran JM, Apostolidis J, Papamichael D, et al. High-dose therapy with autologous haematopoietic support in patients with transformed follicular lymphoma: a study of 27 patients from a single center. *Ann Oncol* 1998;9:865.
112. Williams CD, Harrison CN, Lister TA, et al. High-dose therapy and autologous stem-cell support for chemosensitive transformed low-grade follicular non-Hodgkin's lymphoma: a case-matched study from the European Bone Marrow Transplant Registry. *J Clin Oncol* 2001;19:727.
113. Chen CI, Crump M, Tsang R, et al. Autotransplants for histologically transformed follicular non-Hodgkin's lymphoma. *Br J Haematol* 2001;113:202.
114. Friedberg JW, Neuberg D, Gribben JG, et al. Autologous bone marrow transplantation after histologic transformation of indolent B-cell malignancies. *Biol Bone Marrow Transplant* 1999;5:262.
115. Gribben JG, Freedman AS, Neuberg D, et al. Immunologic purging of marrow assessed by PCR before autologous bone marrow transplantation for B-cell lymphoma. *N Engl J Med* 1991;325:1525.
116. Gribben JG, Neuberg D, Freedman AS, et al. Detection by polymerase chain reaction of residual cells with the bcl-2 translocation is associated with increased risk of relapse after autologous bone marrow transplantation for B-cell lymphoma. *Blood* 1993;81:3449.
117. Williams CD, Goldstone AH, Pearce RM, et al. Purging of bone marrow in autologous bone marrow transplantation for non-Hodgkin's lymphoma: a case-matched comparison with unpurged cases by the European Blood and Marrow Transplant Lymphoma Registry. *J Clin Oncol* 1996;14:2454.
118. Johnson P, Price C, Smith T, et al. Detection of cells bearing the t(14;18) translocation following myeloablative treatment and autologous bone marrow transplantation for follicular lymphoma. *J Clin Oncol* 1994;12:798.
119. Magni M, Di Nichola M, Devizzi L, et al. Successful purging of CD34-containing peripheral blood harvest in mantle cell and indolent lymphoma: evidence for a role of both chemotherapy and rituximab infusion. *Blood* 2000;96:864.

120. Voso MT, Pantel G, Weis M, et al. In vivo depletion of B cells using a combination of high-dose cytosine arabinoside/mitoxantrone and rituximab for autografting in patients with non-Hodgkin's lymphoma. *Br J Haematol* 2000;109:729.
121. Haioun C, Delfau-Larue M, Beaujean F, et al. Efficiency of in vivo purging with rituximab followed by high-dose therapy with autologous peripheral blood stem cell transplantation in B-cell non-Hodgkin's lymphoma. *Blood* 2000;96:184a.
122. Belhadj K, Delfau-Larue M, Elgnoui T, et al. Efficiency of in vivo purging with rituximab followed by high-dose therapy (HDT) with autologous peripheral blood stem cell transplantation (PBSCT) in B-cell lymphomas. A single institution study. *Proc Am Soc Clin Oncol* 2002;21:285a.
123. Lazzarino M, Arcaini L, Bernasconi P, et al. A sequence of immuno-chemotherapy with rituximab, mobilization of in vivo purged stem cells, high-dose chemotherapy, and autotransplant is an effective and non-toxic treatment for advanced follicular and mantle cell lymphoma. *Br J Haematol* 2002;116:229.
124. Morschhauser F, Recher C, Galoin S, et al. Multicenter, phase II trial to evaluate the efficacy and safety of rituximab in patients suffering from follicular non-Hodgkin's lymphoma (FNHL) with residual minimal disease after autologous transplantation of hematopoietic stem cells (M39012 trial). *Proc Am Soc Clin Oncol* 2002;21:267a.
125. Teodorovic I, Pittaluga S, Kluin-Nelemans JC, et al. Efficacy of four different regimens in 64 mantle-cell lymphoma cases: clinicopathologic comparison with 498 other non-Hodgkin's lymphoma subtypes. *J Clin Oncol* 1995;13:2819.
126. Velders GA, Kluin-Nelemans JC, De Boer CJ, et al. Mantle-cell lymphoma: a population-based study. *J Clin Oncol* 1996;14:1269.
127. Zucca E, Roggero E, Pinotti G, et al. Patterns of survival in mantle cell lymphoma. *Ann Oncol* 1996;6:257.
128. Majlis A, Pugh WH, Rodriguez MA, et al. Mantle cell lymphoma: correlation of clinical outcome and biologic features with three histologic variants. *J Clin Oncol* 1997;15:1664.
129. Argatoff LH, Connors JM, Klasa RJ, et al. Mantle cell lymphoma: a clinicopathologic study of 80 cases. *Blood* 1997;89:2067.
130. Oinonen R, Franssila K, Teerenhovi, et al. Mantle cell lymphoma: clinical features, treatment, and prognosis of 94 patients. *Eur J Cancer* 1998;34:329.
131. Vandenberghe E, Ruiz de Elvira C, Isaacson P, et al. Does transplantation improve outcome in mantle cell lymphoma (MCL)? A study from the EBMT. *Blood* 2000;96:482a. [Abstract].
132. Weisenberger DD, Vose JM, Greiner TC, et al. Mantle cell lymphoma. A clinicopathologic study of 68 cases from the Nebraska Lymphoma Study Group. *Am J Hematol* 2000;64:190.
133. Foran JM, Cunningham D, Coiffier B, et al. European phase II study of rituximab (chimeric anti-CD20 monoclonal antibody) for patients with newly diagnosed mantle cell lymphoma, immunocytoma, and small B-cell lymphocytic lymphoma. *J Clin Oncol* 2000;18:317.
134. Howard O, Gribben JG, Neuberg D, et al. Rituximab and CHOP induction therapy for newly diagnosed mantle-cell lymphoma: molecular complete responses are not predictive of progression-free survival. *J Clin Oncol* 2002;20:1288.
135. Stewart DA, Vose JM, Weisenberger DD, et al. The role of high-dose therapy and autologous hematopoietic stem cell transplantation for mantle cell lymphoma. *Ann Oncol* 1995;6:263.
136. Haas R, Brittinger G, Meusers P, et al. Myeloablative therapy with blood stem cell transplantation is effective in mantle cell lymphoma. *Leukemia* 1996;10:1975.
137. Dreger P, von Neuhoff N, Kuse R, et al. Sequential high-dose therapy and autologous stem cell transplantation for treatment of mantle cell lymphoma. *Ann Oncol* 1997;8:401.
138. Ketterer N, Salles G, Espinouse D, et al. Intensive therapy with peripheral blood stem cell transplantation in 16 patients with mantle cell lymphoma. *Ann Oncol* 1997;8:701.
139. Kroger N, Hoffneckht M, Dreger P, et al. Long-term disease-free survival of patients with advanced mantle-cell lymphoma following high-dose chemotherapy. *Bone Marrow Transplant* 1999;21:55.
140. Blay J-Y, Sebban C, Surbiguet C, et al. High-dose chemotherapy with hematopoietic stem cell transplantation in patients with mantle cell or diffuse centrocytic non-Hodgkin's lymphomas: a single center experience on 18 patients. *Bone Marrow Transplant* 1998;21:51.
141. Milpied N, Gaillard F, Moreau P, et al. High-dose therapy with stem cell transplantation for mantle cell lymphoma: results and prognostic factors, a single center experience. *Bone Marrow Transplant* 1998;22:645.

142. Freedman AS, Neuberg D, Gribben JG, et al. High-dose chemoradiotherapy and anti-B-cell monoclonal antibody-purged autologous bone marrow transplantation in mantle cell lymphoma: no evidence for long-term remission. *J Clin Oncol* 1998;16:13.
143. Vose JM, Bierman PJ, Weisenberger DD, et al. Autologous hematopoietic stem cell transplantation for mantle cell lymphoma. *Biol Blood Marrow Transplant* 2000;6:640.
144. Malone JM, Molina A, Stockerl-Goldstein K, et al. High dose therapy and autologous hematopoietic cell transplantation for mantle cell lymphoma: the Stanford / City of Hope experience. *Proc Am Soc Clin Oncol* 2001;20:13a.
145. Khouri IF, Romaguera J, Kantarjian H, et al. Hyper-CVAD and high-dose methotrexate/cytaribine followed by stem cell transplantation: an active regimen for aggressive mantle cell lymphoma. *J Clin Oncol* 1998;16:3803.
146. Romaguera JE, Dang NH, Hagemeister FB, et al. Preliminary report of rituximab with intensive chemotherapy for untreated aggressive mantle cell lymphoma (MCL). *Blood* 2000;96:733a. [Abstract].
147. Decaudin D, Brouse N, Brice P, et al. Efficacy of autologous stem cell transplantation in mantle cell lymphoma: a 3-year follow up study. *Bone Marrow Transplant* 2000;25:251.
148. Lefere F, Delmer A, Suzan F, et al. Sequential chemotherapy by CHOP and DHAP regimens followed by high-dose therapy with stem cell transplantation induces a high rate of complete response and improves event-free survival in mantle cell lymphoma: a prospective study. *Leukemia* 2000;16:587.
149. Hiddemann W, Dreyling M, Pfreundschuh M, et al. Myeloablative radiochemotherapy followed by autologous blood stem cell transplantation leads to a significant prolongation of event-free survival in patients with mantle cell lymphoma (MCL): results of a prospective randomized European Intergroup study. *Blood* 2001;98:861a.
150. Jacquy C, Lambert F, Soree A, et al. Peripheral blood stem cell contamination in mantle cell non-Hodgkin's lymphoma: the case for purging? *Bone Marrow Transplant* 1999;23:681.
151. Anderson NS, Donovan JW, Borus JS, et al. Failure of immunologic purging in mantle cell lymphoma assessed by polymerase chain reaction detection of minimal residual disease. *Blood* 1997;90:4212.
152. Mangel J, Buckstein R, Imrie K, et al. Immunotherapy with rituximab following high-dose therapy and autologous stem-cell transplantation for mantle cell lymphoma. *Semin Oncol* 2002;29(suppl 2):56.
153. Press OW, Eary JF, Gooley T, et al. A phase I/II trial of iodine-131-tositumomab (anti-CD20), etoposide, cyclophosphamide, and autologous stem cell transplantation for relapsed B-cell lymphomas. *Blood* 2000;96:2934.
154. Gopal AK, Rajendran JG, Petersdorf SH, et al. High-dose chemo-radioimmunotherapy with autologous stem cell support for relapsed mantle cell lymphoma. *Blood* 2002;99:3158.
155. Behr TM, Griesinger F, Riggert J, at al. High-dose myeloablative radioimmunotherapy of mantle cell lymphoma with iodine-131-labeled chimeric anti-CD20 antibody C2B8 and autologous stem cell support. *Cancer* 2002;94:1363.
156. Wollner N, Burchenal JH, Liebermann PH, et al. Non-Hodgkin's lymphoma in children: a progress report on the original patients treated with the LSA2L2 protocol. *Cancer* 1979;44:1900.
157. Coleman CN, Picozzi VJ, Cox RS, et al. Treatment of lymphoblastic lymphoma in adults. *J Clin Oncol* 1986;4:1626.
158. Slater DE, Mertelsmann R, Koriner B, et al. Lymphoblastic lymphoma in adults. *J Clin Oncol* 1986;4:57.
159. Milpied N, Ifrah N, Kuentz M, et al. Bone marrow transplantation for adult poor prognosis lymphoblastic lymphoma in first complete remission. *Br J Haematol* 1989;73:82.
160. Santini G, Coser P, Chisesi T, et al. Autologous bone marrow transplantation for advanced stage adult lymphoblastic lymphoma in first complete remission. *Ann Oncol* 1991;2:181.
161. Verdonck LF, Dekker AW, Gast GC, et al. Autologous bone marrow transplantation for adult poor risk lymphoblastic lymphoma in first remission. *J Clin Oncol* 1992;10:644.
162. Sweetenham JW, Liberti G, Pearce R, et al. High-dose therapy and autologous bone marrow transplantation for adult patients with lymphoblastic lymphoma: results of the European Group for Bone Marrow Transplantation. *J Clin Oncol* 1994;12:1358.
163. Jost LM, Jacky E, Dommann-Scherrer C, et al. Short-term weekly chemotherapy followed by high-dose therapy and autologous bone marrow transplantation for lymphoblastic and Burkitt's lymphomas in adult patients. *Ann Oncol* 1995;6:445.

164. Bouabdallah R, Xerri L, Bardou V-J, et al. Role of induction chemotherapy and bone marrow transplantation in adult lymphoblastic lymphoma: A report on 62 patients from a single center. *Ann Oncol* 1998;9:619.
165. Sweetenham JW, Santini G, Qian W, et al. High-dose therapy and autologous stem-cell transplantation versus conventional consolidation/maintenance therapy as postremission therapy for adult patients with lymphoblastic lymphoma: results of a randomized trial of the European Group for Blood and Marrow Transplantation and the United Kingdom Lymphoma Group. *J Clin Oncol* 2001;19:2927.
166. Sweetenham JW, Pearce R, Taghipour G, et al. Adult Burkitt's and Burkitt-like non-Hodgkin's lymphoma—outcome for patients treated with high-dose therapy and autologous stem-cell transplantation in first remission or at relapse: results from the European Group for Blood and Marrow Transplantation. *J Clin Oncol* 1996;14:2465.
167. Magrath I, Adde M, Shad A, et al. Adults and children with small non-cleaved-cell lymphoma have a similar excellent outcome when treated with the same chemotherapy regimen. *J Clin Oncol* 1996;14:925.
168. Mead GM, Sydes MR, Walewski J, et al. An international evaluation of CODOX-M and CODOX-M alternating with IVAC in adult Burkitt's lymphoma: results of United Kingdom Lymphoma Group LY06 study. *Ann Oncol* 2002;13:1264.
169. Bernstein JL, Coleman CN, Strickler JG, et al. Combined modality therapy for adults with small noncleaved cell lymphoma (Burkitt's and non-Burkitt's types). *J Clin Oncol* 1986;4:847.
170. Longo Dl, Duffey PL, Jaffe ES, et al. Diffuse small noncleaved-cell, non-Burkitt's lymphoma in adults: a high-grade lymphoma responsive to ProMACE-based combination chemotherapy. *J Clin Oncol* 1994;12:2153.
171. Soussain C, Patte C, Ostronoff M, et al. Small non-cleaved cell lymphoma and leukemia in adults: a retrospective study of 65 adults treated with the LMB pediatric protocols. *Blood* 1995;85:664.
172. Hoelzer D, Ludwig W-D, Thiel E, et al. Improved outcome in adult B-cell acute lymphoblastic leukemia. *Blood* 1998;87:495.
173. Lee EJ, Petroni GR, Schiffer CA, et al. Brief-duration high-intensity chemotherapy for patients with small noncleaved-cell lymphoma or FAB L3 acute lymphoblastic leukemia: results of Cancer and Leukemia Group B Study 9251. *J Clin Oncol* 2001;19:4014.
174. Thomas DA, Cortes J, O'Brien S, et al. Hyper-CVAD program in Burkitt's type adult lymphoblastic leukemia. *J Clin Oncol* 1999;17:2461.
175. A clinical evaluation of the International Lymphoma Study Group classification of non-Hodgkin's lymphoma: the non-Hodgkin's Lymphoma Classification Project. *Blood* 1997;89:3909.
176. Cheng AL, Chen YC, Wang CH, et al. Direct comparisons of peripheral T-cell lymphoma with diffuse B-cell lymphoma of comparable histologic grades—should peripheral T-cell lymphoma be considered separately? *J Clin Oncol* 1989;7:725.
177. Kwak LW, Wilson M, Weiss LM, et al. Similar outcome of B-cell and T-cell diffuse large-cell lymphomas: the Stanford experience. *J Clin Oncol* 1991;9:1426.
178. Armitage JO, Vose JM, Linder J, et al. Clinical significance of immunophenotype in diffuse aggressive non-Hodgkin's lymphoma. *J Clin Oncol* 1989;7:1783.
179. Melnyk A, Rodriguez A, Pugh WC, et al. Evaluation of the Revised European–American Lymphoma Classification confirms clinical relevance of immunophenotype in 560 cases of aggressive non-Hodgkin's lymphoma. *Blood* 1997;89:4514.
180. Vose JM, Peterson C, Bierman PJ, et al. Comparison of high-dose therapy and autologous bone marrow transplantation for T-cell and B-cell non-Hodgkin's lymphomas. *Blood* 1990;76:424.
181. Blystad AK, Enblad G, Kvaløy S, et al. High-dose therapy with autologous stem cell transplantation in patients with peripheral T-cell lymphomas. *Bone Marrow Transplant* 2001;27:711.
182. Rodriguez J, Munsell M, Yazji S, et al. Impact of high-dose chemotherapy on peripheral T-cell lymphomas. *J Clin Oncol* 2001;19:3766.
183. Rodriguez J, Caballero A, Gutierrez J, et al. Results of high dose chemotherapy and autologous stem cell transplantation in patients with peripheral T-cell lymphoma (PTCL). The Spanish Lymphoma Cooperative Group Experience (GEL/TAMO). *Blood* 2001;98:680a.
184. Fanin R, Silvestri F, Geromin A, et al. Primary systemic CD30 (Ki-1)-positive anaplastic large cell lymphoma of the adult: sequential intensive treatment with F-MACHOP regimen (+/–radiotherapy) and autologous bone marrow transplantation. *Blood* 1996;87:1243.

185. Deconinck E, Lamy T, Foussard C, et al. Autologous stem cell transplantation for anaplastic large-cell lymphomas: results of a prospective trial. *Br J Haematol* 2000;109:736.
186. Jagasia M, Stein R, Kinney M, et al. High dose chemotherapy (HDC) and hematopoietic stem cell transplant (HSCT) in peripheral T-cell (PTCL), NK cell, and Ki-1 anaplastic large cell lymphoma. *Proc Am Soc Clin Oncol* 2001;20:294a.
187. Bakr M, Ketterer N, Rosselet A, et al. High-dose chemotherapy and autologous blood stem cell support in patients with aggressive T-cell lymphomas. *Proc Am Soc Clin Oncol* 2002;21:1147.
188. Stockerl-Goldstein KE, Horning SJ, Negrin RS, et al. Influence of preparatory regimen and source of hematopoietic cells on outcome of autotransplantation for non-Hodgkin's lymphoma. *Biol Blood Marrow Transplant* 1996;2:76.
189. Schmitz N, Linch DC, Dreger P, et al. Randomized trial of filgrastim-mobilised peripheral blood progenitor cell transplantation versus autologous bone marrow transplantation in lymphoma patients. *Lancet* 1996;347:353.
190. Majolino I, Pearce R, Taghipour G, et al. Peripheral blood stem cell transplantation versus autologous bone marrow transplantation in Hodgkin's and non-Hodgkin's lymphomas: a new matched-pair analysis of the European Group for Blood and Marrow Transplantation Registry Data. Lymphoma Working Party of the European Group for Blood and Marrow Transplantation. *J Clin Oncol* 1997;15:509.
191. Brice P, Marolleau JP, Pautier P, et al. Hematologic recovery and survival of lymphoma patients after autologous stem-cell transplantation: comparison of bone marrow and peripheral blood progenitor cells. *Leuk Lymphoma* 1996;22:449.
192. Smith TJ, Hillner BE, Schmitz N, et al. Economic analysis of a randomized clinical trial of to compare filgrastim-mobilised peripheral-blood progenitor-cell transplantation versus autologous bone marrow transplantation in patients with Hodgkin's and on-Hodgkin's lymphoma. *J Clin Oncol* 1997;15:5.
193. Vellenga, E, van Agthoven M, Croockewit AJ, et al. Autologous peripheral blood stem cell transplantation in patients with relapsed lymphoma results in accelerated haematopoietic reconstitution, improved quality of life, and cost reduction compared with bone marrow transplantation: Hovon 22 study. *Br J Haematol* 2001;114:319.
194. Perry AR, Peniket AJ, Watts MJ, et al. Peripheral blood stem cell versus autologous bone marrow transplantation for Hodgkin's disease: equivalent survival outcome in a single-centre matched-pair analysis. *Br J Haematol* 1999;105:280.
195. Narayanasami U, Kanteti R, Morelli J, et al. Randomized trial of filgrastim versus chemotherapy and filgrastim mobilization of hematopoietic progenitor cells for rescue in autologous transplantation. *Blood* 2001;98:2059.
196. Darrington DL, Vose JM, Anderson JA, et al. Incidence and characterization of secondary myelodysplastic syndrome and acute myelogenous leukemia following high-dose chemoradiotherapy and autologous stem-cell transplantation for lymphoid malignancies. *J Clin Oncol* 1994;12:2527.
197. Traweek ST, Slovak ML, Nademanee A, et al. Clonal karyotypic hematopoietic cell abnormalities occurring after autologous bone marrow transplantation for Hodgkin's disease and non-Hodgkin's lymphoma. *Blood* 1994;84:957.
198. André M, Henry-Amar M, Blaise D, et al. Treatment-related deaths and second cancer risk after autologous stem-cell transplantation for Hodgkin's disease. *Blood* 1998;92:1933.
199. Miller JS, Arthur DC, Litz CE, et al. Myelodysplastic syndrome after autologous bone marrow transplantation: an additional late complication of curative cancer therapy. *Blood* 1994;83:3780.
200. Chao NJ, Nademanee AP, Long GD, et al. Importance of bone marrow cytogenetic evaluation before autologous bone marrow transplantation for Hodgkin's disease. *J Clin Oncol* 1991;9:1575.
201. Milligan D, Ruiz de Elvira M, Goldstone A, et al. Secondary leukemia and myelodysplasia after autografting for lymphomas. *Blood* 1998;92:493a.
202. van Leeuwen F, Klokman W, van't Veer M, et al. Long-term risk of second malignancy in survivors of Hodgkin's disease treated during adolescence or young adulthood. *J Clin Oncol* 2000;18:487.
203. Swerdlow A, Barber J, Hudson G, et al. Risk of second malignancy after Hodgkin's disease in a collaborative British cohort: the relation of age to treatment. *J Clin Oncol* 2000;18:498.
204. Tucker MA, Coleman CN, Cox RS, et al. Risk of second cancers after treatment for Hodgkin's disease. *N Engl J Med* 1988;318:76.
205. Oddou S, Vey N, Viens P, et al. Second neoplasms following high-dose chemotherapy and autologous stem cell transplantation for malignant lymphomas: six cases in a cohort of 171 patients from a single institution. *Leuk Lymphoma* 1998;31:187.

206. Jones RJ, Ambinder RF, Piantadosi S, et al. Evidence of a graft-versus-lymphoma effect associated with allogeneic bone marrow transplantation. *Blood* 1998;77:649.
207. van Biesen KW, De Lima M, Giralt SA, et al. Management of lymphoma recurrence after allogeneic transplantation: the relevance of graft-versus-lymphoma effect. *Bone Marrow Transplant* 1997;19:977.
208. Chopra R, Goldstone AH, Pearce R, et al. Autologous versus allogeneic bone marrow transplantation for non-Hodgkin's lymphoma: a case-controlled analysis from the European Bone Marrow Transplant Group Registry data. *J Clin Oncol* 1992;10:1690.
209. Rhondon G, Giralt Sa, Huh Y, et al. Graft-versus-leukemia after allogeneic bone marrow transplantation for chronic lymphocytic leukemia. *Bone Marrow Transplant* 1996;18:669.
210. Collins RH, Shpilberg O, Drobyski WR, et al. Donor leukocyte infusions in 140 patients with relapsed malignancy after bone marrow transplantation. *J Clin Oncol* 1997;15:433.
211. Khouri IF, Keating M, Korbling M, et al. Transplant-lite: induction of graft-versus-malignancy using fludaribine-based nonablative chemotherapy and allogeneic blood progenitor-cell transplantation as treatment for lymphoid malignancies. *J Clin Oncol* 1998;16:2817.
212. Bierman PJ, Sweetenham JW, Loberiza F, et al. Syngeneic hematopoietic stem cell transplantation for non-Hodgkin's lymphoma (NHL): comparison with allogeneic and autologous transplants suggests a role for purging. *Proc Am Soc Clin Oncol* 2001;20:5a.
213. Anderson JE, Litzow MR, Appelbaum FR, et al. Allogeneic, syngeneic, and autologous bone marrow transplantation for Hodgkin's disease: the 21-year Seattle experience. *J Clin Oncol* 1993;11:2342.
214. Milpied N, Fielding AK, Pearce RM, et al. Allogeneic bone marrow transplant is not better than autologous transplant for patients with relapsed Hodgkin's disease. European Group for Blood and Bone Marrow Transplantation. *J Clin Oncol* 1996;14:1291.
215. Gajeweski JL, Phillip T, Carella A, et al. Bone marrow transplants from HLA-identical siblings in advanced Hodgkin's disease. *J Clin Oncol* 1996;14:572.
216. Akpek G, Ambinder SP, Piantadosi S, et al. Long-term results of blood and marrow transplantation for Hodgkin's lymphoma. *J Clin Oncol* 2001;19:4314.
217. Dann EJ, Daugherty CK, Larson RA. Allogeneic bone marrow transplantation for relapsed and refractory Hodgkin's disease and non-Hodgkin's lymphoma. *Bone Marrow Transplant* 1997;20:369.
218. Mendoza E, Territo M, Schiller G, et al. Allogeneic bone marrow transplantation for Hodgkin's and non-Hodgkin's lymphoma. *Bone Marrow Transplant* 1995;15:299.
219. van Besien K, Sobocinski KA, Rowlings PA, et al. Allogeneic bone marrow transplantation for low grade lymphoma. *Blood* 1998;92:1832.
220. Verdonck LF. Allogeneic versus autologous bone marrow transplantation for refractory and recurrent low-grade non-Hodgkin's lymphoma: updated results of the Utrecht experience. *Leuk Lymphoma* 1999;34:129.
221. van Biesen K, Khouri IF, Giralt S, et al. Allogeneic bone marrow transplantation for refractory and recurrent low-grade lymphoma: the case for aggressive management. *J Clin Oncol* 1995;13:1096.
222. Mandigers C, Raemaekers J, Schattenberg A, et al. Allogeneic bone marrow transplantation with T-cell-depleted marrow grafts for patients with poor-risk relapsed low-grade non-Hodgkin's lymphoma. *Br J Haematol* 1998;100:198.
223. Stein RS, Greer JP, Goodman S, et al. High-dose therapy with autologous or allogeneic transplantation as salvage therapy for small cleaved lymphoma of follicular center origin. *Bone Marrow Transplant* 1999;23:227.
224. Toze CL, Shepherd JD, Connors JM, et al. Allogeneic bone marrow transplantation for low-grade lymphoma and chronic lymphocytic leukemia. *Bone Marrow Transplant* 2000;25:605.
225. Forrest D, Matheson K, Couban S, et al. High-dose therapy and allogeneic hematopoietic stem cell transplantation for progressive follicular lymphoma. *Blood* 2001;98:408a.
226. Appelbaum FR, Sullivan KM, Buckner CD, et al. Treatment of malignant lymphoma in 100 patients with chemotherapy, total body irradiation, and marrow transplantation. *J Clin Oncol* 1987;5:1340.
227. Van Biesen KW, Mehra RC, Giralt SA, et al. Allogeneic bone marrow transplantation for poor-prognosis lymphoma: response toxicity, and survival depend on disease histology. *Am J Med* 1996;100:299.
228. Ratanatharathorn V, Uberti J, Karanes C, et al. Prospective comparative trial of autologous versus allogeneic transplantation in patients with non-Hodgkin's lymphoma. *Blood* 1994;84:1050.
229. Stein RS, Greer JP, Goodman S, et al. Intensified preparative regimens and allogeneic transplantation in refractory or relapsed intermediate and high grade non-Hodgkin's lymphoma. *Leuk Lymphoma* 2001;41:343.
230. Khouri IF, Lee M-S, Romaguera J, et al. Allogeneic hematopoietic transplantation for mantle cell lymphoma: molecular remissions and evidence of graft-versus-malignancy. *Ann Oncol* 1999;10:1293.

231. Sohn SK, Bensinger W, Holmberg L, et al. High-dose chemotherapy with allogeneic or autologous stem cell transplantation for relapsed mantle cell lymphoma: the Seattle experience. *Proc Am Soc Clin Oncol* 1997;17:17a. [Abstract].
232. Molina A, Nadenamee A, O'Donnell MR, et al. Autologous and allogeneic stem-cell transplantation for poor-risk mantle cell lymphoma: the City of Hope experience. *Blood* 1998;92:459a. [Abstract].
233. McSweeney PA, Niederweiser D, Shizuru JA, et al. Hematopoietic cell transplantation in older patients with hematologic malignancies: replacing high-dose cytoxic therapy with graft-versus-tumor effects. *Blood* 2001;97:3390.
234. Kottaridis PD, Milligan DW, Chopra R, et al. In vivo CAMPATH-1H prevents graft-versus-host disease following nonmyeloablative stem cell transplantation. *Blood* 2000;96:2419.
235. Perez-Simon JA, Kottaridis PD, Martino, et al. Reduced intensity conditioning (RIC) allogeneic transplantation with or without CAMPATH-1H: comparison between two prospective studies in patients with lymphoproliferative disorders. *Blood* 2001;98:743a. [Abstract].
236. Branson K, Chopra R, Panagiotis D, et al. Role of nonmyeloablative allogeneic stem-cell transplantation after failure of autologous transplantation in patients with lymphoproliferative malignancies. *J Clin Oncol* 2002;20:4022.
237. Khouri IF, Saliba RM, Giralt SA, et al. Nonablative allogeneic hematopoietic transplantation as adoptive immunotherapy for indolent lymphoma: low incidence of toxicity, acute graft-versus-host disease, and treatment-related mortality. *Blood* 2001;98:3595.
238. Carella AM, Cavaliere M, Lerma E, et al. Autografting followed by nonmyeloablative immunosuppressive chemotherapy and allogeneic peripheral-blood hematopoietic stem-cell transplantation as the treatment of resistant Hodgkin's disease and non-Hodgkin's lymphoma. *J Clin Oncol* 2000;18:3918.
239. Robinson SP, Goldstone AH, Mackinnon S, et al. Chemoresistant or aggressive lymphoma predicts for a poor outcome following reduced intensity allogeneic progenitor cell transplantation: an analysis from the Lymphoma Working Party of the European Group for Blood and Marrow Transplantation. *Blood* 2002;100;4310.
240. Khouri IF, Saliba RM, Lee M-S, et al. Nonablative allogeneic stem cell transplantation for non-Hodgkin's lymphoma (NHL): improved outcome with low incidence of acute GVHD and treatment related mortality. *Blood* 2001;98:416a. [Abstract].
241. Spitzer TR, McAfee SL, Dey BR, et al. Durable progression free survival (PFS) following non-myeloablative bone marrow transplantation for chemorefractory diffuse large B-cell lymphoma (B-LCL). *Blood* 2001;98:2813a. [Abstract].
242. Bertz H, Illerhaus G, Veelken H, et al. Allogeneic hematopoietic stem-cell transplantation for patients with relapsed or refractory lymphomas: a comparison of high-dose conventional conditioning versus fludaribine-based reduced-intensity regimens. *Ann Oncol* 2002;13:135.
243. Porter DI, Luger SM, Duffy KM, et al. Allogeneic cell therapy for patients who relapse after autologous stem cell transplantation. *Biol Blood Marrow Transplant* 2001;7:230.
244. Nagler A, Slavin S, Varadi G, et al. Allogeneic peripheral-blood stem cell transplantation using a fludaribine-based low intensity conditioning regimen for malignant lymphoma. *Bone Marrow Transplant* 2000;25:1021.
245. Garcia-Marco, JA, Cabrera R, Perez-Sanz N, et al. Analysis of graft-versus-malignancy effect following nonmyeloabaltive stem cell transplantation in chronic lymphocytic leukemia and non-Hodgkin's lymphoma. *Blood* 2001;98:5237a. [Abstract].
246. Hou JW, Fowler DH, Wilson W, et al. Potent graft-versus-lymphoma effect after a non-myeloablative stem cell transplant in refractory non-Hodgkin's lymphoma: role of rapid complete donor chimerism. *Blood*, 2001;98:1696a. [Abstract].
247. Martino R, Caballero MD, Canals C, et al. Allogeneic peripheral blood stem cell transplantation with reduced-intensity conditioning: results of a prospective multicentre study. *Br J Haematol* 2001;115:653.
248. Mohty M, Fegeux N, Exbrayat C, et al. Reduced intensity conditioning: enhanced graft-versus-tumor effect following dose-reduced conditioning and allogeneic transplantation for refractory lymphoid malignancies after high-dose therapy. *Bone Marrow Transplant* 2001;28:335.
249. Corrandini P, Tarella C, Olivieri A, et al. Reduced-intensity conditioning followed by allografting of hematopoietic cells can produce clinical and molecular remissions in patients with poor-risk hematologic malignancies. *Blood* 2002;99:75.
250. Chakraverty R, Peggs K, Chopra R, et al. Limiting transplantation-related mortality following unrelated donor stem cell transplantation by using a nonmyeloablative conditioning regimen. *Blood* 2002;3:1071.

251. Anderlini P, Giralt S, Anderson B, et al. Allogeneic stem cell transplantation with fludaribine-based, less intensive conditioning regimens as adoptive immunotherapy in advanced Hodgkin's disease. *Bone Marrow Transplant* 2000;26:615.

4 Autologous and Allogeneic Transplantation for Multiple Myeloma

Faith E. Davies, MD *and Kenneth C. Anderson,* MD

Contents

1. AUTOLOGOUS TRANSPLANTATION

The conventional treatment of myeloma frequently results in the achievement of a stable "plateau" phase during which patients have minimal or no symptoms related to their disease; however, during this phase, patients still have a considerable tumor burden. Conventional treatment with melphalan, melphalan and prednisolone, or combination chemotherapy regimens including cyclophosphamide, melphalan, carmustine (BCNU), lomustine (CCNU), adriamycin, vincristine, and prednisolone result in a median survival of between 24 and 36 mo, with approx 50% of patients responding to therapy. However, only a minority (5–10%) of patients attained a true complete remission (CR), with the disappearance of paraprotein and a normal marrow *(1,2)*. Following the introduction of infusional chemotherapy, such as vincristine adriamucin dexamethasone (VAD), the number of patients responding to treatment (70–80%) and the level of response achieved increased, with CR rates of 8–28% *(3,4)*. These responses were often short-lived, and it was with the purpose of improving the duration of response that high-dose therapy (HDT) was introduced *(5)*.

1.1. HDT vs Conventional Therapy

Initial studies using a single large intravenous dose of melphalan (140 mg/m^2) gave encouraging results; however, the treatment was associated with a prolonged myelosuppression period, which resulted in a significant infection risk and a number of procedure-related deaths. Later, this approach was combined with bone marrow (BM) rescue, and its safety improved and a high response rate was noted, with up to 50% of patients attaining a CR *(6)*. In the early 1990s autologous peripheral blood hematopoetic stem cells were reported as an alternative source of support for the high-dose procedure. There are a number of advantages to such a

From: *Stem Cell Transplantation for Hematologic Malignancies*
Edited by: R. J. Soiffer © Humana Press Inc., Totowa, NJ

technique, including ease in collecting stem cells, quicker engraftment times, and a lower transplant-related mortality.

A number of groups have since shown an improvement in response rates and survival using this regimen in both relapsed/refractory and newly diagnosed patients when compared to historical controls *(7,8)*. However, conflicting evidence also suggested that patients who would be potential candidates for HDT but were treated with conventional chemotherapy had similar survival rates to those reported with HDT *(9)* (*see* Table 1). These single-center studies are difficult to assess because patient selection is subject to considerable bias, including young age, good performance status, and normal renal function. Thus, a number of prospective randomized trials have addressed this question by comparing HDT with either peripheral blood stem cell transplantation (PBSCT) or autologous bone marrow transplantation (autoBMT) support to conventional combination therapy. To date, two trials have reported an improved response rate, progression-free survival (PFS), and overall survival (OS) in patients undergoing high-dose treatment *(10,11)*. Two further trials report that despite an increase in response rates in the HDT arms, there was no difference in PFS or OS *(12,13)* (*see* Table 1).

The majority of these trials have set an upper age limit of 65 yr for consideration for HDT. A number of reports from single centers have treated older patients (up to 75 yr of age) who were considered biologically fit, and response rates and survival rates were similar to younger cohorts *(14)*. There are also a number of reports of the use of HDT (in some cases, an attenuated dose of melphalan of 140 mg/m^2 was used) in patients with renal failure, some of who required dialysis. Although in the majority of cases there was no improvement in renal function, the procedure was well tolerated and the renal disease was not a factor influencing OS *(15,16)*.

1.2. Timing of HDT

The relative merits of HDT either early in the disease course or as salvage therapy for relapse after conventional therapy have also been examined in two randomized trials. To date, only one trial has been reported and showed no difference in OS between patients receiving either early or late (relapse) HDT; however, the time without symptoms and toxicity (TwisTT) favored the early-transplant cohort *(17)*. The results of the South West Oncology Group trial are awaited.

Taking these data in the context of the HDT vs conventional trials, the results to date would suggest that all eligible patients should receive HDT. Although the timing of this in the disease course remains unclear, it is probably prudent to collect PBSCs/BM at either diagnosis or at maximum response to ensure that an adequate harvest is available to support a subsequent high-dose procedure.

1.3. Tandem Transplants

In order to improve the response rates and increase the survival, a number of groups are investigating the use of further courses of intensification therapy following the initial high-dose procedure. Results from the Arkansas group have shown that this approach is very effective *(7,18)*. To date, three randomized trials comparing single HDT vs double HDT have reported interim analyses. The approach appears to be feasible with the second HDT being delivered in a timely fashion in approx 75% of patients with a low transplant-related mortality (TRM). One trial reports an improved response rate and prolonged PFS and OS in the double-HDT arm *(19)*. However, the other two trials show similar response rates and OSs in the two arms *(20,21)*. Drawing conclusions from these studies is difficult at present, as results appear to be conflicting and more follow-up is required (*see* Table 2).

Table 1
Autologous Transplantation vs Conventional Chemotherapy for Newly Diagnosed Myeloma

Authors		*Patients (n)*	*CR*[a] *(%)*	*EFS*[a] *(median)*	*OS*[a] *(median)*
Barlogie et al. *(7)*	Conventional[b]	116	—	22 mo	48 mo
	HDT	123	40	49 mo	62 mo
Lenhoff et al. *(8)*	Conventional[b]	274	—		46% at 4 yr
	HDT	274	34	27 mo	61% at 4 yr
Attal et al. *(10)*	Conventional	100	5	18 mo	37 mo
	HDT	100	22	27 mo	52% at 5 yr
Fermand et al. *(12)*	Conventional	96	—	18.7 mo	50.4 mo
	HDT	94	—	24.3 mo	55.3 mo
Blade et al. *(13)*	Conventional	83	11	34.3 mo	66.9 mo
	HDT	81	30	42.5 mo	67.4 mo
Child et al. *(11)*	Conventional	200	8.5	19.6 mo	42.3 mo
	HDT	201	44	31.6 mo	54.8 mo

[a]Abbreviations: CR, complete remission; EFS, event-free survival; OS, overall survival.

[b]Historical controls.

Table 2
Single vs Double Autologous Transplantaion for Newly Diagnosed Myeloma

Authors		*Patients (n)*	*CR (%)*	*EFS (median)*	*OS (median)*
Attal et al. *(19)*	Single	88	50	20% at 5 yr	40% at 5 yr
	Double	92	61	35% at 5 yr	60% at 5 yr
Fermand et al. *(20)*	Single	94	37	No difference	No difference
	Double	99	42		
Cavo et al. *(21)*	Single	81	34	21.5 mo	71% at 4 yr
	Double	97	41	29.5 mo	74% at 4 yr

1.4. Different Conditioning Regimens

A number of groups have since modified the high-dose procedure conditioning regimen of 200 mg/m^2 melphalan by adding total-body irradiation (TBI=8 Gy) and reducing the melphalan dose to 140 mg/m^2. Data from the French Registry comparing high-dose melphalan (HDM) with HDM and TBI showed no improvement in the CR rate, event-free survival (EFS), or OS *(22)*. A randomized trial addressing this question concluded that 200 mg/m^2 melphalan was less toxic and at least as effective as melphalan with TBI, with similar PFS rates for both conditioning regimens *(23)*.

1.5. Contamination of Harvests

One of the major concerns regarding the reinfusion of autologous progenitor cells following a high-dose procedure is contamination of the harvest with myeloma cells and whether these cells have the ability to repopulate the marrow and contribute to relapse of disease. In the majority of myeloma cases (70%), the contamination as measured by flow cytometry and polymerase chain reaction (PCR) is less than 1 tumor cell in 10^3–10^4 normal cells. The cases with high tumor contamination tend to be those with persistent disease within the BM at the time of mobilization *(24)*. Using a more sensitive oligospecific PCR, which is able to detect 1 tumor cell in 10^6 normal cells, there is evidence of contamination in almost 100% of cases *(25)*. Whether these cells are clonogenic is a difficult question to address, but sensitive immunophenotypic tests suggest that the cells within apheresis products have a phenotype similar to myelomatous plasma cells from the BM but express lower levels of syndecan-1 *(26)*. There is no definitive evidence from mouse studies regarding this matter, but, clearly, if these cells are reinfused, they may contribute to disease relapse.

A number of groups have tried to reduce/eliminate the tumor contamination of harvests by either depleting tumor cells or selecting normal hematopoietic progenitor cells by virtue of CD34 expression from autologous bone marrow or peripheral blood stem cells (PBSCs) prior to transplantation *(27,28)*. Although these methods may achieve up to a 5 log depletion of tumor cells without affecting engraftment, their clinical benefit is unproven because residual tumor cells are detectable within both the graft and the patient. For purging to be effective, the major source of contamination must be considered to be from the graft, with the patient being tumor free, and previous trials of induction chemotherapy suggest that this is unlikely. A large randomized study assessing the clinical benefits of CD34 selection in myeloma showed purging resulted in no difference in PFS or OS *(29)*.

1.6. Prognostic Factors

A number of prognostic factors have been identified as important in predicting survival post-HDT. To date, nearly all centers have identified B2 microglobulin (B2m) as the single most important prognostic variable, with patients with a high B2m at diagnosis having a shorter survival post-HDT *(7,10,11)*. Patients with 11q breakpoints or partial/complete deletions of chromosome 13 also fair worse following HDT *(18)*. When both B2m and chromosome 13 abnormalities are taken into account, a group of patients with a particularly poor outlook can be identified *(18,30)*.

The majority of studies have demonstrated that having chemosensitive disease at the time of transplant is also an important prognostic factor *(7,10)*. The introduction of high-dose chemotherapy has resulted in more patients attaining CRs, and, conceptually, attaining a CR is seen as the first step to achieving a cure. It has been suggested that the level of response after high-dose chemotherapy may influence outcome and that patients who achieve a CR may have an improved survival. A number of studies have shown an improved PFS and OS in patients who attain a CR with negative immunofixation *(18,31,32)*, although studies using electrophoresis to define CR are less clear-cut.

1.7. Minimal Residual Disease Detection

Despite the increase in response rates and improvement in survival following HDT, several studies have failed to show a plateau of survival, suggesting that all patients have residual disease, which eventually leads to relapse *(7,10)*.

The use of allogeneic and autologous transplantation has increased the CR rate and OS in patients with myeloma, and in order to accurately assess the effects of such treatments, more sensitive methods to assess residual disease have been introduced. PCR can be used to detect rearrangements of the immunoglobulin heavy-chain region, although a target is only present in approx 80% of patients. Consensus PCR approaches have sensitivities of up to 1 malignant cell in 10^4 normal cells. Clonospecific methods are more sensitive (1 malignant cell in 10^6 normal cells) but can be labor intensive and expensive. Flow cytometry offers a quick and efficient method to detect malignant plasma cells with a sensitivity of greater than 1 in 10^4 and may offer a clinically useful alternative to PCR.

An important question that needs to be fully addressed is whether the application of these technologies can provide additional useful information compared to the simple monitoring of serum or urinary paraprotein levels. A recent report has demonstrated that cases that were immunofixation negative were also IgH PCR negative, using a fluorescent PCR with a sensitivity of 1 in 10^4 *(32)*. Allele-specific oligonucleotide (ASO)-PCR is more sensitive, and although the number of cases studied are small, there is a suggestion that PCR-positive patients have a shorter PFS compared to those patients who become PCR negative *(33,34)*. These data would therefore suggest that there is little additional benefit for using fluorescent IgH PCR to monitor patients who become immunofixation negative and that if PCR monitoring is to be clinically relevant, the more sensitive ASO-PCR approach should be used. Flow cytometry offers an alternative method. A recent study suggests that patients who are immunofixation negative and have sustainable levels of plasma cells with a normal phenotype posttransplantation have an improved survival compared to patients who are immunofixation negative with plasma cells with a malignant phenotype *(35)*.

2. ALLOGENEIC TRANSPLANTATION

2.1. Conventional Allogeneic Transplantation

Allogeneic BMT has not been widely used in the treatment of multiple myeloma because of the high morbidity and mortality (up to 40%) associated with the procedure especially in older patients. Experience drawn from the European Group for Bone Marrow Transplantation (EBMT, 1983–1993 and 1994–1998) on data from 690 patients showed approx 50% of patients achieve a CR, with some of the responses durable *(36,37)*. Residual clonal myeloma cells are, however, still detectable by PCR posttransplantation, consistent with the lack of a plateau in the survival curves and the continued late relapses *(33)*. The stage at diagnosis, preconditioning remission status, extent of previous treatment, and serum β2 microglobulin level were important prognostic factors; males faired less well *(36)*. Importantly, over the two time periods, the

OS at 3 yr rose from 35% to 56% and TRM fell from 40–30%. This is presumed to be the result of better patient selection and improved supportive care with a major reduction in bacterial and fungal infections and interstitial pneumonitis.

The use of peripheral blood (PB) support rather than BM support has also had a major impact on survival following allogeneic transplantation for myeloma. The more rapid engraftment associated with PB has resulted in a reduced infection rate, and, importantly, graft-vs-host disease (GVHD) appears to be manageable despite a greater dose of T cells infused with PB than BM *(37,38)*. Some studies even suggest that this rapid engraftment translates to an improved OS *(38)*.

In the majority of reports, the development of both acute and chronic GVHD has accounted for significant morbidity and mortality, with incidences of up to 50%. T-Cell depletion of grafts offers an approach to reducing the GVHD with a reduction in the associated morbidity and TRM *(39)*. However, there are some theoretical concerns regarding a possible increase in infections and a decrease in the graft-vs-myeloma (GVM) effect.

Despite the high TRM of conventional allogeneic transplantation in myeloma, the assumption that this mode of treatment is most likely to eradicate the myeloma cells and the possibility of a significant GVM effect have encouraged its further consideration. Data from multiple centers have shown that patients with relapsed hematological malignancies after alloBMT can achieve marked clinical responses after infusions of lymphocytes collected from the marrow donor (donor lymphocyte infusion [DLI]) as a result of a graft-vs-leukemia (GVL) effect. A number of recent studies have reported the results of DLI for the treatment of relapsed myeloma after alloBMT *(40,41)*. In one study, there was evidence of response to DLI in 62% of cases, providing further support for a GVM effect; however, GVHD occurred in 66% of patients and contributed to a procedure-related mortality of 15% *(40)*. One approach to maintaining the low TRM but exploiting the GVM effect is to utilize CD8-depleted DLI 6–9 mo after CD6-depleted BMT. Alyea et al. reported the use of this approach in 24 patients with chemoresponsive disease *(41)*. A significant GVM effect was demonstrated following the DLI for persistent disease in 10 patients (6 complete responses and 4 partial responses); unfortunately, this was associated with 50% of patients developing GVHD. Of interest, 10 patients were unable to receive DLI because of transplant-related complications, suggesting that for allogeneic transplantation followed by DLI to be an effective strategy in myeloma, a transplantation regimen with less toxicity is needed (*see* Table 3).

2.2. Low-Intensity Conditioning Regimens

A nonmyeloablative or "miniallogeneic" transplantation approach is currently undergoing evaluation in many centers. The goal of this strategy is to reduce the conditioning-regimen-related toxicity while attempting to take advantage of the GVM effect of allogeneic transplantation. This approach uses immunosupression rather than cytoreduction to induce donor engraftment with minimal toxicity. The approach can be used in older individuals or patients who would otherwise not be eligible for conventional high-dose transplantation because of underlying morbidity. This is particularly important in myeloma patients, as less than 10% of patients are eligible for a conventional allograft (i.e., aged less than 55 yr with a human leukocyte antigen [HLA]-matched sibling) and the TRM, as mentioned earlier, is high. A number of conditioning regimens are being investigated using combinations of low-dose radiotherapy, chemotherapy, and immunosuppressive agents. Initial reports using radiotherapy with mycophenolic acid (MMF) and cyclosporine in end-stage myeloma patients were disap-

Table 3
Representative Studies of Allogeneic Transplantation for Newly Diagnosed Myeloma

	Patients (n)	*TRM (%)*	*CR (%)*	*OS (actuarial)*	*EFS (actuarial)*
Gahrton et al. *(36)*	162	41	44	28% at 84 mo	45% at 60 mo
Bensinger et al. *(42)*	80	44	36	20% at 54 mo	24% at 54 mo
Anderson et al. *(40)*	61[a]	5	28	40% at 36 mo	20% at 38 mo

[a]T-Cell depleted.

Table 4
Representative Studies of Mini-Allogeneic Transplantation in Myeloma[a]

	Conditioning	*n*	*TRM*	*CR*	*Acute GVHD*	*Chronic GVHD*	*PFS*	*OS*
Badros et al. *(44)*	Mel or Mel/TBI/Flu	31	10% early 20% late	CR 61% PR 10%	58%	32%	1 yr, 86%	1 yr, 86%
Kroger et al. *(46)*	PBSCT + Mel/Flu/ATG	17	18%	CR 73% PR 20%	63%	40%	2 yr, 56%	2 yr, 74%
Maloney et al. *(45)*	PBSCT + TBI/MMF/cyc	31	16%	CR 43% PR 31%	45%	55%	—	1 yr, 81%

[a]Nonmyeloablative therapy followed by allogenic peripheral blood stem cell transplantation (PBSCT).

pointing because of poor engraftment and poor response rates. This was thought to be the result of the high tumor burden at the time of transplantation *(43)*. More recent studies have included low-dose chemotherapy and are more encouraging. The Arkansas group report such an approach in 31 patients with myeloma *(44)*. Melphalan, 100 mg/m^2 was used for sibling mini-allogeneic transplantations and 100 mg/m^2 melphalan combined with TBI and fludarabine was used for unrelated mini-allogeneic transplantations. Donor lymphocytes were administered to induce full chimerism or to eradicate residual disease. Transplant-related mortality was 29%, with 58% of patients with acute GVHD and 32% with chronic GVHD. Response rates were very encouraging, with 61% of patients achieving at least a near CR in this heavily pretreated group.

In order to reduce the tumor burden before the mini-allogeneic transplant procedure, a number of groups have been combining its use with a prior autologous transplant using melphalan conditioning *(45,46)*. The procedure is well tolerated, with a TRM of 16–18% and all patients achieving full donor chimerism. Response rates are good, with a high number of patients achieving a CR (up to 73% using stringent criteria); however, the incidence of GVHD is more than 50% (*see* Table 4).

All of these studies have relatively short follow-up, making comments on prolonging OS difficult at this time. However, it remains clear that these approaches are feasible and appear less toxic by reducing the early transplant-related complications and mortality. They also retain the antitumor effect of the conventional transplantation regimen and are able to induce CRs. However, it still remains unclear which is the best conditioning regimen, and modifications are required to reduce the incidence and intensity of GVHD, which is a major problem currently. A number of approaches are under investigation, including combining a low-intensity approach with DLI or reinfusion of subsets of lymphocytes (e.g., CD4) to induce GVM without the GVHD, or including CAMPATH in the conditioning regimen.

3. OTHER STRATEGIES

Although the results from these studies of autografting in myeloma are encouraging, the survival curves show no obvious plateau and suggest that HDT with stem cell support is not a curative procedure. A number of new drugs are being evaluated as part of induction chemotherapy in order to increase the response rate prior to HDT. In many cases, the traditional VAD-like regimens are being substituted by high-dose dexamethasone alone or with drug combinations including thalidomide or the proteasome inhibitor PS-341. In order to target residual malignant plasma cells in the BM at the time of transplant, a number of groups are using antibody therapy during the conditioning; examples include holmium, anti-interleukin-6, and anti-CD138.

One of the major obstacles to curing myeloma is the persistence of minimal residual disease (MRD) after HDT and stem cell transplantation (SCT). Results with previous maintenance therapy regimens have been disappointing. Trials with interferon or prednisolone results in a small prolongation of survival *(47,48)*. A number of approaches are therefore being developed for the generation and enhancement of allogeneic and autologous antimyeloma immunity posttransplantation. These include noncytotoxic approaches utilizing agents such as the thalidomide derivatives, proteasome inhibitors, antibody-directed therapy, and immune-based approaches. The most promising of these include thalidomide or its newer analogs, the immunomodulatory drugs (IMiDs), a variety of vaccination strategies utilizing patient-specific idiotype, RNA, and DNA, immunization with dendritic cells pulsed with patient-specific idiotypic protein or immunization with fusions of myeloma cells with autologous dendritic cells, or the infusion of autologous T cells expanded ex vivo against patient tumor cells.

REFERENCES

1. MacLennan IC, Chapman C, Dunn J, et al. Combined chemotherapy with ABCM versus melphalan for treatment of myelomatosis. The Medical Research Council Working Party for Leukaemia in Adults. *Lancet* 1992;25:200–205.
2. Myeloma Trialists Collaborative Group. Combination chemotherapy versus melphalan plus prednisolone as treatment for multiple myeloma: an overview of 6633 patients from 27 randomised trials. *J Clin Oncol* 1998;16:3832–3842.
3. Samson D, Gaminara E, Newland A, et al. Infusion of vincristine and doxorubicin with oral dexamethasone as first line therapy for multiple myeloma. *Lancet* 1989;2:882–885.
4. Raje N, Powles R, Kullarni S, et al. A comparison of vincristine and doxorubicin infusional chemotherapy with methylprednisolone (VAMP) with the addition of weekly cyclophosphamide (C-VAMP) as induction treatment followed by autografting in previously untreated myeloma. *Br J Haematol* 1997;97:153–160.
5. McElwain TJ, Powles RL. High dose intravenous melphalan for plasma-cell leukaemia and myeloma. *Lancet* 1983;ii:822–824.
6. Gore ME, Selby PJ, Viner C, et al. Intensive treatment of multiple myeloma and criteria for complete remission. *Lancet* 1989;2:879–882.
7. Barlogie B, Jagannath S, Vesole DH, et al. Superiority of tandem autologous transplantation over standard therapy for previously untreated multiple myeloma. *Blood* 1997;89:789–793.
8. Lenhoff S, Hjorth M, Holmberg E, et al. Impact on survival of high does therapy with autologous stem cell support in patients younger than 60 years with newly diagnosed multiple myeloma: a population based study. *Blood* 2000;95:7–11.
9. Blade J, San Miguel JF, Fontanillas M, et al. Survival of multiple myeloma patients who are potential candidates for early high-dose therapy intensification/autotransplantation and who are conventionally treated. *J Clin Oncol* 1996;7:21,667–621,673.
10. Attal M, Harousseau JL, Stoppa AM, et al. Autologous bone marrow transplantation versus conventional chemotherapy in multiple myeloma: a prospective randomised trial. *N Eng J Med* 1996;335:91–97.
11. Child JA, Morgan GJ, Davies FE, et al. High dose therapy with hemotopoietic stem cell rescue for multiple myeloma. *N Engl J Med* 2003; 348:1875–1883.
12. Fermand JP, Ravaud P, Katsahian S, et al. High dose therapy and autologous blood stem cell transplantation versus conventional treatment in multiple myeloma: results of a randomised trial in 190 patients 55–65 years of age. *Blood* 1999;94:396a.
13. Blade J, Sureda A, Ribera JM, et al. High dose therapy autotransplantation/intensification vs continued conventional chemotherapy in multiple myeloma patients responding to initial treatment chemotherapy. Results of a prospective randomised trial from the Spanish Cooperative Group PETHEMA. *Blood* 2001;98 [Abstract 3386].
14. Siegel DS, Desikan KR, Mehta J, et al. Age is not a prognostic variable with autotransplants for multiple myeloma. *Blood* 1999;93:51–54.
15. Badros A, Barlogie B, Siegel E, et al. Results of autologous stem cell transplant in multiple myeloma patients with renal failure. *Br J Haematol* 2001;114:822–829.
16. Sirohi B, Powles R, Mehta J, et al. The implication of comprised renal function at presentation in myeloma: similar outcome in patients who receive high-dose therapy: a single center study of 251 previously untreated patients. *Med Oncol* 2001;18:39–50.
17. Fermand JP, Ravaud P, Chevret S, et al. High dose therapy and autologous blood stem cell transplantation in multiple myeloma: up front or rescue treatment? Results of a multicenter sequential randomised clinical trial. *Blood* 1998;92:3131–3136.
18. Barlogie B, Jagannath S, Desikan KR, et al. Total therapy with tandem transplants for newly diagnosed multiple myeloma. *Blood* 1999;93:55–65.
19. Attal M, Harousseau JL, Facon T, for the IFM. Single versus double transplant in myeloma: a randomised trial of the Intergroupe Francais Myeloma. Proceedings of the VIII International Myeloma Workshop, 2001.
20. Fermand JP, Marolleau JP, Alberti C, et al. Single versus tandem high dose therapy supported with autologous blood stem cell transplantation using unselected or CD34 enriched ABSC: preliminary results of a two by two designed randomized trial in 230 young patients with multiple myeloma. *Blood* 2001;98:815a.

21. Cavo M. Tosi P, Zamagni E, et al. The Bologna 96 clinical trial of single vs double PBSCT transplantation for previously untreated MM: results of an interim analysis. Proceedings of the VIII International Myeloma Workshop, 2001.
22. Harousseau JL, Attal M, Divine M, et al. Autologous stem cell transplantation after first remission induction treatment in multiple myeloma: a report of French Registry on autologous transplantation in multiple myeloma. *Blood* 1995;8:3077–3085.
23. Moreau P, Facon T, Attal M, et al. Comparision of 200 mg/m^2 melphalan and 8 Gy total body irradiation plus 140 mg/m^2 melphalan as conditioning regimens for peripheral blood stem cell transplantation in patients with newly diagnosed multiple myeloma: final analysis of the IFM 9502 randomised trial. *Blood* 2002;99:731–735.
24. Owen RG, Johnson RJ, Rawstron AC, et al. Assessment of IgH PCR strategies in multiple myeloma. *J Clin Pathol* 1996;49:672–675.
25. Corradini P, Voena C, Astolfi M, et al. High dose sequential chemoradiotherapy in multiple myeloma: residual tumor cells are detectable in bone marrow and peripheral blood cell harvests and after autografting. *Blood* 1995;85:1596–1602.
26. Rawstron AC, Owen RG, Davies FE, et al. Circulating plasma cells in multiple myeloma: characterisation and correlation with disease stage. *Br J Haematol* 1997;97:46–55.
27. Johnson RJ, Owen RG, Smith GM, et al. Peripheral blood stem cell transplantation in myeloma using CD34 selected cells. *Bone Marrow Transplant* 1996;17:723–727.
28. Vescio R, Schiller G, Stewart AK, et al. Multicentre phase III trial to evaluate CD34+ selected versus unselected autologous peripheral blood progenitor cell transplantation in multiple myeloma. *Blood* 1999;93:1858–1868.
29. Stewart AK, Vescio R, Schiller G, et al. Purging of autologous peripheral blood stem cells using cell selection does not improve overall or progression free survival after high dose chemotherapy for multiple myeloma: results of a multicenter randomised controlled trial. *J Clin Oncol* 2001;19:3771–3779.
30. Facon T, Avet-Loiseau H, Guillerm G, et al. Chromosome 13 abnormalities identified by FISH analysis and serum B2 microglobulin produce a powerful myeloma staging system for patients receiving high dose therapy. *Blood* 2000;97:1566–1571.
31. Lahuerta JJ, Martinez-Lopez J, Serna JD, et al. Remission status defined by immunofixation vs. electrophoresis after autologous transplantation has a major impact on the outcome of multiple myeloma. *Br J Haematol* 2000;109:438–446.
32. Davies FE, Forsyth PD, Rawstron AC, et al. The impact of attaining a minimal disease state following high dose melphalan and autologous transplantation for multiple myeloma. *Br J Haematol* 2001;112:814–820.
33. Corradini P, Voena C, Tarella C, et al. Molecular and clinical remissions in multiple myeloma: role of autologous and allogeneic transplantation of hematopoeitic cells. *J Clin Oncol* 1999;17:208–215.
34. Martinelli G, Terragna C, Zamagni E, et al. Molecular remission after allogeneic or autologous transplantation of hematopoietic stem cells for multiple myeloma. *J Clin Oncol* 2000;18:2273–2281.
35. Rawstron AC, Davies FE, Dasgupta R, et al. Flow cytometric disease monitoring in multiple myeloma: the relationship between normal and neoplastic plasma cells predicts outcome post-transplantation. *Blood*, 2002; 100:3095–3100.
36. Gahrton G, Tura S, Ljungman P, et al. Prognostic factors in allogeneic bone marrow transplantation for multiple myeloma. *J Clin Oncol* 1995;13:1312–1322.
37. Gahrton G, Svensson H, Cavo M, et al. Progress in allogenic bone marrow and peripheral blood stem cell transplantation for multiple myeloma: a comparison between transplants performed 1983–1993 and 1994–1998 at European Group for Blood and Marrow Transplantation centres. *Br J Haematol* 2001;113:209–216.
38. Bensignger WI, Martin PJ, Storer B, et al. Transplantation of bone marrow as compared with peripheral blood cells from HLA identical relatives in patients with hematologic cancers. *N Engl J Med* 2001;334:175–181.
39. Anderson KC. Plasma cell tumors. In: Cancer Medicine 5th ed. Bast R, Kufe D, Pollock R, Weichselbaum J, Holland J, Frei E, eds. New York: Marcel Dekker, 2000;1257–1276.
40. Lokhorst HM, Schattenberg A, Cornelissen JJ, et al. Donor leucocyte infusions are effective in relapsed multiple myeloma after allogeneic bone marrow transplantation. *Blood* 1997;90:4206–4211.
41. Alyea E, Weller E, Schlossman R, et al. T Cell depleted allogeneic bone marrow transplantation followed by donor lymphocyte infusion in patients with multiple myeloma: induction of graft versus myeloma effect. *Blood* 2001;98:934–939.
42. Bensinger WI, Buckner CD, Anasetti C, et al. Allogeneic marrow transplantation for multiple myeloma: analysis of risk factors on outcome. *Blood* 1996;88:2787–2793.

43. Storb R, Yu C, Sandmaier B, et al. Mixed hematopoietic chimersism after haematopoietic stem cell allografts. *Transplant Proc* 1999;31:677–678.
44. Badros A, Barlogie B, Siegel E, et al. Improved outcome of allogeneic transplantation in high risk multiple myeloma patients after nonmyeloablative conditioning. *J Clin Oncol* 2002;20:1295–1303.
45. Maloney DG, Sahebi F, Stockerl-Goldstein KE, et al. Combining an allogeneic graft vs myeloma effect with high dose autologous stem cell rescue in the treatment of multiple myeoma. *Blood* 2001;98:434a.
46. Kroger N, Schwerdtfeger R, Kiehl M, et al. Autologous stem cell transplantation followed by a dose-reduced allograft induces high complete remission rate in multiple myeloma. *Blood* 2002;100:755–760.
47. The Myeloma Trialists Collaborative Group. Interferon as therapy for multiple myeloma: an individual patient data overview of 24 randomized trials and 4012 patients. *Br J Haematol* 2001;113:1020–1034.
48. Berenson JR, Crowley JJ, Grogan TM, et al. Maintenance therapy with alternative-day prednisone improves survival in multiple myeloma patients. *Blood* 2002;99:3163–3168.

5 Hematopoietic Progenitor Cell Transplantation for Breast Cancer

Yago Nieto, MD *and Elizabeth J. Shpall,* MD

CONTENTS

1. INTRODUCTION

Autologous hematopoietic progenitor cell transplantation (AHPCT), from either the bone marrow or peripheral blood, allows for the administration of chemotherapy with a several-fold increase in the drug doses. High-dose chemotherapy (HDC) achieves a higher tumor-cell kill than standard-dose chemotherapy (SDC), with the goal of improving long-term outcome. In this setting, nonhematopoietic organ toxicities become dose limiting *(1)*. Improvements in supportive care have produced a decrease in the morbidity and mortality associated with HDC to a current toxic death rate of less than 5% in centers where large numbers of these procedures are performed *(2,3)*.

2. DOSE INTENSITY AND BREAST CANCER

Following observations of dose response in vitro, retrospective analyses suggested a clinical correlation between dose intensity of chemotherapy and response rate and outcome in breast cancer, both in the metastatic *(4–6)* and the adjuvant setting *(7,8)*. Prospective studies of conventional chemotherapy in patients with stage IV disease showed that decreasing the dose below the standard range compromised the antitumor effect and palliative effects *(9)*. In contrast, trials testing minor increases in dose intensity of adriamycin *(10)*, paclitaxel *(11)*, or epirubicin *(12–16)* in metastatic breast cancer (MBC) failed to show a progression-free survival (PFS) or overall survival (OS) benefit.

From: *Stem Cell Transplantation for Hematologic Malignancies*
Edited by: R. J. Soiffer © Humana Press Inc., Totowa, NJ

Similar observations have been made in the adjuvant setting. A prospective randomized trial of cyclophosphamide, adriamycin and fluorouracil (CAF) administered to 1572 node-positive patients in three dose intensity levels showed that patients receiving the intermediate and high doses of these drugs had superior disease-free survival (DFS) and OS than those patients who received the lowest dose *(17)*. Although there was no statistically significant differences in outcome between the intermediate and high doses, a trend toward improvement was noted *(18)*. A trial comparing 50–100 mg/m^2 of epirubicin within the FEC regimen 5-fluorouracil/ epirubicin/cyclophosphamide (FEC) regimen, showed improved DFS and OS for the higher dose arm *(19)*. In contrast, other studies have not shown a benefit for increases in the doses of cyclophosphamide *(20,21)* or adriamycin *(22)*, with granulocyte colony-stimulating factor (G-CSF) support, as part of adjuvant treatment.

The use of HDC with AHPCT is based on the hypothesis that major dose escalations within the myeloablative range are needed to overcome tumor cell resistance and produce a meaningful clinical improvement. Stem cell support allows for an increase in the dose well beyond normal bone marrow tolerance (BM), with the goal of maximally capitalizing on the dose–response curve of certain antineoplastic drugs. The first trials of HDC for breast cancer in the mid-1980s were stimulated by the preclinical studies of Emil Frei III and colleagues *(23,24)*. In vitro data and the precedence of other settings where chemotherapy is curative, such as leukemia or lymphoma, supported the use of multidrug combinations over single agents. Alkylating drugs, such as cyclophosphamide (Cy), melphalan, cisplatin, carboplatin, carmustine (BCNU), or thiotepa, were employed in those early trials of HDC for breast cancer, given their steep dose–response effect, non-cross-resistance, and nonoverlapping extramedullary toxicities *(23)*.

3. METASTATIC BREAST CANCER

MBC is incurable in virtually all patients receiving standard-dose chemotherapy *(25,26)*. Median survival after detection of metastatic disease is 18 to 24 mo, ranging from a few months to several years. Around half of a very selected group of chemotherapy-naïve patients (i.e., not previously exposed to adjuvant chemotherapy), with metastatic disease limited to one single site, may be rendered long-term disease-free with conventional multidisciplinary treatment *(27, 28)*. In the vast majority of the cases, however, patients often experience an initial response to standard-dose chemotherapy, but subsequently treatment loses activity as a result of the emergence of resistance.

3.1. Recent Studies of Conventional-Dose Chemotherapy As First-Line Treatment for Metastatic Breast Cancer

Since the appearance of adriamycin three decades ago, there has been minimal or no improvement in outcome resulting from the incorporation to first-line treatment of new drugs, in some cases with remarkable activity, such as the taxanes. The disappointing results of the Intergroup Eastern Cooperative Oncology Group (ECOG) 1193 study illustrate this point *(29)*. This trial compared first-line therapy with single-agent adriamycin, single-agent paclitaxel, or both agents combined with G-CSF support, in 739 patients. The adriamycin/paclitaxel combination improved the response rate, but showed no survival benefit over either drug alone. Recent combinations of docetaxel with adriamycin, the two most active agents for breast cancer, have disappointingly failed to improve outcome *(30,31)*.

The only progress in survival was reported by Slamon et al., who randomized 469 patients to receive chemotherapy (either adriamycin/cyclophosphamide or paclitaxel) with or without anti-HER2 antibody trastuzumab, as first-line treatment for MBC *(32)*. Median survival was superior in the group of patients treated with chemotherapy plus trastuzumab compared to those receiving chemotherapy alone (27 vs 22 mo, p=0.04).

3.2. HDC for MBC: Phase II Studies

The sequential strategies testing HDC for MBC are summarized on Table 1. The initial trials in refractory MBC patients produced higher response rates than those previously reported with standard-dose chemotherapy *(33–36)*. Those responses, however, were short-lived and had no demonstrated impact on OS. Results appeared to improve when HDC was moved upfront as initial therapy for metastatic disease. Peters and colleagues at Duke University, treated 22 patients with newly diagnosed metastases, 64% of whom had previously received adjuvant chemotherapy, with cyclophosphamide/cisplatin/BCNU (STAMP-I regimen) *(37)*. Three patients (14%) were disease free at the time of the initial publication, which was confirmed in the update of this trial, with follow-up longer than 10 yr *(38)*.

In a subsequent step, HDC was used as immediate consolidation after dose-intense adriamycin-based induction chemotherapy, which was administered to maximally cytoreduce the tumor prior to HDC. Several phase II trials testing this strategy, using either STAMP-I or cyclophosphamide/thiotepa (carboplatin, consistently showed a long-term DFS rate of 15–25% (Table 2) *(39–43)*. Because HDC was shown to be most effective at a time of minimal tumor burden, potent induction regimens, such as Aadriamycin/fluorouracil/methotrexate (AFM) *(44)*, were designed to provide substantial cytoreduction prior to HDC. The benefit of posttransplant radiotherapy (RT) to sites of prior bulky disease was later demonstrated *(45)*. Long-term analysis of 212 MBC patients enrolled in prospective trials at the University of Colorado evaluating standard-dose induction (AFM) followed by HDC (STAMP-I) and involved-field RT as first-line therapy for metastatic disease, showed a 22% DFS rate and a 32% OS rate after median and lead follow-up of 7 and 11 yr, respectively (Fig. 1) *(46)*.

In parallel to these advances, the introduction of myeloid growth factors posttransplant, peripheral blood progenitor cells (PBPCs) in place of BM, and other improvements in supportive care, reduced the treatment-related mortality (TRM) rate from the initial 15–20% rate to the current 2–4% expected in experienced transplant units *(2,3)*.

The 15–20% fraction of patients with chemosensitive MBC rendered long-term free of disease in phase II trials of HDC (Table 2) appeared to be substantially higher than the expected long-term DFS of 0–3%, using conventional chemotherapy *(25,47,48)*. These HDC results generated great enthusiasm among physicians and patients for the use of HDC. The rapid transfer of stem cell transplantation (SCT) technology from the academic environment to community hospitals resulted in an explosive growth in the number of breast cancer patients receiving HDC. Unfortunately, many patients received HDC out of a prospectively designed clinical trial, despite the lack of results of randomized studies demonstrating that this approach should be considered the standard of care. From 1992 to 1999, breast cancer was the most common malignancy reported to the American Blood and Marrow Transplant Registry (ABMTR) for which HDC and AHPCT was administered *(2)*.

Detractors of HDC have argued that its promising results could be explained by patient selection (younger age, better performance status), extensive staging bias, and the requirement

Table 1. Sequential strategies of HDC for MBC

Strategy	*Regimen*	*No. of patients*	*Median follow-up mo*	*% Patients transplanted in CR*	*DFS rate*	*%DFS of patients transplanted in CR*	*Ref.*
Refractory disease	STAMP-I	23	–	0	0%	N/A	*33*
	STAMP-V	16	–	0	0%	N/A	*34*
Upfront therapy for untreated MBC	STAMP-I	22	18	0	14%	N/A	*37*
Consolidation after induction	STAMP-I	245	67	25	16%	28	*40*
	Cy/thio	100	62	28	11%	31	*43*
	STAMP-V	62	50	19	21%	31	*41*

HDC, high-dose chemotherapy; MBC, metastatic breast cancer; CR, complete remission; DFS, disease-free Survival; STAMP-I; cyclophosphamide-cisplatin-BCNU. STAMP-V; cyclophosphamide-thiotepa-carboplatin; Cy/thio; cyclophosphamide-thiotepa; N/A, not applicable.

Table 2. Overall Results from Major Phase II Studies of HDC for Breast Cancer.

Setting	*No. of patients*	*High-dose regimen*	*Medianfollow-up (mo)*	*DFS rate*		*Ref.*
4–9 nodes	93	STAMP-I	84	72%		*81*
10+ nodes	85	STAMP-I	120	71%		*80*
	67	HDST	48	57%		*82*
	120	STAMP-I	84	64%		*81*
Inflammatory carcinoma	55	STAMP-I	78	60%		*81*
	46	STAMP-V	27	68%		*88*
	17	Cy/mitox/mel	36	59%		*90*
	22	CAVP/CCVP	46	45%		*91*
	47	Several	27	58%		*92*
				All Patients	CR at transplant	
Metastatic chemosensitive	245	STAMP-I	67	16%	28%	*40*
	100	Cy/TT	62	11%	31%	*43*
	62	STAMP-V	50	21%	31%	*41*
Metastatic NED	60	STAMP-I	62	52%		*56*
	20	Cy/mitox/carbo	28	55%		*60*

(HDC, high-dose chemotherapy; DFS, disease-free survival; STAMP-I; cyclophosphamide (Cy)-cisplatin-BCNU. STAMP-V; Cy-thiotepa-carboplatin; HDST: high-dose sequential therapy using Cy-vincristine-methotrexate-melphalan; CAVP; Cy-adriamycin-VP16; CCVP; Cy-cisplatin-VP16; Cy/TT; Cy-thiotepa, NED, No evidence of disease; CR; complete remission.

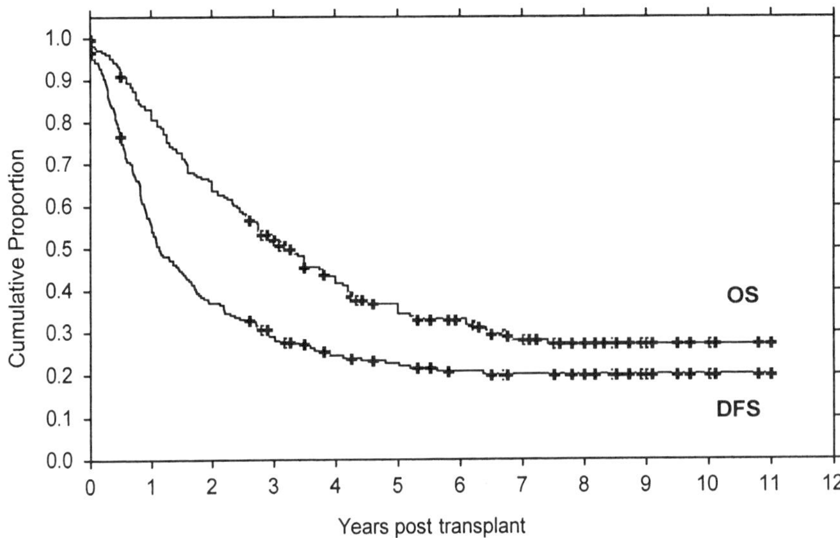

Fig. 1. Combined DFS and OS curves in the prospective phase II trials of HDC (STAMP-I) as first-line therapy for MBC patients (*N*=212) (University of Colorado BMTP).

of proven chemosensitivity *(49,50)*. This controversy clearly underscored the need for mature data from prospective, well-designed and adequately sized, randomized phase III trials.

3.3. Which MBC Patients Are Most Likely to Benefit From HDC?

Although the results from phase II trials of HDC in MBC were encouraging, it became clear that the majority of MBC patients still relapsed after HDC. Several retrospective analyses identified prognostic factors for outcome in this patient population. Dunphy et al. reported that metastases in liver or soft tissues and prior chemotherapy were independent adverse predictors of outcome *(51)*. Ayash et al. observed that one site of disease and attainment of a complete remission (CR) to induction chemotherapy were independent favorable predictors in their series *(52)*. Doroshow et al. reported that patients transplanted in CR, without liver metastases, with less prior chemotherapy, and fewer metastatic sites had improved outcome *(53)*. Rizzieri et al. observed that visceral metastases, prior exposure to adjuvant chemotherapy, shorter disease-free interval from initial diagnosis to metastatic recurrence, and hormone receptor negativity, were adverse predictors *(54)*. Analyses of patients with MBC reported to the ABMTR indicated that chemotherapy responsiveness at transplant, length of initial disease-free interval, central nervous system or liver metastases, number of sites of disease, prior exposure to adjuvant chemotherapy, hormone receptor status, performance status, and age were outcome predictors in this population *(2,55)*. The DFS curves of MBC patients transplanted at Colorado with STAMP-I as first-line therapy based on disease status at transplant and on the specific organ involved are shown on Fig. 2 and 3, respectively.

Overexpression of the HER2/neu oncogene, determined by immunohistochemical study of the primary tumor *(56,57)* or detection of the serum levels of its extracellular domain, *(58)*, has also been identified as an adverse predictor of outcome in this population after HDC.

The hypothesis that good prognosis MBC patients might attain major benefit from HDC early in the course of their disease was prospectively tested at the University of Colorado *(59)*.

Table 3. Randomized Trials in MBC

Trial	Population	*n*	HDC regimen	Follow-up (mo)	EFS rates HDC	EFS rates Control	*p*	OS rates HDC	OS rates Control	*p*
NCIC *(64)*	Responsive	224	CMC	19	38%	24%	0.01	Med: 24 mo	Med: 28 mo	0.9
Philadelphia *(61,62)*	Responsive	184	STAMP-V	67	4%	3%	0.3	14%	13%	0.6
PÉGASE 03 *(65)*	Untreated	180	CT Tandem	48	27% 25%	10% 20%	0.0002	38% 39%	30% 35%	0.7
IBDIS 1 *(66)*	Untreated	110	VIC/CT	42	Med: 14 mo 25%	Med: 9 mo 10% (*)	0.01	Med: 32 mo	Med: 23 mo	0.1
Duke crossover- 1 *(69)*	CR	100	STAMP-I Tandem	75	Med: 9.7 mo	Med: 3.8 mo	0.006	N/E (#)	N/E (#)	N/E (#)
GEBDIS *(68)*	Untreated	92	CME × 2	14	Med: 14 mo	Med: 10 mo	0.05	Med: 28 mo	Med: 25 mo	0.3
Duke crossover-2 *(71)*	HR, Bone only	69	STAMP-I	59	17%	9% (*)	0.001	N/E (#) 30%	N/E (#) 18%	N/E (#)
PÉGASE 04 *(67)*	Responsive	61	CMM	NR	Med: 35 mo	Med: 20 mo	0.06	Med: 43 mo	Med: 20 mo	0.1

MBC, metastatic breast cancer; HDC, high-dose chemotherapy; EFS, event-free survival; OS, overall survival; NCIC; National Cancer Institute of Canada, PÉGASE, Programme d'Étude de la Greffe Autologue dans les Cancers du Sein, IBDIS International Breast Cancer Dose Intensity Study, GEBDIS, German Breast Cancer Dose Intensity Study, CR, complete response, HR, hormone refractory, CMC, cyclophosphamide-mitoxantrone-carboplatin, CT, cyclophosphamide-thiotepa. CME, cyclophosphamide-mitoxantrone-etoposide, VIC, etoposide-ifosfamide-carboplatin, CMM, cyclophosphamide-mitoxantrone-melphalan, NR, Not reported, (*), EFS rates are after salvage HDC in the observation arm, CR, complete response, N/E (#), not evaluable for a direct OS comparison, because of crossover design.

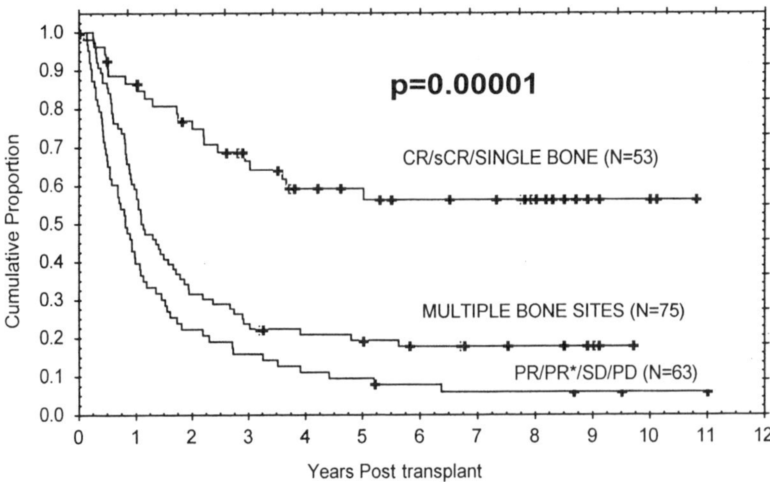

Fig. 2. DFS of MBC patients according to disease status at transplant (p=0.00001). Group 1: CR (complete remission) / surgical NED (no evidence of disease): median DFS not reached. Group 2: multiple bone sites: median DFS 1.2 yr. Group 3: PR (partial remission) / PR* (partial remission + bone lesions) / stable disease (SD): median DFS 0.75 yr (University of Colorado BMTP).

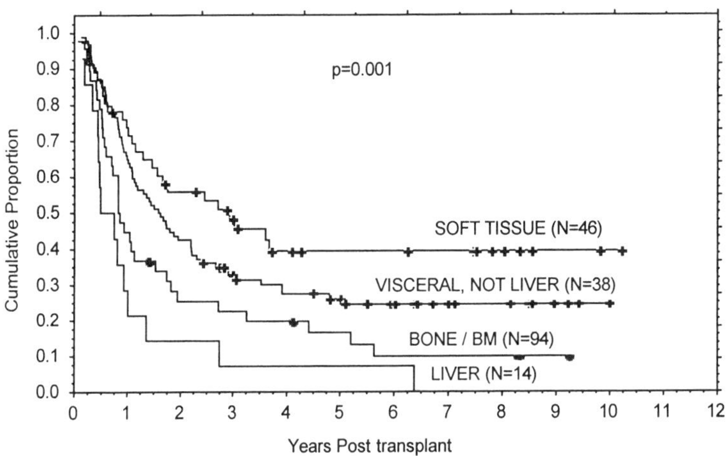

Fig. 3. DFS of MBC patients treated in first line with STAMP-I. Group 1 (soft tissue): median DFS 2.9 years. Group 2 (visceral, not liver): median DFS 1.6 yr. Group 3 (bone/BM): median DFS 0.9 yr. Group 4 (liver): median DFS 0.5 yr (University of Colorado BMTP).

A phase II study of four cycles of adriamycin-based induction therapy followed by HDC with STAMP-I, as first-line therapy for metastatic disease, was conducted in 60 consecutive stage IV patients with oligometastases. These were defined as one or more sites of macroscopic tumor that could be either resected en bloc and/or encompassed within a single RT field, and/or less than 5% of BM involvement. Most patients had received previous adjuvant chemotherapy. At median posttransplant follow-up of 5 yr, the DFS and OS rates were 52 and 62%, respectively, with median DFS and OS times of 4.3 and 6.7 yr, respectively (Fig. 4). HER2/neu negative status and a single metastatic site were independent favorable predictors of outcome *(56)*. Similar results were reported by Abraham et al. using high-dose cyclophoph-

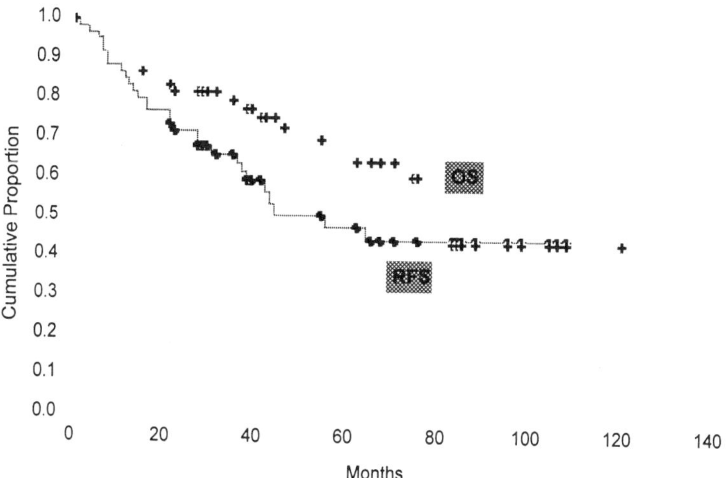

Fig. 4. RFS and OS of stage IV oligometastatic breast cancer patients after STAMP-I (*N*=60) (University of Colorado BMTP).

amide/mitoxantrone/carboplatin in 20 patients with isolated supraclavicular lymph node metastases, with a 55% DFS rate at a median follow-up of 28 mo. *(60)*. These results advocate for closer follow-up after adjuvant treatment for early detection of relapses, and for the use of early HDC in MBC with minimal disease. Randomized trials in this subset of MBC patients should be considered in the future.

Conversely, we are currently able to identify patients with poor prognostic features who are less likely to benefit from the first-generation HDC regimens. Newer high-dose regimens or alternative HDC-based strategies are being explored for these patients.

3.4. Current Status of Randomized Trials Comparing HDC and Standard-Dose Chemotherapy in MBC Patients

The "Philadelphia" PBT-1 study compared HDC with STAMP-V to maintenance conventional chemotherapy with Cyclophosphamide, methotrexate, and 5-fluorouracil (CMF) in 184 MBC patients *(61)*. Stadtmauer and colleagues initially enrolled 553 patients who received induction chemotherapy with CAF (*n*=507) or CMF (*n*=46). Of those, 303 patients (54%) achieved a partial remission (PR) (*n*=247) or a CR (*n*=56). Of the 303 responding patients, 199 were randomized. Of these, 110 were allocated to the STAMP-V arm, and 89 to receive maintenance CMF for 18 mo or until disease progression. After discarding 15 patients who were considered ineligible after randomization, 184 were actually treated in study–101 in the HDC arm and 83 in the CMF arm. In the latest update of this trial with a median follow-up of 67 mo, an intent-to-treat analysis showed no statistically significant differences between the STAMP-V and the CMF arms in PFS rates (4 and 3%, respectively), time to progression (9.6 and 9.1 mo, respectively), or OS rates (14 and 13%, respectively) *(62)*. Several aspects of this trial have been criticized. First, it lacked sufficient power to detect clinically relevant differences: although it was originally designed with an 85% power to detect a doubling in median OS time, it subsequently suffered a 45% dropout rate (34% before and 11% after randomization). Second, only 45 patients in CR were randomized and treated, which confers on this trial only a 20% power to detect a 20% absolute difference in OS between both arms in this patient subset *(63)*. Thus, the Philadelphia trial did not address adequately the value of HDC for patients in CR. This appears to be an important issue, as these patients, as well as those with low tumor burden, seem to be those who may benefit most from HDC. Finally, in the group of 139 patients in PR, the PR to CR conversion rate was surprisingly higher in the maintenance CMF arm (9%) than in the HDC arm (6%). This strikingly low PR to CR conversion rate in the transplant arm of the Philadelphia study is quite different than the vast majority of phase II HDC trials, where PR to CR conversion rates of 20-60% are typically reported *(39–43)*.

In the trial conducted by the National Cancer Institute of Canada, Crump et al. randomized 224 MBC patients responding to four cycles of an anthracycline- or taxane-based regimen to two to four additional cycles or to one to two more cycles followed by HDC with Cy/mitoxantrone/carboplatin *(64)*. In their first analysis at short median follow-up of 19 mo, significant differences in favor of the transplant arm were observed (38 vs 24% DFS rate, p=0.01), with no differences in OS (p=0.9).

Similar observations were made at the time of the first analysis of the French National trial PEGASE-03 *(65)*. Biron and collegues randomized 180 patients who responded to first-line conventional treatment with FEC to high-dose Cy/thiotepa or to observation. At median follow-up of 48 mo, statistically significant and fairly large differences in DFS were observed in favor of HDC compared to the control arm: 1-yr DFS rate of 46 vs 20%, 2-yr DFS rate of 27 vs 10%, with median DFS times of 11 vs 7 mo (p=0.0002). No significant differences in OS were observed yet in this first analysis: 1-yr OS 82% in both groups, 3-yr OS 38 vs 30%, and median OS times of 29 vs 24 mo (p=0.7).

Crown and collaborators from the International Breast Cancer Dose Intensity Study (IBDIS) group treated 110 patients with four cycles of doxorubicin-docetaxel followed by six cycles of CMF , or HDC *(66)*. Patients in the transplant arm received PBPC-supported sequential cycles of ifosfamide (12 g/m2)- carboplatin (AUC 18)-etoposide (1.2 g/m2), followed by Cy (6 g/m^2)-thiotepa (800 mg/m2), 3–6 wk apart. The TRM rates were 4 and 9%, respectively. Overall response and CR rates were higher in the HDC arm (71 and 29%, respectively) than in the control arm (44 and 6, respectively). At median follow-up of 42 mo, the study was positive for its primary endpoint, even-free survival (EFS) (16% in the HDC arm vs 9% in the SDC arm, p=0.01). There was a trend for an OS advantage in the HDC arm in an intent-to-treat analysis (45 vs 37%, p=0.1), which reached significance in an analysis based on actual treatment received (49 vs 35%, p=0.02).

Two other very small studies have been reported. In the French PEGASE-04 trial, Lotz et al. randomized 61 responding MBC patients to additional conventional chemotherapy or HDC with Cy/mitoxantrone/melphalan *(67)*. There appeared to be large differences in favor of the transplant arm in median PFS (35 vs 20 mo), median OS (43 vs 20 mo), and 5-yr OS rates (30 vs 18%), none of which reached statistical significance (p=0.06 and 0.1, respectively)because of the very limited power of the trial.

Schmid et al. reported recently the first analysis of a German trial comparing tandem cycles of high-dose Cy/mitoxantrone/etoposide to conventional treatment with six to nine courses of adriamycin/paclitaxel in 92 untreated MBC patients *(68)*. The CR rate and time to progression were significantly superior in the transplant arm, without significant differences in OS at very short follow-up of 14 months. While a benefit from HDC is suggested in these two trials, their very small sample size clearly limits their ability to detect potentially meaningful differences.

Finally, the Duke University group conducted two small randomized trials with a crossover design, comparing early vs late use of HDC in MBC patients in CR and with bone-only disease, respectively. In the first of those two trials, Peters and colleagues randomized 100 hormone-refractory MBC patients who had achieved CR with AFM to immediate transplant with STAMP-I or to observation *(69)*. Patients in the observation arm were offered HDC at the time of relapse. At median follow-up of 6.3 yr, median DFS times were 9.7 mo for the immediate transplant arm, and 3.8 mo for the observation arm (p=0.006), with 6-yr DFS rates of 25 and 10%, respectively. Median OS times for the immediate transplant and observation arms were 2.34 and 3.57 yr, respectively (p=0.32), with 6-yr OS rates of 33 and 38%, respectively *(70)*.

The second Duke trial randomized 69 patients with hormone-refractory MBC confined to the bones, without prior chemotherapy for metastastic disease, and who did not experience tumor progression after four cycles of AFM, to immediate HDC with STAMP-I followed by RT of all bony metastases, or to RT and observation *(71)*. At median follow-up of 4.9 yr, all 34 patients in the observation arm had progressed, and most of them had subsequently undergone salvage transplant. The PFS rates significantly favored immediate transplant (17 vs 9%, p=0.001). The overall PFS rate for all patients getting HDC (early or late) was 13%. The OS rates were not significantly different between the immediate and late transplant arms (28 vs 22%). The OS was 23% for all transplanted patients.

The lack of a direct comparison between a HDC arm and a non-HDC control arm complicates the interpretation of both of Duke trials. They both showed that early HDC improves DFS or PFS in those populations, but the OS analysis is obviated by the fact that patients in the observation arms were salvaged with HDC.

In summary, currently available results from randomized trials in MBC reported to date are inconclusive. A benefit in DFS in favor of HDC has been noted in seven of the eight trials, with the only exception of the Philadelphia study. In contrast, no OS differences have yet emerged. Because approximately half of all MBC survive at least 2 yr with conventional management, *adequate follow-up is necessary for any OS differences to be noticed.* It is critical that the Canadian and the French PEGASE O3 trials be allowed to mature, before any meaningful conclusions regarding OS are made.

The inadequacy of drawing firm conclusions after preliminary analyses of the randomized studies, particularly with respect to OS, cannot be overemphasized. A large retrospective matched-pair survival comparison underscores this concept. Berry et al. compared the OS of 635 MBC patients enrolled in CALGB trials of SDC with that of 441 MBC patients treated with HDC and registered at the ABMTR *(72)*. This analysis was restricted to patients younger than 65 who had responded to a single chemotherapy regimen in the metastatic setting, with both patient groups being matched for known prognostic factors. No OS differences were observed during the first 2 yr after treatment, and only after the third year of follow-up did significant differences emerge. The 3-yr and 5-yr OS rates in the HDC group (37 and 22%, respectively) were significantly superior to those in the SDC group (27 and 13%, respectively, p=0.01).

The largest randomized HDC trial for MBC, the Canadian study, enrolled just over 220 patients. The small sample size of all these studies contrasts with the large accrual in trials of conventional chemotherapy, where accrual of many hundreds or thousands of patients is the rule. Mature follow-up becomes even more critical when the individual size of the trials is small. No other randomized trials in MBC have been conducted or are currently open in the United States, but several other trials are underway in Europe and may help clarify this crucial issue.

4. HDC FOR HIGH-RISK PRIMARY BREAST CANCER

4.1. Recent Results of Conventional Chemotherapy As Adjuvant Treatment for HRPBC

Most patients with high-risk primary breast cancer (HRPBC), defined by extensive axillary node involvement (four or more positive nodes) or by inflammatory breast disease (IBC), relapse after surgery and conventional-dose adjuvant chemotherapy *(73,74)*. A retrospective analysis by Hryniuk and Levine suggests that dose-intensity may have a greater impact on survival in the adjuvant setting than in patients with MBC *(7)*. However, most prospective trials have failed to show an improved outcome from minor dose escalations, as previously discussed.

Small advantages have been recently achieved with the incorporation of taxanes and the dose-density concept into conventional adjuvant chemotherapy. The large CALGB 9344 trial, enrolling 3170 patients with node-positive disease, showed that the addition of four cycles of paclitaxel to four cycles of adriamycin/cyclophosphamide (AC) resulted in modest but statistically significant improvements in DFS (70 vs 65%, p=0.002) and OS (80 vs 77%, p=0.006) *(22)*. In the similarly designed and sized NSABP B-28 study, which enrolled 3060 node-positive patients, the addition of four courses of paclitaxel after AC four courses of resulted in a comparable small benefit in DFS (73 vs 70%, p=0.008), with no OS impact (p=0.46) at median follow-up of 64 mo *(75)*. In a third study, 524 patients with node-positive breast cancer were randomized to receive four cycles of paclitaxel followed by four or courses of 5-flurouracil/adriamycin/cyclophosphamide (FAC). Thus, the inclusion of paclitaxel, and not the total duration of chemotherapy, was the only variable tested in this trial, in contrast to the previous two studies. At median follow-up of 5 yr, a trend was noted in favor of the paclitaxel arm in terms of DFS (86 vs 83%, p=0.09), without significant differences in OS *(76)*.

The inclusion in the adjuvant therapy armamentarium of docetaxel, arguably the most active single-agent for breast cancer, was evaluated in a multicentric randomized trial *(77)*. In this study, 1491 patients with node-positive disease were randomized to receive six cycles of CAF or docetaxel/adriamycin/cyclophosphamide (TAC). At median follow-up of 33 mo, statistically significant differences in DFS and OS in favor of TAC were noted. Importantly, well-powered and prospectively designed subset analyses according to the number of positive nodes showed that only patients with one to three positive nodes benefited from the addition of docetaxel. No differences in DFS (p=0.3) or OS (p=0.75) were observed between both treatment arms in the HRPBC subset with four or more positive nodes.

A large randomized study tested AC and paclitaxel administered every 3 wk or every 2 wk with G-CSF support in 2005 patients with node-positive disease *(78)*. At median follow-up of 36 mo the dose-dense schedule produced superior DFS (86 vs 81%, p=0.01) and OS (92 vs 89%, p=0.01).

The incorporation of trastuzumab into adjuvant treatment for patients with HER2-positive tumors appears very promising. Several randomized studies are currently testing this approach.

4.2. Phase II Studies of HDC in Patients With Multinode-Positive Breast Cancer

Peters and colleagues at Duke University pioneered the evaluation of HDC in HRPBC patients. These authors conducted the first phase II trial of HDC with STAMP-I in 85 patients with 10 or more involved axillary nodes *(79)*. At the latest update of this trial, at median follow-

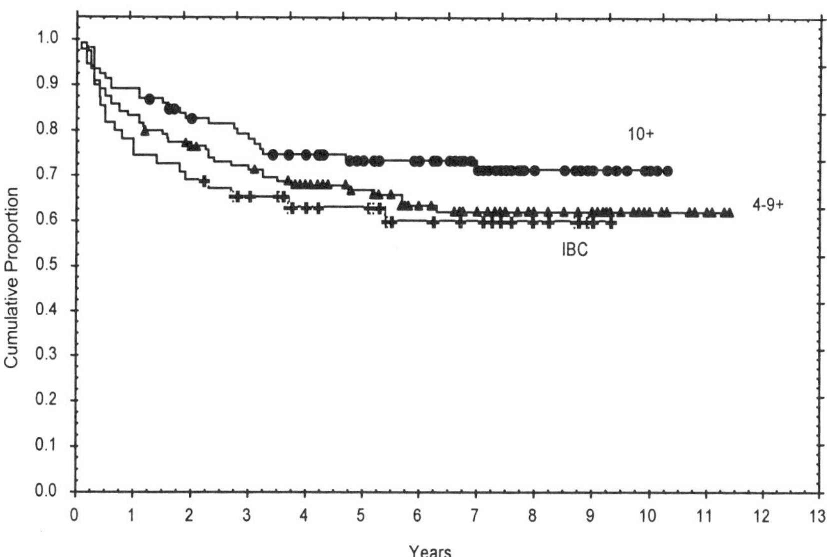

Fig. 5. RFS curves of the prospective trials of HDC for HRPBC conducted at the University of Colorado. Censored patients are indicated by (10 + nodes, *n*=120), ((4-9 + nodes, *n*=93), or ((inflammatory carcinoma, *n*=52).

up of 11 yr, 72% of patients remained diseasefree *(80)*. Long-term analysis of the Colorado phase II trial in this patient group shows similar results with 64% DFS rate in 120 patients analyzed at median follow-up of 7 yr, and lead follow-up of 11.5 yr (Fig. 5) *(81)*.

Gianni and colleagues at the Italian National Cancer Institute in Milan, tested a sequential high-dose single-agent approach with AHPCT in this patient population *(82)*. At a median follow-up of 4 yr, the DFS rate was 57%. In retrospect, this DFS rate appeared to be significantly higher than that observed in the group of patients with 10 or more involved nodes that received the most effective of two adriamycin-based SDC regimens that were compared in a different randomized trial conducted at the same institution using the same selection criteria and pretreatment staging as in Gianni's HDC study *(83)*.

Several investigators have tested HDC for patients with four to nine involved nodes. Bearman et al. conducted a pilot trial in which 54 patients received four cycles of SDC with AC, followed by HDC using STAMP-I *(84)*. In an intent-to-treat analysis, a DFS rate of 71% was seen at a median follow-up of 31 mo. These results have been reproduced by other groups *(85,86)*. In the latest update of patients with four to nine positive nodes transplanted at the University of Colorado with STAMP-I, 72% of 93 patients were alive and free of relapse at median and lead follow-up times of 7 and 10 yr, respectively (Fig. 5) *(81)*.

4.3. Inflammatory Breast Cancer

Patients who present with IBC experience a very aggressive evolution of this disease, with a 5-yr DFS rate of approx 35% following multimodal therapy with doxorubicin-based neoadjuvant chemotherapy, surgery, adjuvant chemotherapy, and locoregional RT *(87)*. In prospective phase II trials at the Dana Farber Cancer Institute *(88)* and the University of Colorado, *(89)* HDC was incorporated into a multimodal approach for this population. These studies included neoadjuvant adriamycin-containing chemotherapy followed in the Dana

Farber study by STAMP-V and posttransplant mastectomy and in the Colorado trial by pretransplant mastectomy and STAMP-I. In both studies, RT and tamoxifen for estrogen receptor (ER)-positive patients were subsequently delivered. The DFS and OS rates in the Dana Farber trial were 64 and 89%, respectively, at follow-up of 27 mo. At a recent update of the Colorado trial with 55 patients enrolled, the DFS and OS rates were 60 and 67%, respectively, at median follow-up of 6 yr and lead follow-up of 9 yr (Fig. 5) *(81)*.

Several other phase II trials of HDC in IBC patients have shown similar DFS rates of 50–60% at median follow-up times of 30 to 46 mo *(90–92)*. Overall, the promising results of these phase II studies suggest a benefit from the inclusion of HDC in the multidisciplinary management of patients with IBC. Randomized trials will be necessary to evaluate the potential benefits of such strategy.

4.4. Predictive Factors for Relapse After HDC for High-Risk Primary Breast Cancer

Somlo et al. analyzed 114 patients treated with two different HDC regimens at City of Hope National Medical Center and followed for a median of 46 months (range: 23–93 mo) *(91)*. These authors observed that the risk of relapse was lower for patients with progesterone receptor (PR)-positive tumors, and higher for patients with IBC, and that OS was better in patients with tumors that were PR positive or ER positive, and worse in high-grade tumors. Of all those, PR positivity was an independent favorable predictor of RFS and OS.

One hundred seventy-six patients treated at the University of Colorado with STAMP-I and followed for a median of 45 mo (range: 12–84 mo), were analyzed for potential adverse predictive factors *(93)*. Tumor size, tumor grade, clinical IBC, ER/PR negativity, and nodal ratio (number of positive nodes/number of sampled nodes) were associated with relapse. Nodal ratio, tumor size, and ER/PR status had independent value, and formed the basis for the following scoring system:

$$\text{Score} = (\text{Nodal Ratio} \times 3.05) + (\text{Tumor Size} \times 0.15) - (\text{ER/PR} \times 1.15)$$

In this formula, tumor size is entered in cm, and ER/PR is assigned "1" if positive (i.e., ER and/or PR are positive) and "0" if negative (both negative). Scores greater than or equal to 2.41 and less than 2.41 allocate patients to a high- or low-risk category, with risks of relapse of 65% and 11%, respectively. The differences in RFS ($p<0.000001$) and OS ($p<0.00005$) were highly significant (Fig. 6A). The model has 60% sensitivity, 90% specificity, 65% positive predictive value; 88% negative predictive value, and 83% accuracy. This predictive model was subsequently validated in an external set of 225 patients treated at Duke University with STAMP-I and followed for a median 46 mo (range: 4–27 mo) (Fig. 6B). The predictive value of the nodal ratio, probably superior to that of the absolute number of positive nodes, has been subsequently confirmed by other authors *(94–96)*. Our model was further validated in a cohort of 71 HRPBC patients, 53 with a low score and 18 with a high score, treated with STAMP-I at our program and followed prospectively since 1997 ($p=0.0004$) *(97)*.

Bitran et al. first reported a correlation between HER2/neu overexpression and risk of relapse in 25 patients with 10 or more positive nodes after high-dose Cy *(98)*. These results were confirmed in a larger analysis of 146 HRPBC patients treated with STAMP-I at the University of Colorado (Fig. 7) *(99)*. In this study, HER2/neu was independent of and complemented the clinical variables that compose the predictive score described earlier.

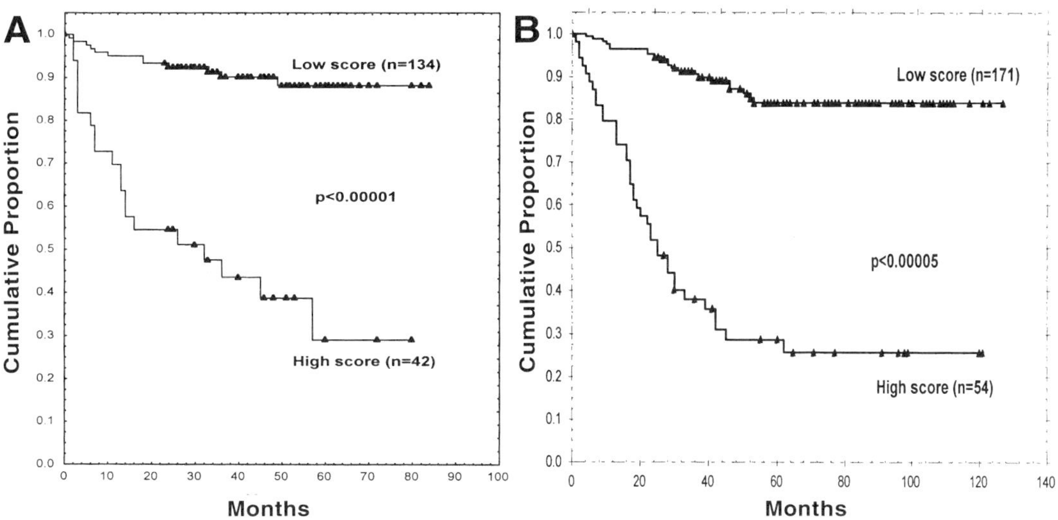

Fig. 6. RFS and OS curves of HRPBC patients treated with HDC (STAMP-I) at Colorado (n=176) (Figure 5A) and Duke (n=225) (Figure 5B), stratified according to their predictive score.

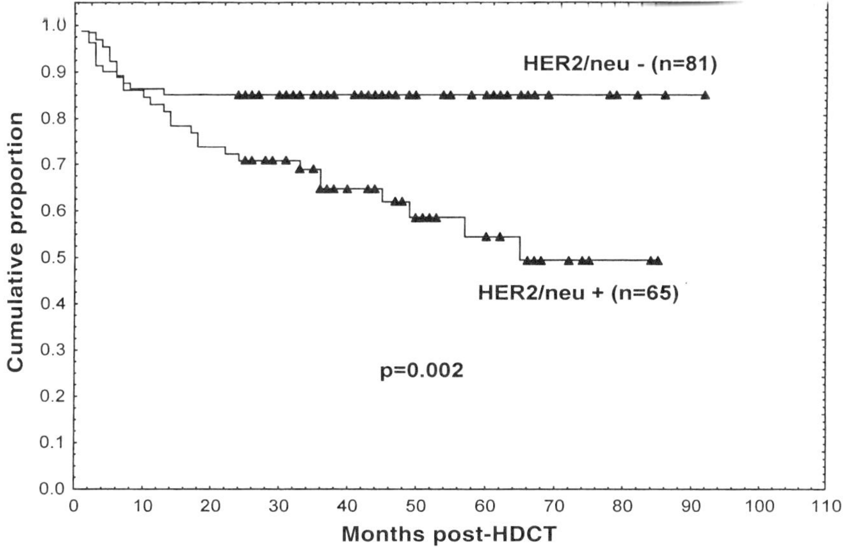

Fig. 7. RFS of HRPBC patients treated with STAMP-I at the University of Colorado BMTP, according to HER2/neu status.

4.5. Current Status of the Randomized Trials of HDC vs SDC for HRPBC

As with MBC, uncontrolled phase II trials in this setting suggested an advantage for recipients of HDC, as compared to historical controls treated with SDC. This apparent improvement in outcome has been attributed by some authors to a stage-migration phenomenon, resulting from extensive pre-HDC staging, and to patient-selection bias *(100,101)*. In contrast, the comparison made by Gianni et al. between their two trials of HDC and SDC, using the same selection criteria and pretreatment staging tests, argues against the relevance of these hypotheses.

The first comparative results came from two very small randomized phase II trials. In the Netherlands Cancer Institute trial conducted by Rodenhuis et al., 81 patients with axillary level III involvement detected by infraclavicular lymph-node biopsy received neoadjuvant FEC, followed by surgery, one postoperative cycle of FEC, and were then randomized to HDC with Cy/thiotepa/carboplatin, or to observation *(102)*. All patients received locoregional RT and tamoxifen. The final intent-to-treat analysis of the trial, at median follow-up of 6.9 yr, did not show significant differences between the HDC and control arms in DFS (49 vs 47.5%, p=0.3) or OS (62.5 vs. 61%, p=0.8). This study employed a nonstandard procedure, an infraclavicular single lymph-node biopsy, to determine eligibility, instead of a standard axillary node dissection to ascertain the number of nodes involved. In the M.D. Anderson Cancer Center trial, Hortobagyi and colleagues randomized 78 patients, with or more 10 positive nodes after upfront surgery or 4 or more positive nodes after preoperative chemotherapy, to eight cycles of FAC, followed by two cycles of dose-intensive Cy, etoposide, and cisplatin (DICEP) or no further therapy *(103)*. Patients in both arms received RT and tamoxifen. At median follow-up of 53 mo range: 7–85 mo), DFS and OS were not significantly different between both arms. This trial was prematurely closed because of slow accrual. The DICEP regimen has been proven to be nonmyeloablative *(104,105)* and is not considered HDC by most experts. It is worthwhile noting that these two small studies were only marginally powered to detect absolute outcome differences of at least 30%, which, if present, would have been of a greater magnitude than the overall impact of adjuvant chemotherapy for breast cancer compared to no treatment at all. Thus, none of these two small studies contribute meaningfully to our understanding of whether HRPBC patients benefit or not from HDC.

Subsequent to these two studies, the first preliminary analyses of larger phase III trials were reported (Table 4). Rodenhuis and colleagues presented the Netherlands Working Party on Autologous Transplantation in Solid Tumors (NWAST) study, which enrolled 885 patients with four or more involved lymph nodes *(106)*. Patients received four cycles of FEC followed by one more cycle of FEC or high-dose CTC (6 g/m^2 cyclophosphamide, 480 mg/m^2 thiotepa, and 1600 mg/m^2 carboplatin) with PBPC support. At median follow-up of 57 mo, there was a trend for an EFS advantage in favor of HDC (65 vs 59%, p=0.09), with no detectable OS differences. The EFS of those patients randomized to HDC who were actually transplanted appeared superior to those in the control arm (p=0.03). Prospectively planned subset analyses showed that HDC improved EFS among patients with 10 or more involved nodes (68 vs 49%, p=0.05). In the four to nine node group, EFS rates were 72% (HDC) vs 65% (SDC) (p=0.5). Other subgroup analyses, which were unplanned, suggested that patients younger than 40 yr old (p=0.05), with HER2-negative disease (p=0.02), or with lower grade tumors (p=0.002) might benefit from HDC.

In the Intergroup CALGB 9082 trial, Peters et al. enrolled patients with 10 or more positive nodes identified after a standard axillary dissection *(107)*. Eligible patients received four cycles of CAF and were randomized to high-dose STAMP-I or to a single cycle of the same three-drug combination at intermediate doses (IDS) with G-CSF support (900 mg/m^2 Cy, cisplatin, and 90 mg/m^2 BCNU [CCB]). This study, designed to detect a 14% absolute difference in DFS at 5 yr, randomized 785 patients, 394 to the HDC arm, and 391 to the ID arm. Twenty-five patients who relapsed on the ID arm (15%) received subsequent salvage HDC. All patients were scheduled to receive locoregional RT, and, if hormone receptor-positive, tamoxifen for 5 yr. Patients in the HDC arm were less likely to initiate RT after systemic therapy than patients allocated to the ID arm (78 vs 89%, p<0.001), because of toxicity asso-

Table 4. Randomized Trials in HRPBC (*N*>300)

	Population			*Follow-up*	*% DFS*			*%OS*		
Trial	*(# + nodes)*	*n*	*HDC regimen*	*(yrs)*	*HDC*	*Control*	*p*	*HDC*	*Control*	*p*
NWAST *(106)*	4	885	CTC	4.75	65	59	0.09	NR	NR	NS
CALGB *(107)*	10	785	STAMP-I	5.1	61	60	0.49	70	72	0.23
Anglo-Celtic *(113)*	4	605	CT	4	51	54	0.6	63	62	0.8
ECOG *(110)*	10	540	CT	6.1	55	48	0.1	58	62	0.3
SBCG *(111)*	>5–8	525	STAMP-V	5	47	52	0.11	56	60	0.29
WSG *(116)*	10	403	Tandem ECT x 2	3.25	60	43	0.001	76	66	0.05
Milan *(117)*	4	382	Sequential single agents	4.3	65	62	NS	77	76	NS
IBCSG *(118)*	10	340	EC × 3	3.9	57	46	0.1	73	64	0.2
PÉGASE 01 *(115)*	>7	314	CMM	2.75	71	55	0.002	84	85	0.33
GABG *(114)*	10	302	CTM	3.7	58	46	0.09	NR	NR	NS

HRPBC, high-risk primary breast cancer; HDC, high-dose chemotherapy; DFS, disease-free survival; OS, overall survival; NWAST, Netherlands Working Party on Autologous Transplantation in Solid Tumors. CALGB, Cancer And Leukemia Group B, ECOG, Eastern Collaborative Oncology Group. SBCG, Scandinavian Breast Cancer Group. WSG, West German Study Group, IBCSG, International Breast Cancer Study Group, GABG, German Autologous Bone Marrow Transplant Group, CTC, cyclophosphamide-thiotepa-carboplatin, ECT, epirubicin-cyclophosphamide-thiotepa, CMM, cyclophosphamide-mitoxantrone-melphalan, CTM, cyclophosphamide-thiotepa-mitoxantrone, NR, not reported, NS, not significant.

ciated with STAMP-I *(108)*. At median follow-up of 5 yr, the intent-to-treat DFS was 61% in the HDC arm and 60% in the ID arm (p=0.5). There were fewer relapses in the HDC arm (32.2% [95% CI, 27–37.8%]) than in the ID arm (42.7.1% [95% CI, 37.1–48.5%]). This represents a 31% relative reduction in the frequency of relapses, consistent with a dose-response effect. However, there were 32 toxic deaths (8.1%) in the HDC arm, most of them in women older than 50, vs none in the ID arm. Centers transplanting more than 50 patients tended to have lower TRM than those performing fewer transplants. Thus, analysis of events was dominated by toxic deaths in the HDC arm and by relapses in the ID arm. No significant difference in OS was observed (70 vs. 72%, p=0.2). At current lead follow-up of 10 yr, the OS in both arms is superior to any previous experience in CALGB or any other study of conventional chemotherapy in this population. Although the outcomes in the HDC arm were as predicted from the pilot phase II study *(79,80)* patients in the ID arm have fared much better than expected during the design of the trial. The reasons for this are unclear, and may include the clinical benefit from the addition of one cycle of G-CSF-supported CCB at the end of treatment, extensive pre-enrollment staging, or the confounding effect from salvage HDC.

A companion study compared quality of life after treatment in 210 patients enrolled in CALGB 9082 (106 on the STAMP-I arm and 104 on the ID arm). There were significant differences in favor of the control arm at the 3-mo time point, but quality-of-life scores were virtually identical between both arms at 1, 2, and 3 yr *(109)*.

Tallman and colleagues from the ECOG randomized 540 patients with 10 or more involved nodes to receive six cycles of CAF with or without consolidation with high-dose Cy (6 g/m^2)–thiotepa (800 mg/m^2) with BM support, and toward the end of the study with PBPC support (110). At median follow-up of 6.1 yr, there were no significant differences between the HDC and the SDC arms in EFS (55 vs 48%, p=0.1) or OS (58 vs 62%, p=0.3). Among patients meeting strict protocol eligibility, EFS appeared higher in the HDC arm (55 vs 45%, p=0.04). There were nine fatal toxicities in the transplant arm, eight of whom had received BM support, and nine cases of secondary leukemia/myelodysplastic syndrome.

Bergh and colleagues from the Scandinavian Breast Cancer Group enrolled 528 patients with either eight or more involved nodes, or five or more involved nodes with an ER-negative and high S-phase fraction tumor *(111)*. Patients were randomized to receive nine cycles of individually tailored dose-intensive FEC, or three cycles of conventional FEC, followed by HDC with STAMP-V. Doses in the tailored dose-intensive FEC arm were escalated to as high as 120 mg/m^2 of epirubicin and 1800 mg/m^2 of Cy per cycle, according to the blood nadir counts of the preceding cycle. All patients in both arms received RT and tamoxifen for 5 yr. None of the usual staging tests in HDC clinical trials were performed before randomization to exclude women with metastatic disease. As it has been pointed out, *(112)*, the total chemotherapy doses in the tailored dose-intensive arm significantly exceeded that of the HDC arm. At median follow-up of 34 mo, the DFS rates in the STAMP-V and the tailored FEC arms were 65 vs 72% (p=0.04), and their respective OS rates were 77 vs 83% (p=0.1). Despite the short follow-up, eight cases of secondary myelodysplastic syndrome/acute leukemia (3.2%) had already been noticed in the tailored FEC arm, and more cases are likely to be detected. Two patients in the STAMP-V arm (0.7%) died from acute regimen-related toxicity. The main question that arises in the interpretation of this trial is deciding which one truly constitutes the higher dose arm, as the "control" arm received doses well above those considered standard, as well as higher total cumulative doses than patients randomized to the HDC arm. Neither this trial nor the CALGB study contained a control arm receiving a chemotherapy regimen that can be considered standard.

In the Anglo-Celtic trial, Crown et al. randomized 605 patients with four or more positive nodes to receive either HDC (Cy/thiotepa) or maintenance CMF, following four cycles of adriamycin at 75 mg/m^2 *(113)*. At median follow-up of 4 yr, no differences were noted between the transplant arm and the control arm in the whole study file in terms of DFS (51 vs 54%, p=0.6) or OS (63 vs 62%, p=0.8). However, an unplanned evaluation of the first 100 patients enrolled revealed fairly large differences in favor of the transplant arm (59 vs 43%).

In the first analysis of the German trial enrolling patients with 10 or more involved nodes, Zander et al. reported a substantial DFS advantage for the transplant arm in those patients with longest follow-up, with 6-yr actuarial DFS rates of 50 and 25%, respectively *(114)*. No DFS or OS differences were noted for the whole study file of 302 patients at median follow-up of 3.7 yr.

The first analyses of the French PEGASE 01 and the West German Study Group (WSG) studies showed large differences in DFS were noted in favor of the transplant arm in both trials. In the first one, Roché and colleagues randomized 314 patients with more than seven involved lymph nodes to receive four cycles of FEC followed by HDC with Cy/mitoxantrone/melphalan or observation *(115)*. At short median follow-up of 33 mo, there were statistically significant differences in DFS (71 vs 55%, p=0.002), but not in OS (84 vs 85%, p=0.3).

Nitz and colleagues from the WSG enrolled 403 patients with 10 or more positive nodes *(116)*. The control arm consisted of a modern dose-dense sequential regimen of four cycles of EC followed by six courses of CMF, all every 2 wk with G-CSF support. The HDC arm included two cycles of EC followed by tandem cycles of epirubicin (90 mg/m2)-Cy (3000 mg/m^2)-thiotepa (400 mg/m^2), administered 4 wk apart with PBPC support. Neither arm had any TRM. At median follow-up of 39 mo, there was clear superiority of the transplant arm in EFS, the primary endpoint of the study (62 vs 48%, p=0.001), with a trend towards improved OS, the secondary endpoint (75.6 vs 66%, p=0.05).

Gianni and colleagues compared their sequential high-dose single-agent approach to conventional chemotherapy in 382 patients with four or more positive nodes *(117)*. High-dose sequential treatment consisted of one cycle of Cy, followed by one course of methotrexate with leucovorin rescue, two cycles of epirubicin and one last course of thiotepa/melphalan, this last one with stem cell support. At median follow-up of 52 mo, no differences in DFS (65 vs 62%) or OS (76 vs 77%) were noted between the high-dose sequential and the control arms. A possible DFS advantage in favor of the HDC arm was suggested in the subset of younger patients and in those with four to nine positive nodes.

Russell and colleagues from the International Breast Cancer Study Group (IBCSG) randomized 344 patients to four cycles AC/EC followed by three cycles CMF, or to a dose-intense arm with three cycles of epirubicin (200 mg/m^2)-Cy (4 g/m^2) every 3 wk with PBPC support *(118)*. Approximately 70% of all patients had 10 or more involved nodes, and 30% had five to nine involved nodes with an ER or a T3 tumor. In its first analysis at a median follow-up of 4 yr, the observed differences in favor of the dose-intense arm did not reach statistical significance for EFS (57 vs 46%, p=0.1) or OS (73 vs 64%, p=0.2).

The controversy about the efficacy of HDC for HRPBC remains far from settled. Once again, we need to bear in mind that the ascertainment of a potential benefit of HDC over SDC requires mature follow-up, and that *premature evaluation of randomized trials can be misleading*. The European Parma study for aggressive non-Hodgkin's lymphoma illustrates this point. Preliminary analyses of this study were negative *(119,120)*, and only after the appropriate duration of follow-up did statistically significant differences become apparent, with 5-yr DFS rates of 46 and 12% for the HDC and control arms, respectively, at the time of the definitive analysis *(121)*.

Median time to relapse of HRPBC patients after SDC is around 2 to 3 yr. In contrast, the majority of relapses after HDC occur within that time period (Fig. 3). Therefore, early analyses will detect most of the relapses in the transplant arms, but only around half the recurrences in the control arms. Furthermore, in the analysis of OS, another 2 yr of median survival after metastatic recurrence need to be considered. All of these facts make *long-term follow-up even more necessary in adjuvant than in metastatic studies.*

5. POTENTIAL LINES OF IMPROVEMENT OF HDC FOR BREAST CANCER

5.1. New HDC Regimens

There is a pressing need to improve HDC for breast cancer. It is unlikely that first-generation high-dose regimens developed 15 yr ago, such as STAMP-I or STAMP-V, would end up being the optimal stem cell-supported high-dose combinations. While the randomized trials, initiated a decade ago, are testing those old HDC regimens, several new strategies are being actively pursued. These include the development of new HDC regimens, tandem or multiple transplants, or combination of HDC with treatments with novel mechanisms of action targeting posttransplant minimal residual disease (MRD).

A critical review of the first generation of high-dose regimens shows that there is ample room for improvement. Although cisplatin and carboplatin are active drugs in first-line treatment for breast cancer, *(122,123)*, they are only escalated twofold above conventional chemotherapy in the STAMP-I and STAMP-V regimens, respectively. Both regimens also include Cy, at doses from 5625 to 6000 mg/m^2, administered over 3d (STAMP-I) or 5d (STAMP-V). Two randomized studies conducted by the National Surgical Adjuvant Breast and Bowel Project (NSABP) tested dose escalations of Cy, combined with adriamycin, in the adjuvant treatment of node-positive patients *(20,21)*. No improvement in DFS or OS were observed from up to fourfold increases in the dose intensity of Cy (2400 mg/m^2 every 3 wk) or its total dose (9600 mg/m^2 over four cycles). The failure of such substantial dose increments of Cy to improve outcome raises serious concerns about its inclusion in high-dose regimens for breast cancer. A possible explanation for why Cy does not show an in vivo dose–response effect, in contrast to the in vitro observations using 4-hydroxy-cyclophosphamide, stems from its pharmacological properties. Cy is a prodrug that requires hepatic activation to 4-hydroxy-cyclophosphamide, a P450-mediated metabolic step that is subject to saturation and multiple drug–drug interactions *(124)*, such as inhibition by high-dose thiotepa when both drugs are given concurrently as a continuous infusions, as in STAMP-V *(125)*. Consequently, this activation step has a high interpatient *(126)* and intrapatient *(127)* variability. Furthermore, intrapatient differences between standard and high doses exist in the metabolic pathways of Cy and its metabolites, with significant increases in the inactivating reactions and reduction of cyclophosphamide bioactivation at high doses, when compared to conventional doses *(128)*.

Current research efforts are testing high-dose combinations using other more potent drugs. Although not alkylating agents, a dose–response effect has been shown with doxorubicin, *(129)* paclitaxel, *(130–132)*, and docetaxel, *(133–135)*, the three most active agents in breast cancer. Although the concern about the potential of doxorubicin for cardiotoxicity has prevented its inclusion in most HDC regimens, Somlo et al. have shown the feasibility and acceptable cardiac tolerance of high-dose doxorubicin (165 mg/m2) in a 96-h continuous infusion, combined with etoposide and Cy *(136)*.

Myelosuppression is dose limiting when paclitaxel *(137)* and docetaxel *(138,139)* are given at conventional doses. In a phase I trial using AHPCT, the MTD of paclitaxel infused over 24 h, in combination with fixed doses of Cy and cisplatin, was established at 775 mg/m^2 *(140)*. This dose of paclitaxel is around threefold higher than its standard maximum tolerated dose (MTD) in 24-h infusions *(141–143)*. Paclitaxel has been subsequently incorporated into other HDC regimens, either as a single *(144,145)* or multiple cycles *(146–148)*.

Docetaxel is currently considered the most active drug for breast cancer *(149)*. In addition, the drug presents a dose-dependent and schedule-independent profile, in contrast to that of paclitaxel *(150,151)*. A phase I trial of stem cell-supported docetaxel in combination with melphalan and carboplatin in patients with chemotherapy-refractory and heavily pretreated disease is currently underway at the University of Colorado *(152)*. This trial has established the MTD of docetaxel at 400 mg/m2, which represents a fourfold increment over its standard dose. Initial evaluation of activity in patients with measurable disease shows a high level of activity in this population with resistant breast cancer (96.5% response rate with 48% complete responses).

Another hypothesis under evaluation speculates that more than one cycle of HDC may be needed to eradicate metastatic disease. Dunphy et al. *(153)* used two cycles of nonmyeloablative dose-intense DICEP, with 25% DFS at 2 yr, which appeared comparable to the outcome after a single cycle of myeloablative HDC. Rapid delivery of multiple cycles of stem cell-supported dose-intense nonmyeloablative chemotherapy has been shown to be feasible *(154,155)*. Several authors have investigated the delivery of tandem cycles of myeloablative HDC with AHPCT after both cycles *(156–158)*. The value of a second cycle of the same regimen remains unclear, because the PR to CR conversion rate appears to decrease substantially from the first to the second cycle of HDC *(158)*.

A different approach involves the sequential use of different noncross-resistant combinations. Ayash et al. *(159)* treated chemosensitive MBC patients with melphalan followed, within a median of 35 d, by STAMP-V. At a median follow-up of 16 mo after the second transplant, their 34% DFS rate did not appear different to results of a single HDC treatment. Preliminary results were reported by Bitran et al. using the reverse sequence of Cy/thiotepa followed by melphalan, with a longer median inter-cycle interval of 105 days *(160)*. The DFS rate was 56% at a median follow-up of 25 mo from the first transplant. Whether the results of both studies are significantly different is unclear, given their short follow-up and the overlapping ranges of DFS rates.

More recent trials have incorporated new drugs to this strategy of sequential noncross-resistant HDC cycles. Vahdat et al. treated 60 chemosensitive MBC patients with three separate high-dose cycles of chemotherapy using sequential paclitaxel, melphalan, and STAMP-V, with 30% DFS and 61% OS rates at median follow-up of 31 mo *(161)*. Elias and colleagues treated 58 patients with MBC previously untreated for metastatic disease with a short and intensive induction treatment with two cycles of single-agent adriamycin, followed by tandem HDC cycles with AHPC support, using STAMP-V preceded (n=32) or followed (n=26) by high-dose melphalan/paclitaxel *(162)*. At median follow-up of 36 mo, the DFS and OS rates were 46 and 66%, respectively, which appeared superior to those reported in previous phase II trials conducted by this group, testing strategies of long induction (four cycles of AFM) followed by one HDC cycle with STAMP-V *(52)* or long induction followed by sequential cycles of high-dose melphalan and STAMP-V *(159)*.

Other authors have reported less promising results with multicycle HDC. Hu et al. treated 55 MBC patients with four cycles of varying combinations of mitoxantrone, paclitaxel, thiotepa, and cyclophosphamide, with AHPCT *(148)*. The actuarial 3-yr DFS rate (15%) did not appear different from that observed in 55 contemporaneous MBC patients treated with a single cycle of STAMP-I (19%).

In parallel with these inconclusive clinical trials, Teicher et al. described the phenomenon of acute in vivo resistance after HDC, after treating tumor-bearing mice with different sequences of several drugs at high doses *(163)*. Tumors became chemoresistant after the first treatment in an inversely proportional fashion to the length of the interval between treatments. Recent in vitro experiments performed by Frei et al. also suggest that the specific sequence of alkylators used may have a substantial influence on response *(164)*. These authors showed that initial treatment with high-dose melphalan generates cross-resistance to subsequent alkylators by increasing tumor-cell concentrations of glutathione and glutathione-*S*-transferase-γ.

5.2. Strategies Targeting Posttransplant Residual Disease

The HER2/neu oncogene is overexpressed in 25–30% of breast cancer patients *(165)*. Trastuzumab (Herceptin®), a humanized monoclonal antibodies targeting the HER2/neu receptor, has shown activity in HER2/neu-positive tumors *(166,167)*. Additionally, preclinical experiments have demonstrated synergy between trastuzumab and cisplatin, carboplatin, docetaxel, etoposide, and thiotepa *(168–171)*. Clinical studies of the combination of this antibody with cisplatin, *(172)* AC, or paclitaxel *(32)* showed an improved outcome compared with the same chemotherapy alone. An early analysis of a pilot study currently underway at the bone marrow transplant programs at Colorado and Duke suggests the safety of concurrent administration of trastuzumab with HDC (STAMP-I), exploiting the synergy observed in vitro, and in the post-transplant setting against MRD *(173)*.

Pilot trials have shown the feasibility of SDC, such as adriamycin or paclitaxel, shortly after recovery from transplant *(174,175)*. Autologous hematopoietic cells may be manipulated in vitro to improve treatment outcomes. It may be possible to genetically modify hematopoietic stem and progenitor cells, for instance, transductions with the multidrug resistance gene MDR-1, to protect them from posttransplant myelotoxic chemotherapy *(176–179)*.

Recent results demonstrate an important prognostic value for early posttransplant lymphocyte recovery in MBC patients *(180,181)*. In these studies, an absolute lymphocyte count on d +15 greater than 500/mm^3 in peripheral blood was an independent favorable predictor of outcome. These observations support the possibility of an important role for the immune system in tumor control after HDC for MBC. The induction of autologous graft-vs-tumor (GVT) effect with cyclosporin and other cytokines has been tested *(182–184)*. Ongoing research efforts are testing innovative immune strategies for breast cancer patients receiving an AHPCT, such as the use of interleukin-2 to increase mobilization of immune effector cells into the graft *(185,186)* or posttransplant reinfusion of ex vivo manipulated dendritic cells *(187,188)* or of autologous lymphocytes with granulocyte-macrophase colony-stimulating factor *(189)*.

Achievement of complete remissions with HDC may allow institution of innovative therapies posttransplant to prevent recurrence by such immunologic approaches, or novel targeted agents. All new therapies will require the scrutiny of controlled clinical trials.

5.3. Purging of Stem Cell Grafts

PBPCs have replaced BM as the primary source of hematopoietic progenitors for AHPCT. Although tumor burden may be lower in PBPC than in BM fractions *(190)*, breast cancer cells can be detected in PBPC fractions of 10–40% of MBC patients, and of 5–20% of stage II–III patients *(191–195)*. Detection of breast cancer cells in the BM at the time of HDC has been correlated with an increased risk of relapse in HRPBC *(196–198)*, but not in MBC *(199)*. Most post-HDC relapses in MBC patients occur in sites of prior disease, suggesting an insufficient cytoreductive capacity of HDC, rather than a direct effect from tumor cells contaminating the graft. Thus, the clinical impact of procedures directed at purging the graft of tumor cells will probably have to be determined in the adjuvant setting.

Negative purging has been tested in patients with BM metastases. Pharmacological purging achieved a mean 2.5-log tumor cell depletion, with a marked engraftment delay *(200)*. Studies using immunomagnetic purging showed a mean 3-log depletion of cancer cells, with no prolongation of the engraftment times compared to historical controls *(201)*. Both procedures combined resulted in a 4.5-log tumor cell depletion, *(202)* at the expense of substantial engraftment delays *(203)*.

Positive selection targets the CD34 antigen, expressed on 0.5–3% of normal BM cells and PBPCs, including both the committed and, probably, the long-term reconstituting progenitor cells. The CD34 antigen does not appear to be expressed on breast cancer cells *(204)*. The University of Colorado BMT Program reported a series of 155 breast cancer patients who received HDC and a BM or PBPC graft that was CD34-selected with the Ceprate immunoadsorption device *(205)*. CD34-selected stem cells effectively reconstituted immediate and long-term hematopoiesis. An average 2-log tumor cell depletion was achieved. Patients receiving CD34-selected PBPCs experienced neutrophil and platelet recovery rates that were comparable to patients who received unmanipulated grafts. Long-term follow-up showed that the durability of engraftment, immune reconstitution, DFS and OS, were comparable to patients receiving unmanipulated hematopoietic cell fractions *(206)*. A subsequent prospective randomized study demonstrated that breast cancer patients who received HDC with an autologous CD34-selected marrow graft had reduced marrow infusion-related toxicity, and comparable neutrophil engraftment times and immune function recovery, and for those who receive greater than or equal to 1.2×10^6 CD34+ cells/kg, comparable time platelet engraftment to women who receive unselected buffy coat fractions of marrow *(207)*.

Similar results were reported by Yanovich et al., who randomized 92 stage II–IV patients who were randomized to receive CD34-selected PBPC, using the Isolex 300/300i device, or an unselected peripheral blood graft *(208)*. In this multicentric trial, there were no significant differences between both groups in neutrophil or platelet engraftment, adverse events, or outcome.

Because most patients still had detectable cancer cells present in their stem cell grafts following CD34-selection, maximally effective purging may require the addition of a second selection procedure. Preclinical studies have demonstrated a larger magnitude of tumor cell depletion using combined positive and negative selection in a sequential fashion than simultaneously (averages 6.38-log and 4.29-log, respectively) *(209)*. Mohr et al. purged the PBPC products of 17 patients with simultaneous positive and negative (immunomagnetic) selection, observing prompt and sustained engraftments *(210)*. Negrin and colleagues transplanted 22 MBC patients with highly purified CD34+ Thy-1+ hematopoetic progenitors, using a combined sequential approach of CD34 selection with the Isolex device followed by CD34+ Thy-

1+ high-speed flow-cytometric cell sorting *(211)*. Tumor cell depletion below the detection of an immunofluorescence-based assay for cytokeratins was accomplished in six patients whose apheresis products contained cytokeratin-positive cells. Hematopoietic engraftment was rapid and sustained.

6. ALLOGENEIC HPCT FOR BREAST CANCER: EARLY RESULTS

Allogeneic BM or PBPC transplantation has been shown to confer an immune GVT effect against hematologic malignancies. Anecdotal reports have suggested the existence of a potential GVT effect in breast cancer *(212,213)*. Ueno and colleagues at M.D. Anderson treated 10 MBC patients with high-dose Cy/thiotepa/BCNU, followed by allogeneic PBPC transplantation from a matched sibling *(214)*. Four patients who experienced tumor progression after transplant had their immunosuppression reduced, and one received a donor lymphocyte infusion. Two of those patients experienced regression of liver metastases in association with exacerbation of acute graft-vs-host disease (GVHD).

A nonmyeloablative "mini-allotransplant" approach is under evaluation for breast cancer at several institutions, incorporating less intense preparative regimens that can provide enough immunosupression to allow engraftment of allogeneic stem cells. The goal is to attain a GVT effect with less toxicity than after a full myeloablative allogeneic transplant. Initial promising results using this approach have been reported in patients with metastatic renal cell carcinoma *(215,216)* Ueno et al. treated seven MBC patients in CR/PR or stable bone-only disease with a reduced intensity "mini-transplant" from a matched sibling donor *(217)*. One patient converted from PR to CR and three patients remained in stable disease at early follow-up. Bregni and colleagues observed two partial responses in six MBC patients, concurrently with the appearance of GVHD *(218)*. Blaise et al. treated eight heavily pretreated MBC patients, none of whom had responded at the time of their initial report *(219)*.

This early and very limited experience, along with that obtained in other solid tumors, suggests the relative safety of nonmyeloablative allogeneic transplantation for patients with MBC. Withdrawal of immunosuppression seems necessary for tumor response. Although different antigens mediate GVHD and GVT in preclinical models, the early clinical experience seems to indicate that occurrence of GVHD is necessary for GVT, which suggests that both events may be mediated by the same allorreactive T cells. More experience with this approach is necessary to determine whether it can be considered a solid therapeutic option for patients without bulky or progressive disease.

7. CONCLUSIONS

High-dose chemotherapy attempts to improve long-term therapeutic results in breast cancer, based on a solid rationale. While results from phase II studies were encouraging, an answer to the important question of its relative merit over standard chemotherapy will only come from the mature results of randomized phase III studies, most of which have only been analyzed in a preliminary fashion with short follow-up. Such data will be forthcoming within the next few years. In the meantime, it is imperative that research be continued to improve HDC regimens and integrate them with novel strategies possessing different and potentially complementary mechanisms of action.

REFERENCES

1. Peters WP, Henner WD, Bast RC, Schnipper L, Frei E III. Novel toxicities associated with high dose combination alkylating agents in autologous bone marrow support. In: Dicke KA, Spitzer G, Zander AR, eds. *Autologous Bone Marrow Transplantation: Proceedings of the First International Symposium*. Houstin, TX: University of Texas Cancer Center, M.D. Anderson Hospital, 1986; pp 231-235.
2. Antman KH, Rowlings PA, Vaughan WP, et al. High-dose chemotherapy with autologous hematopoietic stem-cell support for breast cancer in North America. *J Clin Oncol* 1997; 15: 1870-1879.
3. Damon LE, Hu WW, Stockerl-Goldstein KE, et al. High-dose chemotherapy and hematopoietic stem cell rescue for breast cancer: Experience in California. *Biol Blood Marrow Transplant* 2000; 6:496–505.
4. Hryniuk W, Busch H. The importance of dose intensity in chemotherapy of metastatic breast cancer. *J Clin Oncol* 1984; 2:1281–1288.
5. Hryniuk W, Frei E III, Wright FA. A single scale for comparing dose-intensity of all chemotherapy regimens in breast cancer: Summation dose-intensity. *J Clin Oncol* 1998;16: 3137–3147.
6. Fossati R, Confalonieri C, Torri V, et al. Cytotoxic and hormonal treatment for metastatic breast cancer: A systematic review of published randomized trials involving 31,510 women. *J Clin Oncol* 1998; 16:3439–3460.
7. Hryniuk W, Levine MN. Analysis of dose intensity for adjuvant chemotherapy trials in stage II breast cancer. *J Clin Oncol* 1986; 4:1162–1170.
8. Bonadonna G, Valagussa P. Dose-response effect of adjuvant chemotherapy in breast cancer. *N Eng J Med* 1981; 304:10–15.
9. Tannock IF, Boyd NF, DeBoer G, et al. A randomized trial of two doses of cyclophosphamide, methotrexate and fluorouracil for patients with metastatic breast cancer. *J Clin Oncol* 1988; 6:1377–1387.
10. Hortobagyi GN, Bodey GP, Buzdar AU, et al. Evaluation of high-dose versus standard FAC chemotherapy for advanced breast cancer in protected environment units: A prospective randomized study. *J Clin Oncol* 1987; 5:354–364.
11. Winer E. Berry D, Duggan D, et al. Failure of higher dose paclitaxel to improve outcome in patients with metastatic breast cancer — Results from CALGB 9342. *Proc Am Soc Clin Oncol* 1998; 17:101a.
12. Habeshaw T, Paul R, Jones R, et al. Epirubicin at two dose levels with prednisolone as treatment for advanced breast cancer: The results of a randomized trial. *J Clin Oncol* 1991; 9: 295–304.
13. Bastholt L, Dalmark M, Gjedde SB, et al. Dose-response relationship of epirubicin in the treatment of postmenopausal patients with metastatic breast cancer: A randomized study of epirubicin at four different dose levels performed by the Danish Breast Cancer Cooperative Group. *J Clin Oncol* 1996; 14:1146–1155.
14. Brufman G, Corajort E, Ghilezan N, et al. Doubling epirubicin dose intensity (100 mg/m2 versus 50 mg/m^2) in the FEC regimen significantly increases response rate. An international randomized phase III study in metastatic breast cancer. *Ann Oncol* 1997; 8:155–162.
15. Focan C, Andrien JM, Closon M, et al. Dose-response relationship of epirubicin based first-line chemotherapy for advanced breast cancer: A prospective randomized trial. *J Clin Oncol* 1993; 11:1253–1263.
16. Fountzilas G, Athanassiades A, Giannakkais T, et al. A randomized study of epirubicin monotherapy every four or every two weeks in advanced breast cancer. A Hellenic Cooperative Oncology Group study. *Ann Oncol* 1997; 8:1213–1220.
17. Wood WC, Budman DR, Korzun AH, et al. Dose and dose intensity of adjuvant chemotherapy for stage II, node-positive breast carcinoma. *N Eng J Med* 1994; 330:1253–1259.
18. Budman DR, Berry DA, Cirrincione CT, et al. Dose and dose intensity as determinants of outcome in the adjuvant treatment of breast cancer. *J Natl Cancer Inst* 1999; 91:286–287.
19. Bonneterre J, Roché H, Bremond A, et al. Results of a randomized trial of adjuvant chemotherapy with FEC 50 vs. FEC 100 in high risk node-positive breast cancer patients. Proc Am Soc Clin Oncol 1998; 17:124a.
20. Fisher B, Anderson S, Wickerham DL, et al. Increased intensification and total dose of cyclophosphamide in a doxorubicin-cyclophosphamide regimen for the treatment of primary breast cancer: Findings from National Surgical Adjuvant Breast and Bowel Project B-22. *J Clin Oncol* 1997; 15:1858–1869.
21. Fisher B, Anderson S, DeCillis A, et al. Further evaluation of intensified and increased total dose of cyclophosphamide for the treatment of primary breast cancer: Findings from National Surgical Adjuvant Breast and Bowel Project B-25. *J Clin Oncol* 1999; 17:3374–3388.
22. Henderson IC, Berry D, Demetri G, et al. Improved outcomes from adding sequential paclitaxel but not from escalating doxorubicin in an adjuvant chemotherapy regimen for patients with node-positive primary breast cancer. *J Clin Oncol* 2003; 21:976–983.
23. Frei III E, Canellos GP. Dose: A critical factor in cancer chemotherapy. *The Am J Med* 1980; 69: 585–594.
24. Frei E III, Antman K, Teicher B, et al. Bone Marrow Autotransplantation for solid tumors - Prospects. *J Clin Oncol* 1989; 4:515–526.
25. Falkson G, Gelman RS, Leone L, Falkson CI. Survival of premenopausal women with metastatic breast cancer. Long-term follow-up of Eastern Cooperative Group and Cancer and Leukemia Group B studies. *Cancer* 1990; 66:1621.

26. Greenberg PA, Hortobagyi GN, Smith TL, et al. Long-term follow-up of patients with complete remission following combination chemotherapy for metastatic breast cancer. *J Clin Oncol* 1996; 14:2197–2205.
27. Rivera E, Holmes FA, Buzdar AU, et al. Fluorouracil, doxorubicin, and cyclophosphamide followed by tamoxifen as adjuvant treatment for patients with stage IV breast cancer with no evidence of disease. *Breast J* 2002; 8:2–9.
28. Hortobagyi GN. Can we cure limited metastatic breast cancer? *J Clin Oncol* 2002; 20:620–623.
29. Sledge Jr GW, Neuberg D, Ingle J, et al. Phase III trial of doxorubicin (A) vs. paclitaxel (T) vs. doxorubicin + paclitaxel (A + T) as first-line therapy for metastatic breast cancer (MBC): An intergroup trial. *Proc Am Soc Clin Oncol* 1997; 16:1a.
30. Nabholtz JM, Falkson G, Campos D, et al. A phase III trial comparing doxorubicin (A) and docetaxel (T) (AT) to doxorubicin and cyclophosphamide (AC) as first-line chemotherapy for MBC. *Proc Am Soc Clin Oncol* 1999; 18:127a.
31. Mackey JR, Paterson A, Dirix LY, et al. Final results of the phase III randomized trial comparing docetaxel (T), doxorubicin (A) and cyclophosphamide (C) to FAC as first line chemotherapy (CT) for patients with metastatic breast cancer. *Proc Am Soc Clin Oncol* 2002; 21: 35a.
32. Slamon DJ, Leyland-Jones B, Shak S, et al. Use of chemotherapy plus a monoclonal antibody against HER2 for metastatic breast cancer that overexpresses HER2. *N Engl J Med* 2001; 344:783–792.
33. Peters WP, Eder JP, Henner WD, et al. High-dose combination chemotherapy with autologous bone marrow support: A phase I trial. *J Clin Oncol* 1986; 4:646–654.
34. Eder JP, Antman K, Peters WP, et al. High dose combination alkylating agent chemotherapy with autologous bone marrow support for metastatic breast cancer. *J Clin Oncol* 1986; 4:646–654.
35. Eder JP, Elias A, Shea TC, et al. A phase I-II study of cyclophosphamide, thiotepa, and carboplatin with autologous bone marrow transplantation in solid tumor patients. *J Clin Oncol* 1990; 8:1239–1245.
36. Williams SF, Bitran JD, Kaminer L, et al. A phase I-II study of bialkylator chemotherapy, high-dose thiotepa, and cyclophosphamide with autologous bone marrow reinfusion in patients with advanced cancer. *J Clin Oncol* 1990; 5:260–265.
37. Peters WP, Shpall EJ, Jones RB, et al. High-dose combination chemotherapy with bone marrow support as initial treatment for metastatic breast cancer. *J Clin Oncol* 1988; 6:1368–1376.
38. Peters WP, Dansey R. New Concepts in the treatment of breast cancer using high-dose chemotherapy. *Cancer Chemother Pharmacol* 1997; 40 (Suppl):S88–S93.
39. Jones RB, Shpall EJ, Ross M, et al. AFM induction chemotherapy followed by intensive alkylating agent consolidation with autologous bone marrow support (ABMS) for advanced breast cancer: current results. *Proc Am Soc Clin Oncol* 1990; 7:121.
40. Rizzieri DA, Vredenburgh JJ, Chao NJ, et al. Long term disease free survival for patients with metastatic breast cancer undergoing aggressive induction therapy followed by high dose therapy with hematopoetic support. *Blood* 1998; 92:323a.
41. Antman K, Ayash L, Elias A, et al. A phase II study of high-dose cyclophosphamide, thiotepa, and carboplatin with autologous bone marrow support in women with measurable advanced breast cancer responding to standard-dose therapy. *J Clin Oncol* 1992;10: 102–110.
42. Williams SF, Gilewski T, Mick R, et al. High-dose consolidation therapy with autologous stem cell rescue in stage IV breast cancer: Follow-up report. *J Clin Oncol* 1992; 10:1743–1747.
43. Laport GF, Grad G, Grinblatt DL, et al. High-dose chemotherapy consolidation with autologous stem cell rescue in metastatic breast cancer: a 10-year experience. *Bone Marrow Transplant* 1998; 21:127–132.
44. Jones RB, Shpall EJ, Shogan J, et al. The Duke AFM program. Intensive induction chemotherapy for metastatic breast cancer. *Cancer* 1990; 66:431–436.
45. Carter DL, Marks LB, Bean JM, et al. Impact of consolidation radiotherapy in patients with advanced breast cancer treated with high-dose chemotherapy and autologous bone marrow rescue. *J Clin Oncol* 1999; 17:887–893.
46. University of Colorado BMTP, unpublished observations.
47. Decker DA, Ahman DL, Bisel HF, et al. Complete responders to chemotherapy in metastatic breast cancer. Characterization and analysis. *JAMA* 1979; 242:2075–2079.
48. Powles TJ, Smith IE, Ford HT, et al. Failure of chemotherapy to prolong survival in a group of patients with metastatic breast cancer. *Lancet* 1980; 1:580–582.
49. Smith GA, Henderson IC. High-dose chemotherapy (HDC) with autologous bone marrow transplantation (ABMT) for the treatment of breast cancer: The jury is still out. In Hellman S, and Rosenberg SA, Important Advances in Oncology 1995, pp 201–214, JB Lippincott Company, Philadelphia, 1995.
50. Rahman ZU, Frye DK, Buzdar AU, et al. Impact of selection process on response rate and long-term survival of potential high-dose chemotherapy candidates treated with standard-dose doxorubicin-containing chemotherapy in patients with metastatic breast cancer. *J Clin Oncol* 1997; 15:3171–3177.
51. Dunphy FR, Spitzer G, Rossiter JE, et al. Factors predicting long-term survival for metastatic breast cancer patients treated with high-dose chemotherapy and bone marrow support. *Cancer* 1994; 73:2157–2167.

52. Ayash LJ, Wheeler C, Fairclough D, et al. Prognostic factors for prolonged progression-free survival with high-dose chemotherapy with autologous stem-cell support for advanced breast cancer. *J Clin Oncol* 1995; 13:2043–2049.
53. Doroshow JH, Somlo G, Ahn C, et al. Prognostic factors predicting progression-free and overall survival in patients with responsive metastatic breast cancer treated with high-dose chemotherapy and bone marrow stem cell reinfusion. Proc Am Soc Clin Oncol 14: 319a, 1995.
54. Rizzieri DA, Vredenburgh JJ, Jones RB, et al. Prognostic and predictive factors for patients with metastatic breast cancer undergoing aggressive induction therapy followed by high dose therapy with autologous stem-cell support. *J Clin Oncol* 1999; 17:3064–3074.
55. Rowlings PA, Williams SF, Antman KH, et al. Factors correlated with progression-free survival after high-dose chemotherapy and hematopoietic stem cell transplantation for metastatic breast cancer. *JAMA* 1999; 282:1335–1343.
56. Nieto Y, Nawaz S, Jones RB, et al. Prognostic model for relapse after high-dose chemotherapy with autologous stem-cell transplantation for stage IV oligometastatic breast cancer. *J Clin Oncol* 2002; 20:707–718.
57. Kim YS, Konoplev SN, Montemurro F, et al. HER-2/neu overexpression as a poor prognostic factor for patients with metastatic breast cancer undergoing high-dose chemotherapy with autologous stem cell transplantation. *Clin Cancer Res* 2001; 7:4008–4012.
58. Bewick M, Chadderton T, Conlon M, et al. Expression of C-erbB-2/HER-2 in patients with metastatic breast cancer undergoing high-dose chemotherapy and autologous blood stem cell support. *Bone Marrow Transplant* 1999; 24:377–384.
59. Nieto Y, Cagnoni PJ, Shpall EJ, et al. Phase II trial of high-dose chemotherapy with autologous stem cell transplant for stage IV patients with minimal metastatic disease. *Clin Cancer Res* 1999; 5:1731–1737.
60. Abraham R, Nagy T, Goss PE, Crump M. High dose chemotherapy and autologous blood stem cell support in women with breast carcinoma and isolated supraclavicular lymph node metastases. *Cancer* 2000, 88.790–795.
61. Stadtmauer EA, O'Neill A, Goldstein LJ, et al. Conventional-dose chemotherapy compared with high-dose chemotherapy plus autologous hematopoietic stem-cell transplantation for metastatic breast cancer. *N Engl J Med* 2000; 342:1069–1076.
62. Stadtmauer EA, O'Neill L, Goldstein LJ, et al. Conventional-dose chemotherapy compared with high-dose chemotherapy (HDC) plus autologous stem-cell transplantation (SCT) for metastatic breast cancer: 5-year update of the 'Philadelphia Trial' (PBT-01). *Proc Am Soc Clin Oncol* 2002; 12:43a.
63. Livingston R, Crowley J. Commentary on PBT-1 study of high-dose consolidation versus standard therapy in metastatic breast cancer. *J Clin Oncol* 1999; 17 (11S, November supplement):22–24.
64. Crump M, Gluck S, Stewart D, et al. A randomized trial of high-dose chemotherapy (HDC) with autologous peripheral blood stem cell support (AHPCT) compared to standard chemotherapy in women with metastatic breast cancer: A National Cancer Institute of Canada (NCIC) Clinical Trials Group study. Proc Am Soc Clin Oncol 20: 21a, 2001 (abstr 82).
65. Biron P, Durand M, Roché H, et al. High dose thiotepa (TTP), cyclophosphamide (CPM) and stem cell transplantation after 4 FEC 100 compared with 4 FEC alone allowed a better disease free survival but the same overall survival in first line chemotherapy for metastatic breast cancer. Results of the PEGASE 03 French protocol. *Proc Am Soc Clin Oncol* 2002; 21: 42a.
66. Crown, J, Perey L, Lind M, et al. Superiority of tandem high-dose chemotherapy (HDC) versus optimized conventionally-dosed chemotherapy (CDC) in patients (pts) with metastatic breast cancer (MBC): The International Breast Cancer Dose Intensity Study (IBDIS 1). *Proc Am Soc Clin Oncol* 2003; 22:23a.
67. Lotz J-P, Curé H, Janvier M, et al. Intensive chemotherapy and autograft of hematopoietic stem cells in the treatment of metastatic breast cancer: Results of the national protocol PEGASE 04 [French]. *Hematol Cell Ther* 1999; 41:71–74.
68. Schmid P, Samonigg H, Nitsch T, et al. Randomized trial of up front tandem high-dose chemotherapy (HD) compared to standard chemotherapy with doxorubicin and paclitaxel (AT) in metastatic breast cancer (MBC). *Proc Am Soc Clin Oncol* 2002; 21:43a.
69. Peters WP, Jones RB, Vredenburgh J, et al. A large, prospective, randomized trial of high-dose combination alkylating agents (CPB) with autologous cellular support (ABMS) as consolidation for patients with metastatic breast cancer achieving complete remission after intensive doxorubicin-based induction therapy (AFM). *Proc Am Soc Clin Oncol* 1996;15: 121a.
70. Vredenburgh JJ. Personal communication.
71. Madan B, Broadwater G, Rubin P, et al. Improved survival with consolidation high-dose cyclophosphamide, cisplatin and carmustine (HD-CPB) compared with observation in women with metastatic breast cancer (MBC) and only bone metastases treated with induction adriamycin, 5-fluorouracil and methotrexate (AFM): A phase III prospective randomized comparative trial. *Proc Am Soc Clin Oncol* 2000; 19:48a.
72. Berry D, Broadwater G, Klein JP, et al. High-dose versus standard chemotherapy in metastatic breast cancer: Comparison of Cancer and Leukemia Group B trials with data from the Autologous Blood and Marrow Transplant Registry. *J Clin Oncol* 2002; 20:743–750.

73. Bonadonna G, Valagussa P. Adjuvant systemic therapy for resectable breast cancer. *J Clin Oncol* 1985; 3:259–275.
74. Bonadonna G, Zambetti M, Valagussa P. Sequential or alternating doxorubicin and CMF regimens in breast cancer with more than three positive nodes. Ten-year results. *JAMA* 1995; 273:542–547.
75. Mamounas EP, Bryant J, Lembersky BC, et al. Paclitaxel (T) following doxorubicin/cyclophosphamide (AC) as adjuvant chemotherapy for node-positive breast cancer: Results from NSABP B-28. *Proc Am Soc Clin Oncol* 2003; 22:4a.
76. Buzdar AU, Singletary SE, Valero V, et al. Evaluation of Paclitaxel in adjuvant chemotherapy for patients with operable breast cancer: preliminary data of a prospective randomized trial. Clin Cancer Res 2002; 8:1073–1079.
77. Nabholtz J-M, Pienkowski T, Mackey J, et al. Phase III trial comparing TAC (docetaxel, doxorubicin, cyclophosphamide) with FAC (5-flurouracil, doxorubicin, cyclophosphamide) in the adjuvant treatment of node positive breast cancer patients: Interim analysis of the BCIRG 001 study. *Proc Am Soc Clin Oncol* 2002; 21:36a.
78. Citron ML, Berry DA, Cirrincione C, et al. Randomized trial of dose-dense versus conventionally scheduled and sequential versus concurrent combination chemotherapy as postoperative adjuvant treatment of node-positive primary breast cancer: first report of Intergroup Trial C9741/Cancer and Leukemia Group B Trial 9741. *J Clin Oncol* 2003; 21:1431–1439.
79. Peters WP, Ross M, Vredenburgh JJ, et al. High-dose chemotherapy and autologous bone marrow suppport as consolidation after standard-dose adjuvant therapy for high-risk primary breast cancer. *J Clin Oncol* 1993; 11:1132–1143.
80. Nikcevich DA, Vredenburgh JJ, Broadwater G, et al. Ten year follow-up after high-dose chemotherapy and autologous bone marrow support as consolidation after standard-dose adjuvant therapy for high-risk primary breast cancer. *Proc Am Soc Clin Oncol* 2002; 21:415a.
81. Nieto Y, Shpall EJ, Bearman SI, et al. Long-term analysis of high-risk primary breast cancer patients enrolled in prospective trials of high-dose chemotherapy and autologous hematopoietic progenitor cell transplant. *Biol Blood Marrow Transplant* 2003; 9:72a.
82. Gianni AM, Siena S, Bregni M, et al. Efficacy, toxicity and applicability of high-dose chemotherapy as adjuvant treatment in operable breast cancer with 10 or more involved axillary nodes: Five-year results. *J Clin Oncol* 1997; 15:2312–2321.
83. Buzzoni R, Bonadonna G, Valagussa P, et al. Adjuvant chemotherapy with doxorubicin plus cyclophosphamide, methotrexate and fluorouracil in the treatment of resectable breast cancer with more than three positive nodes. *J Clin Oncol* 1991; 9:2134–2140.
84. Bearman SI, Overmoyer BA, Bolwell BJ, et al. High-dose chemotherapy with autologous peripheral blood progenitor cell support for primary breast cancer in patients with 4-9 involved axillary lymph nodes. *Bone Marrow Transplantation* 1997; 20:931–937.
85. Hussein A, Plummer M, Vredenburgh J, et al. High-dose chemotherapy (HDC) with cyclophosphamide, cisplatin, and BCNU (CPB) and autologous bone marrow and peripheral blood progenitor cells for stage II/III breast cancer involving 4-9 axillary lymph nodes. *Proc Am Soc Clin Oncol* 1996; 15:350a.
86. De Graaf H, Willemse PHB, De Vries EGE, et al. Intensive chemotherapy with autologous bone marrow transfusion as primary treatment in women with breast cancer and more than five involved axillary lymph nodes. *Eur J Cancer* 1994; 30A,150–153.
87. Hortobagyi GN, Singletary SE, Strom EA. Treatment of locally advanced and inflammatory breast cancer. In Diseases of the Breast (JR Harris, editor). Lippincott Williams & Wilkins, Philadelphia, 2000.
88. Ayash L, Elias A, Ibrahim J, et al. High-dose multimodality therapy with autologous stem cell support for stage IIIB breast cancer. *J Clin Oncol* 1998; 16:1000–1007.
89. Cagnoni PJ, Nieto Y, Shpall EJ, et al. High-dose chemotherapy with autologous progenitor cell support as part of combined modality therapy for inflammatory breast cancer. *J Clin Oncol* 1998; 16:1661–1668.
90. Viens P, Penault-Llorca F, Jacquemier J, et al. High-dose chemotherapy and haematopoietic stem cell transplantation for inflammatory breast cancer: pathologic response and outcome. *Bone marrow Transplant* 1998; 21:249–254.
91. Somlo G, Doroshow JH, Forman SJ, et al. High-dose chemotherapy and stem-cell rescue in the treatment of high-risk breast cancer: Prognostic indicators of progression-free and overall survival. *J Clin Oncol* 1997; 15:2882–2893.
92. Adkins D, Brown R, Trinkaus K, et al. Outcomes of high-dose chemotherapy and autologous stem-cell transplantation in stage IIIB inflammatory breast cancer. *J Clin Oncol* 1999; 17:2006–2014.
93. Nieto Y, Cagnoni PJ, Xu X, et al. Predictive model for relapse after high-dose chemotherapy with peripheral blood progenitor cell support for high-risk primary breast cancer. *Clin Cancer Res* 1999; 5:3425–3431.
94. Bolwell BJ, Andresen SW, Pohlman BL, et al. The prognostic importance of the axillary lymph node ratio in autologous transplantation for high-risk stage II-III breast cancer. *Proc Am Soc Clin Oncol* 2000; 19:57a.
95. Prósper F, Sola C, Hornedo J, et al. Prognostic factors for relapse after high-dose chemotherapy (HDC) and stem cell transplant (SCT) in patients with high risk breast cancer (HRBC). *Proc Am Soc Clin Oncol* 2000; 19:147a.

96. Schneeweiss A, Goerner R, Hensel MA, et al. Tandem high-dose chemotherapy in high-risk primary breast cancer: a multivariate analysis and a matched-pair comparison with standard-dose chemotherapy. *Biol Blood Marrow Transplant* 2001; 7:332–342.
97. University of Colorado BMT Program, unpublished observations.
98. Bitran JD, Samuels B, Trujillo Y, et al. Her2/neu overexpression is associated with treatment failure in women with high-risk stage II and stage IIIA breast cancer (>10 involved lymph nodes) treated with high-dose chemotherapy and autologous hematopoietic progenitor cell support following standard-dose adjuvant chemotherapy. *Clin Cancer Res* 1996; 2:1509–1513.
99. Nieto Y, Cagnoni PJ, Nawaz S, et al. Evaluation of the predictive value of HER2/neu overexpression and p53 mutations in high-risk primary breast cancer patients treated with high-dose chemotherapy and autologous stem-cell transplantation. *J Clin Oncol* 2000; 18: 2070–2080.
100. Crump M, Goss PE, Prince M, et al. Outcome of extensive evaluation before adjuvant therapy in women with breast cancer and ten or more positive axillary lymph nodes. *J Clin Oncol* 1996; 14:66–69.
101. García-Carbonero R, Hidalgo M, Paz-Ares L, et al. Patient selection in high-dose chemotherapy trials: Relevance in high-risk breast cancer. J Clin Oncol 15: 3178–3184, 1997.
102. Schrama JG, Faneyte IF, Schornagel JH, et al. Randomized trial of high-dose chemotherapy and hematopoietic progenitor-cell support in operable breast cancer with extensive lymph node involvement: final analysis with 7 years of follow-up. *Ann Oncol* 2002; 13:689–698.
103. Hortobagyi GN, Buzdar AU, Theriault RL, et al. Randomized trial of high-dose chemotherapy and blood cell autografts for high-risk primary breast carcinoma. *J Natl Cancer Inst* 2000; 92:225–233.
104. Dunphy FR, Spitzer G, Buzdar AU, et al. Treatment of estrogen receptor-negative or hormonally refractory breast cancer with double high-dose chemotherapy intensification and bone marrow support. *J Clin Oncol* 1990; 8:1207–1216.
105. Neidhart JE, Kohler W, Stidley C, et al. A phase I study of repeated cycles of high-dose cyclophosphamide, etoposide and cisplatin administered without bone marrow transplantation. *J Clin Oncol* 1990; 8:1728–1738.
106. Rodenhuis S, Bontenbal M, Beex LVAM, et al. High-dose chemotherapy with hematopoietic stem-cell rescue for high-risk breast cancer. *N Engl J Med* 2003; 349:7–16.
107. Peters WP, Rosner G, Vredenburgh J, et al. Updated results of a prospective, randomized comparison of two doses of combination alkylating agents (AA) as consolidation after CAF in high-risk primary breast cancer involving ten or more axillary lymph nodes (LN): CALGB 9082/SWOG 9114/NCIC Ma-13. *Proc Am Soc Clin Oncol* 2001; 20:21a.
108. Marks LB, Fitzgerald TJ, Laurie F, et al. Preliminary analysis of radiotherapy data from CALGB 9082: Variability of treatment fields for local/regional breast cancer and the impact of high dose chemotherapy on the ability to deliver radiation therapy. *Int J Rad Oncol Biol Phys* 1999; 45 (Suppl):195a.
109. Winer EP, Herndon J, Peters WP, et al. Quality of life in patients with breast cancer randomized to high dose chemotherapy with bone marrow support vs. intermediate dose chemotherapy: CALGB 9066 (companion protocol to CALGB 9082). *Proc Am Soc Clin Oncol* 1999; 18:412a.
110. Tallman M, Gray R, Robert N, et al. Conventional adjuvant chemotherapy with or without high-dose chemotherapy and autologous stem-cell transplantation in high-risk breast cancer. *N Engl J Med* 2003; 349:17–26.
111. Bergh J, Wiklund T, Erikstein B, et al. Tailored fluoruracil, epirubicin, and cyclophosphamide compared with marrow-supported high-dose chemotherapy as adjuvant treatment for high-risk breast cancer: a randomised trial. *Lancet* 2000; 356:1384–1391.
112. Antman KH. Critique of the high-dose chemotherapy studies in breast cancer: A positive look at the data. *J Clin Oncol* 1999; 17 (11S, November Supplement):30-35.
113. Crown JP, Lind M, Gould A, et al. High-dose chemotherapy (HDC) with autograft (PBP) support is not superior to cyclophosphamide (CPA), methotrexate and 5-FU (CMF) following doxorubicin (D) induction in patients (pts) with breast cancer and 4 or more involved acillary lymph nodes (4+ LN): The Anglo-Celtic I study. *Proc Am Soc Clin Oncol* 2002; 21:42a.
114. Zander AR, Krüger W, Kröger N, et al. High-dose chemotherapy with autologous hematopoietic stem-cell support (HSCS) vs. standard-dose chemotherapy in breast cancer patients with 10 or more positive lymph nodes: first results of a randomized trial. *Proc Am Soc Clin Oncol* 2002; 21:415a.
115. Roché HH, Pouillart P, Meyer N, et al. Adjuvant high dose chemotherapy (HDC) improves early outcome for high risk (N>7) breast cancer patients: The PEGASE 01 trial. *Proc Am Soc Clin Oncol* 2001; 20:27a.
116. Nitz UA, Frick M, Mohrmann S, et al. Tandem high dose chemotherapy versus dose-dense conventional chemotherapy for patients with high risk breast cancer: Interim results from a multicenter phase III trial. *Proc Am Soc Clin Oncol* 2003; 22:832a.
117. Gianni A, Bonadonna G. Five-year results of the randomized clinical trial comparing standard versus high-dose myeloablative chemotherapy in the adjuvant treatment of breast cancer with >3 positive nodes (LN+). *Proc Am Soc Clin Oncol* 2001; 20:21a.
118. Basser R, O'Neill A, Martinelli G, et al. Randomized trial comparing up-front, multi-cycle dose-intensive chemotherapy (CT) versus standard dose CT in women with high-risk stage 2 or 3 breast cancer (BC): First results from IBCSG trial 15-95. *Proc Am Soc Clin Oncol* 2003; 22:6a.

119. Philip T, Chauvin F, Bron D, et al. PARMA international protocol: Pilot study on 50 patients and preliminary analysis of the ongoing randomized study (62 patients). *Ann Oncol* 1991; 2:57–64.
120. Bron D, Philip T, Guglielmi C, et al. The PARMA international randomized study in relapsed non-Hodgkin's lymphoma. Analysis on the first 153 preincluded patients. *Exp Hematol* 1991; 19(6):546.
121. Philip T, Guglielmi C, Hagenbeek A, et al. Autologous bone marrow transplantation as compared with salvage chemotherapy in relapses of chemotherapy-sensitive non-Hodgkin's lymphoma. *N Engl J Med* 1995; 333:1540–1545.
122. Sledge GW, Loehrer PJ, Roht BJ, Einhorn LH. Cisplatin as first-line therapy for metastatic breats cancer. *J Clin Oncol* 1988; 6:1811–1814.
123. Martín M, Díaz-Rubio E, Casado A, et al. Carboplatin: An active drug in metastatic breast cancer. *J Clin Oncol* 1992; 10:433–437.
124. Tew K, Colvin OM, Chabner BA. Alkylating agents. In: BA Chabner and DL Longo (eds), Cancer Chemotherapy and Biotherapy, 2nd edition, pp 297–332. Philadelphia: Lippincott-Raven, 1996.
125. Huitema ADR, Tibben MM, Kerbusch TH, et al. Simultaneous determination of thiotepa, cyclophosphamide and some metabolites in plasma using capillary gas chromatography. *J Chromatogr* 1998; B 716:177–186.
126. Chen T-L, Passos-Coelho JL, Noe DA, et al. Nonlinear pharmacokinetics of cyclophosphamide in patients with metastatic breast cancer receiving high-dose chemotherapy followed by autologous bone marrow transplantation. *Cancer Res* 1996; 55:810–816.
127. Nieto Y, Xu X, Cagnoni PJ, et al. Nonpredictable pharmacokinetic behavior of high-dose cyclophosphamide in combination with cisplatin and 1,3-bis(2-chloroethyl)-1-nitrosourea. *Clin Cancer Res* 1999; 5:747–751.
128. Busse D, Busch FW, Bohnenstengel F, Eichelbaum M, Fischer P, Opalinska J, Schumacher K, Schweizer E, Kroemer HK. Dose escalation of cyclophosphamide in patients with breast cancer: Consequences for pharmacokinetics and metabolism. *J Clin Oncol* 1997; 15: 1885–1896.
129. Doroshow JH. Anthracyclines and anthracenediones. In: Chabner BA and Longo DL (eds). Cancer Chemotherapy and Biotherapy. Lippincott-Raven, 2nd ed., 1996.
130. Eisenhauer EA, Ten Bokkel Huinink WW, Swenerton KD, et al. European-Canadian randomized trial of paclitaxel in relapsed ovarian cancer: High-dose versus low-dose and long versus short infusion. *J Clin Oncol* 1994; 12:2654–2666.
131. Kohn EC, Sarosy G, Bicher A, et al. Dose intense taxol: High response rate in patients with platinum resistant recurrent ovarian cancer. *J Natl Cancer Inst* 1994; 86:18–24.
132. Raymond E, Hanauske A, Faivre S, et al. Effects of prolonged versus short-term exposure paclitaxel on human tumor colony-forming units. *Anticancer Drugs* 1997; 8:379-385.
133. Hanauske AR, Degen D, Hilsenbeck SG, et al. Effects of Taxotere and Taxol in vitro colony formation of freshly explanted human tumour cells. Anticancer Drugs 3: 121–124, 1992
134. García P, Braguer D, Carkes G, et al. Comparative effects of taxol and taxotere on two different human carcinoma cell lines. *Cancer Chemother Pharmacol* 1994; 34:335–343.
135. Von Hoff DD. The taxoids: same roots, different drugs. *Semin Oncol* 1997; 24(4 Suppl 13):S13–3–S13–10.
136. Somlo G, Doroshow JH, Forman SJ, et al. High-dose doxorubicin, etoposide, and cyclophosphamide with stem cell reinfusion in patients with metastatic or high-risk primary breast cancer. *Cancer* 1994; 15:1678–1685.
137. Donehower RC, Rowinsky EK, Grochow LB,et al. Phase I trial of taxol in patients with advanced cancer. *Cancer Treatment Reports* 1987; 71:1171–1177.
138. Aapro MS, Zulian G, Alberto P, et al. Phase I and pharmacokinetic study of RP 569876 in a new ethanol-free formulation of Taxotere. *Ann Oncol* 1992; 3(Suppl 5):208.
139. Extra JM, Rousseau F, Bruno R, et al. Phase I and pharmacokinetic study of Taxotere (RP 569876; NSC 628503) given as a short intravenous infusion. *Cancer Res* 1993; 53:1037–1042.
140. Stemmer SM, Cagnoni PJ, Shpall EJ, et al. High-dose paclitaxel, cyclophosphamide, and cisplatin with autologous hematopoietic progenitor-cell support: A phase I trial. *J Clin Oncol* 1996; 14:1463–1472.
141. Holmes FA, Walters RS, Theriault RL, et al. Phase II trial of taxol, an active drug in the treatment of metastatic breast cancer. *J Natl Cancer Inst* 1991; 83:1797–1805.
142. Smith RE, Brown AM, Mamounas EP, et al. Randomized trial of 3-hour versus 24-hour infusion of high-dose paclitaxel in patients with metastatic or locally advanced breast cancer: National Surgical Adjuvant Breast and Bowel Project protocol B-26. *J Clin Oncol* 1999; 17: 3403–3411.

143. Buzdar AU, Singletary E, Theriault RL, et al. Prospective evaluation of paclitaxel versus combination chemotherapy with fluorouracil, doxorubicin, and cyclophosphamide as neoadjuvant therapy in patients with operable breast cancer. *J Clin Oncol* 1999; 17:3412–3417.
144. Fields KK, Elfenbein GJ, Perkins JB, et al. High versus standard dose chemotherapy for the treatment of breast cancer. *Annals New York Academy of Sciences* 1995;770: 288–304.
145. Mayordomo JI, Yubero A, Cajal R, et al. Phase I trial of high-dose paclitaxel in combination with cyclophosphamide, thiotepa and carboplatin with autologous peripheral blood stem cell rescue. *Proc Am Soc Clin Oncol* 1997; 16:102a.
146. Vahdat LT, Papadopoulos KP, Balmaceda C, et al. Phase I trial of sequential high-dose chemotherapy with escalating dose paclitaxel, melphalan and cyclophosphamide, thiotepa, and carboplatin with peripheral blood progenitor support in women with responding metastatic breast cancer. *Clin Cancer Res* 1998; 4:1689–1695.
147. Elias AD, Richardson P, Avigan D, et al. A short course of induction chemotherapy followed by two cycles of high-dose chemotherapy with stem cell rescue for chemotherapy naive metastatic breast cancer. *Bone Marrow Transplant* 2001; 27:269–278.
148. Hu WW, Negrin RS, Stockerl-Goldstein K, et al. Four-cycle high-dose therapy with hematopoeitic support for metastatic breast cancer: No improvement in outcomes compared with single-course high-dose therapy. *Biol Blood Marrow Transplant* 2000; 6:58–69.
149. Nabholtz JM, Reese DM, Lindsay MA, Riva A. Docetaxel in the treatment of breast cancer: an update on recent studies. *Semin Oncol* 2002; 29 (3 Suppl 12):28–34.
150. Hanauske AR, Degen D, Hilsenbeck SG, et al. Effects of Taxotere and Taxol in vitro colony formation of freshly explanted human tumour cells. *Anticancer Drugs* 1992; 3:121–124.
151. Garcia P, Braguer D, Carkes G, et al. Comparative effects of taxol and taxotere on two different human carcinoma cell lines. *Cancer Chemother Pharmacol* 1994; 34:335–343.
152. Nieto Y, Cagnoni PJ, Shpall EJ, et al. Phase I trial of docetaxel (DTX) (Taxotere) with peripheral blood progenitor cell (PBPC) support, with melphalan and carboplatin, in refractory advanced cancer. *Proc Am Soc Clin Oncol* 2000; 19:56a.
153. Dunphy FR, Spitzer G, Buzdar AU, et al: Treatment of estrogen receptor-negative or hormonally refractory breast cancer with double high-dose chemotherapy intensification and bone marrow support. *J Clin Oncol* 1990; 8:1207–1216.
154. Crown J, Kritz A, Vahdat L, et al. Rapid administration of multiple cycles of high-dose myelosuppressive chemotherapy in patients with metastatic breast cancer. *J Clin Oncol* 1993; 11:1144–1149.
155. Shapiro CL, Ayash L, Webb IJ, et al. Repetitive cycles of cyclophosphamide, thiotepa, and carboplatin intensification with peripheral-blood progenitor cells and filgrastim in advanced breast cancer patients. *J Clin Oncol* 1997;15:674–683.
156. Ayash LJ, Elias A, Wheeler C, et al. Double dose-intensive chemotherapy with autologous marrow and peripheral-blood progenitor-cell support for metastatic breast cancer: A feasibility study. *J Clin Oncol* 1994; 12:37–44.
157. Rodenhuis S, Westermann A, Holtkamp MJ, et al. Feasibility of multiple courses of high-dose cyclophosphamide, thiotepa, and carboplatin for breast cancer or germ cell cancer. *J Clin Oncol* 1996; 14:1473–1483.
158. Broun ER, Sridhara R, Sledge GW, et al. Tandem autotransplantion for the treatment of metastatic breast cancer. *J Clin Oncol* 1995; 13:2050–2055.
159. Ayash LJ, Elias A, Schwartz G, et al. Double dose-intensive chemotherapy with autologous stem-cell support for metastatic breast cancer: No improvement in progression-free survival by the sequence of high-dose melphalan followed by cyclophosphamide, thiotepa, and carboplatin. *J Clin Oncol* 1996; 14:2984–2992.
160. Bitran JD, Samuels B, Klein L, et al. Tandem high-dose chemotherapy supported by hematopoietic progenitor cells yields prolonged survival in stage IV breast cancer. *Bone Marrow Transplant* 1996; 17:157–162.
161. Vahdat L, Balmaceda C, Papadopoulos K, et al. Phase II trial of sequential high-dose chemotherapy with paclitaxel, melphalan, and cyclophosphamide, thiotepa, and carboplatin with peripheral blood progenitor support in women with responding metastatic breast cancer. *Bone Marrow Transplant* 2002; 30:149–155.
162. Elias AD, Ibrahim J, Richardson P, et al. The impact of induction duration and the number of high-dose cycles on the long-term survival of women with metastatic breast cancer treated with high-dose chemotherapy with stem cell rescue: An analysis of sequential phase I/II trials from the Dana Farber/Beth Israel STAMP program. *Biol Blood Marrow Transplant* 2002; 8:198–205.

163. Teicher BA, Ara G, Keyes SR, et al. Acute in vivo resistance in high-dose therapy. *Clin Cancer Res* 1998; 4:483–491.
164. Frei E III, Ara G, Teicher B, Bunnell C, Richardson P, Wheeler C, Tew K, Elias A. Double high-dose chemotherapy with stem cell rescue (HD-SCR) in patients with breast cancer-effect of sequence. *Cancer Chemother Pharmacol* 2000; 45:239–246.
165. Slamon DJ, Clark G, Wong S, et al. Human breast cancer: correlation of relapse and survival with amplification of the HER2/neu oncogene. *Science* 1987; 2235:177–181.
166. Baselga J, Tripathy D, Mendelsohn J, et al. Phase II study of weekly intravenous recombinant humanized anti-p185HER2 monoclonal antibody in patients with HER2/neu-overexpressing metastatic breast cancer. *J Clin Oncol* 1996; 14:737–744.
167. Cobleigh MA, Vogel CL, Tripathy D, et al. Multinational study of the efficacy and safety of humanized anti-HER2 monoclonal antibody in women who have HER2-over-expressing metastatic breast cancer that has progressed after chemotherapy for metastatic disease. *J Clin Oncol* 1999; 17:2639–2648.
168. Hancock MC, Langton BC, Chan T, et al. A monoclonal antibody against the c-erB-2 protein enhances the cytotoxicity of cis-diamminedichloroplatinum against human breast and ovarian tumor cell lines. *Cancer Res* 1991;51:4575–4580.
169. Arteaga CL, Winnier AR, Poirier MC, et al. p185c-erbB-2 signaling enhances cisplatin-induced cytotoxicity in human breast carcinoma cells: Association between an oncogenic receptor tyrosine kinase and drug–induced DNA repair. *Cancer Res* 1994; 54:3758–3765.
170. Pietras RJ, Fendly BM, Chazin VR, et al. Antibody to HER2 receptor blocks DNA repair after cisplatin in human breast and ovarian cancer cells. *Oncogene* 1994; 9:1829–1838.
171. Slamon DL. Alteration of the HER2/neu gene in human breast cancer: Diagnostic and therapeutic implications. Rosenthal Award Lecture at the 90th Annual Meeting of the American Association for Cancer Research (AACR), Philadelphia, PA, April 10–14, 1999.
172. Pegram MD, Lipton A, Hayes DF, et al. Phase II study of receptor-enhanced chemosensitivity using recombinant humanized anti-p185HER2/neu monoclonal antibody plus cisplatin in patients with HER2/neu-overexpressing metastatic breast cancer refractory to chemotherapy treatment. *J Clin Oncol* 1998; 16:2659–2671.
173. Nieto Y, Vredenburgh JJ, Shpall EJ, et al. Pilot phase II study of concurrent administration of trastuzumab and high-dose chemotherapy in advanced HER2+ breast cancer. *Proc Am Soc Clin Oncol* 2002; 21:416a.
174. De Magalhaes-Silverman M, Bloom E, Lembersky B, et al. High-dose chemotherapy and autologous stem cell support followed by posttransplantation doxorubicin as initial therapy for metastatic breast cancer. *Clin Cancer Res* 1997; 3:193–197.
175. Rahman Z, Kavanagh J, Champlin R, et al. Chemotherapy immediately following autologous stem-cell transplantation in patients with advanced breast cancer. *Clin Cancer Res* 1998; 4:2717–2721.
176. Douer D, Levine A, Anderson WF, Gordon M, Groshen S, Khan A, et al. High-dose chemotherapy and autologous bone marrow plus peripheral blood stem cell transplantation for patients with lymphoma or metastatic breast cancer: use of marker genes to investigate hematopoietic reconstitution in adults. Human Gene Therapy 1996; 7:669–684.
177. Hanania EG, Fu S, Roninson I, Zu Z, Deisseroth AB. Resistance to taxol chemotherapy produced in mouse marrow cells by safety-modified retroviruses containing a human MDR-1 transcription unit. Gene Therapy 1995; 2:279–284.
178. Hanania EG, Fu S, Zu Z, Hegewisch-Becker S, et al. Chemotherapy resistance to taxol in clonogenic progenitor cells following transduction of CD34 selected marrow and peripheral blood cells with a retrovirus that contains the MDR-1 chemotherapy resistance gene. *Gene Therapy* 1995; 2:285–294.
179. Rahman Z, Kavanagh J, Champlin R, et al. Chemotherapy immediately following autologous stem-cell transplantation in patients with advanced breast cancer. *Clin Cancer Res* 1998; 4:2717–2721.
180. Porrata LF, Ingle JN, Litzow MR, Geyer SM, Markovic SN. Prolonged survival associated with early lymphocyte recovery after autologous stem cell transplantation for patients with metastatic breast cancer. *Bone Marrow Transplant* 2001; 28:865-871.
181. Nieto Y, Jones RB, Bearman SI, McNiece IK, McSweeney PA, Shpall EJ. Prognostic analysis of the early lymphocyte recovery in patients with advanced breast cancer receiving high-dose chemotherapy with an autologous hematopoietic progenitor cell transplant. *Biol Blood Marrow Transplant* 2003; 9: 72a.
182. Kennedy MJ, Vogelsang GB, Beveridge RA, et al. Phase I trial of intravenous cyclosporine to induce graft-versus-host disease in women undergoing autologous bone marrow transplantation for breast cancer. *J Clin Oncol* 1993; 11:478–484.
183. Kennedy MJ, Vogelsang GB, Jones RJ, et al. Phase I trial of interferon gamma to potentiate cyclosporine-induced graft-versus-host disease in women undergoing autologous bone marrow transplantation for breast cancer. *J Clin Oncol* 1994; 12:249–257.

184. Stiff PJ, Bayer R, Tan S, et al. High-dose chemotherapy combined with escalating doses of cyclosporin A and an autologous bone marrow transplant for the treatment of drug-resistant solid tumors: a phase I clinical trail. *Clin Cancer Res* 1995;1:1495–1502.
185. Burns LJ, Weisdorf DJ, DeFor TE, et al. Enhancement of the anti-tumor activity of a peripheral blood progenitor cell graft by mobilization with interleukin-2 plus granulocyte colony-stimulating factor in patients with advanced breast cancer. *Exp Hematol* 2000; 28: 96–103.
186. Sosman JA, Stiff P, Moss SM, et al. Pilot trial of interleukin-2 with granulocyte colony-stimulating factor for the mobilization fo progenitor cells in advanced breast cancer patients undergoing high-dose chemotherapy: Expansion of immune effectors within the stem-cell graft and post-stem-cell infusion. *J Clin Oncol* 2001; 19:634–644.
187. Morse MA, Vredenburgh JJ, Lyerly HK. A comparative study of the generation of dendritic cells from mobilized peripheral blood progenitor cells of patients undergoing high–dose chemotherapy. *J Hematother Stem Cell Res* 1999; 8:577–584.
188. Asavaroengchai W, Kotera Y, Mulé J. Tumor lysate-pulsed dendritic cells can elicit an effective antitumor immune response during early lymphoid recovery. *PNAS* 2002; 99:931–936.
189. De Gast GC, Vyth-Dreese FA, Nooijen W, et al. Reinfusion of autologous lymphocytes with granulocyte-macrophage colony-stimulating factor induces rapid recovery of CD4+ and CD8+ T cells after high-dose chemotherapy for metastatic breast cancer. *J Clin Oncol* 2002; 20:58–64.
190. Ross AA, Cooper BW, Lazarus HM, et al: Detection and viability of tumor cells in peripheral blood stem cell collections from breast cancer patients using immunocytochemical and clonogenic assay techniques. *Blood* 1993; 82:2605.
191. Schoenfeld A, Kruger KH, Gomm J, et al. The detection of micrometastases in the peripheral blood and bone marrow of patients with breast cancer using immunohistochemistry and reverse transcriptase polymerase chain reaction for keratin 19. *Eur J Cancer* 1997; 33:854–861.
192. Datta YH, Adams PT, Drobyski WR, Ethier SP, Terry VH, Roth MS. Sensitive detection of occult breast cancer by the reverse-transcriptase polymerase chain reaction. *J Clin Oncol* 1994; 12:475–482.
193. Fields KK, Elfenbein GJ, Trudeau WL. Clinical significance of bone marrow metastases in patients with breast cancer undergoing high-dose chemotherapy and autologous bone marrow transplantation. *J Clin Oncol* 1996; 14:1868–1876.
194. Franklin W, Shpall EJ, Archer P, et al: Immunocytochemical detection of breast cancer cells in marrow and peripheral blood of patients undergoing high dose chemotherapy with autologous stem cell support. Breast Cancer Research and Treatment 41: 1–13, 1996.
195. Sharp JC, Kessinger A, Mann S, et al: Detection and clinical significance of minimal tumor cell contamination of peripheral blood stem cell harvests. *International Journal of Cell Cloning* 1992; 10 (suppl 1):92–94.
196. Vredenburgh J, Silva O, Broadwater G, et al: The significance of tumor contamination in the bone marrow from high-risk primary breast cancer patients treated with high-dose chemotherapy and hematopoietic support. *Biol Blood Marrow Transplantation* 1997;3: 91–97.
197. Umiel T, Moss TJ, Cooper B, et al. The prognostic value of bone marrow micro-metastases in stage II/III breast cancer patients undergoing autologous transplant (ABMT) therapy. Proc Am Soc Clin Oncol 17: 79a, 1998.
198. Solano C, Badia B, Lluch A, et al. Prognostic significance of the immunocytochemical detection of contaminating tumor cells (CTC) in apheresis products of patients with high-risk breast cancer treated with high-dose chemotherapy and stem cell transplantation. *Bone Marrow Transplant* 2001; 27:287–293.
199. Cooper BW, Moss TJ, Ross AA, Ybanez J, and Lazarus HM. Occult tumor contamination of hematopoietic stem-cell product does not affect clinical outcome of autologous transplantation in patients with metastatic breast cancer. *J Clin Oncol* 1998; 16:3509–3517.
200. Shpall EJ, Jones RB, Bast RC, et al: 4-Hydroperoxycyclophosphamide purging of breast cancer from the mononuclear cell fraction of bone marrow in patients receiving high-dose chemotherapy and autologous marrow support: A phase I trial. *J Clin Oncol* 1991; 9:85–93.
201. Shpall EJ, Bast RC, Joines WT, et al: Immunomagnetic purging of breast cancer from bone marrow for autologous transplantation. *Bone Marrow Transplantation* 1991; 7:145–151.
202. Anderson IC, Shpall EJ, Leslie DS, et al. Elimination of malignant clonogenic breast cancer cells from human bone marrow. *Cancer Research* 1989; 15:4659.
203. Vredenburgh JJ, Hussein A, Rubin P, et al: High-dose chemotherapy and immuno-magnetically purged peripheral blood progenitor cells and bone marrow for metastatic breast carcinoma. *Proc Am Soc Clin Oncol* 1996; 15:339.
204. Krause DS, Fackler MJ, Civin CI, and Stratford May W: CD34: Structure, biology and clinical utility. *Blood* 1996; 87:1–13.

205. Shpall EJ, Jones RB, Bearman SI, et al: Transplantation of enriched CD34-positive autologous marrow into breast cancer patients following high-dose chemotherapy: Influence of CD34-positive peripheral-blood progenitors and growth factors on engraftment. *J Clin Oncol* 1994; 12: 28–36.
206. University of Colorado BMT Program, unpublished observations.
207. Shpall EJ, LeMaistre CF, Holland K, et al. A prospective randomized trial of buffy coat versus CD34-selected autologous bone marrow support in high-risk breast cancer patients receiving high-dose chemotherapy. *Blood* 1997; 90:4313–4320.
208. Yanovich S, Mitsky P, Cornetta K, et al. Transplantation of CD34+ peripheral blood cells selected using a fully automated immunomagnetic system in patients with high-risk breast cancer: results of a prospective randomized multicenter clinical trial. *Bone Marrow Transplant* 2000; 25:1165–1174.
209. University of Colorado BMTP, unpublished observations.
210. Mohr M, Hilgenfeld E, Fietz T, et al. Efficacy and safety of simultaneous immuno-magnetic CD34+ cell selection and breast cancer cell purging in peripheral blood progenitor cell samples used for hematopoietic rescue after high-dose therapy. *Clin Cancer Res* 1999; 5:1035–1040.
211. Negrin RS, Atkinson K, Leemhuis T, et al. Transplantation of highly purified CD34+ Thy-1+ hematopoietic stem cells in patients with metastatic breast cancer. *Biol Blood Marrow Transplant* 2000; 6:262–271.
212. Eibl B, Schwaighofer H, Nachbaur D, et al. Evidence for a graft-versus-tumor effect in a patient treated with marrow ablative chemotherapy and allogeneic bone marrow transplantation for breast cancer. *Blood* 1996; 88:1501–1508.
213. Ben-Yosef R, Or R, Nagler A, Slavin S. Graft-versus-tumour and graft-versus-leukaemia effect in patient with concurrent breast cancer and acute myelocytic leukaemia. *Lancet* 1996; 348:1242–1243.
214. Ueno NT, Rondón G, Mirza NQ, et al. Allogeneic peripheral-blood progenitor-cell transplantation for poor-risk patients with metastatic breast cancer. *J Clin Oncol* 1998; 16:986–993.
215. Childs R, Chernoff A, Contentin N, et al. Regression of metastatic renal-cell carcinoma after nonmyeloablative allogeneic peripheral-blood stem-cell transplantation. *N Engl J Med* 2000; 343:750–758.
216. Rini BI, Zimmerman T, Stadler WM, et al. Allogeneic stem-cell transplantation of renal cell cancer after nonmyeloablative chemotherapy: feasibility, engraftment, and clinical results. *J Clin Oncol* 2002; 20:2017–2024.
217. Ueno NT, Cheng YC, Giralt SA, et al. Complete donor chimerism by fludarabine/melphalan in mini-allogeneic transplantation for metastatic renal cell carcinoma (RCC) and breast cancer (BC). *Proc Am Soc Clin Oncol* 2002; 21:415a.
218. Bregni M, Peccatori J, Dodero A, et al. Clinical responses to reduced-intensity allogeneic stem cell transplantation in solid tumors: strong association with graft-vserus-host-disease. *Proc Am Soc Clin Oncol* 2002; 21:417a.
219. Blaise DP, Bay JO, Michallet M, et al. A feasibility study of allogeneic immunotherapy for solid tumors. *Proc Am Soc Clin Oncol* 2002; 21: 417a.

Part II Complications of Transplantion

6 Pathophysiology of Acute Graft-vs-Host Disease

Takanori Teshima, MD, PhD
and James L. M. Ferrara, MD

Contents

1. DEFINITION

The graft-vs-host (GVH) reaction was first noted when irradiated mice were infused with allogeneic marrow and spleen cells. Although mice recovered from radiation injury and marrow aplasia, they subsequently died with "secondary disease," a syndrome consisting of diarrhea, weight loss, skin changes, and liver abnormalities *(1)*. This phenomenon was subsequently recognized as GVH disease (GVHD). The requirements for the development of GVHD was soon formulated *(2)*. First, the graft must contain immunologically competent cells; second, the recipient must be incapable of rejecting the transplanted cells; third, the recipient must express tissue antigens that are not present in the transplant donor

The first requirement of a GVHD reaction, immunocompetent cells, is now recognized as mature T cells *(3)*. In allogeneic bone marrow transplantation (alloBMT), the severity of GVHD correlates with the number of donor T cells transfused *(4)*. The ability of marrow T cells to induce GVHD were much less potent than blood T cells in experimental models *(5)*, therefore, the contamination of bone marrow (BM) with peripheral blood at the time of marrow harvest may be related to the development of GVHD.

The second requirement stipulates that the recipient must be immunocompromised. A patient with a normal immune system will usually reject T cells from a foreign donor. This requirement is most commonly met in allogeneic hematopoietic stem cell transplantation (HSCT), where recipients have usually received very immunosuppressive doses of chemotherapy and/or radiation before stem cell infusion, but it may also be met in other situations, such as solid organ allografts and blood transfusion, where recipients are often immunosuppressed. There are, however, exceptions for this requirement. GVHD can occur in an immunocompetent recipient of tissues from a donor who is homozygous for one of the recipient's haplotypes (e.g., trans-

From: *Stem Cell Transplantation for Hematologic Malignancies*
Edited by: R. J. Soiffer

fusion of blood from an human leukocyte antigen [HLA] homozygous parent to a heterozygous child), even though they are not immunocompromised *(6)*.

The third requirement, the expression of recipient tissue antigens not present in the donor, became the focus of intensive research with the discovery of the major histocompatibility complex (MHC). HLAs are the proteins that are the gene products of the MHC on the cell surfaces of all nucleated cells in the human body, and they are essential to the activation of allogeneic T cells *(7)*. The T cells are selected in the thymus to recognize self-MHC molecules, but when confronted with allogeneic (non-self) MHC molecules, T cells are activated and mount a formidable attack that culminates in the destruction of the allogeneic tissues. In fact, MHC differences between donor and recipient are the most important risk factor for the induction of GVHD. In addition, there are minor histocompatibility antigens (mHAgs), which are derived from the expression of polymorphic genes that distinguish donor and host. Surprisingly, GVH reactions can occur between genetically identical strains and individuals *(8,9)*. These observations have necessitated a revision of the third postulate to include the inappropriate recognition of host self-antigens.

2. PATHOLOGY

Acute GVHD is manifested primarily by the involvement of specific target organs such as the skin, liver, intestine, the immune system, and possibly the lung. In cases of transfusion-associated GVHD, BM aplasia is often observed because the hematopoietic system of the host is targeted. Likewise, marrow aplasia is a serious complication of donor leukocyte infusions (DLIs) given to treat hematologic malignancy in cases involving relapse after an HSC allograft, and it results from a GVH reaction against residual host hematopoietic system.

The pathologic findings of acute GVHD characteristically include epithelial damage that is usually apoptotic in nature *(10)*. In the skin, the epidermis and hair follicles are often destroyed. In the liver, small bile ducts are profoundly affected, and segmental disruption is common. Intestinal crypt destruction results in mucosal ulcerations that may be either patchy or diffuse. A prominent pathologic feature of acute GVHD is the disparity between the severity of tissue destruction and the paucity of the lymphocytic infiltrate. This finding underscores the critical role of cytopathic cytokines in target tissue destruction. During GVHD, MHC class II molecules aberrantly expressed on epithelial and endothelial target cells *(11–13)*, and it has been generally assumed that this aberrant MHC expression is essential for target cell damage in GVHD. However, a recent murine study demonstrated that the aberrant MHC class II expression is the result of tissue inflammation rather than the cause of GVHD *(14)*. This study also demonstrated that direct contact between host target epithelium and donor T cells is often not required for target cell destruction and that soluble mediators of GVHD such as interleukin-1 (IL-1) and tumor necrosis factor (TNF)-α can mediate target injury *(14)*.

3. PATHOPHYSIOLOGY

The development of acute GVHD is proposed to consist of a three-step process in which mononuclear phagocytes and other accessory cells are responsible for both the initiation of a GVH reaction and for the subsequent injury to host tissues after complex interactions with cytokines secreted by activated donor T cells (*see* Fig. 1). The three steps are (1) tissue damage

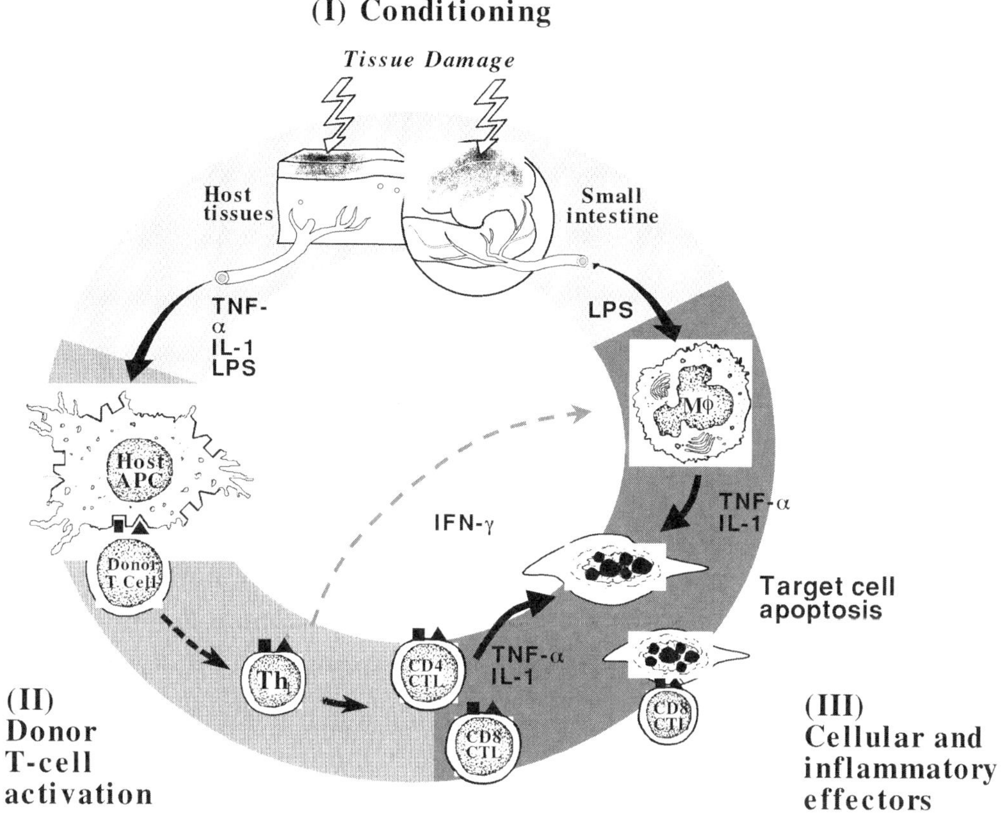

Fig. 1. The immunopathology of GVHD. GVHD pathophysiology can be summarized in a three-step process. In phase 1, the conditioning regimen (irradiation, chemotherapy, or both) leads to the damage and activation of host tissues, especially the intestinal mucosa. This allows the translocation of lipopolysaccharide (LPS) from the intestinal lumen to the circulation, stimulating the secretion of the inflammatory cytokines TNF-α and IL-1 from host tissues, particularly macrophages. These cytokines increase the expression of MHC antigens and adhesion molecules on host tissues, enhancing the recognition of MHC and mHAgs by mature donor T cells. Donor-T-cell activation in phase 2 is characterized by the proliferation of Th1 cells and the secretion of interferfon-γ (IFN-γ), which activates mononuclear phagocytes. The cytoxic T lymphocyte (CTL) damages tissue by perforin/granzyme, FasL, and TNF-α. In phase 3, effector functions of activated mononuclear phagocytes are triggered by the secondary signal provided by LPS and other stimulatory molecules that leak through the intestinal mucosa damaged during phases 1 and 2. This damage results in the amplification of local tissue injury and it further promotes an inflammatory response. Damage to the gastrointestinal tract in this phase, principally by inflammatory cytokines, amplifies LPS release and leads to the "cytokine storm" characteristic of severe acute GVHD.

to the recipient by the radiation/chemotherapy pretransplant conditioning regimen, (2) donor-T-cell activation, and (3) the effector phase. In step 1, the conditioning regimen (irradiation and/or chemotherapy) leads to the damage and activation of host tissues, including intestinal mucosa, liver, and other tissues, and it induces the secretion of inflammatory cytokines TNF-α and IL-1. The consequences of the action of these cytokines are the increased expression of

MHC antigens and other molecules, thus enhancing the recognition of host alloantigens by donor T cells. Donor-T-cell activation in step 2 is characterized by proliferation of donor T cells and secretion of cytokines, including IL-2 and interferon-γ (IFN-γ). The antigen-presenting cell (APC) presents antigen in the form of a peptide–HLA complex to the resting T cells. A second costimulatory signal is required for T-cell activation and the signaling by costimulatory molecules also activates APCs, thus further promoting donor-T-cell activation. IL-2 induces further T-cell expansion, cytotoxic T-lymphocytes (CTL) response, and prime additional mononuclear phagocytes to produce TNF-α and IL-1. These inflammatory cytokines stimulate host tissues to produce inflammatory chemokines, thus recruiting effector cells into target organs. Effector functions of mononuclear phagocytes are triggered through a secondary signal provided by lipopolysaccaride (LPS) that leaks through the intestinal mucosa damaged during step 1. This mechanism may result in the amplification of local tissue injury and further promotion of an inflammatory response, which, together with CTL, leads to target tissue destruction. There is now substantial evidence to implicate the inappropriate production of cytokines, which are the central regulatory molecules of the immune system, as a primary cause for the induction and maintenance of experimental and clinical GVHD *(14,15)*. Dysregulation of this complex cytokine cascade can occur at various steps and eventually results in manifestations of this disease.

3.1. Phase 1: Conditioning

The earliest phase of acute GVHD starts before donor cells are infused. Donor T cells are infused into a host that has been profoundly damaged by underlying disease, infection, and transplant conditioning. These changes activate APCs, thereby enhancing donor-T-cell activation after allogeneic transplantation. Thus, these factors are important variables in the pathogenesis of acute GVHD and explain a number of unique and seemingly unrelated aspects of GVHD. For example, a number of analyses of clinical transplants have noted increased risks of GVHD associated with advanced-stage leukemia, certain intensive conditioning regimens, and histories of viral infections *(16–18)*.

Total-body irradiation (TBI) is particularly important because it activates the host tissue to secrete inflammatory cytokines, such as TNF-α and IL-1 *(19)*, and it also induces endothelial apoptosis in the gastrointestinal (GI) tract followed by epithelial cell damage *(20)*. This gut damage is further amplified by donor-T-cell attack and allows the translocation of immunostimulatory microbial products such as LPS into systemic circulation, leading to further amplification of GVHD. This scenario is in accordance with the observation that an increased risk of GVHD is associated with intensive conditioning regimens that cause extensive injury to epithelial and endothelial surfaces with a subsequent release of inflammatory cytokines and increases in expression of cell surface adhesion molecules. The relationship among conditioning intensity, inflammatory cytokine, and GVHD severity was further supported by animal models *(21)* and clinical observation *(16,17)*.

3.2. Phase 2: Donor-T-Cell Activation

Donor-T-cell activation occurs during the second step of the afferent phase of acute GVHD and it includes antigen presentation, activation of individual T cells, and the subsequent proliferation and differentiation of donor T cells. Murine study demonstrated that host APCs alone are sufficient to stimulate donor T cells *(14,22)* and, thus, this process appears to occur within secondary lymphoid organs such as lymph nodes and the spleen *(23)*. In murine models of

GVHD across MHC disparity, robust donor-T-cell proliferation is observed in the spleen as early as d 3 after BMT, preceding the engraftment of donor BM cells *(14,24–26)*. Although the impact of splenectomy prior to BMT has yet to be conclusively determined in humans, GVHD can readily develop even in the absence of the spleen, suggesting that other secondary lymphoid organs are sufficient to stimulate donor T cells *(27)*.

After allogeneic HSC transplants, both host- and donor-derived APCs are present in secondary lymphoid organs. The T-cell receptor (TCR) of the donor T cells can recognize alloantigens either on host APCs (direct presentation) or donor APCs (indirect presentation). In direct presentation, donor T cells recognize either the peptide bound to allogeneic MHC molecules or allogeneic MHC molecules without peptide *(28)*. During indirect presentation, T cells respond to the peptide generated by degradation of the allogeneic MHC molecules presented on self-MHC *(29)*. A recent murine study demonstrated that APCs derived from the host, rather than from the donor, are critical in inducing GVHD across mHAg mismatch *(22)*. In humans, most cases of acute GVHD developed when both host DCs and donor dendritic cells (DCs) are present in peripheral blood after BMT *(30)*.

CD4 and CD8 proteins are coreceptors for constant portions of MHC class II and MHC class I molecules, respectively. Therefore, MHC class I (HLA-A, -B, -C) differences stimulate CD8+ T cells and MHC class II (HLA-DR, -DP, -DQ) differences stimulate CD4+ T cells *(31)*. Disparities between HLA sequence polymorphisms that are serologically determined are termed "antigen mismatch," whereas those that are identified only DNA typing are termed "allele mismatch." Recent clinical studies demonstrated that allele mismatch is less immunogeneic than antigen mismatch *(32)*, but allele mismatch can be a significant risk factor of GVHD in BMT from unrelated donors *(33)*. In the majority of HLA-identical BMT, GVHD is induced by mHAgs, which are peptides derived from polymorphic cellular proteins that are presented by MHC molecules. Because the manner of protein processing depends on genes outside of the MHC, two siblings will have many different peptides in the MHC groove. In this case, GVHD depends on the recognition of different peptides bound to the same allelic peptide products presented by the same MHC. It remains unclear how many of these peptides behave as mHAgs in humans and mice, although over 50 different mHAg genetic loci have been defined among inbred strains of mice *(34)*. The actual numbers of so-called "major minor" antigens that can potentially induce GVHD are likely to be limited. Recent clinical data suggest that mismatches of mHAgs between HLA-identical donors and recipients are associated with GVHD in adults *(35)*. Of five previously characterized mHAgs (HA-1, -2, -3, -4, -5) recognized by T cells in association with HLA-A1 and HLA-A2, mismatching of HA-1 alone was significantly correlated with acute grade II–IV GVHD and mismatching at HA-1, -2, -4, and -5 was also associated with GVHD. Theoretical models also predict that substantial benefit would be possible if multiple minor loci could be typed *(36)*. One set of proteins that induce minor histocompatiblity responses is encoded on the male-specific Y chromosome. This H-Y antigen is attributed to an increased risk of GVHD when male recipients are transplanted from female donors *(37,38)*. mHAgs with broad or limited tissue expression are potential target antigens for GVHD and graft-vs-leukemia (GVL) reactivity *(39)*, and separation of these activity by using CTLs specific for the hematopoietic system is an area of intense research *(40)*.

The initial binding of T cells with APCs is mediated by the interaction of adhesion molecules (*see* Table 1). When a T cell recognizes specific ligands on an APC, signaling through TCR induces a conformational change in adhesion molecules, resulting in higher-affinity binding *(41)*. T-Cell activation further requires costimulatory signals provided by APCs. Currently,

Table 1
T Cell–APC Interactions

	T cell	*APC*
Adhesion	ICAMs	LFA-1
	LFA-1	ICAMs
	CD2 (LFA-2)	LFA-3
Recognition	TCR/CD4	MHC II
	TCR/CD8	MHCc I
Costimulation	CD28	CD80/86
	CD152 (CTLA-4)	CD80/86
	ICOS	B7H/B7RP-1
	PD-1	PD-L1, PD-L2
	Unknown	B7-H3
	CD154 (CD40L)	CD40
	CD134 (OX 40)	CD134L (OX40L)
	CD137 (4-1BB)	CD137L (4-1BBL)
	HVEM	LIGHT

Abbreviations: HVEM, HSV glycoprotein D for herpesvirus entry mediator; LIGHT, homologous to lymphotoxins, shows inducible expression, and competes with herpes simplex virus glycoprotein D for herpes virus entry mediator (HVEM), a receptor expressed by T lymphocytes.

there are four known CD28 superfamily members expressed on T cells: CD28, cytotoxic T-lymphocyte antigen 4 (CTLA-4), inducible costimulator (ICOS), and programmed death (PD)-1; in addition, there are four TNF receptor family members: CD40 ligand (CD154), 4-1BB (CD137), OX40, and HSV glycoprotein D for herpes virus entry mediator (HVEM) (*see* Table 1). The best characterized costimulatory molecules, CD80 and CD86, deliver positive signals through CD28 that lower the threshold for T-cell activation and promote T-cell differentiation and survival, whereas CTLA-4 delivers an inhibitory signal.

The most potent APCs are DCs; however, the relative contribution of DCs and other semi-professional APCs such as monocytes/macrophages and B cells in inducing GVHD remains to be elucidated. DCs can be matured and activated by (1) inflammatory cytokines, (2) microbial products such as LPS and CpG entering systemic circulation from intestinal mucosa damaged by conditioning, and (3) necrotic cells that were damaged by recipient conditioning. These "danger signals" *(42)* are extremely important because recent reports have suggested that mature DCs induces a T-cell response, whereas immature DCs can induce tolerance *(43)*. In addition, when T cells are exposed to antigens in the presence of an adjuvant such as LPS, T-cell proliferation, migration, and survival are dramatically enhanced in vivo *(44)*. A recent murine study identified the enhanced allostimulatory activity of host APCs in aged mice as one of the important mechanism for this association *(45)*.

The role of natural killer (NK) cells in GVHD is controversial. NK cells are negatively regulated by MHC class I-specific inhibitory receptors; thus, HLA class I mismatched transplants may trigger NK-mediated alloreactivity. Nonetheless, activated NK cells can suppress GVHD through the elimination of host APCs *(46)* or by their tumor growth factor-β (TGF-β) secretion *(47)*. This suppressive effect of alloreactive NK cells on GVHD has been confirmed in humans: HLA class I disparity driving donor NK-mediated alloreactions in the GVH directions mediate potent GVL effects and produce higher engraftment rates without causing severe acute GVHD *(46,48)*. NK cells also produce IFN-γ and TNF-α after stimulation with IL-12 and IL-18 and can thus also participate in the development of GVHD. A recent murine BMT study using mice lacking SH2-containing inositol phosphatase (SHIP), in which the NK compartment is dominated by cells that express two inhibitory receptors capable of binding either self or allogeneic MHC ligands, suggests that host NK cells may play a role in the initiation of GVHD *(49)*.

Subpopulations of donor T cells may be able to suppress GVHD. Repeated stimulation of donor CD4+ T cells with alloantigens in vitro results in the emergence of a population of T-cell clones (T_r1 cells) that secrete high amounts of IL-10 and TGF-β *(50)*. The immunosuppressive properties of these cytokines are explained by their ability to inhibit APC function and to regulate proliferation of T cells directly. The addition of IL-10 or TGF-β to mixed lymphocyte reaction (MLR) cultures induces tolerance *(51)*, with alterations in biochemical signaling similar to costimulatory blockade *(52)*. Transplantation of HLA-mismatched HSCs in patients with severe combined immunodeficiency (SCID) can result in selective engraftment of donor T cells with complete immunologic reconstitution and tolerance in association with the development of donor-derived Tr cells that produce large amount of IL-10 *(53)*. Similarly, so-called "Th3" cells that produce large amount of TGF-β can be regulatory T cells. CD8+ suppressor cells have been identified in both mice and humans *(54–57)*. A specific subpopulation of CD8+ T cells expressing CD57 has been identified as having suppressor function in patients with acute and chronic GVHD *(56,58)*. Natural suppressor (NS) cells suppressed GVHD in a variety of host and donor combinations *(59)*. NK T cells may possess such NS cell functions *(60)*. Peripheral blood NK T cells that are rapidly reconstituted from bone marrow cells after BMT *(61)* as well as marrow NK T cells can suppress GVHD by their IL-4 secretion *(5,60)*. The details of how these three tolerogenic mechanisms interact with each other after allogeneic HSC transplantation is an area of active research that will likely yield future novel therapeutic strategies.

3.3. Phase 2: Cytokines

Antigen presentation induces the activation of individual T cells. This involves multiple, rapidly occurring intracellular biochemical changes, including the rise of cytoplasmic free calcium and activation of protein kinase C and tyrosine kinases *(62,63)*. These pathways in turn activate transcription of genes for cytokines, such as IL-2, IFN-γ, and their receptors. Both IL-2 and IFN-γ are preferentially produced by the T-helper 1 (Thl) subset of T cells *(64)* and mediate acute GVHD by promoting T-cell activation and by inducing additional cellular and inflammatory effectors. The T-cell-activation phase is followed by clonal expansion and differentiation to effector T cells. Activated T cells produce proteins required for specific effector functions, such as the protein esterases required by CTLs *(65)*. The expression of many cell surface molecules, such as adhesion molecules and chemokine receptors, also change the ability of T cells to traffic in vivo *(66)*.

Interleukin-2 has a pivotal role in controlling and amplifying the immune response against alloantigens, representing step 2 of the cytokine cascade that initiates acute GVHD. IL-2 induces the expression of its own receptor (autocrine effect) and stimulates proliferation of other cells expressing the receptor (paracrine effect). IL-2 is secreted by donor CD4+ T cells in the first several days after GVHD induction *(67)*. In some studies, the addition of low doses of IL-2 during the first week after allogeneic BMT enhanced the severity and mortality of

GVHD except when GVHD was induced to MHC class II antigens *(68,69)*. The precursor frequency of alloreactive cells, determined as host-specific IL-2-producing cells (pHTL) predicts the occurrence of clinical acute GVHD *(70–72)*. pHTL cells were detectable as early as d 20 after transplant, often preceding the onset of acute GVHD by approx 2 wk, and persisted until the GVHD resolved. The importance of IL-2 is further underscored by experiments showing that monoclonal antibodies (MAbs) against IL-2 or its receptor are efficient in preventing GVHD in animals or in clinical GVHD when administered shortly after the infusion of T cells *(67,73,74)*. It should be noted, however, that in two clinical trials, the addition of an anti-IL-2 receptor mAb was only moderately successful in reducing the incidence of severe GVHD *(75,76)*. Because of their apparent importance in initiating acute GVHD, IL-2-producing donor T cells have been the primary target to control GVHD. Cyclosporine (CSP) and FK506 are powerful inhibitors of IL-2 production and are effective prophylactic agents against GVHD. The cytokines IL-2 and IL-15 are redundant in stimulating T-cell proliferation. A recent kinetics study of T-cell division demonstrated that IL-15, rather than IL-2, is a critical cytokine in initiating allogeneic T-cell division in vivo *(77)*, and elevated serum levels of IL-15 are associated with acute GVHD in humans *(78)*. IL-15 may therefore be a critical factor in initiating GVHD.

Interferon-γ is a second crucial cytokine that can be implicated in the second step of the pathophysiology of acute GVHD. Increased expression levels of IFN-γ are associated with acute GVHD *(21,79–81)*, and a large proportion of T-cell clones isolated from GVHD patients can produce IFN-γ *(82)*. IFN-γ secretion is also an early event in the cascade leading to GVHD because IFN-γ production in animals with GVHD peaks at d 7 posttransplant before clinical manifestations are apparent. CTLs specific for mHAgs produce IFN-γ and are correlated with the severity of GVH reaction in the skin-explant assay *(40)*. In a small clinical series of patients with GVHD, serum levels of IFN-γ are not significantly increased *(83)*.

Experimental data suggest that IFN-γ is involved in several aspects of the pathophysiology of acute GVHD. First, IFN-γ can increase the expression of numerous important molecules for GVHD, including adhesion molecules, chemokines, MHC, and Fas, resulting in enhanced antigen presentation, the recruitment of effector cells into target organs, and the modulation of target cells so that they are more vulnerable to damage by effector cells. Second, IFN-γ can mediate the development of pathologic processes in the GI tract and skin during GVHD; the administration of anti-IFN-γ MAbs prevents GI GVHD *(84)*, and high levels of both IFN-γ and TNF-α correlate with the most intense cellular damage in skin *(85)*. Third, IFN-γ mediates GVHD-associated immunosuppression in several experimental GVHD systems partly through the induction of nitric oxide (NO) *(86–91)*. Fourth, IFN-γ primes macrophages to produce proinflammatory cytokines and NO in response to LPS *(92,93)*. The inhibition of IFN-γ production after MHC class I or II disparate transplant by injection of polarized donor T cells (which secrete IL-4 but not IFN-γ) results in the downregulation of LPS-triggered TNF-α production and reduced GVHD-related mortality *(94)*. Finally, IFN-γ plays an important role in regulating the death of activated donor T cells by enhancing Fas-mediated apoptosis, thus regulating GVHD *(24,25,95)*.

Cytokines secreted by activated T cells are generally classified as Th1 (secreting IL-2 and IFN-γ) or Th2 (secreting IL-4, IL-5, IL-10, and IL-13) *(64)*. Several factors influence the ability of DCs to instruct naive CD4+ T cell to secrete Th1 or Th2 cytokines, including the type of signal that activates DCs, the duration of DC activation, the ratio of DCs to T cells, as well as varying proportions of DC subsets *(96,97)*. Differential activation of Th1 or Th2 cells has been evoked in the immunopathogenesis of GVHD, as do infectious and autoimmune diseases. Activated Th1 cells (1) amplify T-cell proliferation by secreting IL-2, (2) lyse target cells by Fas/FasL interactions, (3) induce macrophage differentiation in the bone marrow by secreting IL-3 and granulocyte-macrophage colony-stimulating factor (GM-CSF); (4) activate macrophage by secreting IFN-γ and by their CD40–CD40L interactions, (5) activate endothelium to induce macrophage binding and extravasation, and (6) recruit macrophages by secreting monocyte chemoattractant protein-1 (MCP-1). In contrast, GVHD effector mechanisms can be inhibited if donor T cells are activated to produce a Th2 cytokine profile, which downregulates both cell-mediated immune response and the secretion of inflammatory cytokines. Transplantation of Th2 cells (generated in vivo by treating donor mice with a combination of IL-2 and IL-4) into nonirradiated recipients resulted in reduced secretion of TNF-α and protection of recipient mice from LPS-induced TNF-α-mediated lethality *(98)*. Furthermore, cell mixtures of Th2 donor cells with otherwise lethal inocula also protected recipient mice from LPS-induced lethality, demonstrating the ability of Th2 cells to modulate Th1 responses after allogeneic transplantation *(99)*. Similarly, donor Th2 cells polarized in MLR with host cells in the presence of IL-4 failed to induce acute GVHD to MHC class I or class II antigens *(94)*. Pretreatment of BMT donors with granulocyte colony-stimulating factor (G-CSF) can polarize donor T cells toward Th2, resulting in less GVHD *(100)*. Recruitment of CCR5+ T cells, usually Th 1 cells, is associated with hepatic GVHD *(101)*. NK1.1+ T (NKT) cells can suppress GVHD induced by donor T cells through their IL-4 production *(5,60)*. Other studies have shown that GVHD can still occur using donor mice deficient in signal transducer and activator of transcription (STAT) 4, which is crucial to Th1 response, although GVHD induced by STAT4-deficient donors was less severe than GVHD induced by donor cells deficient in STAT6, a molecule critical for Th2 polarization *(102)*. These experiments support the concept that the balance in Th1 and Th2 cytokines is critical for the development of acute GVHD and suggest that Th1 cells produce GVHD more efficiently than Th2 cells, which can be suppressive sometimes. It should be noted, however, that systemic administration of Th2 cytokines IL-4 or IL-10 was tested for its use as a prophylaxis of GVHD and appears to be either ineffective or toxic *(103–105)*.

On the other hand, there are also data suggesting that Th1 cytokines can also reduce GVHD. A brief administration of high doses of exogenous IL-2 early after BMT protects animals from GVHD mortality *(106)*. It has been suggested that IL-2 mediates its protective effect via inhibition of IFN-γ *(79)*. The injection of IFN-γ twice weekly from d 0 to wk 6 prevents the development of experimental GVHD *(107)*, and neutralization of IFN-γ results in accelerated GVHD in lethally irradiated recipients *(89)*. Interestingly, the use of IFN-γ-deficient donor cells can accelerate GVHD in lethally irradiated recipients *(24,108)*, but it results in reduction of GVHD in sublethally irradiated or unirradiated recipients *(109,110)*. These paradoxes may be explained by complex dynamics of the activation, expansion, and contraction of donor T cells. Activation-induced cell death (AICD) is a chief mechanism of clonal deletion, which is largely responsible for the rapid contraction of donor T cells following an initial massive expansion *(111)*. IFN-γ contracts the pool of activated CD4+ T cells by inducing AICD; thus, the complete absence of IFN-γ may result in an unrestrained expansion of activated donor T cells, leading to accelerated GVHD. This phenomenon may, in particular, pertain to recipients of intensified conditioning, which induces greater T-cell activation *(21)*. Similarly, administration of IFN-γ-inducing cytokines such as IL-12 or IL-18 early after BMT protects lethally irradiated recipients from GVHD in a Fas-dependent fashion *(24,25,112,113)*. IL-2 can also prime activated T cells susceptible to AICD. Thus, physiologic and adequate amounts of Th1 cytokine production is critical for GVHD induction, whereas inadequate production (extremely low or high) could modulate GVHD through a breakdown of negative feedback mechanisms for activated donor T cells. Such clonal deletion of host-reactive donor T cells is a critical process for inducing tolerance *(111)*.

3.4. Phase 3: Efferent Phase

The efferent phase of acute GVHD is a complex cascade of multiple effectors. The regulation of effector cell migration into target tissues occurs in a complex millieu of chemotactic signals where several receptors may be triggered simultaneously or successively. Inflammatory chemokines expressed in inflamed tissues upon stimulation by proinflammatory cytokines are specialized for the recruitment of effector cells, such as T cells, neutrophils, and monocytes *(114)*. Chemokine receptors are differentially expressed on subsets of activated/effector T cells. Upon stimulation, T cells can rapidly switch chemokine receptor expression, acquiring a new migratory capacity *(44,115)*. The involvement of inflammatory chemokines and their receptors in GVHD has been recently investigated in mouse models of GVHD. MIP-1α recruits CCR5+ CD8+ T cells into the liver, lung, and spleen during GVHD *(101,116)*, and levels of several chemokines are elevated in GVHD-associated lung injury *(117)*. Further studies will determine whether expression of chemokines and their receptors can explain the unusual cluster of GVHD target organs (skin, gut, and liver) and whether these molecules will prove to be potential targets for modulation of GVHD.

3.4.1. Cellular Effectors

Effector mechanisms of acute GVHD can be grouped into cellular effectors (e.g., CTLs) and inflammatory effectors such as TNF-α, IL-1 and NO. The Fas–Fas ligand (FasL) and the perforin–granzyme (or granule exocytosis) pathways are the principle effector mechanisms used by CTLs and NK cells to lyse their target cells *(118,119)*. Perforin is stored in cytotoxic granules of CTLs and NK cells, together with granzymes and other proteins *(120)*. Following recognition of a target cell through the TCR–MHC interaction, perforin is secreted and inserts itself into the cell-membrane-forming "perforin pores" that allow granzymes to enter the target cells and induce apoptosis through various downstream effector pathways such as caspases *(120)*. Ligation of Fas results in the formation of the death-inducing signaling complex (DISC) and the subsequent activation of caspases *(121)*. A number of ligands on T cells possess the capability to trimerize TNFR-like death receptors (DR), such as TNF-related apoptosis-inducing ligand (TRAIL: DR4,5 ligand) and TNF-like weak inducer of apoptosis (TWEAK: DR3 ligand) *(122–124)*.

The involvement of each of these molecules in GVHD has been tested by utilizing donor cells that are unable to mediate each pathway. Transplantation of perforin deficient T cells results in a marked delay in the onset of GVHD in transplants across mHAg disparities *(125)*, across both MHC and mHAg disparities *(126)*, and across isolated MHC I or II disparities *(127,128)*. However, mortality and clinical and histological signs of GVHD were still induced even in the *absence* of perforin-dependent killing in these studies and, more importantly, demonstrating that the perforin–granzyme pathway plays little role in target organ damage. A role for the perforin–granzyme pathway for GVHD induction is also evident in studies employing donor-T-cell subsets. Perforin- or granzyme B-deficient CD8+ T cells induced significantly less mortality compared to wild-type T cells in experimental transplants across a single

MHC class I mismatch, although this pathway seems to be less important compared to Fas/FasL pathway in CD4-mediated GVHD *(127,129)*. Thus, it seems that CD4+ CTLs preferentially use the Fas–FasL pathway, whereas CD8+ CTLs primarily use the perforin–granzyme pathway.

Fas is a TNF-receptor family member that is expressed by many tissues, including GVHD target organs. Its expression can be upregulated by inflammatory cytokines such as IFN-γ and TNF-α during GVHD *(130)*, and the expression of FasL is also increased on donor T cells *(131–133)*, indicating that FasL-mediated cytotoxicity may be a particularly important effector pathway in GVHD. FasL-defective T cells cause markedly reduced GVHD in the liver, skin and lymphoid organs *(125,134,135)*. The Fas–FasL pathway is particularly important in hepatic GVHD, consistent with the keen sensitivity of hepatocytes to Fas-mediated cytotoxicity in experimental models of murine hepatitis *(136)*. Fas-deficient recipients are protected from hepatic GVHD, but not from other organ GVHD *(137)*, and administration of anti-FasL (but not anti-TNF) MAbs significantly blocked hepatic GVHD damage occurring in murine models *(138)*. Although the use of FasL-deficient donor T cells or the administration of neutralizing FasL MAbs had no effect on the development of intestinal GVHD in several studies *(125,138,139)*, the Fas–FasL pathway may play a role in this target organ, because intestinal epithelial lymphocytes exhibit increased FasL-mediated killing potential *(140)*. Elevated serum levels of soluble FasL and Fas have also been observed in at least some patients with acute GVHD *(141–144)*.

The utilization of a perforin–granzyme and FasL cytotoxic double-deficient (cdd) mouse provides an opportunity to address whether other effector pathways are capable of inducing GVHD target organ pathology. An initial study demonstrated that cdd T cells were unable to induce lethal GVHD across MHC class I and class II disparities after sublethal irradiation *(126)*. However, subsequent studies demonstrated that cytotoxic effector mechanisms of donor T cells are critical in preventing host resistance to GVHD *(145,146)*. Thus, when recipients were conditioned with lethal dose of irradiation, cdd CD4+ T cells produced similar mortality to wild type CD4+ T cells *(146)*. These results were confirmed by a recent study demonstrating that GVHD target damage can occur in mice that lack alloantigen expression on the epithelium, preventing direct interaction between CTLs and target cells (*see* Fig. 1) *(14)*.

3.4.2. Inflammatory Effectors

Inflammatory cytokines synergize with CTLs resulting in the amplification of local tissue injury and further promotion of an inflammation, which ultimately leads to the observed target tissue destruction in the transplant recipient. Macrophages, which had been primed with IFN-γ during step 2, produce inflammatory cytokines TNF-α and IL-1 when stimulated by a secondary triggering signal. This stimulus may be provided through Toll-like receptors (TLRs) by microbial products such as LPS and other microbial particles, which can leak through the intestinal mucosa damaged by the conditioning regimen and gut GVHD. It has recently become apparent that immune recognition through TLRs by the innate immune system also controls activation of adaptive immune responses *(147)*. A recent human study of GVHD suggested the possible association with mutation of TLR genes and severity of GVHD *(148)*. LPS may stimulate gut-associated lymphocytes and macrophages *(93)*. LPS reaching the skin may also stimulate keratinocytes, dermal fibroblasts, and macrophages to produce similar cytokines in the dermis and epidermis. The severity of GVHD appears to be directly related to the level of macrophage priming *(93)*. Injection of small, normally nonlethal amounts of LPSs caused elevated TNF-α serum levels and death in animals with GVHD; this mortality could be prevented with anti-TNF-α serum. These experiments strongly supported the role of mononuclear phagocytes as sources of inflammatory cytokines during the effector phase of acute GVHD. Subsequent murine studies further demonstrated that TNF-α production by donor cells in response to LPS predicts the severity of GVHD *(149)* and that direct antagonism of LPS reduces GVHD *(150)*. Thus, the GI tract plays a major role in the amplification of systemic GVHD and is critical in the propagation of the "cytokine storm" characteristics of acute GVHD *(151)* (*see* Fig. 1). Maintenance of transplant recipients in a germ-free environment (which reduces bacteria in the GI tract) has been shown to be associated with the reduction of GVHD *(152,153)*.

The cytokines TNF-α and IL-1 are produced by an abundance of cell types during processes of both innate and adoptive immunity; they often have synergistic, pleiotrophic, and redundant effects on both afferent and efferent phases of GVHD. A critical role for TNF-α in the pathophysiology of acute GVHD was first suggested almost 15 yr ago because mice transplanted with mixtures of allogeneic BM and T cells developed severe skin, gut, and lung lesions that were associated with high levels of TNF-α mRNA in these tissues *(154,155)*. Target organ damage could be inhibited by infusion of anti-TNF-α MAbs, and mortality could be reduced from 100% to 50% by the administration of the soluble form of the TNF-α receptor (sTNFR), an antagonist of TNF-α *(19)*. Accumulating experimental data further suggest that TNF-α is involved in a multistep process of GVHD pathophysiology. TNF-α (1) can cause cachexia, a characteristic feature of GVHD, (2) maturates DCs, thus enhancing alloantigen presentation, (3) recruits effector T cells, neutrophils, and monocytes into target organs through the induction of inflammatory chemokines, and (4) causes direct tissue damage by inducing apoptosis and necrosis *(156)*. TNF-α also involves in donor-T-cell activation directly through its signaling via TNFR1 and TNFR2 on T cells. TNF–TNFR1 interactions on donor T cells promote alloreactive T-cell responses *(157)* and TNF–TNFR2 interactions are critical for intestinal GVHD *(158)*. In contrast to FasL involvement in hepatic GVHD, TNF-α plays a central role in intestinal GVHD in murine and human studies *(138,154,159)*. TNF-α also seems to be important effector molecules in GVHD in skin and lymphoid tissue *(138,154,160,161)*. TNF-α can also be involved in hepatic GVHD, probably by enhancing effector cell migration to the liver via the induction of inflammatory chemokines: A recent study demonstrated that neutralization of TNF-α and IL-1 prevented lymphocytic infiltration into the liver, resulting in a significant reduction of liver GVHD *(14)*.

An important role for TNF-α in clinical acute GVHD has been suggested by studies demonstrating elevated serum levels or of TNF-α or elevated TNF-α mRNA expression in peripheral blood mononuclear cells in patients with acute GVHD and other endothelial complications, such as hepatic veno-occlusive disease (VOD) *(162–165)*. A phase I–II trial using TNF-α receptor MAbs during the conditioning regimen as a prophylaxis in patients at high risk for severe acute GVHD showed reduction in lesions of the intestine, skin, and liver, however, GVHD flared after discontinuation of treatment *(159)*. These preliminary data, as well as animal and laboratory studies, suggest that approaches to limit TNF-α secretion will be a very important avenue of investigation in allogeneic HSCT.

The second major pro-inflammatory cytokine that appears to play an important role in the effector phase of acute GVHD is IL-1. Secretion of IL-1 appears to occur predominantly during the effector phase of GVHD of the spleen and skin, two major GVHD target organs *(166)*. A similar increase in mononuclear cell IL-1 mRNA has been shown during clinical acute GVHD

(164). Indirect evidence of a role for IL-1 in GVHD was obtained with administration of this cytokine to recipients in an allogeneic murine BMT model *(103)*. Mice receiving IL-1 displayed a wasting syndrome and increased mortality that appeared to be an accelerated form of disease. Investigations of the role of IL-1 in GVHD intensified after the discovery of IL-1 receptor antagonist (IL-1ra) *(167,168)*. Intraperitoneal administration of IL-1ra starting on d 10 posttransplant was able to reverse the development of GVHD in the majority of animals, providing a significant survival advantage to treated animals *(169)*. However, the attempt to use IL-1ra to prevent acute GVHD in a randomized trial was not successful *(170)*.

As a result of activation during GVHD, macrophages also produce NO, which contributes to the deleterious effects on GVHD target tissues, particularly immunosuppression *(91,171)*. NO also inhibits the repair mechanisms of target tissue destruction by inhibiting proliferation of epithelial stem cells in the gut and skin *(172)*. In humans and rats, the development of GVHD is preceded by an increase in serum levels of NO oxidation products *(173,174)*.

The central role of inflammatory cytokines in acute GVHD was confirmed in a murine study by using BM chimeras in which either MHC class I or MHC class II alloantigens were not expressed on target epithelium but on APCs alone *(14)*. GVHD target organ injury was induced in these chimeras even in the absence of epithelial alloantigens and mortality and target organ injury was prevented by the neutralization of TNF-α and IL-1. These observations were particularly true for CD4-mediated acute GVHD but also applied, at least in part, to CD8-mediated disease.

4. EXPERIMENTAL GVHD PREVENTION

Experimental approaches to inhibit phase I include reduced conditioning and protection of the GI tract because intensified conditioning and intestinal damage are critical to the propagation of the "cytokine storm" characteristic of acute GVHD, as discussed earlier. A reduced dose (nonmyeloablative) of conditioning has been used increasingly by many BMT centers *(175)*. In animal models, all cytotoxic conditioning can be eliminated by giving a high dose of MHC-mismatched BM cells followed by costimulatory blockade in vivo *(176,177)*. A recent murine study demonstrated that the pretransplant infusion of alloreactive NK cells obviated the need for intensified conditioning *(46)*. The ability to replace host T-cell depletion with such immunological approaches is encouraging and is an active area of investigation.

"Cytokine shields" are novel experimental approaches to protect GI mucosal barrier from conditioning by cytokines or growth factors such as IL-11, keratinocyte growth factor (KGF), and hepatocyte growth factor (HGF), which have direct protective effects on the GI tract epithelium in various models of gut injury. In experimental mouse models of GVHD, the protective effect of these growth factors on the GI tract resulted in improved survival *(178–181)*. Such strategies to protect the GI tract have reduced GVHD while preserving a GVL effect *(180,182)*. In this regard, blockade of LPS by a LPS antagonist prevents experimental GVHD while preserving GVL effects *(150)*. Unfortunately, a phase I–II clinical study of IL-11 was halted because of severe fluid retention *(183)*.

Current strategies for GVHD prevention or treatment generally interfere with the afferent phase of the GVHD and are primarily targeted at donor T cells. These have included pretreatment of the stem cell donor, in vitro manipulation of the stem cells, and treatment of the patient posttransplant. Calcineurin inhibitors, such as CSP and tacrolimus (FK506), are the most commonly used drugs for GVHD prophylaxis, usually in combination with an inhibitor of nucleotide synthesis, methotrexate or mycophenylate mofetil. CSA and FK506 bind to cyclophilin and FKBP-12, respectively, and inhibit calcineurin, resulting in inhibition of IL-2 gene expression. Thus, the combined use of CSA/FK506 and costimulatory blockade in mice may prevent tolerance induction by inhibiting cell-cycle-dependent T-cell apoptosis by IL-2 and the development of Tr cells *(184)*. In contrast, rapamycin, which does not inhibit IL-2-triggered apoptotic signals, provides strong synergy to costimulatory blockade *(184)*. Glucocorticoids are also widely used as both prophylaxis and treatment for GVHD. Although effects of steroids on GVHD have been attributed primarily to their influence on T cells and monocytes/macrophages, recent studies suggest that steroids can also affect DC functions and may act at the very initiation of the immune response by modulating Tcell–DC interactions *(185,186)*. These different sites of action provide the rationale for the use of drug combinations, and, indeed, the use of pairwise combination of these agents is a more effective prophylaxis against GVHD than any single agent, although they also cause substantial drug-induced toxicity.

One of the important mechanisms of tolerance induction is nondeletional immunoregulation, where alloreactive T cells are not deleted but they no longer respond to an antigenic stimulus. This includes clonal anergy, immune deviation, and active suppression. Such anergy or "paralysis" has been demonstrated clearly in many in vitro systems by blocking critical costimulatory pathways such as B7–CD28 interactions. Such a strategy is attractive, because it would theoretically preserve the functional capacity of the remaining T cells to respond to infectious agents or leukemia cells. Antigen presentation in the absence of costimulation not only fails to prime T cells but can also delete them *(187)*, thus, the blockade of costimulatory pathways has shown great promise in preclinical studies. A soluble form of CD152, CTLA4-Ig, inhibits the interaction of CD80–CD86 with CD28 and partially suppresses GVHD in animal models *(188)* (*see* Table 1). The blockade of this pathway by combined administration of anti-CD80 MAbs and anti-CD86 MAbs is more effective than either agent alone *(189)*. Blockades of other pathways, including the CD40–CD154 *(190,191)* and CD134–CD134L *(192)* have also been shown to prevent GVHD in mice primarily by preventing CD4 help and by aborting the alloresponses of CD8+ T cells. In contrast, the blockade of CD137–CD137L interaction can also regulate CD8-mediated GVHD *(193,194)*. The blockade of LIGHT, which is selectively expressed on immature DCs, by soluble receptor or antibody also ameliorates GVHD in a murine model *(195)*. The ICOS is an important regulatory molecule for Th2-mediated immune responses *(196–198)*. Ex vivo blockade of costimulatory pathways prior to infusion of T cells is an alternative approach. The first clinical study of this approach used CTLA4–Ig with partial success *(199)*. In mice, ex vivo treatment of donor T cells with anti-CD154 MAbs also prevented GVHD in association with the emergence of CD4+ CD25+ regulatory T cells *(200)*. To date, these strategies to inhibit costimulation seem to be partially effective, perhaps because CD4+ and CD8+ T cells require distinct costimulatory pathways for activation *(201)* and costimulation is also essential for the survival of Tr cells *(202)*. Therefore, the blockade of several costimulatory pathways such as the CD40–CD154 pathway that primarily inhibits CD4 response and LIGHT pathway that preferentially inhibits CD8 response may be a promising approach *(203)*.

Suppression of donor-T-cell activation can be achieved by the modulation of host DCs *(22)*. This concept was recently proved by murine studies; administration of alloreactive NK cells reduce GVHD by ablating host APCs *(46)* and administration of Flt3 ligand to recipients prior to BMT alters host DCs and reduces acute GVHD *(26)*.

Finally, strategies to inactivate host DCs are also promising *(22)*. A recent analysis of DC turnover in peripheral blood after allogeneic HSCT demonstrated rapid development of DC chimerism: 80% of DCs are donor origin by d 14 and more than 99% by d 28 after myeloablative HSCT. Thus, donor T cell and host APC interaction early after BMT may be a promising strategy of GVHD prevention. A recent murine study of GVHD suggests a novel strategy that alters host DCs and reduces acute GVHD by the administration of Flt3 ligand to recipients prior to BMT *(26)*.

REFERENCES

1. van Bekkum DW, De Vries MJ. *Radiation Chimaeras*. London: Logos, 1967.
2. Billingham RE. The biology of graft-versus-host reactions. *Harvey Lect* 1966;62:21–78.
3. Korngold R, Sprent J. T cell subsets in graft-vs.-host disease. In: Burakoff SJ, Deeg HJ, Ferrara J, Atkinson K, eds. *Graft-vs.-Host Disease: Immunology, Pathophysiology, and Treatment*. New York: Marcel Dekker, 1990:31–50.
4. Kernan NA, Collins NH, Juliano L, et al. Clonable T lymphocytes in T cell-depleted bone marrow transplants correlate with development of graft-vs-host disease. *Blood* 1986;68:770–773.
5. Zeng D, Lewis D, Dejbakhsh-Jones S, et al. Bone marrow NK1.1(–) and NK1.1(+) T cells reciprocally regulate acute graft versus host disease. *J Exp Med* 1999;189:1073–1081.
6. Anderson KC. Transfusion-associated graft-versus-host disease. In: Ferrara JLM, Deeg HJ, Burakoff SJ, eds. *Graft-vs.-Host Disease*. New York: Marcel Dekker, 1997:587–605.
7. Krensky AM, Weiss A, Crabtree G, et al. T-Lymphocyte-antigen interactions in transplant rejection. *N Engl J Med* 1990;322:510–517.
8. Rappaport H, Khalil A, Halle-Pannenko O, et al. Histopathologic sequence of events in adult mice undergoing lethal graft-versus-host reactions developed across H-2 and/or non-H-2 histocompatibility barriers. *Am J Pathol* 1979;96:121–142.
9. Hess AD, Fischer AC. Immune mechanisms in cyclosporine-induced syngeneic graft-versus-host disease. *Transplantation* 1989;48:895–900.
10. Sale GE, Shulman HM. *The Pathology of Bone Marrow Transplantation*. New York: Masson, 1984.
11. Lampert IA, Suitters AJ, Chisholm PM. Expression of Ia antigen on epidermal keratinocytes in graft-versus-host disease. *Nature* 1981;293:149–150.
12. Mason DW, Dallman M, Barclay AN. Graft-versus-host disease induces expression of Ia antigen in rat epidermal cells and gut epithelium. *Nature* 1981;293:150–151.
13. Barclay AN, Mason DW. Induction of Ia antigen in rat epidermal cells and gut epithelium by immunological stimuli. *J Exp Med* 1982;156:1665–1676.
14. Teshima T, Ordemann R, Reddy P, et al. Acute graft-versus-host disease does not require alloantigen expression on host epithelium. *Nature Med* 2002;8(6):575–581.
15. Antin JH, Ferrara JLM. Cytokine dysregulation and acute graft-versus-host disease. *Blood* 1992;80:2964–2968.
16. Gale RP, Bortin MM, van Bekkum DW, et al. Risk factors for acute graft-versus-host disease. *Br J Haematol* 1987;67:397–406.
17. Clift RA, Buckner CD, Appelbaum FR, et al. Allogeneic marrow transplantation in patients with acute myeloid leukemia in first remission: a randomized trial of two irradiation regimens. *Blood* 1990;76:1867–1871.
18. Ringden O. Viral infections and graft-vs.-host disease. In: Burakoff SJ, Deeg HJ, Ferrara J, Atkinson K, eds. *Graft-vs.-Host Disease*. New York: Marcel Dekker, 1990:467.
19. Xun CQ, Thompson JS, Jennings CD, et al. Effect of total body irradiation, busulfan–cyclophosphamide, or cyclophosphamide conditioning on inflammatory cytokine release and development of acute and chronic graft-versus-host disease in H-2-incompatible transplanted SCID mice. *Blood* 1994;83:2360–2367.
20. Paris F, Fuks Z, Kang A, et al. Endothelial apoptosis as the primary lesion initiating intestinal radiation damage in mice. *Science* 2001;293:293–297.
21. Hill GR, Crawford JM, Cooke KJ, et al. Total body irradiation and acute graft versus host disease. The role of gastrointestinal damage and inflammatory cytokines. *Blood* 1997;90:3204–3213.
22. Shlomchik WD, Couzens MS, Tang CB, et al. Prevention of graft versus host disease by inactivation of host antigen-presenting cells. *Science* 1999;285:412–415.

23. Korngold R, Sprent J. Negative selection of T cells causing lethal graft-versus-host disease across minor histocompatibility barriers: role of the H-2 complex. *J Exp Med* 1980;1114–1123.
24. Yang YG, Dey BR, Sergio JJ, et al. Donor-derived interferon gamma is required for inhibition of acute graft-versus-host disease by interleukin 12. *J Clin Invest* 1998;102:2126–2135.
25. Reddy P, Teshima T, Kukuruga M, et al. Interleukin-18 regulates acute graft-versus-host disease by enhancing Fas-mediated donor T cell apoptosis. *J Exp Med* 2001;194:1433–1440.
26. Teshima T, Reddy P, Lowler KP, et al. Flt3 ligand therapy for recipients of allogeneic bone marrow transplants expands host CD8 alpha(+) dendritic cells and reduces experimental acute graft-versus-host disease. *Blood* 2002;99:1825–1832.
27. Clouthier SG, Ferrara JLM, Teshima T. Graft-versus-host disease in the absence of the spleen after allogeneic bone marrow transplantation. *Transplantation* 2002;73:1679–1681.
28. Newton-Nash DK. The molecular basis of allorecognition. Assessment of the involvement of peptide. *Hum Immunol* 1994;41:105–111.
29. Sayegh MH, Carpenter CB. Role of indirect allorecognition in allograft rejection. *Int Rev Immunol* 1996;13:221–229.
30. Auffermann-Gretzinger S, Lossos IS, Vayntrub TA, et al. Rapid establishment of dendritic cell chimerism in allogeneic hematopoietic cell transplant recipients. *Blood* 2002;99:1442–1448.
31. Sprent J, Schaefer M, Gao EK, et al. Role of T cell subsets in lethal graft-versus-host disease (GVHD) directed to class I versus class II H-2 differences. I. L3T4+ cells can either augment or retard GVHD elicited by Lyt-2+ cells in class I different hosts. *J Exp Med* 1988;167:556–569.
32. Petersdorf EW, Hansen JA, Martin PJ, et al. Major-histocompatibility-complex class I alleles and antigens in hematopoietic-cell transplantation. *N Engl J Med* 2001;345:1794–1800.
33. Sasazuki T, Juji T, Morishima Y, et al. Effect of matching of class I HLA alleles on clinical outcome after transplantation of hematopoietic stem cells from an unrelated donor. Japan Marrow Donor Program. *N Engl J Med* 1998;339:1177–1185.
34. Doolittle DP, Davission MT, Guidi JN, et al. Catalog of mutant genes and polymorphic loci. In: Lyon MF, Rastan S, Brown SDM, eds. *Genetic Variants and Strains of the Laboratory Mouse*. New York: Oxford University Press, 1996:17–854.
35. Goulmy E, Schipper R, Pool J, et al. Mismatches of minor histocompatibility antigens between HLA-identical donors and recipients and the development of graft-versus-host disease after bone marrow transplantation [see comments]. *N Engl J Med* 1996;334:281–285.
36. Martin PJ. How much benefit can be expected from matching for minor antigens in allogeneic marrow transplantation? *Bone Marrow Transplant* 1997;20:97–100.
37. Nash A, Pepe MS, Storb R, et al. Acute graft-versus-host disease: analysis of risk factors after allogeneic marrow transpantation and prophylaxis with cyclosporine and methotrexate. *Blood* 1992;80:1838–1845.
38. Hansen JA, Gooley TA, Martin PJ, et al. Bone marrow transplants from unrelated donors for patients with chronic myeloid leukemia. *N Engl J Med* 1998;338:962–968.
39. Goulmy E. Human minor histocompatibility antigens: new concepts for marrow transplantation and adoptive immunotherapy. *Immunol Rev* 1997;157:125–140.
40. Dickinson AM, Wang XN, Sviland L, et al. In situ dissection of the graft-versus-host activities of cytotoxic T cells specific for minor histocompatibility antigens. *Nature Med* 2002;8:410–414.
41. Dustin ML, Springer TA. T-cell receptor cross-linking transiently stimulates adhesiveness through LFA-1. *Nature* 1989;341:619–624.
42. Matzinger P. The danger model: a renewed sense of self. Science 2002;296:301–305.
43. Roncarolo MG, Levings MK, Traversari C. Differentiation of T regulatory cells by immature dendritic cells. *J Exp Med* 2001;193:F5–F10.
44. Reinhardt RL, Khoruts A, Merica R, et al. Visualizing the generation of memory CD4 T cells in the whole body. *Nature* 2001;410:101–105.
45. Ordemann R, Hutchinson R, Friedman J, et al. Enhanced allostimulatory activity of host antigen-presenting cells in old mice intensifies acute graft-versus-host disease. *J Clin Invest* 2002;109(9):1249–1256.
46. Ruggeri L, Capanni M, Urbani E, et al. Effectiveness of donor natural killer cell alloreactivity in mismatched hematopoietic transplants. *Science* 2002;295:2097–2100.
47. Asai O, Longo DL, Tian ZG, et al. Suppression of graft-versus-host disease and amplification of graft-versus-tumor effects by activated natural killer cells after allogeneic bone marrow transplantation. *J Clin Invest* 1998;101:1835–1842.

48. Ruggeri L, Capanni M, Martelli MF, et al. Cellular therapy: exploiting NK cell alloreactivity in transplantation. *Curr Opin Hematol* 2001;8:355–359.
49. Wang JW, Howson JM, Ghansah T, et al. Influence of SHIP on the NK repertoire and allogeneic bone marrow transplantation. *Science* 2002;295:2094–2097.
50. Jonuleit H, Schmitt E, Schuler G, et al. Induction of interleukin 10-producing, nonproliferating CD4(+) T cells with regulatory properties by repetitive stimulation with allogeneic immature human dendritic cells. *J Exp Med* 2000;192:1213–1222.
51. Zeller JC, Panoskaltsis-Mortari A, Murphy WJ, et al. Induction of CD4+ T cell alloantigen-specific hyporesponsiveness by IL-10 and TGF-beta. *J Immunol* 1999;163:3684–3691.
52. Boussiotis VA, Chen ZM, Zeller JC, et al. Altered T-cell receptor + CD28-mediated signaling and blocked cell cycle progression in interleukin 10 and transforming growth factor-beta-treated alloreactive T cells that do not induce graft-versus-host disease. *Blood* 2001;97:565–571.
53. Bacchetta R, Bigler M, Touraine JL, et al. High levels of interleukin 10 production in vivo are associated with tolerance in SCID patients transplanted with HLA mismatched hematopoietic stem cells. *J Exp Med* 1994;179:493–502.
54. Rolink AG, Gleichmann E. Allosuppressor- and allohelper-T cells in acute and chronic graft-versus-host (GVH) disease. III. Different Lyt subsets of donor T cells induce different pathological syndromes. *J Exp Med* 1983;158:546–558.
55. Hurtenbach U, Shearer GM. Analysis of murine T lymphocyte markers during the early phases of GvH-associated suppression of cytotoxic T lymphocyte responses. *J Immunol* 1983;130:1561–1566.
56. Autran B, Leblond V, Sadat-Sowti B. A soluble factor released by CD8+CD57+ lymphocytes from bone marrow transplanted patients inhibits cell-mediated cytolysis. *Blood* 1991;77:2237–2241.
57. Tsoi MS, Storb R, Dobbs S, et al. Non-specific suppressor cells in patients with chronic graft-versus-host disease after marrow grafting. *J Immunol* 1979;123:1970–1973.
58. Fukuda H, Nakamura H, Tominaga N, et al. Marked increase of CD8+S6F1+ and CD8+CD57+ cells in patients with graft-versus-host disease after allogeneic bone marrow transplantation. *Bone Marrow Transplant* 1994;13:181–185.
59. Strober S. Natural suppressor (NS) cells, neonatal tolerance, and total lymphoid irradiation: exploring obscure relationships. *Annu Rev Immunol* 1984;2:219–237.
60. Lan F, Zeng D, Higuchi M, et al. Predominance of NK1.1+TCR alpha beta+ or DX5+TCR alpha beta+ T cells in mice conditioned with fractionated lymphoid irradiation protects against graft-versus-host disease: "natural suppressor" cells. *J Immunol* 2001;167:2087–2096.
61. Eberl G, MacDonald HR. Rapid death and regeneration of NKT cells in anti-CD3epsilon- or IL-12-treated mice: a major role for bone marrow in NKT cell homeostasis. *Immunity* 1998;9:345–353.
62. Nishizuka Y. Studies and perspectives of protein kinase C. *Science* 1986;233:305–312.
63. Samelson LE, Patel MD, Weissman AM, et al. Antigen activation of murine T cell induces tyrosine phosphorylation of a polypeptide associated with the T cell antigen receptor. *Cell* 1986;46:1083–1090.
64. Mosmann TR, Cherwinski H, Bond MW, et al. Two types of murine helper T cell clone. I. Definition according to profiles of lymphokine activities and secreted proteins. *J Immunol* 1986;136:2348–2357.
65. Weiss A. T lymphocyte activation. In: Paul WE, ed. *Fundamental Immunology*. New York: Raven, 1989:359–384.
66. Forster R, Schubel A, Breitfeld D, et al. CCR7 coordinates the primary immune response by establishing functional microenvironments in secondary lymphoid organs. *Cell* 1999;99:23–33.
67. Via CS, Finkelman FD. Critical role of interleukin-2 in the development of acute graft-versus-host disease. *Int Immunol* 1993;5:565–572.
68. Jadus MR, Peck AB. Lethal murine graft-versus-host disease in the absence of detectable cytotoxic T lymphocytes. *Transplantion* 1983;36:281–289.
69. Malkovsky M, Brenner MK, Hunt R, et al. T Cell-depletion of allogeneic bone marrow prevents acceleration of graft-versus-host disease induced by exogenous interleukin-2. *Cell Immunol* 1986;103:476–480.
70. Theobald M, Nierle T, Bunjes D, et al. Host-specific interleukin-2-secreting donor T-cell precursors as predictors of acute graft-versus-host disease in bone marrow transplantation between HLA-identical siblings. *N Engl J Med* 1992;327:1613–1617.
71. Nierle T, Bunjes D, Arnold R, et al. Quantitative assessment of posttransplant host-specific interleukin-2-secreting T-helper cell precursors in patients with and without acute graft-versus-host disease after allogeneic HLA-identical sibling bone marrow transplantation. *Blood* 1993;81:841–848.

72. Schwarer AP, Jiang YZ, Brookes PA, et al. Frequency of anti-recipient alloreactive helper T-cell precursors in donor blood and graft-versus-host disease after HLA-identical sibling bone-marrow transplantation. *Lancet* 1993;341:203–205.
73. Ferrara JLM, Marion A, McIntyre JF, et al. Amelioration of acute graft-versus-host disease due to minor histocompatibility antigens by in vivo administration of anti-interleukin 2 receptor antibody. *J Immunol* 1986;137:1874–1877.
74. Herve P, Wijdenes J, Bergerat JP, et al. Treatment of corticosteroid-resistant acute graft-versus-host disease by in vivo administration of anti-interleukin-2 receptor monoclonal antibody (B-B10). *Blood* 1990;75:1017–1023.
75. Anasetti C, Martin PM, Hansen JA, et al. A phase I–II study evaluating the murine anti-IL-2 receptor antibody 2A3 for treatment of acute graft-versus-host disease. *Transplantation* 1990;50:49–54.
76. Belanger C, Esperou-Bourdeau H, Bordigoni P, et al. Use of an anti-interleukin-2 receptor monoclonal antibody for GVHD prophylaxis in unrelated donor BMT. *Bone Marrow Transplant* 1993;11:293–297.
77. Li XC, Demirci G, Ferrari-Lacraz S, et al. IL-15 and IL-2: a matter of life and death for T cells in vivo. *Nature Med* 2001;7:114–118.
78. Kumaki S, Minegishi M, Fujie H, et al. Prolonged secretion of IL-15 in patients with severe forms of acute graft-versus-host disease after allogeneic bone marrow transplantation in children. *Int J Hematol* 1998;67:307–312.
79. Szebeni J, Wang MG, Pearson DA, et al. IL-2 inhibits early increases in serum gamma interferon levels associated with graft-versus-host disease. *Transplantation* 1994;58:1385–1393.
80. Wang MG, Szebeni J, Pearson DA, et al. Inhibition of graft-versus-host disease by interleukin-2 treatment is associated with altered cytokine production by expanded graft-versus-host-reactive CD4+ helper cells. *Transplantation* 1995;60:481–490.
81. Troutt AB, Maraskovsky E, Rogers LA, et al. Quantitative analysis of lymphokine expression in vivo and in vitro. *Immunol Cell Biol* 1992;70:51–57.
82. Velardi A, Varese P, Terenzi A, et al. Lymphokine production by T-cell clones after human bone marrow transplantation. *Blood* 1989;74:1665–1672.
83. Niederwieser D, Herold M, Woloszczuk W, et al. Endogenous IFN-gamma during human bone marrow transplantation. *Transplantation* 1990;50:620–625.
84. Mowat A. Antibodies to IFN-gamma prevent immunological mediated intestinal damage in murine graft-versus-host reactions. *Immunology* 1989;68:18–24.
85. Dickinson AM, Sviland L, Dunn J, et al. Demonstration of direct involvement of cytokines in graft-versus-host reactions using an in vitro skin explant model. *Bone Marrow Transplant* 1991;7:209–216.
86. Holda JH, Maier T, Claman NH. Evidence that IFN-g is responsible for natural suppressor activity in GVHD spleen and normal bone marrow. *Transplantation* 1988;45:772–777.
87. Wall DA, Hamberg SD, Reynolds DS, et al. Immunodeficiency in graft-versus-host reaction. I. Mechanism of immune suppression. *J Immunol* 1988;140:2970–2976.
88. Klimpel GR, Annable CR, Cleveland MG, et al. Immunosuppression and lymphoid hypoplasia associated with chronic graft-versus-host disease is dependent upon IFN-g production. *J Immunol* 1990;144:84–93.
89. Wall DA, Sheehan KC. The role of tumor necrosis factor-alpha and interferon gamma in graft-versus-host disease and related immunodeficiency. *Transplantation* 1994;57:273–279.
90. Huchet R, Bruley-Rosset M, Mathiot C, et al. Involvement of IFN-gamma and transforming growth factor-beta in graft-vs-host reaction-associated immunosuppression. *J Immunol* 1993;150:2517–2524.
91. Krenger W, Falzarano G, Delmonte J, et al. Interferon-g suppresses T-cell proliferation to mitogen via the nitric oxide pathway during experimental acute graft-versus-host disease. *Blood* 1996;88:1113–1121.
92. Gifford GE, Lohmann-Matthes M-L. Gamma interferon priming of mouse and human macrophages for induction of tumor necrosis factor production by bacterial lipopolysaccharide. *J Natl Cancer Inst* 1987;78:121–124.
93. Nestel FP, Price KS, Seemayer TA, et al. Macrophage priming and lipopolysaccharide-triggered release of tumor necrosis factor alpha during graft-versus-host disease. *J Exp Med* 1992;75:405–413.
94. Krenger W, Snyder KM, Byon CH, et al. Polarized type 2 alloreactive CD4+ and CD8+ donor T cells fail to induce experimental acute graft-versus-host disease. *J Immunol* 1995;155:585–593.
95. Liu Y, Janeway CA Jr. Interferon gamma plays a critical role in induced cell death of effector T cell: a possible third mechanism of self-tolerance. *J Exp Med* 1990;172:1735–1739.
96. Rissoan MC, Soumelis V, Kadowaki N, et al. Reciprocal control of T helper cell and dendritic cell differentiation. *Science* 1999;283:1183–1186.
97. Reid SD, Penna G, Adorini L. The control of T cell responses by dendritic cell subsets. *Curr Opin Immunol* 2000;12:114–121.

98. Fowler DH, Kurasawa K, Husebekk A, et al. Cells of the Th2 cytokine phenotype prevent LPS-induced lethality during murine graft-versus-host reaction. *J Immunol* 1994;152:1004–1011.
99. Fowler DH, Kurasawa K, Smith R, et al. Donor CD4-enriched cells of Th2 cytokine phenotype regulate graft-versus-host disease without impairing allogeneic engraftment in sublethally irradiated mice. *Blood* 1994;84:3540–3549.
100. Pan L, Delmonte J Jr, Jalonen CK, et al. Pretreatment of donor mice with granulocyte colony-stimulating factor polarizes donor T lymphocytes toward type-2 cytokine production and reduces severity of experimental graft-versus-host disease. *Blood* 1995;86:4422–4429.
101. Murai M, Yoneyama H, Harada A, et al. Active participation of CCR5(+)CD8(+) T lymphocytes in the pathogenesis of liver injury in graft-versus-host disease. *J Clin Invest* 1999;104:49–57.
102. Nikolic B, Lee S, Bronson RT, et al. Th1 and Th2 mediate acute graft-versus-host disease, each with distinct end-organ targets. *J Clin Invest* 2000;105:1289–1298.
103. Atkinson K, Matias C, Guiffre A, et al. In vivo administration of granulocyte colony-stimulating factor (G-CSF), granulocyte-macrophage CSF, interleukin-1 (IL-1), and IL-4, alone and in combination, after allogeneic murine hematopoietic stem cell transplantation. *Blood* 1991;77:1376–1382.
104. Krenger W, Snyder K, Smith S, et al. Effects of exogenous interleukin-10 in a murine model of graft-versus-host disease to minor histocompatibility antigens. *Transplantation* 1994;58:1251–1257.
105. Blazar BR, Taylor PA, Smith S, et al. Interleukin-10 administration decreases survival in murine recipients of major histocompatibility complex disparate donor bone marrow grafts. *Blood* 1995;85:842–851.
106. Sykes M, Romick ML, Hoyles KA, et al. In vivo administration of interleukin 2 plus T cell-depleted syngeneic marrow prevents graft-versus-host disease mortality and permits alloengraftment. *J Exp Med* 1990;171:645–658.
107. Brok HPM, Heidt PJ, van der Meide PH, et al. Interferon-γ prevents graft-versus-host disease after allogeneic bone marrow transplantation in mice. *J Immunol* 1993;151:6451–6459.
108. Murphy WJ, Welniak LA, Taub DD, et al. Differential effects of the absence of interferon-gamma and IL-4 in acute graft-versus-host disease after allogeneic bone marrow transplantation in mice. *J Clin Invest* 1998;102:1742–1748.
109. Ellison CA, Fischer JM, HayGlass KT, et al. Murine graft-versus-host disease in an F1-hybrid model using IFN-gamma gene knockout donors. *J Immunol* 1998;161:631–640.
110. Welniak LA, Blazar BR, Anver MR, et al. Opposing roles of interferon-gamma on CD4+ T cell-mediated graft-versus-host disease: effects of conditioning. *Biol Blood Marrow Transplant* 2000;6:604–612.
111. Li XC, Strom TB, Turka LA, et al. T Cell death and transplantation tolerance. *Immunity* 2001;14:407–416.
112. Sykes M, Szot GL, Nguyen PL, et al. Interleukin-12 inhibits murine graft-versus-host disease. *Blood* 1995;86:2429–2438.
113. Dey BR, Yang YG, Szot GL, et al. Interleukin-12 inhibits graft-versus-host disease through an Fas-mediated mechanism associated with alterations in donor T-cell activation and expansion. *Blood* 1998;91:3315–3322.
114. Moser B, Loetscher P. Lymphocyte traffic control by chemokines. *Nat Immunol* 2001;2:123–128.
115. Sallusto F, Lenig D, Forster R, et al. Two subsets of memory T lymphocytes with distinct homing potentials and effector functions. *Nature* 1999;401:708–712.
116. Serody JS, Burkett SE, Panoskaltsis-Mortari A, et al. T-Lymphocyte production of macrophage inflammatory protein-1alpha is critical to the recruitment of CD8(+) T cells to the liver, lung, and spleen during graft-versus-host disease. *Blood* 2000;96:2973–2980.
117. Panoskaltsis-Mortari A, Strieter RM, Hermanson JR, et al. Induction of monocyte- and T-cell-attracting chemokines in the lung during the generation of idiopathic pneumonia syndrome following allogeneic murine bone marrow transplantation. *Blood* 2000;96:834–839.
118. Kagi D, Vignaux F, Ledermann B, et al. Fas and perforin pathways as major mechanisms of T cell-mediated cytotoxicity. *Science* 1994;265:528–530.
119. Lowin B, Hahne M, Mattmann C, et al. Cytolytic T-cell cytotoxicity is mediated through perforin and Fas lytic pathways. *Nature* 1994;370:650–620.
120. Shresta S, Pham CT, Thomas DA, et al. How do cytotoxic lymphocytes kill their targets? *Curr Opin Immunol* 1998;10:581–587.
121. Krammer PH. CD95's deadly mission in the immune system. *Nature* 2000;407:789–795.
122. Chinnaiyan AM, O'Rourke K, Yu GL, et al. Signal transduction by DR3, a death domain-containing receptor related to TNFR-1 and CD95. *Science* 1996;274:990–992.
123. Chicheportiche Y, Bourdon PR, Xu H, et al. TWEAK, a new secreted ligand in the tumor necrosis factor family that weakly induces apoptosis. *J Biol Chem* 1997;272:32,401–32,410.

124. Pan G, O'Rourke K, Chinnaiyan AM, et al. The receptor for the cytotoxic ligand TRAIL. *Science* 1997;276:111–113.
125. Baker MB, Altman NH, Podack ER, et al. The role of cell-mediated cytotoxicity in acute GVHD after MHC-matched allogeneic bone marrow transplantation in mice. *J Exp Med* 1996;183:2645–2656.
126. Braun YM, Lowin B, French L, et al. Cytotoxic T cells deficient in both functional Fas ligand and perforin show residual cytolytic activity yet lose their capacity to induce lethal acute graft-versus-host disease. *J Exp Med* 1996;183:657–661.
127. Graubert TA, DiPersio JF, Russell JH, et al. Perforin/granzyme-dependent and independent mechanisms are both important for the development of graft-versus-host disease after murine bone marrow transplantation. *J Clin Invest* 1997;100:904–911.
128. Blazar BR, Taylor PA, Vallera DA. CD4+ and CD8+ T cells each can utilize a perforin-dependent pathway to mediate lethal graft-versus-host disease in major histocompatibility complex-disparate recipients. *Transplantation* 1997;64:571–576.
129. Graubert TA, Russell JH, Ley T. The role of granzyme B in murine models of acute graft-versus-host disease and graft rejection. *Blood* 1996;87:1232–1237.
130. Ueno Y, Ishii M, Yahagi K, et al. Fas-mediated cholangiopathy in the murine model of graft versus host disease. *Hepatology* 2000;31:966–974.
131. Shustov A, Nguyen P, Finkelman F, et al. Differential expression of Fas and Fas ligand in acute and chronic graft-versus-host disease: up-regulation of Fas and Fas ligand requires CD8+ T cell activation and IFN-gamma production. *J Immunol* 1998;161:2848–2855.
132. Lee S, Chong SY, Lee JW, et al. Difference in the expression of Fas/Fas-ligand and the lymphocyte subset reconstitution according to the occurrence of acute GVHD. *Bone Marrow Transplant* 1997;20:883–888.
133. Wasem C, Frutschi C, Arnold D, et al. Accumulation and activation-induced release of preformed Fas (CD95) ligand during the pathogenesis of experimental graft-versus-host disease. *J Immunol* 2001;167:2936–2941.
134. Baker MB, Riley RL, Podack ER, et al. Graft-versus-host-disease-associated lymphoid hypoplasia and B cell dysfunction is dependent upon donor T cell-mediated Fas-ligand function, but not perforin function. *Proc Natl Acad Sci USA* 1997;94:1366–1371.
135. Via CS, Nguyen P, Shustov A, et al. A major role for the Fas pathway in acute graft-versus-host disease. *J Immunol* 1996;157:5387–5393.
136. Kondo T, Suda T, Fukuyama H, et al. Essential roles of the Fas ligand in the development of hepatitis. *Nature Med* 1997;3:409–413.
137. van Den Brink MR, Moore E, Horndasch KJ, et al. Fas-deficient lpr mice are more susceptible to graft-versus-host disease. *J Immunol* 2000;164:469–480.
138. Hattori K, Hirano T, Miyajima H, et al. Differential effects of anti-Fas ligand and anti-tumor necrosis factor-α antibodies on acute graft-versus-host disease pathologies. *Blood* 1998;91:4051–4055.
139. Stuber E, Buschenfeld A, von Freier A, et al. Intestinal crypt cell apoptosis in murine acute graft versus host disease is mediated by tumour necrosis factor alpha and not by the FasL-Fas interaction: effect of pentoxifylline on the development of mucosal atrophy. *Gut* 1999;45:229–235.
140. Lin T, Brunner T, Tietz B, et al. Fas ligand-mediated killing by intestinal intraepithelial lymphocytes. Participation in intestinal graft-versus-host disease. *J Clin Invest* 1998;101:570–577.
141. Liem LM, van Lopik T, van Nieuwenhuijze AE, et al. Soluble Fas levels in sera of bone marrow transplantation recipients are increased during acute graft-versus-host disease but not during infections. *Blood* 1998;91:1464–1468.
142. Das H, Imoto S, Murayama T, et al. Levels of soluble FasL and FasL gene expression during the development of graft-versus-host disease in DLT-treated patients. *Br J Haematol* 1999;104:795–800.
143. Kanda Y, Tanaka Y, Shirakawa K, et al. Increased soluble Fas-ligand in sera of bone marrow transplant recipients with acute graft-versus-host disease. *Bone Marrow Transplant* 1998;22:751–754.
144. Kayaba H, Hirokawa M, Watanabe A, et al. Serum markers of graft-versus-host disease after bone marrow transplantation. *J Allergy Clin Immunol* 2000;106:S40–S44.
145. Martin PJ, Akatsuka Y, Hahne M, et al. Involvement of donor T-cell cytotoxic effector mechanisms in preventing allogeneic marrow graft rejection. *Blood* 1998;92:2177–2181.
146. Jiang Z, Podack E, Levy RB. Major histocompatibility complex-mismatched allogeneic bone marrow transplantation using perforin and/or Fas ligand double-defective CD4(+) donor T cells: involvement of cytotoxic function by donor lymphocytes prior to graft-versus-host disease pathogenesis. *Blood* 2001;98:390–397.
147. Schnare M, Barton GM, Holt AC, et al. Toll-like receptors control activation of adaptive immune responses. *Nature Immunol* 2001;2:947–950.

148. Lorenz E, Schwartz DA, Martin PJ, et al. Association of TLR4 mutations and the risk for acute GVHD after HLA-matched-sibling hematopoietic stem cell transplantation. *Biol Blood Marrow Transplant* 2001;7:384–387.
149. Cooke KR, Hill GR, Crawford JM, et al. TNFa production to LPS stimulation by donor cells predicts the severity of experimental acute graft-versus-host disease. *J Clin Invest* 1998;102:1882–1891.
150. Cooke KR, Gerbitz A, Crawford JM, et al. LPS antagonism reduces graft-versus-host disease and preserves graft-versus-leukemia activity after experimental bone marrow transplantation. *J Clin Invest* 2001;107:1581–1589.
151. Hill GR, Ferrara JL. The primacy of the gastrointestinal tract as a target organ of acute graft-versus-host disease: rationale for the use of cytokine shields in allogeneic bone marrow transplantation. *Blood* 2000;95:2754–2759.
152. Vossen JM, Heidt PJ. Gnotobiotic measures for the prevention of acute graft-vs.-host disease. In: Burakoff SJ, Deeg HJ, Ferrara J, Atkinson K, eds. *Graft-vs.-Host Disease: Immunology, Pathophysiology, and Treatment*. New York: Marcel Dekker, 1990:403–413.
153. Storb R, Prentice RL, Buckner CD, et al. Graft-versus-host disease and survival in patients with aplastic anemia treated by marrow grafts from HLA-identical siblings. Beneficial effect of a protective environment. *N Engl J Med* 1983;308:302–307.
154. Piguet PF, Grau GE, Allet B, et al. Tumor necrosis factor/cachectin is an effector of skin and gut lesions of the acute phase of graft-versus-host disease. *J Exp Med* 1987;166:1280–1289.
155. Piguet PF, Grau GE, Collart MA, et al. Pneumopathies of the graft-versus-host reaction. Alveolitis associated with an increased level of tumor necrosis factor MRNA and chronic interstitial pneumonitis. *Lab Invest* 1989;61:37–45.
156. Laster SM, Wood JG, Gooding LR. Tumor necrosis factor can induce both apoptotic and necrotic forms of cell lysis. *J Immunol* 1988;141:2629.
157. Hill GR, Teshima T, Rebel VI, et al. The p55 TNF-alpha receptor plays a critical role in T cell alloreactivity. *J Immunol* 2000;164:656–663.
158. Brown GR, Lee E, Thiele DL. TNF–TNFR2 interactions are critical for the development of intestinal graft-versus-host disease in MHC class II-disparate (C57BL/6J—>C57BL/6J x bm12)F1 mice. *J Immunol* 2002;168:3065–3071.
159. Herve P, Flesch M, Tiberghien P, et al. Phase I-II trial of a monoclonal anti-tumor necrosis factor alpha antibody for the treatment of refractory severe acute graft-versus-host disease. *Blood* 1992;81:1993–1999.
160. Murphy GF, Sueki H, Teuscher C, et al. Role of mast cells in early epithelial target cell injury in experimental acute graft-versus-host disease. *J Invest Dermatol* 1994;102:451–461.
161. Gilliam AC, Whitaker-Menezes D, Korngold R, et al. Apoptosis is the predominant form of epithelial target cell injury in acute experimental graft-versus-host disease. *J Invest Dermatol* 1996;107:377–383.
162. Holler E, Kolb HJ, Moller A, et al. Increased serum levels of tumor necrosis factor alpha precede major complications of bone marrow transplantation. *Blood* 1990;75:1011–1016.
163. Holler E, Kolb HJ, Hintermeier-Knabe R, et al. The role of tumor necrosis factor alpha in acute graft-versus-host disease and complications following allogeneic bone marrow transplantation. *Transplant Proc* 1993;25:1234–1236.
164. Tanaka J, Imamura M, Kasai M, et al. Cytokine gene expression in peripheral blood mononuclear cells during graft-versus-host disease after allogeneic bone marrow transplantation. *Br J Haematol* 1993;85:558–565.
165. Tanaka J, Imamura M, Kasai M, et al. Rapid analysis of tumor necrosis factor-alpha mRNA expression during venoocclusive disease of the liver after allogeneic bone marrow transplantation. *Transplantation* 1993;55:430–432.
166. Abhyankar S, Gilliland DG, Ferrara JLM. Interleukin 1 is a critical effector molecule during cytokine dysregulation in graft-versus-host disease to minor histocompatibility antigens. *Transplantation* 1993;56:1518–1523.
167. Eisenberg SP, Evans RJ, Arend WP, et al. Primary structure and functional expression from complementary DNA of a human interleukin-1 receptor antagonist. *Nature* 1990;343:341.
168. Hannum CH, Wilcox CJ, Arend WP, et al. Interleukin-1 receptor antagonist activity of a human interleukin-1 inhibitor. *Nature* 1990;343:336–340.
169. McCarthy PL, Abhyankar S, Neben S, et al. Inhibition of interleukin-1 by an interleukin-1 receptor antagonist prevents graft-versus-host disease. *Blood* 1991;78:1915–1918.
170. Antin JH, Weisdorf D, Neuberg D, et al. Interleukin-1 blockade does not prevent acute graft-versus-host disease. Results of a randomized, double blinded, placebo-controlled trial of interleukin 1 receptor antagonist in allogeneic bone marrow transplantation. *Blood*, in press.

171. Falzarano G, Krenger W, Snyder KM, et al. Suppression of B cell proliferation to lipopolysaccharide is mediated through induction of the nitric oxide pathway by tumor necrosis factor-a in mice with acute graft-versus-host disease. *Blood* 1996;87:2853–2860.
172. Nestel FP, Greene RN, Kichian K, et al. Activation of macrophage cytostatic effector mechanisms during acute graft-versus-host disease: release of intracellular iron and nitric oxide-mediated cytostasis. *Blood* 2000;96:1836–1843.
173. Weiss G, Schwaighofer H, Herold M. Nitric oxide formation as predictive parameter for acute graft-versus-host disease after human allogeneic bone marrow transplantation. *Transplantation* 1995;60:1239–1244.
174. Langrehr JM, Murase N, Markus PM, et al. Nitric oxide production in host-versus-graft and graft-versus-host reactions in the rat. *J Clin Invest* 1992;90:679–683.
175. Feinstein L, Storb R. Nonmyeloablative hematopoietic cell transplantation. *Curr Opin Oncol* 2001;13:95–100.
176. Wekerle T, Kurtz J, Ito H, et al. Allogeneic bone marrow transplantation with co-stimulatory blockade induces macrochimerism and tolerance without cytoreductive host treatment. *Nature Med* 2000;6:464–469.
177. Durham MM, Bingaman AW, Adams AB, et al. Cutting edge: administration of anti-CD40 ligand and donor bone marrow leads to hemopoietic chimerism and donor-specific tolerance without cytoreductive conditioning. *J Immunol* 2000;165:1–4.
178. Hill GR, Cooke KR, Teshima T, et al. Interleukin-11 promotes T cell polarization and prevents acute graft-versus-host disease after allogeneic bone marrow transplantation. *J Clin Invest* 1998;102:115–123.
179. Panoskaltsis-Mortari A, Lacey DL, Vallera DA, et al. Keratinocyte growth factor administered before conditioning ameliorates graft-versus-host disease after allogeneic bone marrow transplantation in mice. *Blood* 1998;92:3960–3967.
180. Krijanovski OI, Hill GR, Cooke KR, et al. Keratinocyte growth factor separates graft-versus-leukemia effects from graft-versus-host disease. *Blood* 1999;94:825–831.
181. Kuroiwa T, Kakishita E, Hamano T, et al. Hepatocyte growth factor ameliorates acute graft-versus-host disease and promotes hematopoietic function. *J Clin Invest* 2001;107:1365–1373.
182. Teshima T, Hill GR, Pan L, et al. IL-11 separates graft-versus-leukemia effects from graft-versus-host disease after bone marrow transplantation. *J Clin Invest* 1999;104:317–325.
183. Antin JH, Lee SJ, Neuberg D, et al. A phase I/II double-blind, placebo-controlled study of recombinant human interleukin-11 for mucositis and acute GVHD prevention in allogeneic stem cell transplantation. *Bone Marrow Transplant* 2002;29:373–377.
184. Li Y, Li XC, Zheng XX, et al. Blocking both signal 1 and signal 2 of T-cell activation prevents apoptosis of alloreactive T cells and induction of peripheral allograft tolerance. *Nature Med* 1999;5:1298–1302.
185. Piemonti L, Monti P, Allavena P, et al. Glucocorticoids affect human dendritic cell differentiation and maturation. *J Immunol* 1999;162:6473–6481.
186. Rea D, van Kooten C, van Meijgaarden KE, et al. Glucocorticoids transform CD40-triggering of dendritic cells into an alternative activation pathway resulting in antigen-presenting cells that secrete IL-10. *Blood* 2000;95:3162–3167.
187. Critchfield JM, Racke MK, Zuniga-Pflucker JC, et al. T cell deletion in high antigen dose therapy of autoimmune encephalomyelitis. *Science* 1994;263:1139–1143.
188. Blazar BR, Taylor PA, Linsley PS, et al. In vivo blockade of CD28/CTLA4: B7/BB1 interaction with CTLA4-Ig reduces lethal murine graft-versus-host disease across the major histocompatibility complex barrier in mice. *Blood* 1994;83:3815–3825.
189. Blazar BR, Sharpe AH, Taylor PA, et al. Infusion of anti-B7.1 (CD80) and anti-B7.2 (CD86) monoclonal antibodies inhibit murine graft-versus-host disease lethality in part via direct effects on CD4+ and CD8+ T cells. *J Immunol* 1996;157:3250–3259.
190. Durie FH, Aruffo A, Ledbetter J, et al. Antibody to the ligand of CD40, gp39, blocks the occurrence of the acute and chronic forms of graft-vs-host disease. *J Clin Invest* 1994;94:1333–1338.
191. Blazar BR, Taylor PA, Panoskaltsis-Mortari A, et al. Blockade of CD40 ligand-CD40 interaction impairs CD4+ T cell mediated alloreactivity by inhibiting mature donor T cell expansion and function after bone marrow transplantation. *J Immunol* 1997;158:29–39.
192. Tsukada N, Akiba H, Kobata T, et al. Blockade of CD134 (OX40)-CD134L interaction ameliorates lethal acute graft-versus-host disease in a murine model of allogeneic bone marrow transplantation. *Blood* 2000;95:2434–2439.
193. Blazar BR, Kwon BS, Panoskaltsis-Mortari A, et al. Ligation of 4-1BB (CDw137) regulates graft-versus-host disease, graft-versus-leukemia, and graft rejection in allogeneic bone marrow transplant recipients. *J Immunol* 2001;166:3174–3183.

194. Nozawa K, Ohata J, Sakurai J, et al. Preferential blockade of CD8(+) T cell responses by administration of anti-CD137 ligand monoclonal antibody results in differential effect on development of murine acute and chronic graft-versus-host diseases. *J Immunol* 2001;167:4981–4986.
195. Tamada K, Shimozaki K, Chapoval AI, et al. Modulation of T-cell-mediated immunity in tumor and graft-versus-host disease models through the LIGHT co-stimulatory pathway. *Nature Med* 2000;6:283–289.
196. Coyle AJ, Lehar S, Lloyd C, et al. The CD28-related molecule ICOS is required for effective T cell-dependent immune responses. *Immunity* 2000;13:95–105.
197. Dong C, Juedes AE, Temann UA, et al. ICOS co-stimulatory receptor is essential for T-cell activation and function. *Nature* 2001;409:97–101.
198. Tafuri A, Shahinian A, Bladt F, et al. ICOS is essential for effective T-helper-cell responses. *Nature* 2001;409:105–109.
199. Guinan EC, Boussiotis VA, Neuberg D, et al. Transplantation of anergic histoincompatible bone marrow allografts. *N Engl J Med* 1999;340:1704–1714.
200. Taylor PA, Panoskaltsis-Mortari A, Noelle RJ, et al. Analysis of the requirements for the induction of CD4+ T cell alloantigen hyporesponsiveness by ex vivo anti-CD40 ligand antibody. *J Immunol* 2000;164:612–622.
201. Whitmire JK, Ahmed R. Costimulation in antiviral immunity: differential requirements for CD4(+) and CD8(+) T cell responses. *Curr Opin Immunol* 2000;12:448–455.
202. Salomon B, Lenschow DJ, Rhee L, et al. B7/CD28 costimulation is essential for the homeostasis of the CD4+CD25+ immunoregulatory T cells that control autoimmune diabetes. *Immunity* 2000;12:431–440.
203. Tamada K, Tamura H, Flies D, et al. Blockade of LIGHT/LTbeta and CD40 signaling induces allospecific T cell anergy, preventing graft-versus-host disease. *J Clin Invest* 2002;109:549–557.

7 Acute Graft-vs-Host Disease

Uwe Platzbecker, MD *and H. Joachim Deeg,* MD

Contents

1. INTRODUCTION

Hemopoietic stem cell transplantation (HSCT) involves the transfer of cells that produce hemopoietic and lymphoid progeny. For donor cells to accept the host environment as "self" requires that newly developing alloreactive T lymphocytes and mature donor T lymphocytes contained in the transplant inoculum be eliminated or inactivated, and only cells tolerant to the new self be permitted in order to prevent an adverse graft-vs-host (GVH) reaction. Multiple interactions between donor and host cells take place that contribute to the manifestations of this GVH reaction, leading to the clinical picture of GVH disease (GVHD).

2. DEFINITION AND ETIOLOGY

Immunologic identity is expressed in the form of cell surface proteins encoded by genes of the major histocompatibility complex (MHC) and other genes. MHC molecules (termed human leukocyte antigen [HLA] in humans) are critical to the recognition and inactivation or elimination of foreign antigens in immunocompetent individuals. MHC and non-MHC (minor) antigens on transplanted cells are recognized by the recipient's immune system, leading to a host-vs-graft (HVG) reaction. In immunodeficient (or immunosuppressed) recipients, however, transplanted cells are able to survive and, if immunocompetent, to recognize antigens such as HLA in the recipient, and initiate a GVH reaction.

From: *Stem Cell Transplantation for Hematologic Malignancies*
Edited by: R. J. Soiffer © Humana Press Inc., Totowa, NJ

Graft-vs-host reactions were first described in rodents *(1)*. The requirements for the development of GVHD were formulated by Billingham in a classical work *(2)*:

1. The graft must contain immunocompetent cells (T lymphocytes).
2. The host must express "transplantation" antigens not expressed in the donor. HLA differences between donor and recipient represent the strongest risk factor for GVHD; non-MHC (minor) histocompatibility antigens also play a role as illustrated by MHC-identical transplantation. We now know that GVH-like reactions also occur between genetically identical individuals or even with the infusion of autologous marrow, because of modifications of self-antigens or inappropriate self-recognition *(3)*.
3. The host must be unable to mount an effective response against the transplanted cells.

Thus, GVHD is an acute or chronic clinical syndrome initiated by a reaction of donor immunocompetent cells against recipient cells and organs. Although originally distinct acute and chronic forms were described *(4,5)*, such a clear separation may no longer be tenable (see below).

3. CLINICAL SPECTRUM OF GVHD

Acute GVHD usually becomes manifest within 2–5 wk of transplantation. The incidence ranges from 10% to 90% dependent on the degree of histoincompatibility, the number of T lymphocytes transplanted, patient and donor characteristics, and the prophylactic regimen utilized *(6,7)*.

The skin, liver, and gut are the major targets of acute GVHD, but other tissues can be involved (*see* Table 1). GVHD is observed most commonly in the skin as pruritic maculopapular rash, often on palms, soles, shoulders, and ears, and may progress to total-body erythroderma. Separation at the dermo-epidermal junction may lead to bullae formation and desquamation. Even with clinically normal skin, biopsies may reveal histological evidence of GVHD (subclinical GVHD).

Nausea, vomiting, diarrhea, pain, and paralytic ileus are signs of involvement of the intestinal tract. Hyperbilirubinemia and elevations of alkaline phosphatase and transaminases may indicate liver involvement. Hepatic failure and metabolic encephalopathy are rare and are more likely the result of causes such as veno-occlusive disease and infections.

Histological findings confirm the diagnosis of GVHD *(9)*. Primarily undifferentiated epithelial cells serve as targets. Epidermis and skin appendages lose their integrity. Damage is prominent at the tips of the rete ridges. Small bile ducts may show segmental disruption. The intestinal mucosa shows ulcerations and crypt destruction, most severe at the basis. Conjunctival, vaginal, oral, and esophageal mucosae are less frequently involved. There may be subtle mononuclear cell infiltrates or severe inflammation. Target cell destruction may be mediated by tumor necrosis factor-α (TNF-α), perforin or Fas ligand (FasL) without direct contact between lymphocytes and epithelial target cells *(10,11)*. Histological staging is generally not used in the grading of acute GVHD.

Current grading systems of GVHD score clinical manifestations in the skin, upper and lower intestinal tract, and liver *(4,12)*. Martin et al. have shown that for practical purposes, International Bone Marrow Transplant Registry (IBMTR) levels A, B, C and D roughly correspond to Glucksberg grades I, II, III, and IV, respectively *(13)*. Assessment of GVHD, especially of the intestinal tract and liver, is difficult and shows considerable interobserver variation *(13–16)*. Simplified "consensus" schemes for functional GVHD grading have been proposed *(17,18)*

Table 1
Targets and Manifestation of Acute and Chronic GVHD

Target organ	*Acute GVHD*	*Chronic GVHD*
Skin and appendages	Pruritus, maculopapular rash, generalized eythroderma, bullae	Erythematous papular rash (lichenoid) or thickened, tight, fragile skin (sclerodermatous), hair loss, nail changes such as vertical ridging
Liver	Cholestasis	Cholestasis, hypoalbuminemia
Intestinal tract	Hypersecretory diarrhea, cramps, bleeding, vomiting, ileus	Abnormal motility, strictures, diarrhea, cramps, malabsorption
Mucous membranes	Acute inflammation	Dryness, plaques, ulcerations, secondary malignancies
Airways	Not specific	Bronchiolitis obliterans with chronic obstructive lung disease, fibrosis, chronic sinopulmonary syndrome, high risk for *Pneumocystis carinii* pneumonia
Hematopoietic and immune system	Immunodeficiency	Cytopenias, eosinophilia, profound immunodeficiency, functional asplenia
Eyes	Conjunctivitis	Sicca syndrome with dryness, photophobia, and corneal ulcers
Others		Virtually all manifestations of autoimmune disease, including serositis, nephrotic syndrome, neuropathy, fasciitis

Source: Adapted from ref *8*.

including grading on the basis of outcome (i.e., taking into account the patient's entire course rather than considering only one time-point) *(15)*.

Chronic GVHD is likely a different entity than acute GVHD *(19–21)*. Chronic GVHD has been recognized as early as d 31, although the median day of diagnosis is 201 after hematopoietic stem cell transplantation (HSCT) from HLA-identical siblings, 159 d after HSCT from HLA-nonidentical related donors, and 133 d after HSCT from unrelated donors *(22)*. Overall, 50% of patients develop chronic GVHD, 65% with unrelated donors *(22–25)*. Chronic GVHD resembles an autoimmune disease with clinical manifestations in the liver, gut, eyes, lung, and skin (*see* Table 1) *(26)*. The skin is most frequently involved, showing lichenoid papules, areas of hypopigmentation, and areas of hyperpigmentation. With extensive chronic GVHD, sclerodermiform changes and generalized subcutaneous fibrosis may develop. Alopecia and dystrophic nail changes are common. Liver involvement presents as obstructive jaundice reflecting bile duct abnormalities. If the liver is the only organ involved, the disease may be self-limited and immunosuppressive therapy may not be necessary *(23)*. Alkaline phosphatase levels are often markedly increased and a good parameter for the course. Histological findings include fibrosis with hyalinization of portal triads, obliteration of bile ducts, and extensive cholestasis. Lichen planus-like plaques, ulcerations, and dryness of the oral mucosa are common. A sicca syndrome with dryness of the eyes and oral mucosa is commonly quantitated with a Schirmer's test. Artificial tears or patching of the eye to protect the corneal surface may be required. Gut involvement, less prominent than with acute GVHD, may lead to abdominal pain, diarrhea, anorexia, nausea, and vomiting. Bronchiolitis obliterans is highly correlated with chronic GVHD in other organs *(27–29)*. Symptoms and findings include obstructive lung disease, cough, dyspnea, and, in advanced cases, pneumothorax. Profound immunodeficiency accompanies chronic GVHD. Patients may have functional asplenia and are at high risk for sepsis. Fungal infections and, in the absence of prophylaxis, *Pneumocystis carinii* pneumonia are not infrequent. Eosinophilia and thrombocytopenia can also be present after transplant, with the latter being associated with poor prognosis *(30,31)*.

4. PROGNOSTIC SIGNIFICANCE

Mild to moderate acute GVHD (grades I or II by Glucksberg) is associated with low morbidity, but it is a significant risk factor for the development of chronic GVHD *(24,25)*. Grades III and IV acute GVHD carry a grave prognosis; with grade IV, mortality approaches 100%. Increased mortality with severe chronic GVHD is generally related to infections and organ failure. Progressive obstructive airway disease also may prove fatal. On the other hand, GVHD, particularly in its chronic form, is associated with a graft-vs-leukemia (GVL) effect and a decreased risk of relapse in patients transplanted in advanced disease *(32,33)*.

Recent observations in patients transplanted with nonmyeloablative regimens ("minitransplants") have shown changes in the kinetics of GVHD. Clinical features of acute GVHD may develop several months after HSCT and may not have the same impact on survival as in patients in whom GVHD occurs early posttransplant. In these patients, the historic classification into acute GVHD (onset before d 100) and chronic GVHD (onset after d 100) no longer satisfies clinical needs. These insights need to be incorporated into new grading schemes (*see* Fig. 1).

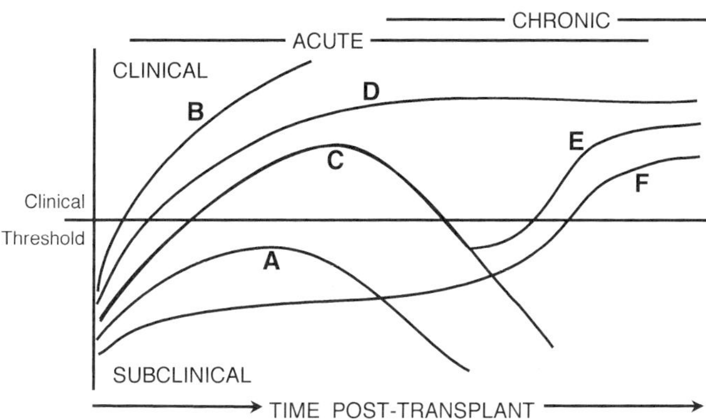

Fig. 1. Kinetics and patterns of GVHD: (**A**) no clinical evidence of GVHD; (**B**) rapidly progressive acute GVHD; (**C**) acute GVHD resolving spontaneously or with therapy; (**D**) acute GVHD progressing to chronic GVHD; (**E**) chronic GVHD after a quiescent phase following acute GVHD; (**F**) *de novo*-onset chronic GVHD or delayed-onset acute GVHD.

5. PATHOPHYSIOLOGY

Ferrara et al. have proposed a model in which initial damage to host tissue, induced by the transplant conditioning regimen, is followed by donor-T-cell activation, adhesion to and interaction with host tissue and costimulatory signals, and amplification of the cytokine network *(34)*. The effector phase leads to host cell destruction via inflammatory signals, cytolytic effects, and programmed cell death. Inflammatory cytokines are released primarily in the gut, and endotoxins/lipopolysaccharides (LPSs), transferred into the circulation, lead to macrophage activation (*see* Fig. 2). Amplification of cytokines such as TNF-α and interleukin (IL)-1 follows *(35,36)*, and leads to target cell death. Expression of costimulatory molecules (e.g., CD80, CD86 and MHC class II antigens on dendritic cells [DCs], T-cell stimulation, and upregulation of Th1 cytokines [IL-2, interferon-α {IFN-α}]) will lead to effector cell expansion *(37,38)*. The blockade of LPS-mediated signals (via CD14) may be effective in reducing the incidence/severity of GVHD, in part by way of reduction of TNF-α levels *(39)*.

The efferent arm of acute GVHD involves cytotoxic T cells that cause damage in tissues with high numbers of antigen-presenting cells (APCs) *(40)* such as the skin, liver, and gut *(41)*. A recent study showed that host DCs play a central role in the development of GVHD *(42)*. In murine models, CD4+ cells have been shown to induce GVHD across MHC class II, and CD8+ cells across MHC class I barriers *(43)*. In MHC-identical transplants (non-MHC barriers), GVHD was induced by either subset of T cells *(44,45)*. However, signals mediating the GVH effect may differ by organs *(46)*. Fas/FasL-mediated signals play a central role in hepatic injury *(47,48)*, TNF-α/TNF receptor signals in intestinal GVHD, and both TNF-α and FASL in skin manifestations. Perforin-mediated cytotoxicity may be more important in mediating a GVL effect *(10)*. However, even T cells from mice doubly deficient in Fas-L and perforin/granzyme can cause GVHD when aggressive conditioning is used *(49)*. The actions of different cytokines, effector cells (e.g., large granular lymphocytes), and regulatory cells are still incompletely understood. Regulatory T cells with a CD25+ CD4+ phenotype, functionally reminiscent of the classic "suppressor T cell," have recently been shown to play a pivotal role in the development of GVHD *(50)*.

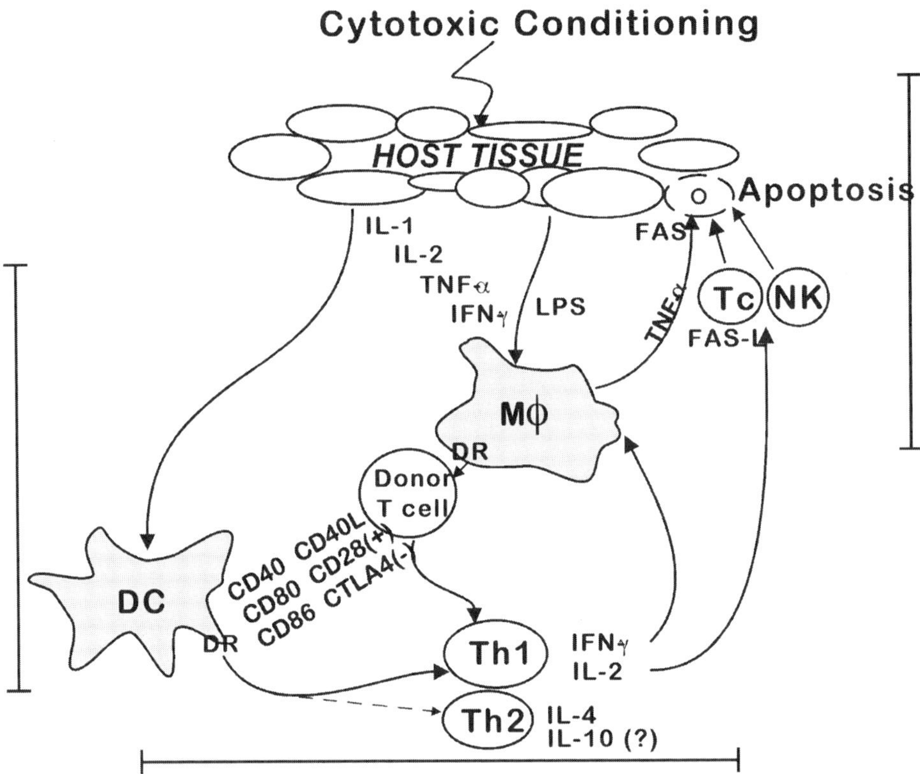

Fig. 2. Three components of GVHD immunopathophysiology: (1) Conditioning with cytotoxic regimens results in tissue damage and the release of cytokines. (2) Allorecognition: Antigen-presenting cells, monocytes (macrophage [M∅]), or dendritic cells (DCs), present host antigen in the form of an HLA-(DR) peptide complex to donor T cells. Antigen-presenting cells also supply costimulatory signals (e.g., CD80, interleukin-1 [IL-1]). These and additional costimulatory interactions lead to (3) T-cell activation, particularly in the direction of Th1 (rather than Th2) cells, and further amplification (in particular by IL-2) and secretion of cytokines (such as interferon-γ [IFN-γ]), which amplify the function of antigen-presenting cells. The function of DCs is enhanced by the CD40 ligand on activated T cells. The expression of cytokines leads to maturation of cytotoxic T cells (Tc) and activation of natural killer (NK) cells. Along with factors such as tumor necrosis factor-α (TNF-α), these cause and further amplify host tissue damage (predominantly via apoptosis) and lead to the clinical manifestations of GVHD. DR, HLA-DR; Th1, CD4+ T cells type 1; Th2, CD4+ T cells type 2; Fas, death receptor CD95; FasL, Fasligand. CD28+ provides a costimulatory signal, CTLA4 may have a tolerogenic effect. The function of IL-10 is not clear and may be time dependent.

The role of costimulatory molecules such as CD80/86, CD40L/CD40, CD28, and CTLA4 and vascular cellular adhesion molecule 1/intercellular adhesion molecule 1 (VCAM-1/ICAM-1) (CD54), E-selectin, OX40 (CD134)/CD134L, and others is still being defined *(51–53)*. Signals transmitted via CTLA4 appear to have tolerogenic effects, whereas signals through CD28 will lead to activation *(54)*.

The pathophysiology of chronic GVHD is less well understood, and only some observations are summarized here. In certain mouse strains, transplantation of low numbers of allogeneic T cells is more likely to result in chronic than in acute GVHD *(55,56)*. There is evidence that although Th1 cells are deficient, the activity of Th2 cells is increased *(57)*. Consistent with that notion is a recent report that shows an increase in chronic GVHD in mice transplanted from IFN-γ knockout donors *(58)* and an earlier report indicating that both acute and chronic GVHD were Th2 cytokine dependent *(59)*. Conversely, increased IFN-γ mRNA levels have been documented in skin biopsies of patients with chronic GVHD *(60)*. Data by Chen et al. suggest that the presence of recipient CD4+ T cells is also required for chronic GVHD to develop *(61)*. The current opinion is that various features of GVHD (acute and chronic) are dependent on the subsets of donor T cells activated *(62,63)*. An interesting but poorly understood phenomenon is that sensitization of recipients with donor antigen via the oral route alleviates manifestations of chronic GVHD *(64)*.

Impairment of thymic function as a result of the preparative regimen, acute GVHD, or age-related involution may allow for the development of autoreactive T cells, which may eventually lead to the autoimmune manifestations of chronic GVHD. This may also be one reason why older patients experience more GVHD *(25)*. Additionally, a recent study in mice suggested that APCs from older animals have a higher capacity to stimulate donor T cells than those from young recipients *(65)*. Conceivably, these host cells are also involved in the mechanism of oral sensitization, as described earlier *(64)*. That recipient APCs play a central role in triggering GVHD has been shown convincingly by Shlomchik et al. *(42)*. The role of Fas and FasL *(66)* as well as CD40-L and other factors is not clear *(67–70)*.

The use of peripheral blood stem cells (PBSCs) mobilized either by means of chemotherapy or hemopoietic growth factors (e.g., granulocyte colony-stimulating factor [G-CSF] or stem cell factor), or both, is associated with rapid hemopoietic reconstitution *(71)*. Murine studies suggest that G-CSF may polarize donor cells toward Th2 cells and thereby favor the development of tolerance *(72)*.

Results of several clinical studies, some of them randomized *(71,73,74)* suggest that the incidences of acute GVHD in patients transplanted with marrow or PBSCs are similar, whereas the incidence of chronic GVHD appears to be increased with PBSCs *(75)*. A meta-analysis of 5 randomized controlled trials and 11 cohort studies suggests that both acute and chronic GVHD are more common with PBSCs *(76)*. An additional factor in these studies may also be differences in the GVHD prophylactic regimen. Of note, a higher incidence of GVHD with PBSCs may not be associated with increase mortality. In fact, particularly in patients with "high-risk" disease, survival appears to be improved in comparison to patients given marrow, possibly because of an enhanced GVL effect *(71,73)*.

Whether the fact that monocytes from G-CSF mobilized PBSCs show increased production of IL-10, decreased levels of TNF-α, and reduced expression of costimulatory molecules and MHC class II results in downregulation of alloreactivity and a tolerogenic effect is controversial at present.

Cord blood cells have low GVHD potential *(77–80)*. Kurtzberg et al. *(81)* reported results on 25 consecutive patients, mostly children transplanted with cord blood. Among these, 24 were discordant for one to three HLA antigens. In 23 of the 25 patients, engraftment was achieved, and 11 of 21 evaluable patients developed acute GVHD of grades II–IV. Gluckman et al. *(78)* presented results on 143 transplants carried out at 45 centers. GVHD of grades II–IV occurred in 9% of HLA-identical transplants and in 50% of HLA-mismatched transplants. Stimulating capacity *(82)* and intracytoplasmatic signaling (following T-cell-receptor engagement) in cord blood T cells differs from that in adult T cells *(83)*. Also, cord blood monocytes express low levels of MHC class II, CD86, and ICAM-1 and produce lower levels of IL-10 and

IFN-α. Most cytotoxicity of cord blood is mediated by natural killer (NK) type cells (rather than CD3+ T cells).

6. RISK FACTORS

Risk factors for acute GVHD in clinical transplantation are listed in Table 2. The probability of developing acute GVHD grades II–IV with HLA genotypically identical sibling transplants may be less than 30%, but 60–90% with mismatched related and with unrelated transplants (35% grades III–IV GVHD). Progress in HLA typing has allowed in recent years for selection of unrelated donors on the basis of molecular matching *(84–86)*, which is reflected in improved results. In a study of patients with chronic myelogenous leukemia (CML) in chronic phase, DRB1 allele mismatching was associated with a significant increase in grades III–IV acute GVHD and inferior survival. HLA-DPB1 also had an effect on GVHD if two alleles were mismatched. MHC class I allele mismatches had a negative impact on engraftment, but did not significantly affect GVHD *(86)*. Similar results on the impact of molecular typing have been obtained in patients with aplastic anemia *(87)*.

Omission of GVHD prophylaxis significantly increases the risk of GVHD *(88)*. Allosensitization of (female) donors for male recipients is associated with a twofold to threefold higher risk of GVHD than with nonsensitized donors *(89)*. The intensity of the GVHD prophylactic regimen inversely correlates with the incidence of acute GVHD *(90,91)*. Recent data by several teams indicate that the incorporation of antithymocyte globulin (ATG), specifically thymoglobulin, into the transplant conditioning regimen or administered early after transplantation not only facilitates engraftment but also reduces the incidence of GVHD *(92,93)*.

Infusion of viable donor buffy coat cells in earlier studies and, more recently, viable donor lymphocytes for the reinduction of remission in patients whose leukemia recurred after HSCT *(94)* is associated with an increased risk of GVHD. The impact of PBSCs was discussed earlier *(95,96)*. In one analysis of risk factors for acute GVHD after allogeneic PBSC transplantation, the type of GVHD prophylaxis and CD34 cell dose were the only two independent variables noted *(97)*, although it is currently not clear what the optimal CD34 dose should be.

High IL-10 production by peripheral blood mononuclear cells pretransplant has been correlated with a low incidence of GVHD and transplant-related mortality (TRM) *(98)*. Certain polymorphic alleles in the IFN-γ, TNF, and IL-10 genes have been associated with severe acute GVHD after HLA-identical sibling HSCT and polymorphisms for IL-6 with chronic GVHD *(99–102)*. Mismatching for CD31 (PECAM-1, platelet-endothelial cell adhesion molecule) has been reported to increase the risk of acute GVHD *(103,104)*.

The role of antiviral immunity *(105)* and certain HLA alleles has remained controversial. In a retrospective IBMTR study of 751 patients with CML in chronic phase transplanted from HLA-identical family members, the presence of HLA-A3 increased, and HLA-DR1 decreased, the risk of acute GVHD *(106)*. Attempts aimed at determining whether in vitro tests (e.g., skin explant models in which patient skin and donor lymphocytes are cocultured) identify groups of patients who are at risk of developing GVHD have met with only limited success.

The main risk factor for chronic GVHD is acute GVHD, as discussed earlier (*see* Table 2) *(25)*. The use of PBSCs appears to be associated with an increased incidence of chronic GVHD *(76)*, particularly when higher doses of CD34+ cells (> 8.0×10^6/kg) are transplanted *(107)*. G-CSF decreases IFN-γ and increases IL-4 production *(108)*, and other reports show that the numbers of T helper 2-inducing dendritic cells (pre-DC2s) are increased in G-CSF-mobilized

Table 2
Risk Factors for the Development of Acute and Chronic GVHD

Acute GVHD	*Chronic GVHD*
Histoincompatibility	Prior acute GVHD
Allosenzitation of donor	Histoincompatibility
Patient age	Patient age
Stem cell source (PBSC)?	Stem cell source (PBSC)
Number of CD34+ cells infused with PBSC	Number of CD34+ cells infused with PBSC
Infusion of viable donor leukocytes	Infusion of viable donor leukocytes
Donor age	Steroid dependence
Gender mismatch	
Omission of GVHD prophylaxis	
Type of GVHD prophylaxis	
Intensity of conditioning regimen (irradiation)	
Cytokine polymorphisms (IFN-α, TNF-α, IL-6, IL-10)	
Serum cytokine levels	
Donor cytomegalovirus (herpes simplex virus) seropositivity	

allografts *(109)*. Whether the prolongation of CSP prophylaxis lowers the incidence of chronic GVHD is controversial *(110–113)*. The relevance of herpes immunity in either the donor or recipient for GVHD development is not clear *(114,115)*.

7. PROPHYLAXIS

Strategies for GVHD prevention have focused on eliminating donor T cells or preventing T-cell activation (i.e., the afferent limb) (*see* Table 3). The deciphering of numerous cytokine and chemokine signals involved in clinical GVHD has also drawn attention to the efferent limb. When designing and evaluating GVHD trials, both efficacy and toxicity need to be considered because net improvements in survival are likely to be achieved only if GVHD prevention does not negatively affect other end points such as relapse. Overviews of prophylactic and therapeutic trials have recently been presented *(6,116)*.

7.1. In Vivo Prophylaxis

Classic studies by Uphoff *(117)* used the antimetabolite α-aminopterin for posttransplant GVHD prevention. Methotrexate (MTX) was beneficial in dogs and monkeys, and cyclophosphamide was beneficial in rats. Corticosteroids and ATG have also been used. In 1978, cyclosporine (CSP) was added *(118)*, and tacrolimus (FK506) *(119,120)*, thalidomide, mycophenolate mofetil (MMF), and rapamycin followed more recently.

The mechanisms of action of these agents differ. MTX, for example, blocks dihydrofolate reductase and prevents division and expansion of T cells already activated. Corticosteroids are lympholytic and repress gene transcription. CSP and FK506 bind to cyclophilin and FK binding protein (FKBP), respectively. The resulting complexes interfere with the serine/threonine phosphatase calcineurin and block the activity of NF-ATp, thereby downregulating IL-2 transcription *(121)*. Rapamycin binds to FKBP (and in vitro is a competitive inhibitor of FK506), but interacts with the mammalian TOR protein. The result is p70 S6 kinase inactivation and

Table 3
Agents and Modalities Used for Prevention and Treatment of GVHD

In vivo	*In vivo or in vitro*	*In vitro*
Methotrexate	Glucocorticoids	Elutriation
Cyclosporine	Monoclonal antibodies	Soybean and sheep red blood cell agglutination
FK506 (tacrolimus)	Immunotoxins	Column fractionation
Mycophenolate mofetil	Phototherapy	
	PUVA	
	Photopheresis	
Rapamycin (sirolimus)		
Antithymocyte globulin (ATG)		
Thalidomide		
Gnotobiosis		
Cytokine antagonists		
Receptor fusion proteins		
CTLA4Ig		
TNFR-Ig		

inhibition of cell cycle progression in the late G1 phase *(122)*. MMF is activated to mycophenolic acid, which blocks inosine monophosphate dehydrogenase (IMPDH) and thereby interferes with purine biosynthesis *(123)*.

CTLA4Ig, a fusion protein that interferes with costimulatory signals by blocking B7–CD28 and B7–CTLA4 interactions *(124,125)* has been tested in pilot trials. Recent data indicate that although the blockade of CD28 signals is beneficial in the prevention of GVHD, CTLA4-mediated signals facilitate the establishment of tolerance and, hence, may be desirable. Monoclonal antibodies to TNF-α or IL-2 or their receptors and the IL-1 antagonist IL-1RA block cytokine signals *(126)*. Peptides with high affinity for MHC may block T-cell activation *(127,128)* and the polarization of CD4+ T cells from a Th1 to a Th2 phenotype *(72,129)*. Monoclonal antibody to CD40L *(130)*, CD80 and CD86 *(131)*, CD95L (FasL) *(48)*, CD134L *(51)*, TAK-603, a new quinolone that selectively suppresses Th1 cytokine production *(132)*, a rationally designed Janus kinase (JAK) 3 inhibitor WHI-P131 *(133)*, and peptides exhibiting the same molecular sequence as a portion of the CDR3-like region in domain 1 of the CD4 molecule *(134)* all represent interesting recent developments.

A randomized study comparing GVHD prophylaxis with no prophylaxis has never been done. Single-arm studies indicate, however, that prophylaxis is beneficial. Single-agent (MTX or CSP) prophylaxis was considered standard until the early 1980s *(6,135)*. More recently, two- or three-drug combinations were tested *(119,120,136)*, and results indicate that combinations such as MTX + CSP or FK506 + MTX offer more effective prophylaxis than any single agent. However, improved GVHD prophylaxis was not necessarily reflected in superior survival (*see* Table 4). A combination of MTX, CSP, and corticosteroids, for example, reduced the incidence of acute GVHD grades II–IV to 9%, but survival was identical to that in patients given CSP plus prednisone only *(144)*. Combination regimens are also associated with more toxicity and higher probability of leukemic relapse, which may be preventable, however, by utilizing lower drug doses *(148,151,152)*. The addition of corticosteroids to CSP resulted in an increased incidence of chronic GVHD *(145)* and an increased risk of infection *(153)*. Results from three randomized trials comparing the combination of CSP + MTX with CSP, MTX, and methylprednisone were inconsistent and hence inconclusive *(110,143,154)*. In a prospective, randomized multicenter trial, the combination of FK506 and MTX was superior in preventing acute GVHD grades II–IV compared to CSP and MTX in recipients of T-cell-replete, HLA-identical HSCT from unrelated donors (56% vs 74%) *(120)*. The FK506 and MTX-treated patients also required less corticosteroids, but there was no difference in the incidence of chronic GVHD, and overall survival did not differ.

7.2. T-Cell Depletion

The most effective method of GVHD prevention is T-cell depletion of the donor marrow or peripheral blood cells before infusion *(155,156)*. T-Cell depletion is accomplished in the form of either positive (elimination of T cells) or negative selection (enrichment for hemopoietic precursor cells, leaving T cells behind *(156)*. T Cells are either killed by a toxin (e.g., ricin A chain) conjugated to anti-T-cell antibody or by incubating donor cells with antibody and complement, which then lyses the antibody-coated T cells. Some rat antibodies (e.g., Campath-1) activate the patient's own complement. These techniques allow for 90–99.9% T-cell elimination. A more selective approach involves depletion of donor T cells reactive with host tissues (alloreactive) by sensitizing donor T cells to host tissues and then depleting T cells that now

Table 4
Drug Combinations for GVHD Prophylaxis

Center/(ref.)	Diagnosis	Regimen[a] (no. of patients)	Incidence of acute GVHD[b]	p-Value	Incidence of chronic GVHD[b]	p-Value	Overall survival	p-Value
Minneapolis (218)	Hematological-malignancies	MTX (35)	48%	0.01	43%	NA[a]	45%	NS[a]
	Aplastic anemia	MTX+PDN+ATG (32)	21%		25%	50%		
Seattle (91)	Acute and chronic myeloid leukemia	CSA (50)	54%	0.014	58%	NS	55%	0.042
		MTX+CSA (43)	33%	46%	80%			
Seattle (137)	Aplastic anemia	MTX (24)	53%	0.012	42%	NS	60% (p=0.062)	NS
	MTX+CSA (22)	18%	47%	82%				
City of Hope (138)	Acute and chronic myeloid	MTX+PDN (53)	47%	<0.05	NA	NA	48% leukemia	NA
		CSA+PDN (54)	28%	68%				
Baltimore (139)	Hematological malignancies, aplastic anemia	Cy+PDN (40)	68%	0.005	35%	NS	20%	NS
		CSA+PDN (42)	32%	68%	38%			
Stockholm (140)	Hematological malignancies, aplastic anemia	CSA (45)	31%	0.02	40%	NS	67%	NS
		MTX (66)	25%	42%	57%			
		MTX+CSA (29)	8%	31%	79%			
Pesaro (141)	Children with thalassemia	CSA (22)	41%	<0.05	40%	NA	86%	NS
		CSA+Cy+MTX (22)	15%	12%	77%			
Seattle (142)	Hematological malignancies	Standard MTX (44)	25%	0.0001	33%	NS	66%	0.024[c]
		Short MTX (40)	59%	51%	55%			
		Standard MTX+DBC (25)	82%	44%	36%			

(continued on next page)

Table 4
Drug Combinations for GVHD Prophylaxis

Center/(ref.)	*Diagnosis*	*Regimen*[a] *(no. of patients)*	*Incidence of acute GVHD*[b]	*p-Value*	*Incidence of chronic GVHD*[b]	*p-Value*	*Overall survival*	*p-Value*
Seattle *(143)*	Hematological malignancies	MTX+CSA (74) MTX+CSA+PDN (73)	36%	0.28	40%	0.01	54%	NS
			45%	62%	53%			
Stanford *(144)*	Hematological malignancies	CSA+PDN (74) CSA+PDN+MTX (75)	23%	0.02	60%	NS	59%	NS
				9%	57%	64%		
Seattle *(145)*	Hematological malignancies	CSA (59) CSA+PDN (61)	74%	0.01	21%	0.02	26%	NS
			60%	44%	23%			
Multicenter *(146)*	Hematological malignancies	MTX+CSA (164) MTX+FK506 (165)	44%	0.01	49%	NS	57%	0.02
			32%	56%	47%[d]			
Genoa *(147)*	Acute myeloid leukemia	Low-dose CSA (28) Low-dose CSA+low-dose MTX (32)	61%	0.02	82%	NS	68%	NS
			34%	70%	74%			
Multicenter *(148)*	Aplastic anemia	CSA (34) CSA+short-term MTX (37)	38% 30%	NS 44%	30% 94%	NS	78%	0.05
Helsinki *(149)*	Hematological malignancies	MTX+CSA+PDN (53) MTX+CSA (55)	13%	0.005	36%	NS	60%	NS
			36%	48%	51%			
Multicenter *(120)*	Hematological malignancies, aplastic anemia	Short-term MTX+FK506 (90) Short-term MTX+CSA (90)	56%	0.0002	76%	NS	54%	NS
			74%	70%	50%			
Multicenter *(150)*	Hematological malignancies, aplastic anemia	FK506 (66)+MTX (56) CSA (65)+MTX (56)	18%	<0.0001	47%	NS	63%	NS
			48%	43%	65%			

[a]Abbreviations: ATG, antithymocyte globulin; CSA, cyclosporine A; Cy, cyclophosphamide; DBC, donor buffy coat; MTX, methotrexate; PDN, prednisone or other glucocorticoid; NS, not significant; NA, not available.
[b]Acute GVHD grades II–IV and overall chronic GVHD.
[c]For standard versus standard plus DBC.
[d]More advanced diseases in FK506 arm.

express activation markers (e.g., IL-2R, CD25, CD69, CD71, or HLA-DR) *(157–159)*. Ex vivo incubation of donor marrow with host cells and CTL4Ig *(160)* was beneficial in one study, but results have not been confirmed. It now appears that CTLA4-mediated signals may actually facilitate the establishment of tolerance *(161,162)*.

Intensive GVHD prophylaxis may also cause problems. T-Cell depletion by certain methods is associated with higher rates of graft failure (subsets of T cells mediate a graft-facilitating effect) and an increased incidence of relapse *(163,164)*. Therefore, more recent trials used selective depletion of T-cell subsets, specifically CD4, CD6, or CD8 cells *(165–167)*. Although engraftment was generally achieved, survival was not significantly different from that among patients transplanted with broadly T-cell-depleted marrow. Thus, although T-cell depletion leads to reduced morbidity and mortality related to GVHD, disease-free survival (DFS) was generally not improved.

Conversely, the development of GVHD conveys a lower probability of leukemic relapse than seen in patients without GVHD *(32,142)*. Importantly, even patients transplanted from allogeneic donors who do not develop GVHD have a lower probability of relapse than do syngeneic transplant recipients. Unfortunately, attempts to separate GVHD from a GVL effect have, so far, been unsuccessful in the clinic *(168)*. In HLA-identical transplants, Goulmy and colleagues have shown in vitro that such a separation is conceivable by using cytotoxic T cells specific for minor histocompatibility antigens expressed on hemopoietic cells *(169)*. After HLA-mismatched transplantation, the utilization of donor-vs-recipient NK-cell alloreactivity mediated by killer cell immunoglobulinlike receptors (KIR) might be a promising approach *(170)*. The selective application of ligands like perforin or TRAIL (TNF-related apoptosis-inducing ligand), known to be primarily involved in antitumor effects of T and NK cells, could be another strategy *(10,11,171)*.

Methods of T-cell engineering aim at preserving functional T cells to assure engraftment and provide a GVL effect but then eliminate those cells if evidence of GVHD develops. This involves the transduction of donor lymphocytes with a so-called suicide gene (e.g., the herpes virus thymidine kinase), which allows one to inactivate the suicide gene (e.g., with ganciclovir) *(172–174)*.

7.3. Reduced-Intensity Conditioning and Mixed Chimerism

In murine models, mixed chimerism can be achieved by design with modified conditioning regimens without jeopardizing the eradication of leukemia *(175)*. In a canine model, similarly mixed chimerism without GVHD was achieved in recipients conditioned with only 200 cGy of TBI, transplanted with histocompatible marrow, and given postgrafting CSP and MMF *(176)*. This led to low-intensity clinical conditioning regimens (fludarabine plus low-dose [200 cGy] TBI or other combinations). This approach allows one to reduce early posttransplant toxicity and mortality but still achieve engraftment of donor cells *(177)*. However, this approach does not prevent GVHD in humans, although the manifestations may be less severe and may become clinically apparent only months after transplantation.

7.4. Gnotobiosis

Gnotobiosis (i.e., the maintenance of transplant recipients in a germ-free environment) has been successful in rodent models but less so in clinical studies, presumably because of incomplete decontamination of patients. Nevertheless, in patients with severe aplastic anemia (conditioned with cyclophosphamide only) and transplanted in laminar airflow isolation, the incidence of GVHD was reduced, and survival improved *(178,179)* Some investigators have further pursued this technique in larger studies in patients with malignant disorders and have reported improved outcome *(180)*.

8. THERAPY

Dependent on various parameters, 10–90% of patients develop acute GVHD requiring therapy. The probability of survival depends on the response to therapy *(181–183)*. Many drugs used for GVHD prevention were first tested for therapy of GVHD. Generally, these drugs are more effective for prevention, presumably because of limited expansion of donor cells. Furthermore, our understanding of the effector limb of the GVH reaction is rather incomplete, rendering rational design of treatment regimens difficult.

Corticosteroids (e.g., methylprednisolone, 2 mg/kg/d for 7 or 14 d or longer) are the mainstay of acute (and chronic) GVHD therapy. Complete responses occur in 20% of patients and useful responses in about 40% of patients. A prospective randomized study comparing 2 mg/kg/d of methylprednisolone to 10 mg/kg/d failed to show any advantage of the higher dose for any end point studied *(184)*. "Nonabsorbable" oral beclomethasone is effective in a proportion of patients to treat acute intestinal GVHD *(185,186)*.

CSP is useful in patients who have not received CSP prophylaxis. Tacrolimus is effective in some patients who have failed CSP prophylaxis *(187)*, although retrospective data showed a benefit only in patients who were switched because of central nervous system toxicity on CSP *(188)*. A combination of tacrolimus and ATG has yielded promising results in one study *(189)*. MMF might be effective in combination with CSP and prednisolone *(190)*. A recent trial with rapamycin in 21 patients showed a response rate of more than 50% and suggested improved survival compared to historic controls *(191)*.

Antithymocyte globulins of horse or rabbit origin are potent anti-T-cell agents, achieving responses in 20–30% of patients even after steroid failure *(183,192–194)*. However, infections and thrombocytopenia are common complications, and in some trials, patient survival was as low as 10% *(195)*.

Monoclonal antibodies in murine or humanized form, with pan T or T-subset reactivity have been used, often as a secondary therapy for GVHD. Responses have been observed with anti-CD2, anti-CD3, anti-CD5, and other antibodies *(196–198)*. More than half of the patients with steroid-refractory acute GVHD responded to the anti-CD147 antibody ABX-CBL, and survival was superior to that observed in historical controls treated with horse ATG *(199)*. Intriguing results have been obtained with HuM291, a humanized antibody directed at the T-cell-receptor zeta chain *(200)*. Among 15 patients with steroid-refractory GVHD, 7 achieved complete remission and 8 achieved partial remission. Sustained remissions were achieved with a single dose. Many patients experienced a rise in plasma titers of Epstein–Barr virus (EBV) DNA, which was controlled with anti-CD20 antibody.

Another strategy involves antibodies against cytokine receptors. A monoclonal antibody to IL-2R (B-B10) was effective experimentally and clinically *(201)*. Monoclonal antibody specific for Tac, the α-subunit of the IL-2R (anti-TAC, daclizumab), showed responses in about 40% of patients who had failed to respond to corticosteroids *(202,203)*. One clinical report suggested efficacy of an anti-TNF-α monoclonal antibody (infliximab) in steroid-refractory acute GVHD *(204)*. Toxin-conjugated monoclonal antibodies have also shown encouraging results *(205)*, although only a marginally significant effect was observed in a randomized trial with a ricin A-conjugated anti-CD5 antibody *(206)*.

Photosensitization with 8-methoxypsoralen and ultraviolet A (PUVA) irradiation is effective in the treatment of acute and chronic GVHD of the skin in some patients. Extracorporeal exposure of the recipient's peripheral blood mononuclear cells to the photosensitizing effect of 8-methoxypsoralen and UV light (photopheresis) and their subsequent reinfusion is effective in treating acute (and chronic) GVHD refractory to conventional treatment *(207–209)*.

Chronic GVHD responds differently than acute GVHD to treatment. Alternate-day CSP and prednisone is currently the treatment of choice for patients with newly diagnosed extensive chronic GVHD *(210)*, although a recent randomized trial failed to show a survival benefit with the addition of CSP *(211)*. Patients in whom CSP fails might benefit from a switch to tacrolimus *(212)*. Intriguing results with thalidomide were reported by Vogelsang et al. *(213)* and Parker et al. *(214)* for primary and salvage treatment of patients with chronic GVHD. Subsequent randomized studies, however, failed to show significant benefit *(215,216)*. Improvements of skin and liver have been reported with PUVA therapy *(217–219)* and low-dose total-body irradiation (TBI; 100 cGy) has been shown to improve symptoms in some patients *(220)*. MMF in combination with CSP or FK506 *(221–223)* as salvage treatment showed promising results and allowed for a reduction of corticosteroid doses. The recombinant soluble TNF receptor Enbrel® has also yielded encouraging results *(224)*. All patients with chronic GVHD need antimicrobial prophylaxis especially directed against *Pneumocystis carinii* and encapsulated bacteria. Overall chronic GVHD management should involve a multidisciplinary approach.

9. FUTURE CONSIDERATIONS

Future attempts at prophylaxis and therapy are likely to exploit results derived from ongoing research in cellular and molecular biology. The genetic cloning of receptors for multiple growth factors and for cell surface proteins will allow new insights into cell proliferation (e.g., CD28 and CTLA4) and migration. The availability of small molecules that block antigen presentation, lymphocyte activation, or both will be further advanced by the identification of peptides that are critical to receptor function. The discovery of cytosolic proteins that control protein folding and lymphocyte activation is likely to provide the rationale for the use of drugs that interfere with these processes. Adoptive transfer of T cells reactive to minor histocompatibility antigens has been shown to cause no GVHD, but to mediate a curative antileukemic response *(225)*. The role of CD25+ CD4+ regulatory T cells remains to be defined in the clinical setting. Intriguing are also the observations by Velardi and colleagues *(226)* showing that with appropriate conditioning, T-cell depletion and mismatching for the relevant KIR ligands, non-HLA-identical stem cells can be transplanted successfully and without the development of GVHD.

REFERENCES

1. van Bekkum DW, de Vries MJ. *Radiation Chimaeras*. London: Logos, 1967.
2. Billingham RE. The biology of graft-versus-host reactions. In: *The Harvey Lectures*. New York: Academic, 1966:21–78.
3. Hess AD. The immunobiology of syngeneic/autologous graft-versus-host disease. In: Ferrara JLM, Deeg HJ, Burakoff SJ, eds. *Graft-vs.-Host Disease*, 2nd ed., revised and expanded. New York: Marcel Dekker, 1997:561–586.
4. Glucksberg H, Storb R, Fefer A, et al. Clinical manifestations of graft-versus-host disease in human recipients of marrow from HLA-matched sibling donors. *Transplantation* 1974;18:295–304.
5. Sullivan KM. Acute and chronic graft-versus-host disease in man [review]. *Int J Cell Cloning* 1986;4(suppl 1):42–93.

6. Chao NJ, Deeg HJ. In vivo prevention and treatment of GVHD. In: Ferrara JLM, Deeg HJ, Burakoff S, eds. *Graft-vs.-Host Disease*, 2nd ed., revised and expanded. New York: Marcel Dekker, 1997:639–666.
7. Ringdén O, Deeg HJ. Clinical spectrum of graft-versus-host disease. In: Ferrara JLM, Deeg HJ, Burakoff S, eds. *Graft-vs.-Host Disease*, 2nd ed., revised and expanded. New York: Marcel Dekker, 1997:525–559.
8. Vogelsang GB. How I treat chronic graft-versus-host disease. *Blood* 2001;97:1196–1201.
9. Sale GE, Shulman HM, Hackman RC. Bone marrow. In: Colvin RB, Bhan AK, McCluskey RT, eds. *Diagnostic Immunopathology*, 2nd ed. New York: Raven, 1995:435–453.
10. Schmaltz C, Alpdogan O, Horndasch KJ, et al. Differential use of Fas ligand and perforin cytotoxic pathways by donor T cells in graft-versus-host disease and graft-versus-leukemia effect. *Blood* 2001;97:2886–2895.
11. Tsukada N, Kobata T, Aizawa Y, et al. Graft-versus-leukemia effect and graft-versus-host disease can be differentiated by cytotoxic mechanisms in a murine model of allogeneic bone marrow transplantation. *Blood* 1999;93:2738–2747.
12. Rowlings PA, Przepiorka D, Klein JP, et al. IBMTR Severity Index for grading acute graft-versus-host disease: retrospective comparison with Glucksberg grade. *Br J Haematol* 1997;97:855–864.
13. Martin P, Nash R, Sanders J, et al. Reproducibility in retrospective grading of acute graft-versus-host disease after allogeneic marrow transplantation. *Bone Marrow Transplant* 1998;21:273–279.
14. Atkinson K, Horowitz MM, Gale RP, et al. Consensus among bone marrow transplanters for diagnosis, grading and treatment of chronic graft-versus-host disease. *Bone Marrow Transplant* 1989;4:247–254.
15. Martin PJ, Schoch G, Gooley T, et al. Methods for assessment of graft-versus-host disease [letter]. *Blood* 1998;92:3479–3481.
16. Hings IM, Severson R, Filipovich AH, et al. Treatment of moderate and severe acute GVHD after allogeneic bone marrow transplantation. *Transplantation* 1994;58:437–442.
17. Pan L, Delmonte J Jr, Jalonen CK, et al. Pretreatment of donor mice with granulocytc colony-stimulating factor polarizes donor T lymphocytes toward type-2 cytokine production and reduces severity of experimental graft versus host disease. *Blood* 1995;86:4422–4429.
18. Przepiorka D, Weisdorf D, Martin P, et al. Consensus conference on acute GVHD grading. *Bone Marrow Transplant* 1995;15:825–828.
19. Saurat JH, Gluckman E, Bussel A, et al. The lichen planus-like eruption after bone marrow transplantation. *Br J Dermatol* 1975;93:675–681.
20. Siimes MA, Johansson E, Rapola J. Scleroderma-like graft-versus-host disease as late consequence of bone-marrow grafting [letter]. *Lancet* 1977;2:831–832.
21. Hood AF, Soter NA, Rappeport J, et al. Graft-versus-host reaction. Cutaneous manifestations following bone marrow transplantation. *Arch Dermatol* 1977;113:1087–1091.
22. Sullivan KM, Agura E, Anasetti C, et al. Chronic graft-versus-host disease and other late complications of bone marrow transplantation. *Semin Hematol* 1991;28:250–259.
23. Sullivan KM, Shulman HM, Storb R, et al. Chronic graft-versus-host disease in 52 patients: adverse natural course and successful treatment with combination immunosuppression. *Blood* 1981;57:267–276.
24. Storb R, Prentice RL, Sullivan KM, et al. Predictive factors in chronic graft-versus-host disease in patients with aplastic anemia treated by marrow transplantation from HLA-identical siblings. *Ann Intern Med* 1983;98:461–466.
25. Atkinson K, Horowitz MM, Gale RP, et al. Risk factors for chronic graft-versus-host disease after HLA-identical sibling bone marrow transplantation. *Blood* 1990;75:2459–2464.
26. Shulman HM, Sullivan KM, Weiden PL, et al. Chronic graft-versus-host syndrome in man. A long-term clinicopathologic study of 20 Seattle patients. *Am J Med* 1980;69:204–217.
27. Roca J, Granena A, Rodriquez-Roison R, et al. Fatal airway disease in an adult with chronic graft-versus-host disease. *Thorax* 1982;37:77–78.
28. Wyatt SE, Nunn P, Hows JM, et al. Airways obstruction associated with graft-versus-host disease after bone marrow transplantation. *Thorax* 1984;39:887–894.
29. Ralph DD, Springmeyer SC, Sullivan KM, et al. Rapidly progressive air-flow obstruction in marrow transplant recipients: possible association between obliterative bronchiolitis and chronic graft-versus-host disease. *Am Rev Respir Dis* 1984;129:641–644.
30. Sullivan KM. Graft-versus-host-disease. In: Thomas ED, Blume KG, Forman SJ, eds. *Hematopoietic Cell Transplantation*, 2nd ed. Boston: Blackwell Science, 1999:515–536.
31. Wingard JR, Piantadosi S, Vogelsang GB, et al. Predictors of death from chronic graft versus host disease after bone marrow transplantation. *Blood* 1989;74:1428–1435.

32. Horowitz MM, Gale RP, Sondel PM, et al. Graft-versus-leukemia reactions after bone marrow transplantation. *Blood* 1990;75:555–562.
33. Weiden PL, Flournoy N, Thomas ED, et al. Antileukemic effect of graft-versus-host disease in human recipients of allogeneic-marrow grafts. *N Engl J Med* 1979;300:1068–1073.
34. Ferrara JL, Levy R, Chao NJ. Pathophysiologic mechanisms of acute graft-vs.-host disease [review]. *Biol Blood Marrow Transplant* 1999;5:347–356.
35. Hill GR, Teshima T, Gerbitz A, et al. Differential roles of IL-1 and TNF-alpha on graft-versus-host disease and graft versus leukemia. *J Clin Invest* 1999;104:459–467.
36. Xun CQ, Tsuchida M, Thompson JS. Delaying transplantation after total body irradiation is a simple and effective way to reduce acute graft-versus-host disease mortality after major H2 incompatible transplantation. *Transplantation* 1997;64:297–302.
37. Hill GR, Crawford JM, Cooke KR, et al. Total body irradiation and acute graft-versus-host disease: the role of gastrointestinal damage and inflammatory cytokines. *Blood* 1997;90:3204–3213.
38. Hill GR, Ferrara JL. The primacy of the gastrointestinal tract as a target organ of acute graft-versus-host disease: rationale for the use of cytokine shields in allogeneic bone marrow transplantation [review]. *Blood* 2000;95:2754–2759.
39. Cooke K, Olkiewicz K, Clouthier S, et al. Critical role for CD14 and the innate immune response in the induction of experimental acute graft-versus-host disease. *Blood* 2001;98(suppl 1):776a, [Abstract #3229].
40. Janossy G, Bofill M, Poulter LW, et al. Separate ontogeny of two macrophage-like accessory cell populations in the human fetus. *J Immunol* 1986;136:4354–4361.
41. Hakim FT, Mackall CL. The immune system: effector and target of graft-versus-host disease. In: Ferrara JLM, Deeg HJ, Burakoff SJ, eds. *Graft-vs.-Host Disease*, 2nd ed., revised and expanded. New York: Marcel Dekker, 1997:257–290.
42. Shlomchik WD, Couzens MS, Tang CB, et al. Prevention of graft versus host disease by inactivation of host antigen-presenting cells. *Science* 1999;285:412–415.
43. Korngold R, Sprent J. Murine models for graft-versus-host disease. In: Thomas ED, Blume KG, Forman SJ, eds. *Hematopoietic Cell Transplantation*, 2nd ed. Boston: Blackwell Science, 1999:296–304.
44. Baker MB, Riley RL, Podack ER, et al. Graft-versus-host-disease-associated lymphoid hypoplasia and B cell dysfunction is dependent upon donor T cell-mediated Fas- ligand function, but not perforin function. *Proc Natl Acad Sci USA* 1997;94:1366–1371.
45. Graubert TA, DiPersio JF, Russell JH, et al. Perforin/granzyme-dependent and independent mechanisms are both important for the development of graft-versus-host disease after murine bone marrow transplantation. *J Clin Invest* 1997;100:904–911.
46. Hiroyasu S, Shiraishi M, Koji T, et al. Analysis of Fas system in pulmonary injury of graft-versus-host disease after rat intestinal transplantation. *Transplantation* 1999;68:933–938.
47. Mori T, Nishimura T, Ikeda Y, et al. Involvement of Fas-mediated apoptosis in the hematopoietic progenitor cells of graft-versus-host reaction-associated myelosuppression. *Blood* 1998;92:101–107.
48. Hattori K, Hirano T, Miyajima H, et al. Differential effects of anti-Fas ligand and anti-tumor necrosis factor alpha antibodies on acute graft-versus-host disease pathologies. *Blood* 1998;91:4051–4055.
49. Jiang Z, Podack E, Levy RB. Major histocompatibility complex-mismatched allogeneic bone marrow transplantation using perforin and/or Fas ligand double-defective CD4(+) donor T cells: involvement of cytotoxic function by donor lymphocytes prior to graft-versus-host disease pathogenesis. *Blood* 2001;98:390–397.
50. Taylor PA, Lees CJ, Blazer BR. The infusion of ex vivo activated and expanded CD4(+)CD25(+) immune regulatory cells inhibits graft-versus-host disease lethality. *Blood* 2002;99:3493–3499.
51. Buhlmann JE, Gonzalez M, Ginther B, et al. Cutting edge: sustained expansion of CD8+ T cells requires CD154 expression by Th cells in acute graft versus host disease. *J Immunol* 1999;162:4373–4376.
52. Saito K, Sakurai J, Ohata J, et al. Involvement of CD40 ligand–CD40 and CTLA4–B7 pathways in murine acute graft-versus-host disease induced by allogeneic T cells lacking CD28. *J Immunol* 1998;160:4225–4231.
53. Tsukada N, Akiba H, Kobata T, et al. Blockade of CD134 (OX40)–CD134L interaction ameliorates lethal acute graft-versus-host disease in a murine model of allogeneic bone marrow transplantation. *Blood* 2000;95:2434–2439.
54. Zhou P, Szot G, Guo Z, et al. Role of STAT6 signaling in the induction and long-term maintenance of tolerance mediated by CTLA4-Ig. *Transplant Proc* 2001;33:214–216.
55. Allen RD, Staley TA, Sidman CL. Differential cytokine expression in acute and chronic murine graft-versus-host disease. *Eur J Immunol* 1993;23:333–337.

56. De Wit D, Van Mechelen M, Zanin C, et al. Preferential activation of Th2 cells in chronic graft-versus-host reaction. *J Immunol* 1993;150:361–366.
57. Kataoka Y, Iwasaki T, Kuroiwa T, et al. The role of donor T cells for target organ injuries in acute and chronic graft-versus-host disease. *Immunology* 2001;103:310–318.
58. Ellison CA, Bradley DS, Fischer JM, et al. Murine graft-versus-host disease induced using interferon-gamma-deficient grafts features antibodies to double-stranded DNA, T helper 2-type cytokines and hypereosinophilia. *Immunology* 2002;105:63–72.
59. Rus V, Svetic A, Nguyen P, et al. Kinetics of Th1 and Th2 cytokine production during the early course of acute and chronic murine graft-versus-host disease. Regulatory role of donor CD8+ T cells. *J Immunol* 1995;155:2396–2406.
60. Ochs LA, Blazar BR, Roy J, et al. Cytokine expression in human cutaneous chronic graft-versus-host disease. *Bone Marrow Transplant* 1996;17:1085–1092.
61. Chen F, Maldonado MA, Madaio M, et al. The role of host (endogenous) T cells in chronic graft-versus-host autoimmune disease. *J Immunol* 1998;161:5880–5885.
62. Ferrara JL, Krenger W. Graft-versus-host disease: the influence of type 1 and type 2 T cell cytokines [review]. *Transfusion Med Rev* 1998;12:1–17.
63. Parkman R. Clonal analysis of murine graft-vs-host disease. I. Phenotypic and functional analysis of T lymphocyte clones. *J Immunol* 1986;136:3543–3548.
64. Ilan Y, Gotsman I, Pines M, et al. Induction of oral tolerance in splenocyte recipients toward pretransplant antigens ameliorates chronic graft versus host disease in a murine model. *Blood* 2000;95:3613–3619.
65. Ordemann R, Hutchinson R, Friedman J, et al. Enhanced allostimulatory activity of host antigen-presenting cells in old mice intensifies acute graft-versus-host disease. *J Clin Invest* 2002;109:1249–1256.
66. Shustov A, Nguyen P, Finkelman F, et al. Differential expression of Fas and Fas ligand in acute and chronic graft-versus-host disease: up-regulation of Fas and Fas ligand requires CD8+ T cell activation and IFN-gamma production. *J Immunol* 1998;161:2848–2855.
67. Durie FH, Aruffo A, Ledbetter J, et al. Antibody to the ligand of CD40, gp39, blocks the occurrence of the acute and chronic forms of graft-vs-host disease. *J Clin Invest* 1994;94:1333–1338.
68. Tamada K, Tamura H, Flies D, et al. Blockade of LIGHT/LTbeta and CD40 signaling induces allospecific T cell anergy, preventing graft-versus-host disease. *J Clin Invest* 2002;109:549–557.
69. Via CS, Rus V, Gately MK, Finkelman FD. IL-12 stimulates the development of acute graft-versus-host disease in mice that normally would develop chronic, autoimmune graft-versus-host disease. *J Immunol* 1994;153:4040–4047.
70. Okamoto I, Kohno K, Tanimoto T, et al. IL-18 prevents the development of chronic graft-versus-host disease in mice. *J Immunol* 2000;164:6067–6074.
71. Powles R, Mehta J, Kulkarni S, et al. Allogeneic blood and bone-marrow stem-cell transplantation in haematological malignant diseases: a randomised trial. *Lancet* 2000;355:1231–1237.
72. Krenger W, Snyder KM, Byon JC, et al. Polarized type 2 alloreactive CD4+ and CD8+ donor T cells fail to induce experimental acute graft-versus-host disease. *J Immunol* 1995;155:585–593.
73. Bensinger WI, Martin PJ, Storer B, et al. Transplantation of bone marrow as compared with peripheral-blood cells from HLA-identical relatives in patients with hematologic cancers. *N Engl J Med* 2001;344:175–181.
74. Schmitz N, Beksac M, Hasenclever D, et al. A randomised study from the European Group for Blood and Marrow Transplantation comparing allogeneic transplantation of filgrastim-mobilised peripheral blood progenitor cells with bone marrow transplantation in 350 patients (pts) with leukemia. *Blood* 2000;96(Pt 1):481a [Abstract 2068].
75. Storek J, Gooley T, Siadak M, et al. Allogeneic peripheral blood stem cell transplantation may be associated with a high risk of chronic graft-versus-host disease. *Blood* 1997;90:4705–4709.
76. Cutler C, Giri S, Jeyapalan S, et al. Acute and chronic graft-versus-host disease after allogeneic peripheral-blood stem-cell and bone marrow transplantation: a meta-analysis. *J Clin Oncol* 2001;19:3685–3691.
77. Rubinstein P, Carrier C, Scaradavou A, et al. Outcomes among 562 recipients of placental-blood transplants from unrelated donors. *N Engl J Med* 1998;339:1565–1577.
78. Gluckman E, Rocha V, Boyer-Chammard A, et al. Outcome of cord-blood transplantation from related and unrelated donors. *N Engl J Med* 1997;337:373–381.
79. Broxmeyer HE, Smith FO. Cord blood stem cell transplantation. In: Thomas ED, Blume KG, Forman SJ, eds. *Hematopoietic Cell Transplantation*, 2nd ed. Boston: Blackwell Science, 1999:431–443.

80. Gluckman E, Broxmeyer HE, Auerbach AD, et al. Hematopoietic reconstitution in a patient with Fanconi's anemia by means of umbilical-cord blood from an HLA-identical sibling. *N Engl J Med* 1989;321:1174–1178.
81. Kurtzberg J, Laughlin M, Graham ML, et al. Placental blood as a source of hematopoietic stem cells for transplantation into unrelated recipients. *N Engl J Med* 1996;335:157–166.
82. Apperley JF. Umbilical cord blood progenitor cell transplantation. The International Conference Workshop on Cord Blood Transplantation, Indianapolis, November 1993 [see comments]. *Bone Marrow Transplant* 1994;14:187–196.
83. Miscia S, Di Baldassarre A, Sabatino G, et al. Inefficient phospholipase C activation and reduced Lck expression characterize the signaling defect of umbilical cord T lymphocytes. *J Immunol* 1999;163:2416–2424.
84. Petersdorf E, Anasetti C, Servida P, et al. Effect of HLA matching on outcome of related and unrelated donor transplantation therapy for chronic myelogenous leukemia [review]. *Hematol–Oncol Clin North Am* 1998;12:107–121.
85. Petersdorf EW, Gooley T, Malkki M, et al. The biological significance of HLA-DP gene variation in haematopoietic cell transplantation. *Br J Haematol* 2001;112:988–994.
86. Petersdorf EW, Hansen JA, Martin PJ, et al. Major-histocompatibility-complex class I alleles and antigens in hematopoietic-cell transplantation. *N Engl J Med* 2001;345:1794–1800.
87. Deeg HJ, Seidel K, Casper J, et al. Marrow transplantation from unrelated donors for patients with severe aplastic anemia who have failed immunosuppressive therapy. *Biol Blood Marrow Transplant* 1999;5:243–252.
88. Sullivan KM, Deeg HJ, Sanders J, et al. Hyperacute graft-vs-host disease in patients not given immunosuppression after allogeneic marrow transplantation [concise report]. *Blood* 1986;67:1172–1175.
89. Gale RP, Bortin MM, van Bekkum DW, et al. Risk factors for acute graft-versus-host disease. *Br J Haematol* 1987;67:397–406.
90. Hagglund H, Bostrom L, Ringden O, et al. Risk factors for acute graft-versus-host disease in 325 consecutive bone marrow recipients. *Transplant Proc* 1994;26:1821–1822.
91. Storb R, Deeg HJ, Whitehead J, et al. Methotrexate and cyclosporine compared with cyclosporine alone for prophylaxis of acute graft versus host disease after marrow transplantation for leukemia. *N Engl J Med* 1986;314:729–735.
92. Remberger M, Storer B, Ringden O, et al. Association between pretransplant thymogloblulin and reduced non-relapse mortality rate after marrow transplantation from unrelated donors. *Bone Marrow Transplant* 2002;29:391–397.
93. Bacigalupo A, Oneto R, Lamparelli T, et al. Pre-emptive therapy of acute graft-versus-host disease: a pilot study with antithymocyte globulin (ATG). *Bone Marrow Transplant* 2001;28:1093–1096.
94. Kolb HJ, Schattenberg A, Goldman JM, et al. Graft-versus-leukemia effect of donor lymphocyte transfusions in marrow grafted patients. European Group for Blood and Marrow Transplantation Working Party Chronic Leukemia. *Blood* 1995;86:2041–2050.
95. Dreger P, Schmitz N. Allogeneic transplantation of peripheral blood stem cells. *Baillière's Best Pract Clin Haematol* 1999;12:261–278.
96. Bensinger WI, Clift R, Martin P, et al. Allogeneic peripheral blood stem cell transplantation in patients with advanced hematologic malignancies: a retrospective comparison with marrow transplantation. *Blood* 1996;88:2794–2800.
97. Przepiorka D, Smith TL, Folloder J, et al. Risk factors for acute graft-versus-host disese after allogeneic blood stem cell transplantation. *Blood* 1999;94:1465–1470.
98. Holler E, Roncarolo MG, Hintermeier-Knabe R, et al. Prognostic significance of increased IL-10 production in patients prior to allogeneic bone marrow transplantation. *Bone Marrow Transplant* 2000;25:237–241.
99. Cavet J, Middleton PG, Segall M, et al. Recipient tumor necrosis factor-alpha and interleukin-10 gene polymorphisms associated with early mortality and acute graft-versus-host disease severity in HLA-matched sibling bone marrow transplants. *Blood* 1999;94:3941–3946.
100. Middleton PG, Taylor PRA, Jackson G, et al. Cytokine gene polymorphisms associating with severe acute graft-versus-host disease in HLA-identical sibling transplants. *Blood* 1998;92:3943–3948.
101. Cullup H, Dickinson AM, Jackson GH, et al. Donor interleukin 1 receptor antagonist genotype associated with acute graft versus-host disease in human leucocyte antigen-matched sibling allogeneic transplants. *Br J Haematol* 2001;113:807–813.
102. Bacigalupo A, Soracco M, Vassallo F, et al. Donor lymphocyte infusions (DLI) in patients with chronic myeloid leukemia following allogeneic bone marrow transplantation. *Bone Marrow Transplant* 1997;19:927–932.

103. Grumet FC, Hiraki DD, Brown BWM, et al. CD31 mismatching affects marrow transplantation outcome. *Biol Blood Marrow Transplant* 2001;7:503–512.
104. Balduini CL, Frassoni F, Noris P, et al. Donor–recipient incompatibility at CD31-codon 563 is a major risk factor for acute graft-versus-host disease after allogeneic bone marrow transplantation from a human leucocyte antigen-matched donor. *Br J Haematol* 2001;114:951–953.
105. Broers AEC, van der holt R, van Esser JWJ, et al. Increased transplant-related morbidity and mortality in CMV-seropositive patients despite highly effective prevention of CMV disease after allogeneic T-cell-depleted stem cell transplantation. *Blood* 2000;95:2240–2245.
106. Clark RE, Hermans J, Madrigal A, et al. HLA-A3 increases and HLA-DR1 decreases the risk of acute graft-versus-host disease after HLA-matched sibling bone marrow transplantation for chronic myelogenous leukaemia. *Br J Haematol* 2001;114:36–41.
107. Zaucha JM, Gooley T, Bensinger WI, et al. CD34 cell dose in granulocyte colony-stimulating factor-mobilized peripheral blood mononuclear cell grafts affects engraftment kinetics and development of extensive chronic graft-versus-host disease after human leukocyte antigen-identical sibling transplantation. *Blood* 2001;98:3221–3227.
108. Sloand EM, Kim S, Maciejewski JP, et al. Pharmacologic doses of granulocyte colony-stimulating factor affect cytokine production by lymphocytes in vitro and in vivo. *Blood* 2000;95:2269–2274.
109. Arpinati M, Green CL, Heimfeld S, et al C. Granulocyte-colony stimulating factor mobilizes T helper 2-inducing dendritic cells. *Blood* 2000;95:2484–2490.
110. Ruutu T, Volin L, Elonen E. Low incidence of severe acute and chronic graft-versus-host disease as a result of prolonged cyclosporine prophylaxis and early aggressive treatment with corticosteroids. *Transplant Proc* 1988;20:491–493.
111. Lönnqvist B, Aschan J, Ljungman P, et al. Long-term cyclosporin therapy may decrease the risk of chronic graft-versus-host disease. *Br J Haematol* 1990;74:547–548.
112. Bacigalupo A, Maiolino A, Van Lint MT, et al. Cyclosporin A and chronic graft versus host disease. *Bone Marrow Transplant* 1990;6:341–344.
113. Kansu E, Gooley T, Flowers MED, et al. Administration of cyclosporine for 24 months compared with 6 months for prevention of chronic graft-versus-host disease: a prospective randomized clinical trial [brief report]. *Blood* 2001;98:3868–3870.
114. Boström L, Ringdén O, Gratama JW, et al. The impact of pretransplant herpesvirus serology on acute and chronic graft-versus-host disease. *Transplant Proc* 1990;22:206
115. Ljungman P, Niederwieser D, Pepe MS, et al. Cytomegalovirus infection after marrow transplantation for aplastic anemia. *Bone Marrow Transplant* 1990;6:295–300.
116. Vogelsang GB. Advances in the treatment of graft-versus-host disease [review]. *Leukemia* 2000;14:509–510.
117. Uphoff DE. Alteration of homograft reaction by A-methopterin in lethally irradiated mice treated with homologous marrow. *Proc Soc Exp Biol Med* 1958;99:651–653.
118. Powles RL, Clink HM, Spence D, et al. Cyclosporin A to prevent graft-versus-host disease in man after allogeneic bone-marrow transplantation. *Lancet* 1980;1:327–329.
119. Nash RA, Pineiro LA, Storb R, et al. FK506 in combination with methotrexate for the prevention of graft-versus-host disease after marrow transplantation from matched unrelated donors. *Blood* 1996;88:3634–3641.
120. Nash RA, Antin JH, Karanes C, et al. Phase 3 study comparing methotrexate and tacrolimus with methotrexate and cyclosporine for prophylaxis of acute graft-versus-host disease after marrow transplantation from unrelated donors. *Blood* 2000;96:2062–2068.
121. Pai SY, Fruman DA, Leong T, et al. Inhibition of calcineurin phosphatase activity in adult bone marrow transplant patients treated with cyclosporine A. *Blood* 1994;84:3974–3979.
122. Vander Woude AC, Bierer BE. Immunosuppression and immunophilin ligands: cyclosporin A, FK506, and rapamycin. In: Ferrara JLM, Deeg HJ, Burakoff SJ, eds. *Graft-vs.-Host Disease*. New York, NY: Marcel Dekker, 1997:111–149.
123. Hughes SE, Gruber SA. New immunosuppressive drugs in organ transplantation [review]. *J Clin Pharmacol* 1996;36:1081–1092.
124. Blazar BR, Taylor PA, Linsley PS, et al. In vivo blockade of CD28/CTLA4: B7/BB1 interaction with CTLA4-Ig reduces lethal murine graft-versus-host disease across the major histocompatibility complex barrier in mice. *Blood* 1994;83:3815–3825.
125. Lin H, Wei RQ, Gordon D, et al. Review of CTLA4Ig use for allograft immunosuppression. *Transplant Proc* 1994;26:3200–3201.

126. Antin JH, Weinstein HJ, Guinan EC, et al. Recombinant human interleukin-1 receptor antagonist in the treatment of steroid-resistant graft-versus-host disease. *Blood* 1994;84:1342–1348.
127. Ferrara JL. Pathogenesis of acute graft-versus-host disease: cytokines and cellular effectors [review]. *J Hematother Stem Cell Res* 2000;9:299–306.
128. Schlegel PG, Aharoni R, Chen Y, et al. A synthetic random basic copolymer with promiscuous binding to class II major histocompatibility complex molecules inhibits T-cell proliferative responses to major and minor histocompatibility antigens in vitro and confers the capacity to prevent murine graft-versus-host disease in vivo. [erratum appears in *Proc Natl Acad Sci USA* 1996;93(16):8796]. *Proc Natl Acad Sci USA* 1996;93:5061–5066.
129. Zeng D, Dejbakhsh-Jones S, Strober S. Granulocyte colony-stimulating factor reduces the capacity of blood mononuclear cells to induce graft-versus-host disease: impact on blood progenitor cell transplantation. *Blood* 1997;90:453–463.
130. Blazar BR, Taylor PA, Panoskaltsis-Mortari A, et al. Blockade of CD40 ligand-CD40 interaction impairs CD4+ T cell-mediated alloreactivity by inhibiting mature donor T cell expansion and function after bone marrow transplantation. *J Immunol* 1997;158:29–39.
131. Blazar BR, Sharpe AH, Taylor PA, et al. Infusion of anti-B7.1 (CD80) and anti-B7.2 (CD86) monoclonal antibodies inhibits murine graft-versus-host disease lethality in part via direct effects on CD4+ and CD8+ T cells. *J Immunol* 1996;157:3250–3259.
132. Lu Y, Sakamaki S, Kuroda H, et al. Prevention of lethal acute graft-versus-host disease in mice by oral administration of T helper 1 inhibitor, TAK-603. *Blood* 2001;97:1123–1130.
133. Cetkovic-Cvrlje M, Roers BA, Waurzyniak B, et al. Targeting Janus kinase 3 to attenuate the severity of acute graft-versus-host disease across the major histocompatibility barrier in mice. *Blood* 2001;98:1607–1613.
134. Townsend RM, Gilbert MJ, Korngold R. Combination therapy with a CD4–CDR3 peptide analog and cyclosporin A to prevent graft-vs-host disease in a MHC-haploidentical bone marrow transplantation model. *Clin Immunol Immunopathol* 1998;86:115–119.
135. Deeg HJ, Storb R, Thomas ED, et al. Cyclosporine as prophylaxis for graft-versus-host disease: a randomized study in patients undergoing marrow transplantation for acute nonlymphoblastic leukemia. *Blood* 1985;65:1325–1334.
136. Storb R, Deeg HJ, Pepe M, et al. Methotrexate and cyclosporine versus cyclosporine alone for prophylaxis of graft-versus-host disease in patients given HLA-identical marrow grafts for leukemia: Long-term follow-up of a controlled trial. *Blood* 1989;73:1729–1734.
137. Storb R, Deeg HJ, Farewell V, et al. Marrow transplantation for severe aplastic anemia: methotrexate alone compared with a combination of methotrexate and cyclosporine for prevention of acute graft-versus-host disease. *Blood* 1986;68:119–125.
138. Forman SJ, Blume KG, Krance RA, et al. A prospective randomized study of acute graft-v-host disease in 107 patients with leukemia: methotrexate/prednisone vs cyclosporine A/prednisone. *Transplant Proc* 1987;19:2605–2607.
139. Santos GW, Tutschka PJ, Brookmeyer R, et al. Cyclosporine plus methylprednisolone versus cyclophosphamide plus methylprednisolone as prophylaxis for graft-versus-host disease: a randomized double-blind study in patients undergoing allogeneic marrow transplantation. *Clin Transplant* 1987;1:21–28.
140. Tollemar J, Ringdén O, Heimdahl A, et al. Decreased incidence and severity of graft-versus-host disease in HLA matched and mismatched marrow recipients of cyclosporine and methotrexate. *Transplant Proc* 1988;20:470–479.
141. Galimberti M, Polchi P, Lucarelli G, et al. A comparative trial of posttransplant immunosuppression in patients transplanted for thalassemia. Cyclosporine alone versus cyclosporine, cyclophosphamide, and methotrexate. *Transplantation* 1988;45:566–569.
142. Sullivan KM, Storb R, Buckner CD, et al. Graft-versus-host disease as adoptive immunotherapy in patients with advanced hematologic neoplasms. *N Engl J Med* 1989;320:828–834.
143. Storb R, Pepe M, Anasetti C, et al. What role for prednisone in prevention of acute graft-versus-host disease in patients undergoing marrow transplants? *Blood* 1990;76:1037–1045.
144. Chao NJ, Schmidt GM, Niland JC, et al. Cyclosporine, methotrexate, and prednisone compared with cyclosporine and prednisone for prophylaxis of acute graft-versus-host disease. *N Engl J Med* 1993;329:1225–1230.
145. Deeg HJ, Lin D, Leisenring W, et al. Cyclosporine or cyclosporine plus methylprednisolone for prophylaxis of graft-versus-host disease: a prospective, randomized trial. *Blood* 1997;89:3880–3887.

146. Ratanatharathorn V, Nash RA, Przepiorka D, et al. Phase III study comparing methotrexate and tacrolimus (Prograf, FK506) with methotrexate and cyclosporine for graft-versus-host-disease prophylaxis after HLA-identical sibling bone marrow transplantation. *Blood* 1998;92:2303–2314.
147. Zikos P, Van Lint MT, Frassoni F, et al. Low transplant mortality in allogeneic bone marrow transplantation for acute myeloid leukemia: a randomized study of low-dose cyclosporin versus low-dose cyclosporin and low-dose methotrexate. *Blood* 1998;91:3503–3508.
148. Locatelli F, Bruno B, Zecca M, et al. Cyclosporin A and short-term methotrexate versus cyclosporin A as graft versus host disease prophylaxis in patients with severe aplastic anemia given allogeneic bone marrow transplantation from an HLA-identical sibling: results of a GITMO/EBMT randomized trial. *Blood* 2000;96:1690–1697.
149. Ruutu T, Volin L, Parkkali T, et al. Cyclosporine, methotrexate, and methylprednisolone compared with cyclosporine and methotrexate for the prevention of graft-versus-host disease in bone marrow transplantation from HLA-identical sibling donor: a prospective randomized study. *Blood* 2000;96:2391–2398.
150. Hiraoka A, Ohashi Y, Okamoto S, et al. Phase III study comparing tacrolimus (FK506) with cyclosporine for graft-versus-host disease prophylaxis after allogeneic bone marrow transplantation. Japanese FK506 BMT Study Group. *Bone Marrow Transplant* 2001;28:181–185.
151. Bacigalupo A, Van Lint MT, Occhini D, et al. Increased risk of leukemia relapse with high-dose cyclosporine A after allogeneic marrow transplantation for acute leukemia. *Blood* 1991;77:1423–1428.
152. Carlens S, Ringden O, Remberger M, et al. Factors affecting risk of relapse and leukemia-free survival in HLA-identical sibling marrow transplant recipients with leukemia. *Transplant Proc* 1997;29:3147–3149.
153. Sayer HG, Longton G, Bowden R, et al. Increased risk of infection in marrow transplant patients given methylprednisolone for graft-versus-host disease prevention. *Blood* 1994;84:1328–1332.
154. Atkinson K, Biggs J, Concannon A, et al. A prospective randomised trial of cyclosporin and methotrexate versus cyclosporin, methotrexate and prednisolone for prevention of graft-versus-host disease after HLA-identical sibling marrow transplantation for haematological malignancy. *Aust NZ J Med* 1991;21:850–856.
155. Martin PJ, Kernan NA. T-cell depletion for GVHD prevention in humans. In: Ferrara JLM, Deeg HJ, Burakoff SJ, eds. *Graft-vs.-Host Disease*, 2nd ed. New York: Marcel Dekker, 1997:615–637.
156. Ho VT, Soiffer RJ. The history and future of T-cell depletion as graft-versus-host disease prophylaxis for allogeneic hematopoietic stem cell transplantation [review]. *Blood* 2001;98:3192–3204.
157. Harris DT, Sakiestewa D, Lyons C, et al. Prevention of graft-versus-host disease (GVHD) by elimination of recipient-reactive donor T cells with recombinant toxins that target the interleukin 2 (IL-2) receptor. *Bone Marrow Transplant* 1999;23:137–144.
158. van Dijk AM, Kessler FL, Stadhouders-Keet SA, et al. Selective depletion of major and minor histocompatibility antigen reactive T cells: towards prevention of acute graft-versus-host disease. *Br J Haematol* 1999;107:169–175.
159. Fehse B, Frerk O, Goldmann M, et al. Efficient depletion of alloreactive donor T lymphocytes based on expression of two activation-induced antigens (CD25 and CD69). *Br J Haematol* 2000;109:644–651.
160. Guinan EC, Boussiotis VA, Neuberg D, et al. Transplantation of anergic histoincompatible bone marrow allografts. *N Engl J Med* 1999;340:1704–1714.
161. Yu X-Z, Martin PJ, Anasetti C. Role of CD28 in acute graft-versus-host disease. *Blood* 1998;92:2963–2970.
162. Yu XZ, Bidwell SJ, Martin PJ, et al. CD28-specific antibody prevents graft-versus-host disease in mice. *J Immunol* 2000;164:4564–4568.
163. Hughes WT. Use of dapsone in the prevention and treatment of Pneumocystis carinii pneumonia: a review [review]. *Clin Infect Dis* 1998;27:191–204.
164. Papadopoulos EB, Carabasi MH, Castro-Malaspina H, et al. T-cell-depleted allogeneic bone marrow transplantation as postremission therapy for acute myelogenous leukemia: freedom from relapse in the absence of graft-versus-host disease. *Blood* 1998;91:1083–1090.
165. Martin PJ, Rowley SD, Anasetti C, et al. A phase I–II clinical trial to evaluate removal of CD4 cells and partial depletion of CD8 cells from donor marrow for HLA-mismatched unrelated recipients. *Blood* 1999;94:2192–2199.
166. Nimer SD, Giorgi J, Gajewski JL, et al. Selective depletion of CD8+ cells for prevention of graft-versus-host disease after bone marrow transplantation. A randomized controlled trial. *Transplantation* 1994;57:82–87.
167. Soiffer RJ, Weller E, Alyea EP, et al. CD6+ donor marrow T-cell depletion as the sole form of graft-versus-host disease prophylaxis in patients undergoing allogeneic bone marrow transplant from unrelated donors. [erratum appears in *J Clin Oncol* 2001;19(9):2583]. *J Clin Oncol* 2001;19:1152–1159.

168. Truitt RL, Johnson BD, McCabe CM, et al. Graft versus leukemia. In: Ferrara JLM, Deeg HJ, Burakoff SJ, eds. *Graft-vs.-Host Disease*, 2nd ed., revised and expanded. New York: Marcel Dekker, 1997:385–423.
169. Dickinson AM, Wang XN, Sviland L, et al. In situ dissection of the graft-versus-host activities of cytotoxic T cells specific for minor histocompatibility antigens. *Nature Med* 2002;8:410–414.
170. Ruggeri L, Capanni M, Urbani E, et al. Effectiveness of donor natural killer cell alloreactivity in mismatched hematopoietic transplants. *Science* 2002;295:2097–2100.
171. Takeda K, Hayakawa Y, Smyth MJ, et al. Involvement of tumor necrosis factor-related apoptosis-inducing ligand in surveillance of tumor metastasis by liver natural killer cells. *Nature Med* 2001;7:94–100.
172. Tiberghien P, Ferrand C, Lioure B, et al. Administration of herpes simplex-thymidine kinase-expressing donor T cells with a T-cell-depleted allogeneic marrow graft. *Blood* 2001;97:63–72.
173. Munshi NC, Govindarajan R, Drake R, et al. Thymidine kinase (TK) gene-transduced human lymphocytes can be highly purified, remain fully functional, and are killed efficiently with ganciclovir. *Blood* 1997;89:1334–1340.
174. Bonini C, Ferrari G, Verzeletti S, et al. HSV-TK gene transfer into donor lymphocytes for control of allogeneic graft-versus-leukemia. *Science* 1997;276:1719–1724.
175. Sykes M. Mixed chimerism and transplant tolerance [review]. *Immunity* 2001;14:417–424.
176. Storb R, Yu C, Wagner JL, et al. Stable mixed hematopoietic chimerism in DLA-identical littermate dogs given sublethal total body irradiation before and pharmacological immunosuppression after marrow transplantation. *Blood* 1997;89:3048–3054.
177. Maris M, Niederwieser D, Sandmaier B, et al. Nonmyeloablative hematopoietic stem cell transplants (HSCT) using 10/10 HLA antigen matched unrelated donors (URDs) for patients with advanced hematologic malignancies ineligible for conventional HSCT. *Blood* 2001;98(Pt 1):858a [Abstract 3563].
178. Storb R, Prentice RL, Buckner CD, et al. Graft-versus-host disease and survival in patients with aplastic anemia treated by marrow grafts from HLA-identical siblings. Beneficial effect of a protective environment. *N Engl J Med* 1983;308:302–307.
179. Heidt PJ, Vossen JM. Experimental and clinical gnotobiotics: influence of the microflora on graft-versus-host disease after allogeneic bone marrow transplantation [review]. *J Med* 1992;23:161–173.
180. Beelen DW, Elmaagacli A, Muller KD, et al. Influence of intestinal bacterial decontamination using metronidazole and ciprofloxacin or ciprofloxacin alone on the development of acute graft-versus-host disease after marrow transplantation in patients with hematologic malignancies: final results and long-term follow-up of an open-label prospective randomized trial. *Blood* 1999;93:3267–3275.
181. Martin PJ, Schoch G, Fisher L, et al. A retrospective analysis of therapy for acute graft-versus-host disease: initial treatment. *Blood* 1990;76:1464–1472.
182. Weisdorf D, Haake R, Blazar B, et al. Treatment of moderate/severe acute graft-versus-host disease after allogeneic bone marrow transplantation: an analysis of clinical risk features and outcome. *Blood* 1990;75:1024–1030.
183. Martin PJ, Schoch G, Fisher L, et al. A retrospective analysis of therapy for acute graft-versus-host disease: secondary treatment. *Blood* 1991;77:1821–1828.
184. Van Lint MT, Uderzo C, Locasciulli A, et al. Early treatment of acute graft-versus-host disease with high- or low-dose 6-methylprednisolone: a multicenter randomized trial from the Italian Group for Bone Marrow Transplantation. *Blood* 1998;92:2288–2293.
185. McDonald GB, Bouvier M, Hockenbery DM, et al. Oral beclomethasone dipropionate for treatment of intestinal graft-versus-host disease: a randomized, controlled trial. *Gastroenterology* 1998;115:28–35.
186. Bertz H, Afting M, Kreisel W, et al. Feasibility and response to budesonide as topical corticosteroid therapy for acute intestinal GVHD. *Bone Marrow Transplant* 1999;24:1185–1189.
187. Ohashi Y, Minegishi M, Fujie H, et al. Successful treatment of steroid-resistant severe acute GVHD with 24-h continuous infusion of FK506. *Bone Marrow Transplant* 1997;19:625–627.
188. Furlong T, Storb R, Anasetti C, et al. Clinical outcome after conversion to FK 506 (tacrolimus) therapy for acute graft versus-host disease resistant to cyclosporine or for cyclosporine-associated toxicities. *Bone Marrow Transplant* 2000;26:985–991.
189. Mollee P, Morton AJ, Irving I, et al. Combination therapy with tacrolimus and anti-thymocyte globulin for the treatment of steroid-resistant acute graft-versus-host disease developing during cyclosporine prophylaxis [erratum appears in *Br J Haematol* 2001;115(1):235]. *Br J Haematol* 2001;113:217–223.
190. Basara N, Blau WI, Romer E, et al. Mycophenolate mofetil for the treatment of acute and chronic GVHD in bone marrow transplant patients. *Bone Marrow Transplant* 1998;22:61–65.

191. Benito AI, Furlong T, Martin PJ, et al. Sirolimus (Rapamycin) for the treatment of steroid-refractory acute graft-versus-host disease. *Transplantation* 2001;72:1924–1929.
192. Storb R, Gluckman E, Thomas ED, et al. Treatment of established human graft-versus-host disease by antithymocyte globulin. *Blood* 1974;44:57–75.
193. MacMillan ML, Weisdorf DJ, Davies SM, et al. Early antithymocyte globulin therapy improves survival in patients with steroid-resistant acute graft-versus-host disease. *Biol Blood Marrow Transplant* 2002;8:40–46.
194. Hsu B, May R, Carrum G, et al. Use of antithymocyte globulin for treatment of steroid-refractory acute graft-versus-host disease: an international practice survey. *Bone Marrow Transplant* 2001;28:945–950.
195. Khoury H, Kashyap A, Brewster C, et al. Anti-thymocyte globulin (ATG) for steroid-resistant acute graft-versus-host disease after allogeneic hematopoietic stem cell transplantation: a costly therapy with limited benefits. *Blood* 1999;94(suppl 1):668a [Abstract 2962].
196. Martin PJ, Remlinger K, Hansen JA, et al. Seattle Marrow Transplant Team. Murine monoclonal anti-T cell antibodies for treatment of refractory acute graft-versus-host disease (GVHD). *Transplant Proc* 1984;16:1494–1495.
197. Hebart H, Ehninger G, Schmidt H, et al. Treatment of steroid-resistant graft-versus-host disease after allogeneic bone marrow transplantation with anti-CD3/TCR monoclonal antibodies. *Bone Marrow Transplant* 1995;15:891–894.
198. Przepiorka D, Phillips GL, Ratanatharathorn V, et al. A phase II study of BTI-322, a monoclonal anti-CD2 antibody, for treatment of steroid-resistant acute graft-versus-host disease. *Blood* 1998;92:4066–4071.
199. Deeg HJ, Blazar BR, Bolwell BJ, et al. Treatment of steroid-refractory acute graft-versus-host disease with anti-CD147 monoclonal antibody, ABX-CBL. *Blood* 2001;98:2052–2058.
200. Carpenter PA, Appelbaum FR, Corey L, et al. A humanized non-FcR-binding anti-CD3 antibody, visilizumab, for treatment of steroid-refractory acute graft-versus-host disease. *Blood* 2002;99:2712–2719.
201. Hervé P, Wijdenes J, Bergerat JP, et al. Treatment of corticosteroid resistant acute graft-versus-host disease by in vivo administration of anti-interleukin-2 receptor monoclonal antibody (B-B10). *Blood* 1990;75:1017–1023.
202. Anasetti C, Hansen JA, Waldmann TA, et al. Treatment of acute graft-versus-host disease with humanized anti-Tac: an antibody that binds to the interleukin-2 receptor. *Blood* 1994;84:1320–1327.
203. Przepiorka D, Kernan NA, Ippoliti C, et al. Daclizumab, a humanized anti-interleukin-2 receptor alpha chain antibody, for treatment of acute graft-versus-host disease. *Blood* 2000;95:83–89.
204. Kobbe G, Schneider P, Rohr U, et al. Treatment of severe steroid refractory acute graft-versus-host disease with infliximab, a chimeric human/mouse antiTNFalpha antibody. *Bone Marrow Transplant* 2001;28:47–49.
205. van Oosterhout YV, van Emst L, Schattenberg AV, et al. A combination of anti-CD3 and anti-CD7 ricin A-immunotoxins for the in vivo treatment of acute graft versus host disease. *Blood* 2000;95:3693–3701.
206. Martin PJ, Nelson BJ, Appelbaum FR, et al. Evaluation of a CD5-specific immunotoxin for treatment of acute graft-versus-host disease after allogeneic marrow transplantation. *Blood* 1996;88:824–830.
207. Greinix HT, Volc-Platzer B, Kalhs P, et al. Extracorporeal photochemotherapy in the treatment of severe steroid-refractory acute graft-versus-host disease: a pilot study. *Blood* 2000;96:2426–2431.
208. Besnier DP, Chabannes D, Mahé B, et al. Treatment of graft-versus-host disease by extracorporeal photochemotherapy: a pilot study. *Transplantation* 1997;64:49–54.
209. Dall'Amico R, Rossetti F, Zulian F, et al. Photopheresis in paediatric patients with drug-resistant chronic graft-versus-host disease. *Br J Haematol* 1997;97:848–854.
210. Sullivan KM, Mori M, Witherspoon R, et al. Alternating-day cyclosporine and prednisone (CSP/PRED) treatment of chronic graft-vs-host disease (GVHD): predictors of survival. *Blood* 1990;76(suppl 1):568a [Abstract].
211. Koc S, Leisenring W, Flowers MED, et al. Therapy of chronic graft-versus-host disease: a randomized trial comparing cyclosporine plus prednisone versus prednisone alone. *Blood*, 2002;100:48–51.
212. Tzakis AG, Abu-Elmagd K, Fung JJ, et al. FK 506 rescue in chronic graft-versus-host-disease after bone marrow transplantation. *Transplant Proc* 1991;23:3225–3227.
213. Vogelsang GB, Farmer ER, Hess AD, et al. Thalidomide for the treatment of chronic graft versus host disease. *N Engl J Med* 1992;326:1055–1058.
214. Parker PM, Chao N, Nademanee A, et al. Thalidomide as salvage therapy for chronic graft-versus-host disease. *Blood* 1995;86:3604–3609.
215. Koc S, Leisenring W, Flowers MED, et al. Thalidomide for treatment of patients with chronic graft-versus-host disease. *Blood* 2000;96:3995–3996.

216. Arora M, Wagner JE, Davies SM, et al. Randomized clinical trial of thalidomide, cyclosporine, and prednisone versus cyclosporine and prednisone as initial therapy for chronic graft-versus-host disease. *Biol Blood Marrow Transplant* 2001;7:265–273.
217. Eppinger T, Ehninger G, Steinert M, et al. 8-Methoxypsoralen and ultraviolet A therapy for cutaneous manifestations of graft-versus-host disease. *Transplantation* 1990;50:807–811.
218. Aubin F, Humbert P. Immunomodulation induced by psoralen plus ultraviolet A radiation [review]. *Eur J Dermatol* 1998;8:212–213.
219. Greinix HT, Volc-Platzer B, Rabitsch W, et al. Successful use of extracorporeal photochemotherapy in the treatment of severe acute and chronic graft-versus-host disease. *Blood* 1998;92:3098–3104.
220. Socié G, Devergie A, Cosset JM, et al. Low-dose (one gray) total-lymphoid irradiation for extensive, drug-resistant chronic graft-versus-host disease. *Transplantation* 1990;49:657–658.
221. Mookerjee B, Altomonte V, Vogelsang G. Salvage therapy for refractory chronic graft-versus-host disease with mycophenolate mofetil and tacrolimus. *Bone Marrow Transplant* 1999;24:517–520.
222. Busca A, Saroglia EM, Lanino E, et al. Mycophenolate mofetil (MMF) as therapy for refractory chronic GVHD (cGVHD) in children receiving bone marrow transplantation. *Bone Marrow Transplant* 2000;25:1067–1071.
223. Basara N, Blau WI, Kiehl MG, et al. Efficacy and safety of mycophenolate mofetil for the treatment of acute and chronic GVHD in bone marrow transplant recipient. *Transplant Proc* 1998;30:4087–4089.
224. Chiang KY, Abhyankar S, Bridges K, et al. Recombinant human tumor necrosis factor receptor fusion protein as complementary treatment for chronic graft-versus-host disease. *Transplantation* 2002;73:665–667.
225. Fontaine P, Roy-Proulx G, Knafo L, et al. Adoptive transfer of minor histocompatibility antigen-specific T lymphocytes eradicates leukemia cells without causing graft-versus-host disease [see comments.]. *Nature Med* 2001;7:789–794.
226. Ruggeri L, Capanni M, Urbani E, et al. Kir epitope incompatibility in the GvH direction predicts control of leukemia relapse after mismatched hematopoietic transplantation. *Bone Marrow Transplant* 2001;27(suppl 1):S11 [Abstract OS78].

8 Chronic Graft-vs-Host Disease After Transplantation

Georgia B. Vogelsang, MD
and Colleen H. McDonough, MD

Contents

1. INTRODUCTION

Chronic graft-vs-host disease (GVHD) is one of the most common and significant problems affecting long-term survivors of allogeneic bone marrow transplantation (alloBMT). Despite recent and ongoing advances in the treatment of acute GVHD, the incidence of chronic GVHD continues to rise. Factors associated with this increase include changes in patient demographics and changes in transplant procedures. As our ability to support patients through alloBMT improves, older patients who are at an increased risk for chronic GVHD are undergoing transplantation. Furthermore, whereas vigorous T-cell depletion was employed in recent decades, most centers have moved away from this method of GVHD prophylaxis because it has been associated with higher rates of graft failure and relapse and no improvement in overall survival (OS) *(1)*. Alternative donors, including unrelated donors mismatched at a single human lymphocyte antigen (HLA) allele and haplo-identical related donors, are being used with increasing frequency in the nonmyeloablative transplant setting and in pediatric patients. Additionally, the use of donor lymphocyte infusion (DLI) to prevent or to treat disease relapse is contributing the higher rates of chronic GVHD. Finally, although peripheral blood stem cell transplant (PBSCT) has resulted in equivalent or reduced rates of acute GVHD, most trials have shown that the incidence of chronic GVHD in this setting is increased *(2)*.

From: *Stem Cell Transplantation for Hematologic Malignancies*
Edited by: R. J. Soiffer © Humana Press Inc., Totowa, NJ

The incidence of chronic GVHD is estimated at 25–60% of patients surviving more than 4 mo after allogeneic transplantation. Clinical risk factors for the development of chronic GVHD include older age, history of acute GVHD, and a positive skin or oral biopsy at d 100 post-BMT without signs or symptoms of GVHD. Transplant methods, including unrelated or mismatched donors, DLIs, and PBSCT, are all associated with higher rates of chronic GVHD. Chronic GVHD is an important cause of morbidity and mortality in transplant patients. In a recently published study of quality of life (QOL) post-BMT, chronic GVHD was one of three factors associated with poor QOL scores *(3)*. Extensive GVHD affected vocational and domestic environmental functioning most profoundly, but it was also associated with reduced interest in extended family and leisure activities. The disease and its treatment are associated with profound and long-lasting immunosuppression with an inherent risk of overwhelming infection and death. Chronic GVHD therefore remains a major obstacle facing the field of blood and marrow transplantation.

2. PATHOGENESIS

The pathophysiology of chronic GVHD is incompletely defined. Clinical studies of chronic GVHD are difficult, in part because the disease presents months after BMT, after many patients have left the direct care of the transplant center. The early presenting signs of chronic GVHD may be misdiagnosed by a local physician and referral back to the transplant center delayed or deferred. Although animal models of allogeneic chronic GVHD do exist, they are expensive and time-consuming to develop and maintain. These obstacles have hampered the investigation of pathophysiology in animal models.

The main murine model employed to study chronic GVHD used a parent into F1 hybrid in which the main manifestations, including severe nephritis, more closely resemble lupus than GVHD. This model has not been validated by confirmatory human studies of chronic GVHD. Nonetheless, even with this limitation, this model has led to several important observations. First, chronic GVHD appears to be primarily mediated by Th2 cells and cytokines, whereas acute GVHD is mediated by Th1 cells and cytokines. However, this delineation may not be as clear as initially thought. Several cytokines, such as interleukin (IL)-18, were initially thought to be important primarily as pro-inflammatory cytokines. However, they now appear to play a role in preventing chronic GVHD and reversing the disease if established, suggesting a therapeutic role for IL-18. The timing of administration of cytokines is critical in determining their effects, evidence that the cytokine milieu also strongly influences the cytokine effect. These very provocative findings highlight the limitations of the model, namely that most of these effects have been measured in antibody production and loss of donor B cells. The relevance to clinical human GVHD is not yet known.

Another model of chronic GVHD is that of autologous GVHD induced by cyclosporine A (CSA). Although CSA has potent immunosuppressive activity, it also inhibits thymic-dependent clonal deletion of autoreactive T cells, thereby paradoxically disrupting self-tolerance *(4)*. Administration of CSA after autologous or syngeneic BMT elicits a T-cell-dependent autoimmune syndrome in both human and rodent models that presents with signs and symptoms of chronic GVHD, including scleroderma, sicca syndrome, and wasting *(5,6)*. Using CSA after syngeneic BMT, murine systems can be manipulated to study factors affecting the course and severity of GVHD. Variables including the CD4+ to CD8+ lymphocyte number and ratio, type of recipient immunosuppression, thymic damage, age of donors and recipients, use of prior chemotherapy and irradiation, and the presence or absence of infection have been found to influence the clinical manifestations of autologous GVHD *(5–7)*.

The pathological changes seen in chronic GVHD, including pulmonary fibrosis, skin scleroderma, esophageal dismotility, and increased autoantibody production to thyroid, muscle, and red blood cells, suggest similarities between chronic GVHD and autoimmune disease *(8)*. These similarities to autoimmune disease further highlight the differences between acute and chronic GVHD. Because of decreased negative selection, reduced extrathymic generation, and/or acceleration of the normal thymic aging process with chronic GVHD *(9)*, patients have a concurrent increase in peripheral autoreactive T lymphocytes. These autoreactive T lymphocytes act with interferon (IFN)-γ to produce the increased collagen deposition seen histopathologically in chronic GVHD *(10)*.

3. CLASSIFICATION OF CHRONIC GVHD

Chronic GVHD can be classified according to the type of onset, the clinical manifestations, or the extent of disease. The majority of patients with chronic GVHD have had prior acute GVHD. Their disease may evolve directly from acute GVHD and is labeled as progressive, or it may follow a period of recovery and be labeled as quiescent GVHD. A smaller subset of patients may develop chronic GVHD with no history of prior acute GVHD and are labeled *de novo*. A fourth type of onset, explosive GVHD, is associated with the abrupt onset of multisystem involvement and manifestations of both acute and chronic GVHD. Both explosive GVHD and progressive GVHD carry poor prognoses.

Alternatively, a classification system based on clinical manifestations classifies the cutaneous findings as lichenoid or sclerodermatous. The lichenoid form is more common, occurs earlier after BMT, and may evolve into sclerodermatous GVHD. The most commonly employed classification system stratifies patients by extent of disease into two groups: those with limited disease and those with extensive disease. This staging system was published in 1980 and was based on the outcome of 20 patients *(11,12)*. Localized skin involvement, with or without hepatic dysfunction, is classified as limited disease. Patients with generalized skin involvement or with limited skin involvement in association with eye involvement, oral involvement, hepatic dysfunction with abnormal liver histology, or involvement of any other target organ are considered to have extensive disease. Although this staging system is highly reproducible among transplant centers, it provides little information about prognosis and is therefore of limited clinical utility.

More recently, researchers at Johns Hopkins Oncology Center have developed a grading system for chronic GVHD that stratifies patients into risk categories according to clinical characteristics *(13)*. Using a data base of 151 patients with chronic GVHD, three variables were found to be risk factors for shortened survival by multivariate analysis: extensive skin GVHD involving greater than 50% of the body surface area, platelet count of less than 100,000/μL, and progressive-type onset. This model was validated using data from 1108 patients from the International Blood Marrow Transplant Registry (IBMTR) ($n = 711$), Fred Hutchinson Cancer Center ($n = 188$), the University of Nebraska ($n = 60$), and the University of Minnesota ($n = 149$) *(14)*. Despite significant heterogeneity of the data, the proposed grading system identified three prognostic groups, each with different survival outcomes. Because this grading system is highly predictive of outcome, it may help to improve clinical management, trial design, and communication among transplant centers.

4. CLINICAL MANIFESTATIONS

The diagnosis of chronic GVHD is usually made after d 100 posttransplant and before d 500, although exceptions on either end are possible. The median time of diagnosis is 201 d after human leukocyte antigen (HLA)-identical sibling transplant, 159 d after mismatched related transplant, and 133 d after unrelated donor transplant *(15)*. Clinical manifestations are summarized in Table 1 and described in more detail in the following subsections. The skin is the most commonly involved organ in chronic GVHD, but isolated oral, ocular, hepatic, or pulmonary disease may occur.

4.1. Skin

Chronic GVHD of the skin can be lichenoid or sclerodermatous. Lichenoid GVHD presents as an erythematous, papular rash that resembles lichen planus and has no typical distribution pattern. Keratoconjuctivitis sicca and salivary dysfunction causing dry eyes and dry mouth are commonly seen in association with lichenoid GVHD.

Sclerodermatous GVHD may involve the dermis and/or the muscular fascia and is clinically similar to systemic sclerosis. The skin is thickened, tight, and fragile, with very poor wound-healing capacity. Alteration in pigmentation, either hypopigmentation or hyperpigmentation, may occur. In severe cases, the skin may become blistered or ulcerated. Because the sclerosis affects the dermis, hair loss and destruction of sweat glands are common.

Isolated fascial scleroderma with musculoskeletal manifestations is discussed in more detail. It manifests as decreased mobility with normal skin and is particularly debilitating when joint areas are involved. It is important to distinguish between skin and fascial scleroderma because treatment decisions may be affected. In addition to systemic therapy, skin chronic GVHD benefits from aggressive moisturization with petroleum jelly, strict sun protection, and prompt treatment of local infections.

4.2. Nails

Fingernails and toenails may be affected by chronic GVHD. Nails develop vertical ridges and cracking and are very fragile. The diagnosis is made clinically and local treatment with nail polish may help prevent problematic fragmentation of the nail.

4.3. Musculoskeletal System

Fascial involvement in sclerodermatous GVHD is common. It is most frequently associated with skin changes, but may develop with normal overlying skin. Fasciitis causes significant limitations in range of motion, especially if joint areas are involved. Patients should undergo regular evaluation by a physical therapist and begin a rigorous physical therapy program should fasciitis develop.

Muscular cramping in patients with chronic GVHD is common, although the pathophysiology is not well understood. Myositis, with tender muscles and elevated muscle enzymes, is rare and does not explain the frequent cramping in most patients. Because many patients with chronic GVHD have received steroids for prophylaxis and treatment and because hormone levels are often low posttransplant, osteoporosis may occur. Regular bone density evaluation and the use of bisphosphatase to treat and/or prevent degenerative disease are recommended.

4.4. Eyes

Ocular GVHD manifests most commonly as Sjogregn's syndrome, or dry eyes. Destruction of the lacrimal glands results in dryness, photophobia, and burning. Regular ophthalmologic evaluation with Schirmer's test to measure tear production is important so that asymptomatic disease can be treated before it progresses to corneal damage. Local therapy involves preservative-free tears and ointment and placement of punctal plugs by an experienced ophthalmologist. Conjunctival GVHD is a rare manifestation of severe chronic GVHD and is associated with a poor prognosis.

4.5. Mouth

Simultaneous involvement of the mouth and eyes is common. Early oral GVHD commonly causes xerostomia (dryness of the mouth) and/or sensitivity to minty, spicy, and acidic foods. More advanced disease may cause odynophagia (pain with swallowing) and lichenoid changes of the buccal mucosa. Physical exam in mild disease reveals only erythema. Lichenoid changes of more advanced disease cause whitish plaques resembling thrush or lichen planus. Worsening erythema with ulcerations and atrophy of the mucosa and gums may develop. Because dental damage can occur secondary to gum atrophy and decreased secretions, regular dental care with appropriate endocarditis prophylaxis is recommended. Diagnosis of salivary gland and mucosal involvement is made by biopsy. Secondary infections with viruses (especially herpes simplex) and yeasts are common and may make diagnosis difficult. Changes in symptoms may occur with local infections; therefore, cultures are warranted at the time chronic GVHD is diagnosed and for worsening of symptoms.

4.6. Respiratory Tract

Bronchiolitis obliterans is an uncommon but serious manifestation of chronic GVHD. Patients typically present with a cough 3–20 mo posttransplant *(16)*, and progress to develop dyspnea, wheezing, and respiratory failure. Chest computed tomography (CT) may be normal or may show hyperinflation with or without interstitial pneumatosis, bronchial dilatation, or consolidation. Pulmonary function testing reveals an obstructive pattern and lung biopsy is usually diagnostic. The onset may be insidious or more acute with rapid progression. Overall, patients with bronchiolitis obliterans have minimal response to therapy and a very poor prognosis.

Patients with chronic GVHD are also at risk for chronic sinuopulmonary disease, chronic cough, and bronchospasm. Severe scleroderma of the torso may cause restrictive lung disease though restriction of chest wall movement. Sinus infections and pneumonia should be treated with appropriate antibiotics and referral to an otolaryngologist may be indicated.

4.7. Gastrointestinal Tract

Many patients with chronic GVHD have signs and symptoms involving the gastrointestinal (GI) tract, including gastroesophageal reflux, dysphagia, esophageal strictures or webs, and substernal chest pain. Malabsorption resulting in chronic diarrhea is seen. However, in most patients, these symptoms are attributable to other disease states including acute GVHD, infection, dysmotility, pancreatic insufficiency, and drug-related side effects *(17)*. In a retrospective review of the intestinal biopsies of 40 patients with chronic GVHD and persistent GI symptoms, histopathologic evidence of chronic GVHD was found in only 11 patients. The majority of these patients had evidence of both acute and chronic GVHD, with only three patients (7%) found to have isolated chronic GVHD. This study illustrated that although chronic GVHD alone may involve the GI tract, it may be difficult to diagnosis and is seldom seen without concurrent acute GVHD.

Table 1
Clinical Manifestations of Chronic GVHD

Organ	*Clinical manifestations*	*Evaluation*	*Supportive care*
Skin	Lichenoid: papular rash Sclerodermatous: thick, taut, fragile skin; poor wound healing	Clinical and/or skin biopsy	Moisturization (petroleum jelly) Treatment of local infections Protection from sun/trauma
Nails	Vertical ridging, cracking, fragility	Clinical	Nail polish may help prevent further damage
Sweat glands	Inflammation and destruction, risk of hyperthermia	Clinical	Avoidance of excessive heat
Hair	Complete or partial alopecia; thin, fragile hair		
Eyes	Dryness, photophobia, blurring Progression to corneal abrasion	Opthamalogic evaluation, Schirmer's test	Preservative-free tears and ointment
Mouth	Dryness, sensitivity Plaques resembling lichen plauns Erythema, painful ulceration Mucosal slceroderma	Dental evaluation Viral/fungal cultures at diagnosis and with worsening	Avoidance of spicy foods and toothpastes Regular dental care with endocarditis prophylaxis
Respiratory tract	Bronchiolitis obliterans (BO) with dyspnea, wheezing, and cough; Chronic sinopulmonary symptoms and infections	Pulmonary function tests (FEV_1, FVC, DLCO, helium lung volume) Chest CT in symptomatic patients Lung biopsy if clinically indicated	IgG replacement may decrease incidence of infections; Investigational therapy for BO
Gastrointestinal tract (GI)	Abnormal motility, strictures Diarrhea, malabsorption, weight loss	Nutritional evaluation Upper GI, endoscopy if clinically indicated	Early nutritional intervention Correction of strictures

(continued on next page)

Table 1
Clinical Manifestations of Chronic GVHD

Organ	*Clinical manifestations*	*Evaluation*	*Supportive care*
Liver	Cholestasis with increased serum bilirubin and alkaline phosphatase	Liver function tests Liver biopsy necessary for isolated hepatic involvement	FK506 may have better liver concentration
Musculoskeletal system	Fascitis with decreased range of motion, myositis rare	Physical and occupational therapy evaluations	Aggressive physical and occupational therapy programs
	Osteoporosis possible secondary to steroid use or hormonal deficit	Bone density evaluation	
Immune system	Profound immunodeficiency; functional asplenia, variable IgG levels	Assume severe immunocompromise in all patients	PCP prophylaxis for 6 mo after resolution of cGVHD; lifetime pneumococcal prophylaxis; IgG replacement to keep > 500 mg/dL
Hematopoietic system	Variable cytopenias, eosinophilia	Complete blood count with differential, antineutrophil, and antiplatelet antibody studies	Systemic treatment of chronic GVHD

Malnutrition in patients with chronic GVHD is common, with one recent report describing malnutrition in 43% of patients and severe malnutrition with body mass index less than 18.5 in 14% *(18)*. The mechanisms of wasting are not fully defined but may include increased catabolic rate as a result of elevated resting energy expenditure and high cytokine levels, especially tumor necrosis factor (TNF-α) *(18)*. Although full nutritional evaluation and interventions are recommended, many patients with active GVHD continue to lose weight despite adequate caloric intake. Symptoms often improve with successful systemic treatment of GVHD.

4.8. Liver

Hepatic disease typically presents as cholestasis, with laboratory evaluation revealing elevated alkaline phosphatase and elevated serum bilirubin. Isolated hepatic chronic GVHD is uncommon, but has been observed with increased frequency with the use of DLI *(19)*. Liver biopsy is required to confirm the diagnosis and is especially important if the patient has no other symptoms of chronic GVHD, because viral infection and drug toxicity may mimic GVHD. Most patients with hepatic GVHD are asymptomatic until the disease is extensive.

4.9. Immune System

Chronic GVHD, both the disease and its therapies, results in profound immunosuppression. In fact, most chronic GVHD deaths are attributable to infection. Functional asplenia with an increased susceptibility to encapsulated bacteria is common, and circulating Howell–Jolly bodies may be seen on peripheral blood smear. Patients are also at risk for invasive fungal infections and *Pneumocystis carinii* pneumonia (PCP). Routine prophylaxis against PCP should continue for 6 mo after resolution of GVHD and patients should receive pneumococcal prophylaxis for life *(20)*. Immunoglobulin levels should be monitored and patients with frequent infections should be supplemented with intravenous IgG for levels less than 500 mg/dL. Vaccinations, including Prevnar, should be delayed for 6 mo after resolution of GVHD and discontinuation of immunosuppressive medications. Patients vaccinated before that time should have titers monitored prevaccination and postvaccination so that an adequate immune response can be documented.

4.10. Hematopoietic System

Cytopenias are seen commonly in chronic GVHD patients. This may be a result of stromal damage, but autoimmune neutropenia, anemia, and/or thrombocytopenia are also seen. Antineutrophil and antiplatelet antibody studies may be helpful in making this diagnosis. Thrombocytopenia at the time of chronic GVHD diagnosis has been associated with a poor prognosis *(13,21)*. Eosinophilia is occasionally seen with chronic GVHD. The exact etiology is unknown, but the eosinophilia usually resolves with adequate systemic treatment of GVHD.

5. EVALUATION OF SUSPECTED CHRONIC GVHD

The accurate and timely diagnosis of chronic GVHD is an important step in its successful treatment. Many patients have returned to the care of their primary oncologist when chronic GVHD develops and its signs and symptoms may therefore be overlooked or misdiagnosed. However, not every rash or GI complaint represents GVHD. In a series of 123 patients referred to Johns Hopkins for the management of refractory chronic GVHD, 9 patients never had chronic GVHD and 26 patients had inactive disease *(22)*. Because the therapies for chronic GVHD are highly immunosuppressive, it is important to confirm the diagnosis before initiating therapy. Alternatively, more subtle manifestations of chronic GVHD may go undiagnosed for months and this delay may make successful treatment and rehabilitation difficult. The diagnosis of fascitis without skin changes, for example, may be a difficult diagnosis to establish. Because it may be rapidly progressive and significantly impede the range of motion of the joints, timely initiation of GVHD therapy and physical therapy is crucial.

If a diagnosis of chronic GVHD is suspected, histologic confirmation of at least one organ system is recommended. Review by a pathologist experienced in GVHD diagnosis is also helpful. After histologic confirmation is made, the extent of involvement should be ascertained. A comprehensive evaluation of all organ systems that may be affected by GVHD should be undertaken to assess the extent of disease and to help guide therapy.

Ophthalmologic evaluation should include Schirmer's test to assess tear production. Tear production of less than 5 mL in 5 min represents a positive test and probable involvement with GVHD. Fundal examination for infections and corneal examination for cataracts secondary to total-body irradiation or chronic steroid use is also important.

The mouth should be carefully examined for involvement with chronic GVHD. Findings may include mild erythema, plaque formation, ulcerations, or sclerodermatous changes. Cultures for herpes simplex virus (HSV) and yeast should be obtained at the time of diagnosis and if oral signs and symptoms worsen. Dental pathologies should be treated to minimize infectious risk and trauma to the buccal mucosa.

To assess for pulmonary involvement of GVHD, pulmonary function tests with spirometry and diffusing capacity (DLCO) are advisable. In early stages of bronchiolitis obliterans (BO), abnormal pulmonary function testing with evidence of obstructive lung disease may be the only finding. A suspected diagnosis of BO should be confirmed pathologically, as treatment and prognosis will be affected.

From a GI perspective, evaluation should include nutritional assessment and liver function tests. Hepatic GVHD is usually asymptomatic and elevated alkaline phosphatase and bilirubin levels may be the only sign of disease.

Finally, thorough evaluations by physical and occupational therapists are very important in determining the extent of skin and fascial involvement of GVHD. Range of motion, strength, and functional ability should be carefully measured and followed over time with the initiation and continuation of systemic therapy. A rigorous physical therapy program may help maintain or improve mobility and prevent further functional limitations.

6. TREATMENT OF CHRONIC GVHD

The successful treatment of chronic GVHD involves the participation of a multidisciplinary team. Members of the team should have expertise in the diagnosis and management of chronic GVHD and should include the following participants: transplant physician and nurse, social worker, physical and occupational therapists, dermatologist, ophthalmologist, gastroenterologist, and nutritionist. Patients should be encouraged to return to the transplant center for evaluation by this multidisciplinary team. Enrollment of patients onto treatment protocols is desirable, as we have much to learn about the pathophysiology and optimal treatment of chronic GVHD.

6.1. Primary Therapy

The most widely employed first line therapies for treatment of chronic GVHD are CSA and prednisone, administered on alternating days. This recommendation stems from work performed primarily in Seattle and published by Sullivan et al. in 1988 *(21,23)*. In two studies published simultaneously, Sullivan and colleagues reported that prednisone alone is superior to prednisone plus azathioprine for primary treatment of patients with standard-risk extensive chronic GVHD. However, in patients classified as high risk on the basis of platelet counts less than 100,000/µL, treatment with prednisone alone resulted in only a 26% 5-yr survival. When a similar group of patients was treated with alternating-day CSA and prednisone, 5-yr survival exceeded 50%. With the publication of these promising results, the combination of CSA and prednisone became standard frontline therapy for the treatment of patients with chronic GVHD, with or without thrombocytopenia.

More recent work, however, calls into question the use of this treatment regimen in patients with newly diagnosed standard-risk chronic GVHD. In a report from Seattle currently under review, prednisone alone was compared to prednisone plus CSA in patients with platelet counts greater than 100,000/µL (Martin, personal communication). Two hundred eighty-seven patients with extensive GVHD were randomized. The authors found no statistically significant difference in nonrelapse death at 5 yr or in cumulative incidence of secondary therapy at 5 yr. When patients were observed over the entire length of follow-up, however, a trend suggesting a lower probability of survival without relapse in the CSA plus prednisone arm was found (HR=0.70, p=0.06). Patients treated with prednisone alone did have a higher incidence of avascular necrosis. The findings of this study suggest that CSA may confer no treatment advantage over prednisone alone other than potentially decreasing steroid related toxicities. This uncertainty regarding the choice of frontline therapy further emphasizes the importance of enrolling patients on clinical trials so that fundamental questions about the pathogenesis and treatment of chronic GVHD may be answered.

The CSA plus prednisone regimen starts with daily prednisone at 1 mg/kg/d and daily CSA at 10 mg/kg/d divided BID. CSA dosing is based on the lower of actual and ideal body weight. If the disease is nonprogressive after 2 wk, prednisone is tapered by 25% per week to a target dose of 1 mg/kg every other day. After successful completion of this steroid taper, CSA is reduced by 25% per week to alternate-day dosing of 10 mg/kg/d divided BID, every other day. Researchers at Johns Hopkins have found that 90% of all responders have done so by 3 mo, and thus are re-evaluated for response at 3 mo *(24)*. If the disease has completely resolved, patients are slowly weaned from both medications, with dose reductions approximately every 2 wk. Patients with incomplete response are kept on therapy for an additional 3 mo and then re-evaluated. After maximal response is achieved, CSA and prednisone are continued for another 3 mo and then tapered. If patients fail to respond by 3 mo or demonstrate progressive disease, salvage regimens are warranted.

6.2. Alternative Therapies

6.2.1. Tacrolimus and Mycophenolate Mofetil

Tacrolimus (FK506) and mycophenolate mofetil (MMF) are reasonable alternatives to CSA and prednisone in patients in patients diagnosed with chronic GVHD while receiving these medications or in whom this first-line therapy fails. FK506 was studied by Tzakis et al. in steroid refractory patients *(25)*. Of 17 patients with extensive chronic GVHD, 6 showed an unequivocal beneficial response. FK506 concentrates in the liver and may therefore be more efficacious than CSA for the treatment of hepatic GVHD. It should be dosed starting at 1 mg twice a day for adults, with dosages adjusted according to serum levels. Trough levels of 5–15 ng/mL are desirable and should be achieved within 3–4 wk.

Mycophenolate mofetil is a potent, reversible inhibitor of eukaryotic inosine monophosphate dehydrogenase that has been used extensively in recipients of renal allografts. Recent reports have shown promising results for the treatment of chronic GVHD. Basara and colleagues reported a response to MMF in 7 of 11 patients with limited chronic GVHD *(26)*. In a series of 15 pediatric alloBMT patients, Busca et al. reported an overall response rate of 60% when MMF was employed as salvage therapy for extensive chronic GVHD *(27)*. Patients were dosed with 15–40 mg/kg/d, most often in combination with other immunosuppressive medications.

Tacrolimus and MMF may also be used in combination. A retrospective review of 26 patients treated with this regimen at Johns Hopkins showed a response rate of almost 50% and a low incidence of side effects *(28)*. A prospective phase II study of tacrolimus and MMF for the treatment of refractory chronic GVHD is currently underway. A phase III multi-institutional trial comparing CSA and FK506 with or without MMF is also in progress. Standard MMF dosing is 1 g orally twice a day in adults. In children, the suspension is dosed at 600 mg/m^2/dose twice daily or a 750-mg capsule may be administered twice daily for children 1.25–1.5 m^2. Children over 1.5 m^2 should receive adult dosing.

6.2.2. Thalidomide

Thalidomide has been reported to have immunosuppressive properties and to be active against chronic GVHD. The first prospective trial of thalidomide for refractory or high-risk chronic GVHD was conducted at Johns Hopkins and published in 1992 *(29)*. Forty-four patients participated in the trial, 23 with refractory disease and 21 with high-risk disease. The overall response rate was 59% and the actuarial survival of all enrolled patients was 76%. The drug was particularly effective in patients with refractory chronic GVHD, with a survival rate of 76%. Side effects in this trial were mild.

Subsequent trials, however, have not confirmed the efficacy or tolerability of thalidomide. A prospective randomized clinical trial of CSA and prednisone with or without thalidomide found no clinical benefit with the addition of thalidomide *(30)*. A similar trial conducted in Seattle was unable to evaluate the activity of thalidomide because the majority of patients discontinued the medication because of severe neurotoxicity *(31)*. Although the drug is now commercially available, patients with pre-existing neuropathies should not be considered for thalidomide therapy.

6.2.3. Etretinate and Acetretin

Etretinate is a synthetic retinoid that has been used to treat patients with systemic scleroderma. Based on reports of response in this patient population, it has been used to treat patients with sclerodermatous and fascial chronic GVHD. The initial report of its use was published in 1999 and described 32 patients with refractory disease treated with etretinate *(32)*. Twenty-seven patients completed a 3-mo trial of the drug and, of these, 20 showed an improvement in their skin lesions and/or range of motion. Side effects include skin erythema, dryness, and peeling of the palms, soles, and lips. Liver toxicity may also develop and the drug is a known teratogen. Etretinate is not currently commercially available, and acetretin, a more rapidly cleared derivative, has been used in its place. Acetretin may be added to immunosuppressive medications to increase the cutaneous response in patients with sclerodermatous GVHD.

6.2.4. Plaquenil and Clofazimine

Clofazimine, an antimycobacterial drug used to treat leprosy and *Mycobacterium avium* complex, has anti-inflammatory activity in a number of chronic autoimmune skin disorders. Based on the success of treatment in these disorders, it was studied in 22 patients with chronic GVHD *(33)*. More than half of the patients with sclerodermatous disease showed improvement in skin involvement, flexion contractures, or oral manifestations. In this study, the drug was dosed at 300 mg orally once daily for the first 90 d, and then lowered to 100 mg/d. Clofazimine was generally well tolerated except for GI side effects and transient skin hyperpigmentation.

Plaquenil (hydroxychloroquine) is an antimalarial drug used in the treatment of autoimmune diseases. It interferes with antigen presentation and cytokine production and is synergistic with CSA and tacrolimus in vitro *(34)*. Based on preclinical data and promising results in a phase II trial *(34)*, Plaquenil is now being studied in a Children's Oncology Group Phase III randomized placebo-controlled trial. Patients with extensive chronic GVHD are being randomized to receive CSA and prednisone, with or without Plaquenil. Plaquenil will be dosed at 12 mg/kg/d orally (up to 1000 mg/d) divided BID.

6.2.5. Nonpharmacologic Approaches

Photosensitization with 8-methoxypsoralen and ultraviolet A irradiation (PUVA) is an attractive treatment option in patients with lichenoid chronic GVHD. PUVA was originally reported in the mid-1980s, and since that time, it has been extensively employed. In a study undertaken at our institution, 40 patients with refractory or high-risk GVHD were treated with PUVA *(35)*. Of the 11 patients with isolated cutaneous disease, 5 obtained a complete response. Of the 22 patients with multiorgan chronic GVHD, 17 showed improvement in their skin disease. PUVA had no effect on the noncutaneous manifestations of GVHD. PUVA is not indicated for sclerodermatous GVHD, but it may be beneficial to patients with extensive or refractory lichenoid cutaneous chronic GVHD. Theoretically, this approach should be associated with less global immunosuppression and may be particularly attractive in patients in whom a maximal graft-vs-leukemia effect is desired.

Low-dose total lymphoid irradiation (TLI) has also been used to treat drug-resistant chronic GVHD. A dose of 100 cGy of thoraco-abdominal irradiation resulted in clinical benefit in 6 of 11 patients in one report *(36)*.

Extracorporeal photochemotherapy (ECP) represents a third nonpharmacological approach to the treatment of chronic GVHD. With ECP, peripheral blood mononuclear cells are collected by aphaeresis and exposed to the photosensitizing compound PUVA prior to reinfusion. ECP has been used to treat cutaneous T-cell lymphoma, some autoimmune diseases, and solid-organ rejection. More recently, it has been successfully employed in the treatment of both acute and chronic GVHD. One report published by Greinix et al. describes 21 patients treated with ECP *(37)*. Of these, 15 patients had extensive chronic GVHD, in most cases involving more than one organ system. Cutaneous chronic GVHD improved in 80% of cases, and complete resolution of hepatic GVHD was seen in 7 of the 10 patients with liver involvement. Oral mucosal lesions resolved completely and some improvement was seen in the knee and elbow contractures associated with sclerodermatous GVHD. ECP in this series was not associated with any significant side effects.

6.3. Supportive Care

Supportive care seeks to reduce the morbidity associated with chronic GVHD by preventing infections, treating symptoms, and encouraging physical activity. Although systemic therapy directed against GVHD is crucial, these measures may help to improve the length and quality of life of patients with chronic GVHD.

6.3.1. Infection Prophylaxis

Infection is the leading cause of death among patients with chronic GVHD. Infection prophylaxis with antimicrobials and prompt treatment of suspected and documented infections are important means of reducing infection-associated morbidity and mortality. Prophylaxis against *P. carinii* should be administered to all patients undergoing treatment of chronic GVHD for 6 mo after discontinuation of immunosuppressive medications. These patients also have lifelong splenic dysfunction and should therefore receive prophylaxis against encapsulated bacteria for life. The guidelines published by the American Heart Association for endocarditis prophylaxis should be followed when patients are undergoing dental or other invasive procedures.

Routine systemic antifungal prophylaxis is not required. However, patients receiving topical steroid therapy for oral GVHD should be treated with clotrimazole troches or nystatin swishes. Oral thrush unresponsive to these measures should be treated with systemic antifungal therapy. Likewise, systemic prophylaxis against viral infections is unnecessary. However, HSV outbreaks should be promptly and adequately treated with Famvir, and patients with recurrent episodes may benefit from daily Famvir prophylaxis. Patients at risk for cyclomegalovirus (CMV) reactivation should receive frequent monitoring with CMV surveillance cultures or antigenemia testing. A positive antigenemia test should be treated preemptively with ganciclovir, and patients with evidence of CMV disease should receive both ganciclovir and CMV-specific immunoglobulin.

Intravenous IgG should be administered to patients with hypogammaglobulinemia and recurrent infections to keep IgG levels greater than 500 mg/dL. Vaccination series should be delayed until 1 yr after the completion of GVHD therapy because most patients will not mount an immune response with active disease or while receiving immunosuppressive medications. Posttransplant vaccination guidelines are available on the Centers for Disease Control and Prevention website (www.cdc.gov/mmwr/mmwr_rr).

6.3.2. Symptom Management

Chronic GVHD of the skin may cause severe dryness and pruritis. Aggressive lubrication with a perfume-free, preservative-free ointment such as petroleum jelly is recommended. Sunburn and trauma should be avoided, and patients should be advised to wear sunscreen (SPF > 30) and a wide-brimmed hat outside. Patients with affected sweat glands should avoid overheating and be aware that they are at risk for heat exhaustion and heat stroke. Patients with sicca syndrome may be managed with preservative-free artificial tears and artificial saliva. Careful ophthalmologic follow-up is important so that long-term damage to the eyes is avoided. Patients with dry mouth are at increased risk for dental caries and should be followed closely by a dentist. In women, vaginal dryness and strictures may be a manifestation of chronic GVHD. Topical steroids and hormone replacement therapy may help relieve these symptoms.

Malnutrition and wasting are common in patients with GVHD. The etiology is most likely multifactorial, with increased caloric requirement, altered taste, oral and esophageal disease, and malabsorption likely contributing. Patients with weight loss should be followed carefully by a nutritionist and enteral supplements encouraged. In patients who are unable to maintain adequate caloric intake, parenteral nutrition or enteral feeds through a gastrostomy tube may be required. Often, wasting and malnutrition persist despite adequate caloric intake and resolve when the underlying GVHD is successfully treated.

6.3.3. Physical and Occupational Therapy

Patients with sclerodermatous GVHD and restricted range of motion may benefit tremendously from the management of a physical therapist. Although little data exist about its efficacy, our observations have been encouraging. Physical therapy may serve to decrease pain and to increase and maintain strength, range of motion, and mobility. Occupational therapy helps patients maximize their functional abilities in activities of daily living, employment opportunities, and sexual satisfaction. All patients with chronic GVHD should receive full physical and occupational therapy evaluations as part of their initial workup. Personal exercise and activity plans should be prescribed with formal re-evaluations every 3–4 mo.

6.3.4. Psychosocial Considerations

Chronic GVHD is a multisystem disease. Skin and fascial involvement may cause significant pain and disfigurement. Intestinal involvement often results in anorexia, nausea, diarrhea, and weight loss. Mucosal disease can cause extreme discomfort when the mouth, eyes, or vagina are involved. In addition, the treatment of chronic GVHD may result in side effects, including infections requiring aggressive therapy and hospitalization. It is, in summary, a disease that impacts immensely on a patient's quality of life. Recognition of the psychosocial stressors associated with chronic GVHD is mandatory. Patients should be followed closely by an oncology social worker when possible and patients showing signs of depression or anxiety should be referred to a psychiatrist. Antidepressant medications are likely underprescribed in patients with chronic GVHD.

7. FUTURE DIRECTIONS

Efforts to prevent the development of chronic GVHD have been unsuccessful. A report published in 1996 found no effect on the incidence or mortality from chronic GVHD with the prophylactic administration of IVIgG following BMT *(38)*. A more recent trial of prolonged administration of CSA found no difference in chronic GVHD or mortality when CSA was given for 24 mo rather than 6 mo *(39)*. Current transplantation practices, including the use of DLIs and PBSCs, older patient age, and the increasing use of unrelated and mismatched marrow donors make the challenges facing physicians who care for patients with chronic GVHD even greater.

Chronic GVHD remains the most significant late complication of alloBMT. Ongoing research to further characterize the pathogenesis of this disease is crucial to the development of new therapeutic approaches. Several new therapies are currently under evaluation, including the antineoplastic and immunosuppressive drug pentostatin, daclizumab, a soluble interleukin-2 (IL-2) receptor antagonist, and infliximab, an anti-TNF-α monoclonal antibody. New strategies may employ a sequential approach to therapy so that each phase of the GVHD cascade, including patient conditioning, donor T-cell activation, and effector cell stimulation, is effectively targeted. Particularly intriguing are animal models showing that some of the newly identified cytokines, including IL-18 and inducible costimulator, may play a protective and/or therapeutic role in chronic GVHD. Transplant centers and referring physicians must work closely together to identify patients with chronic GVHD and to deliver the multidisciplinary care that they require.

REFERENCES

1. Ho VT, Soiffer RJ. The history and future of T-cell depletion as graft-versus-host disease prophylaxis for allogeneic hematopoietic stem cell transplantation. *Blood* 2001;98:3192–3204.
2. Korbling M, Anderlini P. Peripheral blood stem cell versus bone marrow allotransplantation: does the source of hematopoietic stem cells matter? *Blood* 2001;98:2900–2908.
3. Chiodi S, Spinelli S, Ravera G, et al. Quality of life in 244 recipients of allogeneic bone marrow transplantation. *Br J Haematol* 2000;110:614–619.
4. Chen W, Thoburn C, Hess AD. Characterization of the pathogenic autoreactive T cells in cyclosporine-induced syngeneic graft-versus-host disease. *J Immunol* 1998;161:7040–7046.
5. Glazier A, Tutschka PJ, Farmer ER, et al. Graft-versus-host disease in cyclosporine A treated rats after syngeneic and autologous bone marrow reconstitution. *J Exp Med* 1983;158:1–8.
6. Hess AD, Thoburn CJ. Immunobiology and immunotherapeutic implications of syngeneic/autologous graft-versus-host disease. *Immunol Rev* 1997;157:111–123.
7. Krenger W, Ferrara JL. Graft-versus-host disease and the Th1/Th2 paradigm. *Immunol Res* 1996;15:50–73.
8. Gaziev D, Galimberti M, Lucarelli G, et al. Chronic graft-versus-host disease: is there an alternative to the conventional treatment? *Bone Marrow Transplant* 2000;25:689–696.
9. Weinberg K, Annett G, Kashyap A, et al. The effect of thymic function on immunocompetence following bone marrow transplantation. *Biol Blood Marrow Transplant* 1995;1:18–23.
10. Parkman R. Chronic graft-versus-host disease. *Curr Opin Hematol* 1998;5:22–25.
11. Shulman HM, Sullivan KM, Weiden PI, et al. Chronic graft-versus-host syndrome in man: a long-term clinicopathologic study of 20 Seattle patients. *Am J Med* 1980;69:204–217.
12. Sullivan KM, Shulman HM, Storb R, et al. Chronic graft-versus-host disease in 52 patients: adverse natural course and successful treatment with combination immunosuppression. *Blood* 1981;57:267–276.
13. Akpek G, Zahurak ML, Piantadosi S, et al. Development of a prognostic model for grading chronic graft-versus-host disease. *Blood* 2001;97:1219–1226.
14. Akpek G, Lee SJ, Flowers ME, et al. Multi-center validation of a prognostic grading in chronic graft-versus-host disease. *Blood* 2001;98:3086 [Abstract].
15. Sullivan K, Agura E, Anasetti C. Chronic graft-versus-host disease and other late complications of bone marrow transplantation. *Semin Hematol* 1991;28:250–259.
16. Ratanatharathorn V, Ayash L, Lazarus HM, et al. Chronic graft-versus-host disease: clinical manifestation and therapy. *Bone Marrow Transplant* 2001;28:121–129.
17. Akpek G, Chinratanalab W, Hallick JP, et al. Gastrointestinal involvement in chronic graft-versus-host disease: a clinicopathologic study. *Blood* 2001;98:1666 [Abstract].
18. Jacobsohn DA, Margolis J, Doherty J, et al. Weight loss and malnutrition in patients with chronic graft-versus-host disease. *Bone Marrow Transplant* 2002;29:231–236.
19. Arai A, Anders V, Lee LA, et al. Graft-versus-host disease after donor lymphocyte infusion presenting as an acute hepatitis. *Blood* 2001;98:5228 [Abstract].
20. Vogelsang GB. How I treat chronic graft-versus-host disease. *Blood* 2001;97:1196–1201.
21. Sullivan KM, Witherspoon RP, Storb R, et al. Alternating-day cyclosporine and prednisone for treatment of high-risk chronic graft-versus-host disease. *Blood* 1988;72:556–561.
22. Jacobsohn DA, Montross S, Anders V, et al. Clinical importance of confirming or excluding the diagnosis of chronic graft-versus-host disease. *Bone Marrow Transplant* 2001;28:1047–1051.
23. Sullivan KM, Witherspoon RP, Storb R, et al. Prednisone and azathioprine compared with prednisone and placebo for treatment of chronic graft-versus-host disease: prognostic influence of prolonged thrombocytopenia after allogeneic marrow transplantation. *Blood* 1988;72:546–554.
24. Wingard JR, Piantadosi S, Vogelsang GB, et al. Predictors of death from chronic graft-versus-host disease after bone marrow transplantation. *Blood* 1989;74:1428–1435.
25. Tzakis AG, Abu-Elmagd K, Fung JJ, et al. FK-506 rescue in chronic graft-versus-host disease after bone marrow transplantation. *Transplant Proc* 1991;23:3225–3227.

26. Basara N, Kiehl MG, Blau W, et al. Mycophenolate mofetil in the treatment of acute and chronic GVHD in hematopoietic stem cell transplant patients: four years of experience. *Transplant Proc* 1991;33:2121–2123.
27. Busca A, Saroglia EM, Lanino E, et al. Mycophenolate mofetil (MMF) as therapy for refractory chronic GVHD in children receiving bone marrow transplantation. *Bone Marrow Transplant* 2000;25:1067–1071.
28. Mookerjee B, Altomonte V, Vogelsang G. Salvage therapy for refractory chronic graft-versus-host disease with mycophenolate mofetil and tacrolimus. *Bone Marrow Transplant* 1999;24:517–520.
29. Vogelsang GB, Farmer ER, Hess AD, et al. Thalidomide for the treatment of chronic graft-versus-host disease. *N Engl J Med* 1992;326:1055–1058.
30. Arora M, Wagner JE, Davies SM, et al. Randomized clinical trial of thalidomide, cyclosporine and prednisone versus cyclosporine and prednisone as initial therapy for chronic graft-versus-host disease. *Biol Blood Marrow Transplant* 2001;7:265–273.
31. Koc S, Leisenring W, Flowers ME, et al. Thalidomide for treatment of patients with chronic graft-versus-host disease. *Blood* 2000;96:3995–3996.
32. Marcellus DC, Altomonte VL, Farmer ER, et al. Etretinate therapy for refractory sclerodermatous chronic graft-versus-host disease. *Blood* 1999;93:66–70.
33. Lee SJ, Wegner SA, McGarigle CJ, et al. Treatment of chronic graft-versus-host disease with clofazimine. *Blood* 1997;89:2298–2302.
34. Gilman AL, Chan KW, Mogul A, et al. Hydroxychloroquine for the treatment of chronic graft-versus-host disease. *Biol Blood Marrow Transplant* 2000;6:327–334.
35. Vogelsang GB, Wolff D, Altomonte V, et al. Treatment of chronic graft-versus-host disease with PUVA. *Bone Marrow Transplant* 1996;17:1061–1067.
36. Socie G, Devergie A, Cosset J, et al. Low dose total lymphoid irradiation for extensive, drug resistant chronic graft-versus-host disease. *Transplantation* 1990;49:657–658.
37. Greinix HT, Volc-Platzer B, Rabitsch W, et al. Successful use of extracorporeal photochemotherapy in the treatment of sever acute and chronic graft-versus-host disease. *Blood* 1998;92:3098–3104.
38. Sullivan KM, Storek J, Kopecky KJ, et al. A controlled trial of long-term administration of intravenous immunoglobulin to prevent late infection and chronic graft-versus-host disease after marrow transplantation: clinical outcome and effect on subsequent immune recovery. *Biol Blood Marrow Transplant* 1996;2:44–53.
39. Kansu E, Gooley T, Flowers ME, et al. Administration of cyclosporine for 24 months compared with 6 months for prevention of chronic graft-versus-host disease: a prospective randomized clinical trial. *Blood* 2001;98:3868–3870.

9 Immune Reconstitution After Allogeneic Transplantation

Carolyn A. Keever-Taylor, PhD

CONTENTS

1. INTRODUCTION

Allogeneic hematopoietic stem cell transplantation (alloHSCT) is an effective and curative treatment for a number of hematological malignancies, immune system or genetic disorders, and even solid tumors. AlloHSCT allows marrow lethal treatment of the primary disorder as well as providing immunotherapy in the form of a graft-vs-tumor (GVT) effect. Despite more than 30 yr of experience with HSCT, the major barriers to this treatment have remained the same. These include graft-vs-host disease (GVHD) in both the acute and chronic forms and the rather prolonged period of immune incompetence that occurs as the immune system redevelops. Approaches to reduce GVHD often result in exacerbation of immune incompetence or cause problems with engraftment, whereas attempts to speed engraftment and immune reconstitution have often exacerbated GVHD. Thus, a better understanding of the forces affecting each of these barriers is needed such that the right balance can be achieved to improve HSCT outcome.

Both autologous HSCT (autoHSCT) and alloHSCT are followed by a period during which the immune system redevelops both by a process of peripheral expansion of transferred mature precursors and via reconstitution from immature progenitors. Physically, the major cellular elements of the immune system recover relatively early and in a fairly predictable pattern in nearly all patients. This is followed by a more prolonged and variable period of functional recovery and maturation of the complex cellular interactions required for full immune competence. The recovery of immune function is further complicated in alloHSCT because of the need for immune suppression to permit engraftment and prevent or treat GVHD. Despite

From: *Stem Cell Transplantation for Hematologic Malignancies*
Edited by: R. J. Soiffer

numerous advances in supportative care, morbidity and mortality resulting from infectious complications secondary to this procedure remain a serious problem. Better antimicrobial drugs, especially antiviral agents, have reduced early transplant mortality but may have in some cases served to delay infections to a later time period. Late infection (> 50 d) remains one of the leading causes of death following HSCT, most especially in recipients of grafts from unrelated donors *(1,2)*.

The immune deficiencies that occur post-HSCT have been extensively characterized by sequential studies of patient blood sampled at intervals posttransplant. These studies have identified patient, donor, and graft variables that appear to affect the rate of immune reconstitution primarily and, to a lesser extent, the pattern of reconstitution. Studies such as these have proven useful, as they have allowed for the prediction of an expected pattern and rate of immune reconstitution for subgroups of transplant patients. Assessments that fall below the expected parameters of immune reconstitution for a given time posttransplant may signal that the patient is at higher risk for infectious complications, thus warranting intervention. In a similar fashion, certain immune phenotypes may be diagnostic of posttransplant events, such as graft rejection *(3)* or cytomegalovirus (CMV) reactivation *(4–6)*. Knowledge of the kinetics of immune reconstitution and of the patient, donor, or graft variables that affect immune reconstitution can provide insights into the function of the immune system as well as provide useful information relevant to patient care.

This chapter will review the expected pattern of cellular and humoral immune reconstitution following alloHSCT describing both classical and newer methods to evaluate immune function. Some of the more important variables that affect the tempo of immune reconstitution will be identified and some of the newer approaches that might serve to promote a faster or more complete immune reconstitution in these patients will be described.

2. PATTERNS OF IMMUNE RECONSTITUTION

2.1. Neutrophil and Monocyte Recovery

Neutrophils are essential as a first line of defense against bacterial and fungal infection. Until recently, patients were conditioned for transplant using myeloablative doses of chemotherapy with or without irradiation. The patient invariably experienced a period of 1 wk or more of nearly absolute neutropenia, during which there is a high risk of infection. Without a HSCT rescue, the patient would not be expected to recover hematopoiesis. The kinetics of neutrophil engraftment are influenced primarily by the graft source, dose of $CD34^+$ progenitor cells, use of hematopoietic growth factors, the use of posttransplant GVHD chemoprophylaxis, and to a lesser extent by the underlying disease *(7)*. In general, recipients of mobilized peripheral blood progenitor cell (PBPC) grafts from both related and unrelated donors engraft neutrophils and platelets earlier than do recipients of bone marrow (BM) *(8–11)*. This may be the result not only of a larger dose of CD34+ progenitors in PBPCs, but also to the more mature status of peripheral progenitors compared to BM. There is a dose–response increase in the rate of neutrophil engraftment up to a threshold amount of CD34+ cells (approx 2.0×10^6/kg) in most studies *(12)*. CD34+ cell dose can be somewhat controlled using PBPCs as a source for HSCT by collecting until a predetermined dose is achieved, but it is less controllable when BM is the graft source. Hematopoietic growth factors (primarily granulocyte colony-stimulating factor [G-CSF] and granulocyte-macrophage colony-stimulating factor [GM-CSF]) have been widely used to enhance the kinetics of neutrophil engraftment *(13)* but may be associated under certain circumstances with a delay in platelet engraftment *(7)*. Drugs such as methotrexate that are widely used to prevent acute GVHD are marrow suppressive and may further delay neutrophil engraftment even when growth factors are used *(14)*. Antiviral agents such as ganciclovir may likewise be myelosuppressive. The patient's primary disease may also affect the rate of neutrophil recovery. One study showed that patients transplanted with T-cell-replete BM for aplastic anemia engrafted neutrophils more quickly than patients transplanted for acute leukemia or chronic myelogenous leukemia (CML) *(15)*. However, even under the most optimal conditions, one can expect from 9 to 16 d during which the absolute neutrophil count (ANC) is below 0.5×10^9/L. Once engraftment occurs, the ANC generally rises to protective levels above 10^9/L fairly rapidly

Most studies have found that neutrophil function returns early post-HSCT. Neutrophil chemotaxis normalizes by 4 mo posttransplant unless the patient is experiencing active GVHD or infection, whereas other functions appear to normalize more quickly *(16–19)*. Zimmerli et al. *(18)* demonstrated that patients who subsequently developed pyogenic infections had lower neutrophil function than those who did not. In this study, defective skin window migration or combined defects were predictive for late pyogenic infections. Neutrophil migration may be further reduced during infusion of GM-CSF *(20)*. It is during the early period of neutropenia that supportative care is of most importance in preventing infection. The more recent use of nonmyeloablative conditioning regimens for alloHSCT has modified this pattern somewhat in that, depending on the protocol, patients experience few or no days of neutropenia, thus lessening the risks for early infectious complications *(21,22)*.

The kinetics of monocyte recovery post-HSCT are similar to neutrophils. BM-grafted patients have shown mostly normal monocyte phagocytic and killing function, although impairment in tissue-derived macrophages and in monocyte adherence early after transplant is seen *(23–25)*. Antigen-presenting capacity for immunoglobulin (Ig) synthesis likewise appears to be intact *(26)*, and engrafted monocytes produce normal levels of interleukin (IL)-1 *(27)*. Monocytes from a minority of patients exhibit suppressor activity in several systems, especially with nonphysiologic ratios of monocytes to T cells or B cells *(26)*. Early post-HSCT, there is evidence of monocyte activation marked by increased measures of respiratory burst and higher than normal levels of neopterin. Serum neopterin and tumor necrosis factor (TNF) levels were greater than twice normal at regeneration and remained raised for up to 6 wk after alloHSCT. This increase was not associated with GVHD or veno-occlusive disease and may represent a nonspecific activation state because of exposure to infectious agents during this period *(28)*. Indeed, multivariate analysis has shown that below normal monocyte counts or low B-cell counts at d 80, rather than a low ANC, predicts a higher incidence of infection from d 100 to d 365 in BM-grafted patients *(29)*. Consistent with this finding, recipients of T-cell-replete alloPBPCs who recover normal absolute monocytes by 1 mo experience few early or late posttransplant infections *(9,30)*.

The essential role of monocytes in immune reconstitution has been strikingly demonstrated in recipients of CD34+ cell-selected haploidentical HSCT who were given G-CSF to promote neutrophil engraftment *(31)*. In this study, G-CSF was shown to interfere with the ability of engrafted monocytes to produce IL-12. This defect, in turn, delayed reconstitution of CD4+ T cells with T helper 1 (Th1) activity and skewed T cells to a T helper 2 (Th2) phenotype. The production by Th2 T cells of IL-4 and IL-10 inhibited monocyte maturation into dendritic cells (DCs), resulting in an overall long-term impairment of immune function beyond that expected. When transplants were performed without using G-CSF, neutrophil engraftment was delayed, but not prevented. In the absence of G-CSF the defect in monocyte IL-12 production was corrected and the recovery of Th1-type CD4+ T cells was greatly improved. Although defects are seen in monocyte function in G-CSF-mobilized PBPC donors, these do not seem to translate into clinical immune deficits, likely the result of the larger number of hematopoic cells and the short duration of the therapy *(32)*. Monocytes contained within PBPC products have been shown to produce a large amount of IL-10 and to suppress alloreactive T-cell responses *(33)*. This finding may explain why allogeneic PBPC HSCT have not been associated with higher rates of acute GVHD despite the nearly 10-fold larger dose of T cells infused *(10,11)*.

2.2. Natural Killer Cells

Natural killer (NK) cells, like monocytes and neutrophils, provide a first-line defense against infection without the need for immunologic memory or human leukocyte antigen (HLA) restriction (reviewed in ref. *34*). Most cells mediating NK activity express the CD56 surface antigen; coexpress the Fcγ receptor, CD16, and lack CD3 and T-cell receptor (TCR) αβ expression. A subset of NK cells dimly express CD8 (αα homodimer), and some may bear TCRγδ. NK cells mediate cytotoxicity both through direct recognition of the infected target (intracellular bacteria, parasites, or virus) or transformed target cell and indirectly via antibody-dependent cellular cytotoxicity (ADCC). In addition to lytic activity, NK cells post-HSCT have been shown to produce IL-2, interferon (IFN)-γ, TNF-α, and B-cell differentiation factors both spontaneously and after stimulation and may play a role in the regeneration of B-cell function during the early posttransplant period *(35)*. The degree of killing and the spectrum of targets that can be recognized by NK cells are greatly increased when the cells are activated by cytokine exposure. The most potent NK-cell activator is IL-2, although IL-12, IL-15, IFN-γ and IL-18 can all activate NK cells. NK cells may play a role not only in the restoration of posttransplant immunity but may also mediate graft rejection, participate in GVHD reactions, as well as serve as GVT effectors (reviewed in ref. *36*).

Natural killer cells have two types of receptor: those that trigger the cells to lysis and those that inhibit lysis. The killer inhibitory receptors (KIR) deliver a negative signal when recognizing the appropriate intact self-HLA class I allele even if ligands for the killer-cell activating (KAR) receptors are present. Although KIRs from different families may be coexpressed by NK cells, in any given individual's NK repertoire there are cells that express a single KIR. Such NK cells can be triggered to kill targets that do not express class I, express defective class I, or lack the specific class I ligand they recognize, provided the target also expresses the appropriate costimulatory and adhesion molecules to allow triggering of the KAR receptors *(36)*. Some recent data from the Perugia group have shown that NK cells from HLA haploidentical donors who express unique KIR receptors are highly effective in killing patient-derived myeloid leukemia blast targets. Indeed, the relapse incidence in patients with acute myelogenous leukemia (AML) who received HSCT from donors with a unique KIR family was significantly lower than in recipients of grafts from donors who shared the same KIR families *(37,38)*.

Similar to neutrophils and monocytes, the number and function of donor-derived NK cells appear to normalize or even to exceed normal levels quite early after nearly all forms of HSCT *(39–46)*. During the first 3–4 mo, NK cells may be the dominant lymphocyte population, especially in recipients of grafts that have been depleted of mature T cells *(42,47)*, irrespective of HLA match *(48)*. This includes allogeneic recipients of highly purified CD34+ cell-selected grafts *(45)*. Indeed, during the earliest engraftment period, a lymphocyte phenotype devoid of NK cells is a hallmark for pending rejection *(3)*. These data together with the fact that NK cells do not rapidly reappear in patients who are rendered cytopenic with chemotherapy without stem cell rescue *(49)* indicate that the rapid NK-cell redevelopment post-HSCT predominately occurs from thymus-independent mechanisms. Many of these findings are illustrated in the upper left panel of Fig. 1 from our own studies of recipients of conventional T-cell-replete BM grafts and partially T-cell-depleted (TCD) BM grafts. Here, it can be seen that even during the first 2 mo post-HSCT, the median absolute NK-cell count is within or near the normal range, and NK recovery is not much affected by patient age, extensive chronic GVHD, or T-cell depletion.

Natural-killer-cell lytic function is normal to high early posttransplant, and in contrast to most other immunological functions, NK activity may be increased in patients with acute GVHD, perhaps secondary to activation from the cytokines produced during this reaction *(50–52)*. Even in the absence of GVHD, NK-cell function is activated during the early post-HSCT period *(49,53)*. Although not initiators of GVHD reactions, NK cells may participate in the pathology of GVHD lesions either directly or via cytokine release *(54,55)*. Bulk culture studies have shown that NK cells readily respond to further activation by IL-2 even at the earliest times tested post-HSCT (18 d) and achieve maximal levels of activation sooner than normal controls through the first 5 mo posttransplant, a finding that may also reflect a state of endogenous activation *(53)*. Limiting dilution studies showed a lower precursor frequency of NK cells induced to activated killing compared to normal donors through the first 2 mo posttransplant before rising to normal levels, further indicating a heightened responsiveness to activation rather than an overabundance of precursors *(52)*. Even without the benefit of the release from inhibition of killing by KIR differences, reconstituting IL-2-activated NK cells from HLA-identical donors are capable of lysing fresh leukemia targets, and in the setting of chronic myelogenous leukemia (CML), the presence of this activity may be associated with a decreased likelihood to relapse in recipients of a TCD HSCT *(56,57)*.

The heightened response of reconstituting NK cells to IL-2 activation may be explained by the results of several detailed studies of NK-cell phenotype post-HSCT. Most NK cells in normal donors are CD3– and express low levels of CD56 and high levels of CD16 (CD56^{dim}CD16^{bright}) with a subset of these cells, approx 20%, expressing low-density CD8. CD3–CD56^{dim}CD16^{bright} NK cells have the highest degree of resting lytic activity *(34)*. Approximately 2% of normal lymphocytes express high levels of CD56 (CD56^{bright}) and low or no CD16. These cells have NK activity but to a lesser degree than CD56^{dim}CD16^{bright} cells and represents the NK population most responsive to activation and expansion by IL-2 *(34)*. The majority of patients reconstitute with the normal CD56^{dim}CD16^{bright} NK subset. However, a subset of patients (35%) receiving autologous or allogeneic non-TCD grafts have shown an overrepresentation of CD56^{bright}CD16– cells through 4 mo posttransplant *(58)*. As expected, these cells displayed poor lytic activity when tested fresh, but they were highly lytic after culture with IL-2 *(59)*. Consistent with the ready response to IL-2, the CD56^{bright}CD16– cells express high levels of the IL-2-receptor β-chain and coexpress CD26, an activation antigen *(59)*. The endogenously activated NK activity described post-HSCT may reflect the presence of these minor subsets of CD16– or CD16^{dim} NK cells that have developed as a result of acute GVHD secondary to the encounter with infectious agents.

In contrast to most studies, Shenoy et al. *(30)* have reported lower than normal NK cell recovery and impaired lytic activity during the first year posttransplant of allogeneic PBPCs. The absolute numbers were highest during the first month and gradually declined over the year follow-up period. Conversely, other comparative studies have shown similar rapid and sustained recovery of NK numbers and function in PBPC or BM recipients *(11,60,61)*. This occurs

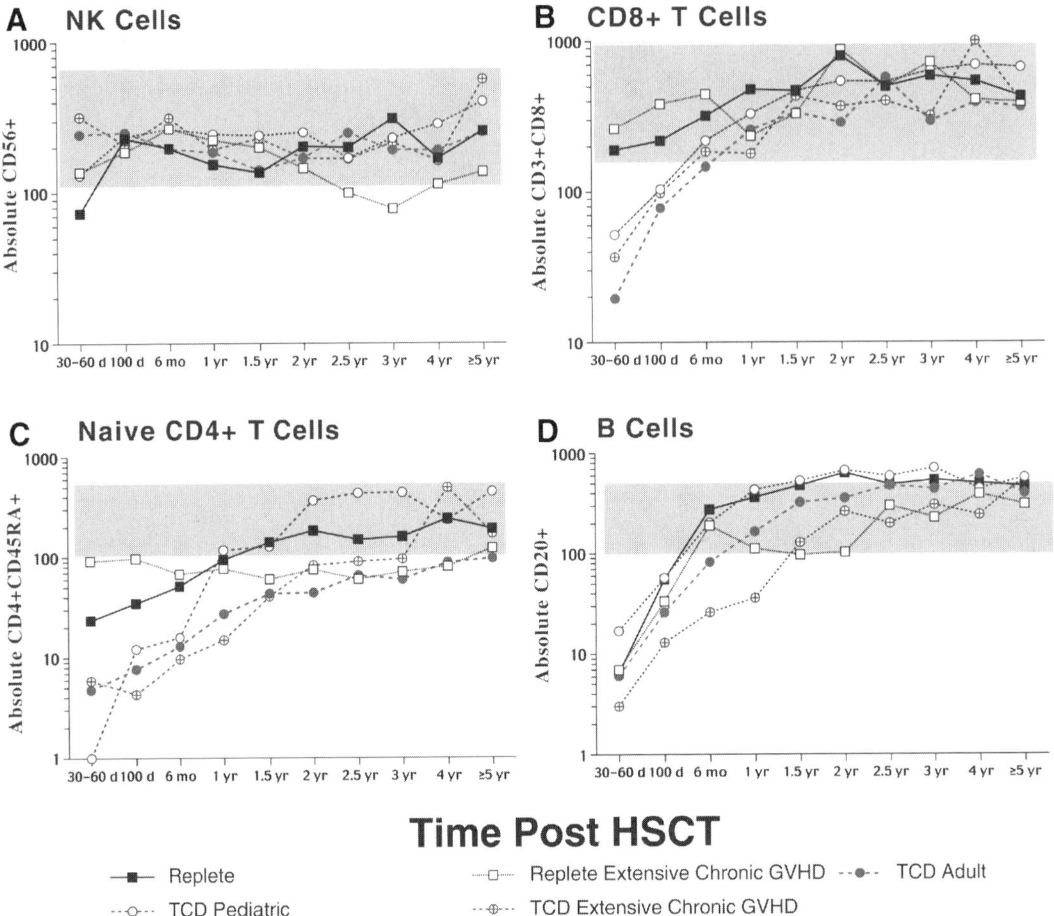

Fig. 1. Effect of TCD, age, and extensive chronic GVHD on lymphocyte subset recovery following HSCT. The median absolute cell counts of CD56^{+} NK cells (**A**), CD3+CD8+ T cells (**B**), CD45RA+ naïve CD4+ T cells (**C**), and CD20+ B cells (**D**) for patients tested at or near the indicated time following BM HSCT are shown. Patients studied in each group include the following: T-cell-replete (solid squares), $N = 49$ (20 under 18 yr); T-cell-replete with extensive chronic GVHD (open squares), $N = 9$ (1 under 18 yr); adult (>18 yr) TCD (solid circles), $N = 241$; pediatric (18 yr) TCD (open circles), $N = 181$; and TCD with extensive chronic GVHD (crossed circles), $N = 51$ (8 under 18 yr). Not all patients were tested at each interval, but a given patient was tested only once during an interval. All recipients of TCD transplants received grafts purged by complement-mediated lysis using T10B9-1A1 monoclonal antibody, resulting in 1.8 ± 0.4 logs TCD. Recipients of TCD grafts were treated for the first 3 mo with cyclosporine A for additional GVHD prophylaxis, then tapered through 6 mo provided they were not experiencing GVHD at that time. TCD data represent matched sibling donors, unrelated matched donors, and unrelated or related HLA-mismatched donor's data are combined because the median absolute cell counts for these groups did not differ, as shown for CD4+ T cells in Fig. 2. The shaded area represents the 5th to 95th percentile of absolute values from 49 normal adult donors.

despite the fact that G-CSF-mobilized products show decreased mature NK-cell numbers and activity as well as fewer CD34+ NK-cell progenitors *(62)*. Like mobilized PBPCs, NK-cell activity in cord blood is also very low, although the precursor frequency of IL-2-activated NK cells is normal to increased *(63)*. Here, too, NK cells and their function rapidly reconstitute following allogeneic cord blood transplantation *(46,64–66)*. Moreover, NK-cell recovery and function does not appear to be hindered by growth factor use post-HSCT and may be increased if GM-CSF is used *(36,67)*.

The rapid redevelopment of NK cells post-HSCT is consistent with current knowledge of lymphoid development (reviewed in ref. *68*). T Cells and NK cells likely share a common precursor but with different sites of differentiation. Whereas T cells normally mature and develop in the thymus, a structure that is mostly atrophied in adult transplant recipients and takes considerable time to recover, NK cells primarily develop in the BM *(69)*. It might be expected then, that NK cells would repopulate the host before T cells, which must develop in a less optimal site.

2.3. T Cells

The recovery of T cells and T-cell function post-HSCT has been extensively studied. For it is here that the most profound and long-lasting deficiency in immune function is found. Much data support the concept that in contrast to neutrophils, monocytes, and NK cells that rapidly reconstitute from progenitors, early T-cell reconstitution is largely derived from mature cells contained in the graft responding to the antigenic environment of the host. T-Cell reconstitution is further impaired in allograft recipients because therapies for the prevention or treatment of GVHD are nearly all targeted at T cells. Furthermore, GVHD itself can directly hinder T-cell reconstitution by damaging lymphoid organs, including the thymus, that are needed for T-cell redevelopment from stem cell precursors *(70,71)*.

For recipients of T-cell-replete allogeneic BM HSCT, absolute T-cell counts gradually recover over the first year to nearly normal levels by approx 9 mo. Recovery is more delayed in the setting of TCD based on the degree of TCD and the type of posttransplant therapy used *(42,45,72–75)*. Even when absolute T-cell counts recover, there remain marked deficiencies in subset composition. Recovery of CD4+ T cells is more prolonged than CD8+ T cells, resulting in an inverse ratio of CD4 : CD8+ T cells that may last for 2 or more years in recipients of some types of TCD transplant *(75,76)*. Small et al. *(73)* demonstrated that adult recipients of a TCD transplant who received antithymocyte globulin (ATG) and methylprednisolone rapidly engrafted neutrophils, yet experienced an early delay in T-cell reconstitution, more prominent subset deficiencies, and a functional recovery that was delayed compared to recipients who did not receive this therapy. Similar results were reported by Kook et al. *(72)* in pediatric patients where both T- and B-cell reconstitution was severely delayed in patients receiving ATG during the engraftment period. These data confirm the added effect of posttransplant therapy on the rate of T-cell reconstitution.

CD4+ T cells recover faster in children, eventually reaching normal levels in most studies, likely the result of the presence of more functional thymic tissue *(73,77)*. In contrast to children, residual deficiencies in adults may never fully resolve *(78,79)*. Patients with extensive chronic GVHD have the most profound deficiencies in T-cell reconstitution with a resultant increased risk for viral infections and late bacterial infections *(80)*. For reasons that are not fully clear, adult but not pediatric recipients of rigorous TCD grafts (3–4 logs) from unrelated donors had slower T-cell reconstitution than did their counterparts receiving grafts from sibling donors *(74)*. One possible speculation involved possible defects in migration to the thymus and subsequent maturation as a result of undetected HLA disparity.

Significant differences in T-cell-immune reconstitution between sibling and unrelated or HLA-mismatched related donors has not been seen in our own patient series representing a less rigorous TCD method (average 1.8 logs), which might explain the difference. These findings are illustrated in Figs. 1 and 2. Figure 2A compares the median recovery of CD4+ T cells in recipients of T-cell-containing BM grafts from matched sibling donors, with adult (>18 yr) or pediatric (age 18 yr) recipients of TCD BM from a matched sibling (RM), a matched unrelated donor (UR) or a partially HLA-matched donor (PM). As can be seen, recipients of T-cell-replete BM have a median of 200 CD4+ T cells by 6 mo and are at the lower level of normal by 1 yr, whereas adult recipients of TCD grafts reach a median of 200 CD4+ T cells only at 1 yr and the lower limits of normal by 2 yr. Pediatric recipients of TCD grafts in contrast recover CD4+ T cells at a rate very similar to T-cell-replete patients. Neither donor relationship nor HLA matching affected CD4+ T-cell recovery in either age group. Extensive chronic GVHD (mostly adults in our series) with or without TCD did cause additional delays in CD4+ T-cell recovery as shown in Fig. 2B. The recovery of naïve CD4+ T cells is most affected by TCD, in agreement with other studies, and also recovers faster in children. In the absence of extensive chronic GVHD, the absolute CD4+CD45RA+ T-cell count in children is near low normal levels by 1 yr, similar to recipients of T-cell-replete grafts (Fig. 1C). CD8+ T cells (Fig. 1B) recover fastest in patients receiving T-cell-replete grafts with little effect from extensive chronic GVHD or patient age on the rate of recovery. Nearly all patients in our study had low normal numbers of CD8+ T cells by 6 mo post-HSCT.

Consistent with the concept that T cells initially recover because of peripheral expansion of T cells infused with the graft, recipients of PBPC grafts who receive 10-fold more T cells than BM recipients recover T cells and especially CD4+ T cells faster than recipients of BM allografts *(11,60,81)*. The opposite occurs with extensive TCD in that CD4+ T cells in particular are extremely slow to reconstitute. Of interest in this regard, Soiffer et al. *(76)* reported on 40 HLA-identical sibling recipients of BM TCD using complement-mediated lysis with antibody to CD6, an antigen normally expressed on 95% of CD3+ T cells. Although T-cell reconstitution was rapid in this group who did not require additional posttransplant immune suppression to prevent GVHD, most of the patients exhibited a substantial proportion of CD6– T cells as long as 2 yr posttransplant. The majority of the CD6–CD3+ T cells were CD8+CD45RO+ (a memory phenotype) and likely expanded from the cells spared by the treatment for TCD.

The most rigorous methods of TCD employ a highly purified selection of CD34+ progenitor cells from PBPCs, resulting in infusion of fewer than 5×10^4 T cells/kg (approx 4.0 log depletion). The detrimental effects on T-cell recovery and especially CD4+ T-cell recovery are profound. For recipients of allogeneic transplant, this degree of T-cell depletion was initially used in the setting of haploidentical HSCT. Handgretinger et al. *(82)* achieved engraftment with virtually no GVHD and without the need for post-HSCT immune suppression with this approach. CD4+ T-cell recovery was very delayed, but given the pediatric patient population, those who survived eventually did recover T-cell numbers and function *(83,84)*. T Cells recovered fastest in patients who received 20×10^6/CD34+ cells/kg or more, a dose that often required more than one donor aphaeresis to achieve *(85)*. Early infectious deaths were increased in this series, and attempts to decrease the high relapse rate in this high-risk patient group with add-back of donor T cells resulted in clinically significant GVHD in some patients *(85)*. Improved immune reconstitution in recipients of rigorously TCD CD34+ cell-selected grafts was seen when G-CSF was eliminated from the post-HSCT supportive care regimen

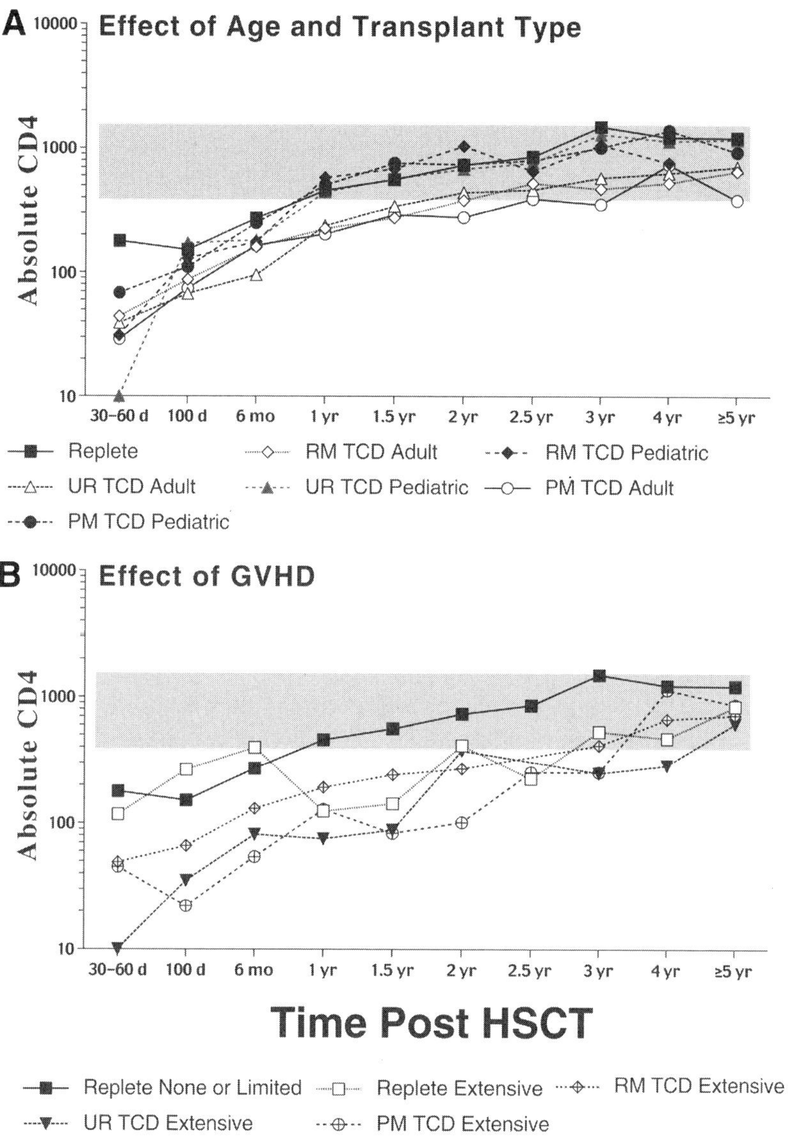

Fig. 2. Effect of patient age, transplant type, and GVHD on CD4+ T-cell recovery post-HSCT. The median absolute CD4+ T-cell counts are shown for patients tested at or near the indicated time following BM HSCT. **A** shows the effect of transplant type and age on CD4+ cell recovery for patients with no or limited chronic GVHD. Patients studied in each group include the following: T-cell-replete (solid squares), $N = 49$ (20 under 18 yr) related matched (RM) TCD adults (open diamonds), $N = 132$; RM TCD pediatric (solid diamonds), $N = 25$; unrelated matched (UR) TCD adults (open triangles), $N = 48$; UR TCD pediatric (solid triangles), $N = 41$; partially matched (PM) TCD adults (open circles), $N = 63$; PM TCD pediatric (solid circles), $N = 106$. **B** shows the effects of extensive chronic GVHD. Patients studied in each group include the following: T-cell-replete (solid squares), $N = 49$ (20 under 18 yr) T-cell-replete extensive GVHD (open squares), $N = 9$; RM TCD extensive GVHD (crossed diamonds), $N = 16$; UR TCD extensive GVHD (solid inverted triangles), $N = 16$; PM TCD extensive GVHD (crossed circles), $N = 39$. PM represents both related and unrelated donors. Not all patients were tested at each interval, but a given patient was tested only once during an interval. The shaded area represents the 5th to 95th percentile of absolute values from 49 normal adult donors.

(31). Delayed T-cell reconstitution was also reported by Beelen et al. *(45)* in a series of 10 adult CML patients who received rigorous TCD CD34+ cell-selected grafts from HLA-identical sibling donors. These patients were given G-CSF but 4 of the 10 patients also received low-dose donor leukocyte infusion (DLI) to treat molecular or cytogenetic relapse. None of the patients died from infection during the first year, perhaps the result of less genetic disparity and a potential benefit from the T cells infused with the DLI. These results are superior to those seen for patients receiving CD34+ grafts from HLA-identical siblings who were conditioned for transplant using Campath-1H, an antibody that may have resulted in additional TCD of the infused product. This group had an extremely high early mortality (8 deaths in 11 cases) because of infection that was not seen in identically conditioned patients who received a less rigorous TCD graft *(86)*. The problems with high infection rates and profoundly delayed CD4+ T-cell recovery have not been seen in patients receiving allogeneic CD34+ cell-selected grafts that contain on average of 5×10^5 CD3+ cells/kg, showing the important role of T-cell dose rather than the method of TCD on outcome *(87–89)*. Interestingly in this study, CD34+ cell doses greater than 3×10^6/kg appeared to be associated with a worse treatment-related mortality *(89)*, unlike the experience in the more rigorous TCD haploidentical transplant studies *(85)*. Clearly, care must be taken in using approaches that may result in extreme TCD, especially in patients receiving grafts from HLA-disparate donors such that there are insufficient donor T cells to provide protection while new T cells develop from the thymus.

A more limited diversity in T-cell response may be one consequence of T-cell repopulation by peripheral expansion of T cells in the graft. Gorski et al. *(90,91)* at our center performed one of the earliest studies of overall T-cell repertoire recovery in recipients of partial TCD grafts. He found a pattern of early limited diversity that persisted in patients with chronic GVHD or active infections, whereas longer-term patients without GVHD had diverse repertoires. Repertoire deficiencies have also been described in recipients of T-cell-replete grafts, although to a lesser extent than recipients of TCD grafts *(92,93)*. As might be predicted, recovery of T-cell repertoire diversity is most rapid in recipients of PBPC HSCT who receive larger T-cell infusions *(94)*. A broader T-cell repertoire is largely associated with the presence of CD4+CD45RA+ T cells as determined by analysis of separated populations *(95)*. DLI given following TCD BM HSCT for the treatment of relapse appears to have variable effects on the incomplete T-cell repertoire, with some patients showing more diversity, some more skewing, and others essentially unchanged *(96)*. This finding may well depend on the timing and dose of T cells given in the DLI.

T-Cell reconstitution may be additionally affected by the increased tendency of both CD4+ and CD8+ T cells to undergo enhanced spontaneous apoptosis in short-term culture for up to 1 yr post-HSCT *(97)*. This effect is seen most prominently in the CD8+CD45RO+ subset and is associated with upregulation of Fas expression and a decrease in the level of the *bcl-2* gene product (an antiapoptotic protein) but not Bax (a proapoptotic protein), resulting in a change in the Bcl-2 : Bax ratio that leads to apoptosis *(98)*. The high apoptosis rate decreases in conjunction with the appearance of naïve T cells from the thymus. This phenomenon may help explain the additional delay in T-cell recovery sometimes seen following HLA-disparate or unrelated HSCT as well as that secondary to GVHD, as both situations result in higher rates of spontaneous T-cell apoptosis *(99)*. NK cells appeared to be relatively resistant to apoptosis in this study *(99)*.

2.3.1. CD8+ T-Cell Reconstitution

The first T cells to appear following BM or PBPC grafts with or without TCD are predominately CD8+, and these remain the predominant population well past the first year. Total CD8+ populations were very early observed to be highest in patients with viral infections, especially CMV infection *(100)*. In addition, the CD8+ T cells in HSCT patients may, at times, be skewed toward a number of abnormal phenotypic variations in subtypes that are only rarely seen in normal donors and that may result in impaired immune function.

A subset of CD8+ T cells that coexpress CD57 may be dominant (up to 75% of CD8+ T cells) in CMV+ HSCT recipients, especially in association with viral reactivation *(4)*. Normal individuals express only low levels of CD8+CD57+ T cells (7%±5%). The CD8+CD57+ T-cell subset suppresses T-cell functions and does not itself proliferate well to mitogen stimulation, but it is capable of mediating cytotoxicity *(101,102)*. TCR analysis of the expanded CD8+CD57+ subset in HSCT patients has shown a limited clonality *(6,103)*. However, oligoclonal CD8+CD57+ T cells are also found in normal donors and may represent a normal response to antigen *(104)*. Indeed, CD8+CD57+ T cells from individuals that are CMV+ have been shown to contain a high frequency of CMV-specific cells as measured by cloning or by IFN-γ and TNF-α production in response to CMV *(105,106)*. Although blood from HSCT patients with high percentages of CD8+CD57+ cells proliferated well to autologous CMV-infected fibroblasts, there was only low CMV-specific cytolytic capacity compared to blood from patients with few CD8+CD57+ T cells *(6)*. The exact function of this CD8+ T-cell subset post-HSCT is unknown. Clearly, it expands in response to CMV, but whether it represents an immune response to the virus or a mechanism by which CMV suppresses the immune response to itself is unclear. Dolstra et al. *(5)* found a lower relapse rate in recipients of lymphocyte-depleted HSCT with high levels of CD8+CD57+ T cells, suggesting an additional role of this subset in mediating a graft-vs-leukemia (GVL) effect. Our own studies in recipients of TCD grafts support the role of CMV in the expansion of CD3+CD57+ T cells post-HSCT. The number of CD3+CD57+ T cells was normal by d 100 in patients who were CMV+ at the time of transplant and rapidly rose and remained at above normal levels throughout the posttransplant course (Fig. 3B). In contrast, CD3+CD57+ T cells gradually rose to normal numbers by 6 mo and stayed in the normal range thereafter in CMV– patients (Fig. 3A).

Other abnormalities commonly described in post-HSCT CD8 populations include an overexpression of HLA-DR without CD25 coexpression in contrast to truly activated T cells that express both HLA-DR and CD25 *(100)*. There is also skewed coexpression of CD28 and CD11b on the CD8+ T cells from HSCT patients. Approximately 25–50% of normal adult CD8+ T cells express CD28, whereas a largely reciprocal subset of approx 50% CD8+ T cells express the β2 intergrin antigen CD11b *(107)*. Early posttransplant, less than 5% of patient CD8+ T cells express CD28 and there is an concurrent increase in the percent coexpressing CD11b that slowly normalizes over the first year. In normal donors as well as HSCT patients, the CD8+CD11b+ subset appears to primarily display suppressor activity, whereas the CD28+ subset mediates cytotoxicity. The patient-derived CD8+CD11b+ T cells suppress pokeweed mitogen (PWM) stimulated immunoglobulin production both early and late posttransplant *(108)*. They have further been shown to be highly suppressive to IL-2 production by CD4+ T cells, resulting in reduced T-cell proliferation *(109,110)*. CD8+CD11b+ T cells may also express CD57 and have been shown to produce high levels of IFN-γ and low levels of IL-2, in

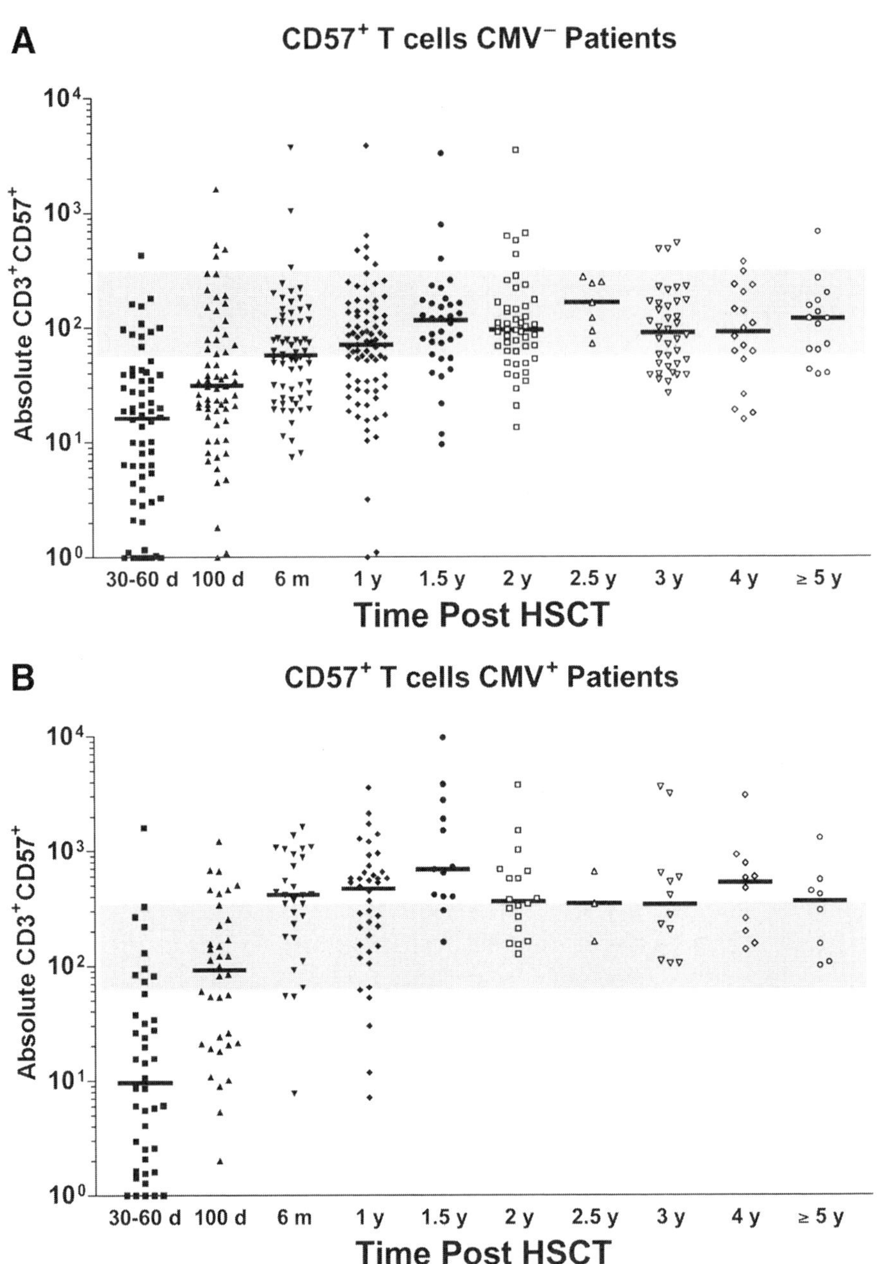

Fig. 3. Effect of CMV sero-status at the time of transplant on the recovery of CD3+CD57+ T cells post-HSCT. The absolute numbers of CD3+CD57+ T cells are shown for patients tested at or near the indicated time following BM HSCT for patients who were CMV seronegative (**A**) or CMV seropositive (**B**) at the time of transplant are shown. All data are from recipients of a TCD transplant and represent 301 (143 under 18 yr) CMV seronegative patients and 172 (46 under 18 yr) CMV seropositive patients. Not all patients were tested at each interval, but a given patient was tested only once during an interval. The shaded area represents the 5th to 95th percentile of absolute values from 49 normal adult donors of unknown CMV sero-status.

contrast to the CD8+CD57–CD11b– subset in HSCT patients *(111)*. High levels of circulating CD8+CD11b+ T cells at 2 mo post-HSCT was associated with low levels of serum IgM and IgA compared to patients with high levels of CD8+CD11b+ CD56+ NK cells, suggesting that suppressor of Ig production by this subset occurs in vivo *(112)*. CD3+ T cells lacking expression of CD5 have been described to be predominately in the CD8+CD3+ subset early posttransplant and may be seen in patients with GVHD *(113)*. These CD5– T cells produce IL-2 and mediate lytic activity, but their potential role in posttransplant events has not been further described. This CD3+CD5– T-cell subset has not been seen in our own patient studies (data not shown).

2.3.2. CD4+ T-Cell Recovery

The major phenotypic abnormality seen in CD4+ T cells post-HSCT other than their slower rate of recovery is the predominance of CD4+ T cells with the CD45RO phenotype. Memory T cells have undergone clonal expansion after antigen encounter and characteristically express the CD45RO isoform. However, this phenotype is not strictly associated with memory, rather with activation, thus naïve cells can reversibly acquire CD45RO expression. The CD45RA isoform is predominately expressed on naïve T cells that have not yet encountered antigen since their differentiation in the thymus. A recently described methodology for detection of naïve T cells uses quantitative real-time polymerase chain reaction (PCR) to estimate the number of T cells in a sample with excised DNA fragments left over from the TCR rearrangement that occurs during thymus maturation. These fragments, called TCR rearrangement excision circles (Trec) remain in the cytoplasm and are diluted in number as the T cell divides. Therefore, the proportion of T cells with Trec in a population is a measure of recent thymic activity *(114)*. Although there is a general correlation of Trec with CD45RA+ phenotype, the Trec assay is more specific for the detection of recent thymus emigrates. Thus far, the best in vitro correlate of immune competence in HSCT patients seems to be the development of new CD4+ T cells in the thymus, making this assay especially useful. Trec levels have been found to correlate with TCR diversity, the ability to mount specific immune responses, and recipient age. Children with an intact thymus show faster overall immune reconstitution as well as higher levels of Trec than do adult recipients *(69)*. Still, in the absence of chronic GVHD, most adult recipients do eventually recover Trec, although with a more prolonged time-course that may extend as long as 20 yr post-HSCT *(79)*. The appearance of Trec in the CD8+ compartment in general correlates with CD4, although the thymus may not be absolutely required. A 15-yr-old child who was transplanted postthymectomy was found to recover CD8+CD45RA+ cells (presumed to be Trec+) in parallel to similarly treated children who were not thymectomized but failed to recover detectable CD4+CD45RA+ T cells even by 2 yr *(115)*. These data suggest an additional extrathymic pathway for recovery of CD8+ T cells that may explain their earlier appearance post-HSCT.

CD134 (OX-40) is an activation-associated antigen that functions as a costimulatory receptor for CD4+ T cells. CD134 is expressed in 1–8% of CD4+ T cells in normal donors but is up-regulated with activation. Lamb et al. *(116)* described the early appearance of a population of CD4+CD134+ cells in patients without GVHD that rose to 40–50% of CD4+ T cells by 1 mo after TCD HSCT. Neither the relative percentage nor the absolute number of CD4+CD134+ T cells predicted the onset of GVHD, but a decline in this subset did foretell the clinical response to GVHD therapy. CD4+ T cells that coexpress HLA-DR and CD38 are also increased early post-HSCT, further suggesting CD4+ T-cell activation during the recovery period *(117)*.

As for CD8+ T cells, there does not appear to be a significant coexpression of CD25 during this same time period and the number of activated CD4+ T cells is not clearly correlated with clinical events. Therefore, the role of activated CD4+ T cells in post-HSCT clinical events is unclear.

Some interesting differences are seen when cord blood is used as the HSCT source. Studies have shown that overall T-cell reconstitution is similar to recipients of TCD BM or PBPC grafts, likely reflecting the low number of T cells in the infusion as well as the nearly total lack of memory T cells in either the CD4+ or CD8+ subsets *(63)*. Unlike the usual fast recovery of the CD8+ T-cell subset seen in PBPC and BM transplants, CD4+ T cells were found to be equal to or greater than CD8+ T cells, with a CD4 : CD8 ratio above 1.0 by the second month following a cord blood HSCT *(46,64)*. Cord blood recipients did exhibit a highly abnormal T-cell repertoire the first year following transplant, similar to BM recipients, but attained a higher level of diversity by 2 yr as measured both by TCR CDR3 diversity and by Trec analysis *(118)*. The effect of these differences on clinical events in recipients of cord blood transplants has not yet been fully described.

2.3.3. TCRγδ+ T-Cell Recovery

T Cells can express one of two forms of the TCR in association with CD3. Approximately 98% of T cells use the αβ TCR in normal adult T cells with nearly all TCRαβ+ cells expressing either CD4 or CD8. T cells with the γδ TCR range from 1% to 3% of lymphocytes in normal adults and are mostly CD4–CD8–, although a minority will express CD8αα homodimers. The normal function of TCRγδ+ T cells include the recognition of bacterial or vial pathogens, control of immune reactivity by downregulation of activated macrophages, and as antitumor effectors (reviewed in refs. *119* and *120*). In the setting of HSCT, TCRγδ+ T cells in the graft may help to promote engraftment and do not appear to play a causative role in GVHD *(121–124)*. Gratama et al. *(125)* were the first to describe TCRγδ+ T-cell recovery post-HSCT and found that in contrast to the TCRαβ+ subset, TCRγδ+ T cells recovered at nearly equal rates in recipients of TCD and T-cell-replete BM grafts. There was no effect of CMV infection on the rate of TCRγδ+ T-cell recovery in this study. However, in the setting of solid-organ transplants, overexpression of TCRγδ+ T cells has been seen in association with CMV infection *(126)*. Consistent with this observation, Cela et al. *(127)* described a series of recipients of TCD HSCT who showed two patterns of TCRγδ+ T-cell reconstitution. One group gradually recovered TCRγδ+ T cells over the first year, although still not reaching control levels, and the second group exhibited unusually high absolute TCRγδ+ T cells on one or more occasions posttransplant. This second group was distinguished by a high rate of fungal or viral infections during this time period, suggesting that the increase in TCRγδ+ T cells may have been in response to these infections. Vilmer et al. *(128)* described an unusual recipient of a TCD HSCT with delayed immune reconstitution and a predominance of TCRγδ+ T cells with suppressor activity. TCRγδ+ T cells from a second patient showing overexpansion did not display suppressor activity but were of a γδ-receptor subtype that differed from the first patient *(129)*. Analysis of V-region gene usage during TCRγδ+ T-cell repopulation was performed by van der Harst et al. *(130)* and included four patients with an overexpression of TCRγδ+ T cells through 4 mo post-HSCT. Here, they found nearly exclusive use of Vγ9Vδ2 during the first month, followed by Vδ1. In normal donors, TCRγδ+ T cells with Vγ9Vδ2 are the majority population, whereas thymic TCRγδ+ T cells express mostly Vδ1, suggesting that the early-appearing TCRγδ+ T cells may have expanded from the cells transferred in the graft.

Lamb et al. *(131)* described a subset (10 of 43) of recipients of haploidentical TCD HSCT with high percentages of TCRγδ+ T cells (more than 10% of total lymphocytes) at one or more examinations from 60 to 270 d posttransplant. The antibody used for TCD in this series, T10B9-1A1, depletes TCRαβ+ T cells to a greater degree than TCRγδ+ T cells, so the over-expanded cells may have been graft derived. Patients with high TCRγδ+ T cells, had significantly better disease-free survival than patients without TCRγδ+ T-cell overshoot. In contrast, this investigator did not find a similar increase in patients with increased TCRγδ+ T cells following HSCT TCD using a different antibody (OKT3) that purged TCRγδ+ T cells as well as TCRαβ+ T cells *(132)*. Our own studies have included 396 recipients of BM TCD using T10B9-1A1 and have found only 9 patients with 10% or more of TCRγδ+ T cells on one or more occasions during the first year. However, of the nine patients, only one subsequently relapsed at 2 yr posttransplant, and two died of infection; the remainder are alive and disease free. Our recipients of T-cell-replete grafts recovered normal numbers of TCRγδ+ T cells by 6 mo, similar to pediatric recipients of TCD grafts. The recovery of TCRγδ+ T cells in adult recipients of TCD grafts was more delayed and did not reach normal control numbers until the fourth or fifth year of the testing period with relatively little effect of extensive chronic GVHD on recovery (*see* Fig. 4). Abnormally expanded populations of TCRγδ+ T cells appear to play a varied role in posttransplant events that may, in part, be determined by the subset that expands. Given the faster recovery of absolute TCRγδ+ T cells in TCD pediatric patients, the thymus may play a role in the reconstitution of this T-cell subset.

2.4. Recovery of T-Cell Function

T Cells function in the immune system as a balanced network of subsets that provide help to other cells (including T cells), regulate immune response, and serve as effectors through soluble mediators and by cell-mediated cytotoxic killing. The striking imbalance in T-cell subsets revealed by the above-described phenotypic studies predicts that there will be a period during which the functional activity of T cells in HSCT patients is abnormal. A number of such functional defects have been described in both isolated T cells and in mixed mononuclear cell populations sampled early post-HSCT. These T-cell functional defects may be responsible for the increased susceptibility of HSCT recipients to viral infection, particularly reactivation of viruses in the Herpes family, including CMV *(133)*, herpes simplex virus (HSV), human herpes virus (HHV)-6 *(134,135)*, Epstein–Barr virus (EBV) *(136)*, and varicella zoster virus (VZV) *(137)* during this period *(138)*.

2.4.1. Proliferative Response

When stimulated through the TCR, T cells initially proliferate and then clonally expand. This is trigged primarily via the CD3 antigen secondary to TCR engagement, but may also be stimulated via alternative pathways, such as through CD2. Stimulation of the TCR/CD3 complex by T-cell mitogens bypasses the need for specific antigen and triggers nearly all normal T cells to proliferate through a series of intracellular events initiated by the membrane perturbation. The T-cell proliferative response in HSCT patients appears to lag behind the recovery of total T-cell numbers and is most depressed in patients with extensive chronic GVHD *(139)*. Stimulation via CD3, the CD2 pathway, and T-cell mitogens are all depressed 1 yr or longer even in patients who do not receive post-HSCT immune suppression *(42,76,140)*. The proliferative response to alloantigen recovers somewhat faster (approx 6 mo) and seems to be less affected in patients with GVHD than are mitogen responses. The proliferative response to viral

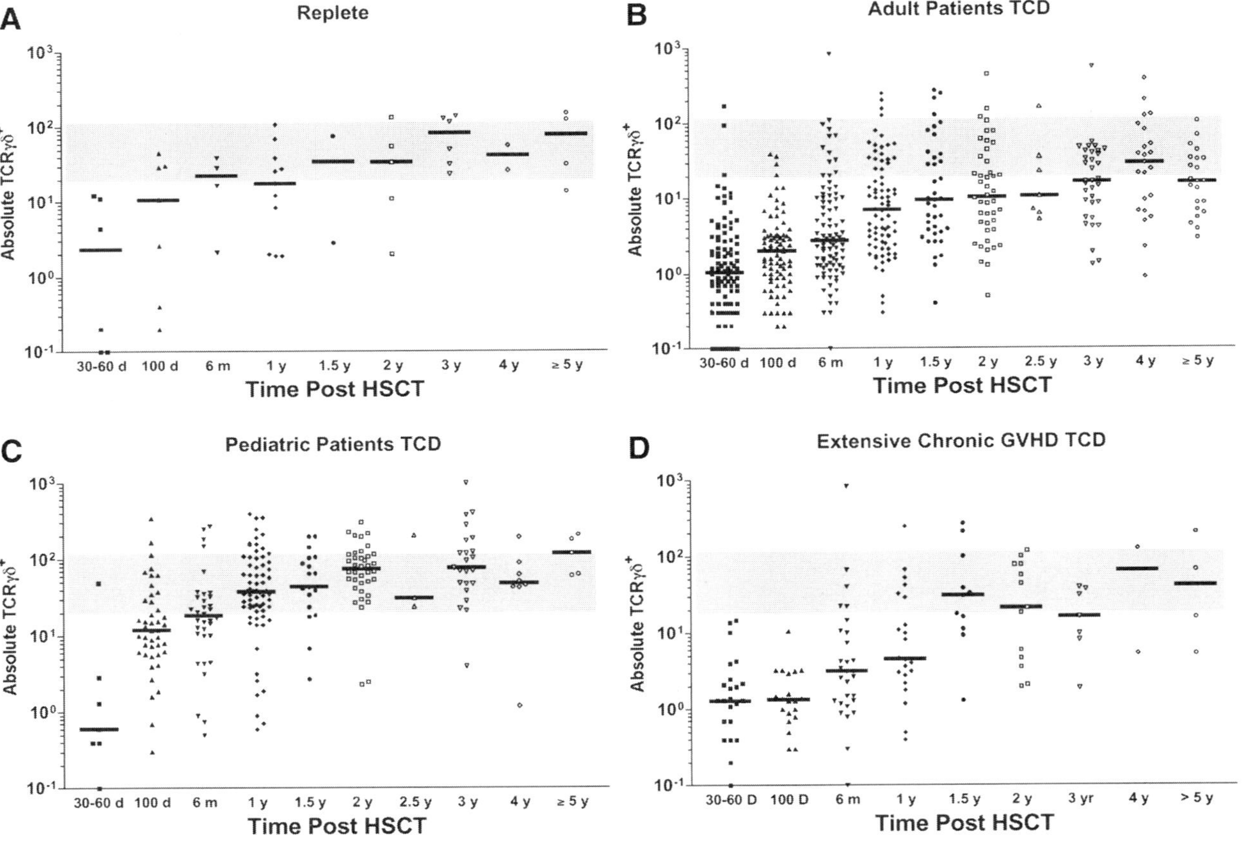

Fig. 4. Effect of transplant type, patient age, and GVHD on recovery of TCRγδ+ T cells following HSCT. The absolute numbers of CD3+TCRγδ+ T cells are shown for patients tested at or near the indicated time following BM HSCT for recipients of T-cell-replete grafts (**A**), adult recipients of TCD grafts (**B**). pediatric recipients of TCD grafts (**C**) and recipients of TCD grafts with extensive chronic GVHD (**D**). Not all patients were tested at each interval, but a given patient was tested only once during an interval. The shaded area represents the 5th to 95th percentile of absolute values from 49 normal adult donors. TCRγδ antibodies were added to the immune reconstitution panel at a date later than the other assessments shown; thus, fewer patients in each category were tested than indicated in Fig. 1.

antigens such as HSV and VZV is most depressed during the first 3 mo after HSCT when susceptibility to viral infection is high *(141,142)*. Indeed, in one study, patients who developed detectable proliferative response to VZV or HSV following infection were less likely to experience second infections. Treatment with acyclovir during the initial infection inhibited the development of specific proliferative responses and those patients were more likely to have second infections *(143)*. For CMV-specific cytotoxic T lymphocyte (CTL) viral immunity to be effective, patients must also recover or be provided with helper T cells that proliferate to viral antigens *(144)*. The poor antigen-nonspecific T-cell proliferative response may involve defects in transmembrane calcium flux, but this has not explained the results in most studies that have been reported *(76,145,146)*. Most likely, the poor proliferative response involves T-cell subset imbalances together with a decreased ability of post-HSCT T cells to produce IL-2, as described in Subheading 2.4.3.

2.4.2. Cytotoxic Response

The ability to generate normal CTL response to alloantigen is less delayed than proliferative responses with detectable activity by the third month in patients without GVHD *(147)*. As for virus-specific proliferative response, CTL response to viral antigens recovers in a similar time frame that coincides with the period during which patients are most susceptible to viral infection. The recovery of CTL and proliferative responses to viral antigens during this period is strongly correlated with protection against infection with CMV *(133,148)*. Ganciclovir usage has significantly reduced the previously seen high early mortality as a result of CMV infection *(149)*. A consequence of suppression of the virus during this period is a delay in the recovery of CMV-specific CTL immunity, thus predisposing patients to more late CMV infection *(150,151)*. CMV disease remains a significant problem for patients after alloHSCT *(152)*. Monitoring CMV-specific T-cell immunity post-HSCT may be a useful tool to detect patients in need of intervention to prevent CMV disease using some of the newer methods to enhance immunity post-HSCT discussed *(148,153–155)*. Although PBPC grafts and nonmyeloablative stem cell transplant (NST) are associated with faster T-cell reconstitution, the risk of CMV reactivation remains. NST is associated with less CMV antigenemia, viremia, and disease in CMV+ patients with CMV+ donors prior to the first year, compared with controls receiving myeloablative HSCT. By 1 yr, the overall incidence of CMV disease became similar in both groups, although with a delayed onset among NST patients *(156)*.

Unlike CMV, major histocompatibility complex (MHC) unrestricted cytotoxicity may contribute to protection against EBV infection prior to the redevelopment of T-cell-specific immunity *(157)*. However, the critical nature of the T-cell response to EBV is indicated by the markedly increased risk of posttransplant lymphoproliferative disease (PTLD) associated with delayed T-cell recovery *(158)*, especially if the graft used for HSCT contains B cells *(159)*. There is poor CTL response to EBV during the first 3 mo in recipients of TCD grafts, with recovery in most patients by 6 mo *(160)*. Patients without EBV-specific CTL precursors were at increased risk for PTLD in this study.

2.4.3. Cytokine Production

The failure of T cells early post-HSCT to produce normal amounts of IL-2 was one of the first T-cell functional defects described. Like total T-cell recovery, this response is most deficient during the first 100 d and the kinetics of recovery are strongly correlated with the number of T cells infused in the graft *(27,161–164)*. Defective IL-2 production is not restored by bypassing the need for accessory cells through stimulation of the cells with phorbol ester and ionophore *(165)*. Addition of IL-2 into proliferation assays during the period of deficient IL-2 production enhances but does not always fully correct the above-described proliferative defects *(163,164)*. The overrepresentation of T-cell subsets that either produce low levels of IL-2 or directly inhibit IL-2 production, such as $CD8^+CD11b^+$ T cells and $CD8^+CD57^+$ T cells in the cultures are likely responsible. In the absence of GVHD, IL-2 production appears to return to normal levels at or near 6 mo in most patients, provided T-cell recovery has occurred.

Other cytokines, such as IFN-γ, TNF-α, IL-3, IL-4, IL-5, IL-6, and IL-7 appear to be produced early after transplant, with any reduction in amount related to the T-cell content of the sample being tested or to samples from patients with extensive chronic GVHD *(166–168)*. One recent study found a lower number of IFN-γ-producing T cells and total naïve T cells in recipients of PBPC grafts who subsequently relapsed compared to those who did not relapse *(169)*.

3. B-CELL RECONSTITUTION

The absolute number of B cells is usually low during the first 100 d post-HSCT with or without TCD. Most patients rapidly recover B cells to normal levels after d 100, whereas the absolute B-cell count in children and recipients of T-cell-replete BM grafts may exceed normal once recovery is complete *(42,170,171)*. Failure to recover normal B-cell and monocyte numbers in the expected time post-HSCT has been shown to correlate in multivariate analysis to a higher probability for infection after transplant *(29)*. Prolonged treatment with corticosteroids delays B-cell reconstitution to a greater extent than T-cell reconstitution and was found to be associated with a higher infection rate in those patients whose B cells did not recover by d 100 *(172)*. Comparative studies of B cells from T-cell-replete and TCD patients using a T-cell-independent B-cell mitogen showed IgM production by 4–6 mo and recovery of IgG production to control levels by 1 yr, with only quantitative differences in the TCD group *(42,170)*. These data suggest there are some intrinsic B-cell defects during the first year post-HSCT. Other studies of in vitro B-cell function have used the T-cell-dependent PWM Ig production system that reveals defects both in T helper cells and B cells *(173)*. PWM-induced Ig production is highly sensitive to inhibition by suppressor T cells of either the CD4+ or CD8+ subsets *(174)*. CD3+CD8+CD11b+ cells are particularly inhibitory to Ig production in these systems *(108)*. Most helper-T-cell defects and increased suppressor activity occur during the first 4–6 mo post-HSCT but persist in patients with chronic GVHD. Studies to determine the nature of the defects in humoral immunity point to problems with B-cell activation early post-HSCT, problems with Ig switching and production later after transplant, and both types of problem in patients with chronic GVHD *(175)*. B-Cell reconstitution was found to proceed with the expected pattern as described earlier in our study of T-cell-replete and partial TCD transplants in adults and children. As shown in Fig. 1C, the rate of B-cell recovery in recipients of T-cell-replete grafts and in pediatric patients without extensive chronic GVHD was nearly identical and rapid, with median absolute numbers in the normal range by 6 mo. Adult recipients of TCD grafts lagged slightly behind but were recovered by 1 yr, whereas extensive GVHD delayed recovery of B cells in the TCD group until 18 mo and resulted in lowered B-cell numbers in recipients of T-cell-replete grafts.

Intrinsic B-cell defects may be marked by abnormal phenotypes, such as the presence of CD5+ B cells, a phenotype usually seen in fetal life *(40,170)*. The early reconstituting B cells may also coexpress other fetal-restricted antigens, including CD38, CD71, CD1c, and CD23 *(170,171)*. B Cells appear to be a source of autoantibodies and display other abnormal functions post-HSCT *(176)*. Ig gene rearrangement studies show less diversity in the Ig gene repertoire even at 1–2 yr post-HSCT, with patterns not unlike those seen in fetal ontogeny *(177,178)*. Oligoclonal expansions in the IgM and IgG repertoires are revealed by CDR3 spectra-typing. Skewed IgM repertories normalized by 3–4 mo, whereas the IgG compartment remained restricted for 9 or more months *(179)*. Even with repertoire normalization at the gene level, there is less diversity from somatic hypermutation during the first year post-HSCT compared to normal donors *(180)*. This factor combined with a defect in class switching and clonal dominance may help explain the defects in mounting a specific immune response during the first year post-HSCT.

In concurrence with B-cell recovery, serum IgM becomes normal by 2–6 mo and IgG1 and IgG3 reach normal levels by 9–12 mo post-HSCT *(175)*. In contrast, IgG2, IgG4, and both serum and secretory IgA levels are deficient for several years *(139,181)* and are not corrected by infusion of intravenous Ig *(182)*. Chronic GVHD results in more profound defects in secretory and serum IgA *(183)*. Children have lower IgA levels at 3 and 6 mo post-HSCT than do adults *(184)*. The failure to respond normally to encapsulated organisms with an IgG2 or IgA response may contribute to the increase in bacterial infections seen after the first posttransplant year. These defects may reflect a deficiency in B cells capable of undergoing isotype switch and are characteristic of B cells in fetal life and infancy *(185)*. Serum IgE may be increased during the first 100 d in patients with grade II or higher acute GVHD *(186)* or active infection *(187)*.

There is evidence from a number of studies showing that humoral immunity can be transferred from donor to host. These include the demonstration of antibody to recall antigens such as tetanus toxoid (TT), diphtheria, and measles during the first 100 d *(188,189)*. However, transfer of immunity is best demonstrated in patients who were sero-negative pretransplant to nonlatent virus such as measles, mumps, or rubella, to which the donor was immune. Many such patients demonstrate a virus-specific antibody response for up to 1 yr post-HSCT *(190)*. Transferred immunity is more likely to occur if the donor is immunized prior to harvest and is most likely to occur when both donor and patient are immunized *(191,192)*. TT-specific helper T cells sharing a predominant donor clonotype are found to be nearly exclusively responsible for early TT responses. These, too, are more likely to be present if the donor is immunized prior to transplant *(193,194)*. Transferred donor Ig can not only be detected in the serum but also in the secretions with peak IgA activity during the first 2–3 wk that then declines until 2 mo, when levels rise again *(195,196)*. Transfer of humoral immunity also occurs in recipients of TCD grafts *(197)*. Unfortunately, transferred immunity eventually declines, requiring that the patient be vaccinated to remain protected from these common pathogens *(198)*.

The data support the need for immunization post-HSCT, and a number of studies have been performed to optimize how this should be best performed. The ability to mount a specific humoral response to a neo-antigen is nearly absent until after d 100 in recipients of T-cell-replete BM grafts. The response to neo-antigen recovers to nearly normal levels by d 180, except, of course, in patients with chronic GVHD, who may take much longer or never fully recover *(199)*. Most clinical studies would support immunization at 1 yr for patients not suffering from extensive chronic GVHD. The best responses are seen to immunizations with protein antigens, with much poorer response to polysaccharide antigens, as might be expected in patients with prolonged IgG2 and IgG4 deficiencies. For patients immunized at 2 yr post-HSCT, fewer than 12% responded to a pure polysaccharide pneumococcal vaccine, whereas there was an 80% response after two immunizations with a protein-conjugated pneumococcal vaccine *(200)*. In a similar fashion, children vaccinated with measles, mumps, and rubella vaccine responded well to vaccines given 2 yr after matched sibling HSCT *(201)*. The timing and number of vaccine doses to achieve an optimal response has also been studied. Responses to TT were best when vaccination was begun after immune reconstitution was more complete. Patients vaccinated early and repeatedly during the early posttransplant period had more oligoclonal responses and lower antibody titers than those vaccinated later *(202)*. Likewise, vaccination to influenza virus is ineffective at 6 mo, with increasingly better responses with time post-HSCT. A single dose of TT vaccine at 2 yr post-HCST was highly effective, even for patients with chronic GVHD *(203)*. Response to polio vaccine differs somewhat in that patients vaccinated as early as 6 mo received some benefit from two to three sequential doses of inactivated vaccine *(204,205)*.

4. DENDRITIC-CELL RECONSTITUTION

Only recently have studies of circulating DCs and monocyte-derived DCs been studied in HSCT patients. Early studies looked at the recovery of Langerhans cells (LCs) in skin biopsies at intervals over the first year posttransplant *(18,206,207)*. Nearly all patients showed very low numbers of LCs through the first 4 mo that subsequently normalized. In most patients, LCs were of host origin through d 49 and in some up to d 120. Through the first year, LC chimerism gradually became all donor in the majority of patients. Patients with GVHD had a more prolonged recovery, suggesting that poor antigen-presenting capacity in the skin may contribute to the pathology of this disorder. A lack of skin resident LCs may also explain why patients with chronic GVHD exhibit poor delayed-type hypersensitivity reactions to challenge with neo-antigens and recall antigens, unlike patients without chronic GVHD *(208)*. In contrast, peripheral blood DCs of donor origin reconstitute rapidly following both ablative and NST HSCT, with approx 80% being donor derived by d 14 and 95% or more by d 56 *(209)*. Purified DCs in this study were shown to be capable of stimulating an allogeneic mixed-lymphocyte culture response to a much greater degree than peripheral blood mononuclear cells (PBMC), indicating functional competence *(209)*.

Graft-vs-host disease is thought to be initiated by the presentation of host alloantigens by host DCs to donor-derived T cells *(210)*. DCs (and LCs) express the CD52 antigen recognized by Campath and are effectively depleted by preparative treatment with Campath-1G at a time when host-type DCs remain in patients not conditioned with Campath-1G *(211)*. Host DC depletion during conditioning may contribute to the low rate of acute GVHD in Campath-1G-treated patients *(212)*. Campath-1G conditioning did not affect the tempo of donor-derived DC recovery compared to untreated patients. DC1 (CD11c+) recovered more rapidly than DC2 (CD11c–) in this group; however, DC numbers were only half of those of normal donors by 1 yr *(211)*.

5. APPROACHES TO ENHANCE POST-HSCT IMMUNE RECONSTITUTION

Attempts to significantly enhance immune reconstitution post-HSCT have thus far had only modest success. Many programs have now switched to peripheral blood as the primary stem cell source for transplant, and although this does improve the early rate of T-cell reconstitution, the issues of immune suppression as a result of GVHD have not been fully solved. This is especially true because recipients of PBPC grafts may be more likely to suffer from extensive chronic GVHD and all of the associated immune suppression *(213)*. The recent increase in the use of NST has further decreased the period of neutropenia early post-HSCT, but here, too, there are problems with GVHD, and even with faster T-cell immune reconstitution, a period of immune deficiency still exists *(22,214)*. In order to transplant patients who lack a HLA-matched donor, centers have turned to approaches that rigorously deplete T cells so as to allow larger doses of CD34+ cells to facilitate engraftment of haploidentical grafts. Here, GVHD has not been a significant problem, but the recovery of T-cell immunity, specifically CD4+ T cells, is profoundly delayed, resulting in increased early transplant-related mortality because of infection. Approaches to enhance immune reconstitution in this setting have been attempted, and a number of new approaches that appear to have great promise are currently in clinical study or are in the preclinical stages of testing.

5.1. Cytokine Therapy

5.1.1. Hematopoietic Growth Factors

Both G-CSF and GM-CSF have been widely used after alloHSCT to decease the period of neutropenia with the hope that there would be fewer early infections. Neutrophil engraftment is enhanced in most studies by 2–4 d, resulting in a reduced incidence of very early infection *(215,216)*. Nonetheless, these effects have not translated to improved outcome and add considerable expense to the transplant procedure if growth factors are used routinely *(217)*. Furthermore, G-CSF, at least in the setting of CD34+ cell-selected haploidentical transplants, may actually decrease the rate of CD4+ T-cell recovery. Volpi et al. *(31)* described the reconstitution of Th2-inducing DCs that fail to produce IL-12, resulting in a skewing to Th2 CD4+ cells that produced high levels of IL-4 and IL-10 in patients who received G-CSF to enhance engraftment. In a series of patients who did not receive G-CSF, there was no difference in neutrophil engraftment, but there was faster recovery of CD4+ T cells displaying a more protective Th1 phenotype. The use of growth factors to treat neutropenia in association with infection later posttransplant may be more useful than their use during the engraftment period.

5.1.2. Interleukin-2

Because IL-2 is a T-cell growth factor and production early after transplant is severely depressed in nearly all BM recipients, administration of IL-2 was among the earliest clinical interventions to improve posttransplant immunity. The major concern in initiating this treatment was that acute GVHD would be exacerbated. This was not the case; regrettably, neither did IL-2 administration result in enhancement of T cell immunity. Rather, the predominant effect was to further activate NK cells *(218–220)*. Continuous infusion of low doses of IL-2 are better tolerated that higher-dose bolus injections. In spite of this, the enhancing effects of IL-2 on NK activity rapidly declines when infusions are discontinued and this approach offers no real general long-lasting advantage in reconstituting immunity *(218,219)*.

5.1.3. Interleukin-7

Interleukin-7 is a stromal cell-derived cytokine that has major effects on lymphopoiesis and thymopoiesis (reviewed in ref. *221*). Preclinical studies using IL-7 in murine models are very exciting and hold promise that this cytokine may truly enhance thymic function even following TCD HSCT and thus improve T-cell recovery post-HSCT *(222–225)*. Thus far, this appears to be the case, and in most models, there has been no increase in GVHD or loss of GVL reactions as a result of IL-7 administration *(226)*. IL-7 appears to enhance immune reconstitution by increasing thymic output and by increasing antigen-driven peripheral expansion, possibly through upregulation of bcl-2 *(225,227)*. Clinical trials are pending the availability of sufficient quantities Good Manufacturing Practices (GMP)-grade recombinant IL-7 *(221)*.

5.1.4. Neuroendocrine Hormones

Preclinical work is also underway to evaluate the potential effects of several neuroendocrine hormones that have shown stimulatory activity on immune reconstitution post-HSCT *(228)*. Among these are growth hormone (GH) and insulin-like growth factor-1 (IGF-1). Treatment with neuroendocrine hormones is attractive in part because of their limited toxicity after systemic administration *(228)*. Exogenous GH has pleiotropic effects on the thymic microenvironment, including the enhanced production of secretory products like cytokines and hormones (thymulin) *(229)*. GH treatment enhances the proliferation of thymic epithelial cells (TECs) and thymocyte proliferation. Mice with a genetic deficiency in GH show an increase in thymic size and the reappearance of CD4+CD8+ cells within the thymus of treated animals *(230)*. Injections of GH into aging mice increased total thymocyte number and the percentage of circulating CD3+ T cells, as well as thymocyte mitogen response and IL-6 production *(231)*. GH has also been shown to stimulate intrathymic T-cell traffic, an effect that is at least partially mediated by extracellular matrix-mediated interactions *(232)*. In a HSCT setting, GH augments the overall speed of hematopoietic cell recovery in a murine model *(233)*. Additional data indicate that IGF-1 is involved in several effects of GH in the thymus, including the modulation of thymulin secretion, TEC proliferation, as well as thymocyte/TEC adhesion *(234)*. IGF-1 is produced by TECs and thymocytes. Treatment of mice with IGF-1 following HSCT resulted in markedly enhanced recovery of B lymphocytes, and treatment of intact animals enhanced both T- and B-lymphocyte production and function *(235,236)*. Both GH and IGF-1 receptors have been identified in human thymus, making human use of these neuroendocrine hormones particularly attractive *(237,238)*.

5.2. T-Cell Add-Back

5.2.1. Donor Leukocyte Infusion

The first attempts at T-cell add-back used increasing doses of buffy coat cells from BM donors infused following with a T-cell-replete BM HSCT to promote engraftment in immunized patients transplanted for aplastic anemia. Engraftment was enhanced, but patients at even the lowest doses experienced an unacceptably high rate of extensive chronic GVHD *(239)*. Data from experimental systems and from a long experience using DLI to reinduce patients into remission who have relapsed post-HSCT have shown us that donor leukocytes can be tolerated if added back at a later period posttransplant, and in smaller doses *(240)*. Small et al. *(74)* have recently described a series of patients who received prophylactic DLI for the prevention of PTLD that resulted in a significant improvement in immune function, especially in T-cell recovery. However, here too, some patients experienced severe GVHD, even with delayed addition of low numbers of intact T cells *(241)*. DLI for immune reconstitution may be safer if the T cells are engineered with a suicide gene such as herpes simplex virus thymidine kinase such that they can be killed should GVHD occur. Such infusions (at very low doses) have been attempted very early after TCD HSCT and appear to be safe, although no data on the effects on immune reconstitution were reported *(242)*.

5.2.2. CD8-Depleted Donor Peripheral Blood Lymphocytes (PBL)

Several centers have used CD8+ cell-depleted donor peripheral blood infusions for DLI with the hope of more safely restoring antileukemia CTL activity by providing missing T-cell help *(243–245)*. Here, the incidence of GVHD was found to be significantly lower than standard DLI and the infusions did result in GVL responses. The use of planned infusions of CD8-depleted DLI for immune reconstitution is currently undergoing assessment in several institutions and may be a promising approach. The optimal dose and timing of the infusions need to be determined. The assumption is that the reconstituting CD8+ T cells can function to provide immunity to virus if provided exogenous T-cell help in a manner less likely to cause acute GVHD.

5.2.3. LLME-Treated Donor PBL

Haploidentical recipients of rigorously TCD CD34-selected grafts most often have class II as well as class I differences with their donors; therefore, for this group, the use of DLI with removal of only the CD8+ subset may be more risky. L-Leucyl-L-leucine methyl ester (LLME) is a lysosomotrophic agent that is incorporated into lymphocytes by a dipeptide-facilitated transport mechanism and is converted by the acyl transferase activity of the granule enzyme dipeptidyl peptidase I into hydrophobic polymerization products with membranolytic properties *(246,247)*. LLME is selective in its action to cells with cytotoxic potential, such as granulocytes, monocytes, NK cells, and cytotoxic T cells both of the CD4+ and CD8+ phenotype. LLME induces cell death via apoptosis *(248)*. In MHC-disparate murine models, LLME-treated progenitor cell grafts did not mediate GVHD *(249)*. Disappointingly, this agent could not be used in humans for primary treatment of the stem cell graft because of toxicity to hematopoietic cell precursors at the concentrations needed to deplete cytotoxic T cells *(250,251)*. However, LLME is well suited to selectively deplete cytotoxic CD8+ and CD4+ cells while sparing CD4+ helper T cells in peripheral blood cells to be used for DLI. Phase I dose-escalation clinical trials are currently underway in Philadelphia to test this hypothesis (Flomenberg, personnel communication) and are soon to begin at our center, among others. The goal is to enhance the recovery of CD4+ T cells in recipients of grafts rigorously depleted of T cells without causing clinically significant GVHD.

5.2.4. Antigen-Specific T-Cell Lines or Clones

An effective, but somewhat labor-intensive, approach to improve immune reconstitution post-HSCT involves the add-back of T-cell populations that are enriched for cells specific for viral pathogens. The earliest studies were designed to provide CMV immunity for both the prevention and treatment of CMV disease and have included the use of donor-derived CMV-specific T-cell clones or lines *(252–255)*. Such passive immunity can protect against disease without completely suppressing virus, thus allowing for the redevelopment of the patient's own immune response to CMV. The studies of Riddell and Greenberg have also demonstrated the importance of both CD8+ T-cell and CD4+ T-cell immunity to CMV to protect against disease during this period post-HSCT *(144)*. CD4+ and CD8+ CMV-specific clones have been successfully used and were shown to be safe but may not be required for this approach, given the recent encouraging results using CMV-specific T-cell lines for prevention or treatment of disease in patients who have reactivated CMV after TCD HSCT *(256,257)*.

As with CMV, approaches to overcome the function immune deficiency to EBV in patients at high risk for PTLD involve the use of donor-derived EBV-specific T cell lines as prophylaxis during the susceptible period post-HSCT *(258)* or for treatment once PTLD is diagnosed *(259)*. This approach appears to be effective, even in HLA-mismatched recipients, and is safer than using direct infusion of unenriched donor PBMCs, a treatment associated with a high risk of GVHD *(241)*. Several investigators have explored methods to generate lines with specificity for more than one virus in a single culture, such as EBV + CMV or EBV + adenovirus *(254,260)*. However, no clinical trials of such lines have yet been reported. Adenovirus, in particular, is an infection of concern especially in pediatric recipients of TCD HSCT and new approaches to treating early infections are needed *(261)*.

Neither the use of antigen-specific T-cell clones nor T-cell lines post-HSCT has been associated with the induction or exacerbation of GVHD. Because normal donors with previous immunity to CMV or EBV possess relatively high viral-specific T-cell precursors, generating highly lytic active and specific T-cell lines has not been a difficult task. Antigen-specific therapy for viruses with a lower T-cell frequency or for fungal infections, another major cause of post-HSCT morbidity, may be more difficult to develop. Although effective, this approach may not be readily exportable given the need for dedicated laboratory facilities of a level beyond those of most transplant centers.

6. SUMMARY AND CONCLUSIONS

There are many combinations of factors relating to the patient, the donor, and the graft that affect immune reconstitution following alloHSCT. Nevertheless, an overall theme emerges that allows prediction of the rate at which immune reconstitution will occur. For granulocytes, monocytes, dendritic cells, and NK cells, the cellular reconstitution is rapid and occurs with relatively few defects regardless of the combination of factors. For T-cell and B-cell reconstitution, the story is more complex. During the first year after transplant, T cells primarily derive from those cells that were infused with the graft. The degree of graft TCD is inversely correlated with the speed of T-cell reconstitution in this period. Add in immune suppression and there are further delays in T-cell recovery. Younger patients with more functional thymus tissue recover faster, and GVHD impairs recovery both by targeting thymic regeneration and secondary to the immune suppression required to control it. T-cell-Helper function recovers more slowly than cytotoxic T-cell function and there is a period during which CD8+ T cells with suppressor function may predominate. Recipients of unrelated donor grafts or grafts from HLA-disparate related donors are more likely to suffer GVHD and may require more intense conditioning to allow engraftment, which together may explain the higher rate of post-HSCT infection that these patients experience *(48,262)*. Because B-cell function is T-cell dependent, B-cell reconstitution suffers from some of the same effects as T-cell reconstitution. In addition, there are intrinsic B-cell defects that take time to resolve. Like T cells, much of the early humoral immunity is transferred from the donor and eventually declines until a new system develops from the graft progenitor cells. Recently, genetic factors have even been identified that may additionally predispose HSCT recipients to infection *(263)*. Although we now understand many of the forces that affect immune reconstitution, the challenge remains to try and improve it and thus allow more patients to benefit from the potentially curative therapy of HSCT. Some exciting new approaches to enhancing thymic recovery are in development and we anxiously await their introduction into the clinic.

REFERENCES

1. Ochs L, Shu XO, Miller J, et al. Late infections after allogeneic bone marrow transplantations: comparison of incidence in related and unrelated donor transplant recipients. *Blood* 1995;86:3979–3986.
2. Kernan NA, Bartsch G, Ash RC, et al. Analysis of 462 transplantations from unrelated donors facilitated by the National Marrow Donor Program. *N Engl J Med* 1993;328:593–602.

3. Bordignon C, Keever CA, Small TN, et al. Graft failure after T-cell-depleted human leukocyte antigen identical marrow transplants for leukemia: II. In vitro analyses of host effector mechanisms. *Blood* 1989;74:2237–2243.
4. Wursch AM, Gratama JW, Middeldorp JM, et al. The effect of cytomegalovirus infection on T lymphocytes after allogeneic bone marrow transplantation. *Clin Exp Immunol* 1985;62:278–287.
5. Dolstra H, Preijers F, Van de Wiel-van Kemenade E, et al. Expansion of CD8$^+$CD57$^+$ T cells after allogeneic BMT is related with a low incidence of relapse and with cytomegalovirus infection. *Br J Haematol* 1995;90:300–307.
6. Rowbottom A, Garland R, Lepper M, et al. Functional analysis of the CD8$^+$CD57$^+$ cell population in normal healthy individuals and matched unrelated T-cell-depleted bone marrow transplant recipients. *Br J Haematol* 2000;110:315–321.
7. Keever-Taylor CA, Klein JP, Eastwood D, et al. Factors affecting neutrophil and platelet reconstitution following T cell-depleted bone marrow transplantation: differential effects of growth factor type and role of CD34$^+$ cell dose. *Bone Marrow Transplant* 2001;27:791–800.
8. Bernstein SH, Nademanee AP, Vose JM, et al. A multicenter study of platelet recovery and utilization in patients after myeloablative therapy and hematopoietic stem cell transplantation. *Blood* 1998;91:3509–3517.
9. Bensinger WI, Storb R. Allogeneic peripheral blood stem cell transplantation. *Rev Clin Exp Hematol* 2001;5:67–86.
10. Korbling M, Anderlini P. Peripheral blood stem cell versus bone marrow allotransplantation: does the source of hematopoietic stem cells matter? *Blood* 2001;98:2900–2908.
11. Elmaagacli AH, Basoglu S, Peceny R, et al. Improved disease-free-survival after transplantation of peripheral blood stem cells as compared with bone marrow from HLA-identical unrelated donors in patients with first chronic phase chronic myeloid leukemia. *Blood* 2002;99:1130–1135.
12. Weaver C, Hazelton B, Birch R, et al. An analysis of engraftment kinetics as a function of the CD34 content of peripheral blood progenitor cell collections in 692 patients after the administration of myeloablative chemotherapy. *Blood* 1995;86:3961–3969.
13. Lazarus HM. Recombinant cytokines and hematopoietic growth factors in allogeneic and autologous bone marrow transplantation. *Cancer Treat Res* 1997;77:255–301.
14. Martin-Algarra S, Bishop MR, Tarantolo S, et al. Hematopoietic growth factors after HLA-identical allogeneic bone marrow transplantation in patients treated with methotrexate-containing graft-vs.-host disease prophylaxis. *Exp Hematol* 1995;23:1503–1508.
15. Atkinson K, Downs K, Ashby M, et al. Recipients of HLA-identical sibling marrow transplants with severe aplastic anemia engraft more quickly, and those with chronic myeloid leukemia more slowly, than those with acute leukemia. *Bone Marrow Transplant* 1989;4:23–27.
16. Clark RA, Johnson FL, Klebanoff SJ, et al. Defective neutrophil chemotaxis in bone marrow transplant patients. *J Clin Invest* 1976;58:22–31.
17. Sosa R, Weiden PL, Storb R, et al. Granulocyte function in human allogenic marrow graft recipients. *Exp Hematol* 1980;8:1183–1189.
18. Zimmerli W, Zarth A, Gratwohl A, et al. Neutrophil function and pyogenic infections in bone marrow transplant recipients. *Blood* 1991;77:393–399.
19. Territo MC, Gale RP, Cline MJ. Neutrophil function in bone marrow transplant recipients. *Br J Haematol* 1977;35:245–250.
20. Peters WP, Stuart A, Affronti ML, et al. Neutrophil migration is defective during recombinant human granulocyte–macrophage colony-stimulating factor infusion after autologous bone marrow transplantation in humans. *Blood* 1988;72:1310–1315.
21. Slavin S, Nagler A, Naparstek E, et al. Nonmyeloablative stem cell transplantation and cell therapy as an alternative to conventional bone marrow transplantation with lethal cytoreduction for the treatment of malignant and nonmalignant hematologic diseases. *Blood* 1998;91:756–763.
22. Barrett J, Childs R. Non-myeloablative stem cell transplants. *Br J Haematol* 2000;111:6–17.
23. Brochu S, Perreault C, Belanger R. Evaluation of Fc-dependent monocyte–macrophage function in bone marrow transplant recipients. *Exp Hematol* 1989;17:948–951.

24. Winston DJ, Territo MC, Ho WG, et al. Alveolar macrophage dysfunction in human bone marrow transplant recipients. *Am J Med* 1982;73:859–866.
25. Zander AR, Reuben JM, Johnston D, et al. Immune recovery following allogeneic bone marrow transplantation. *Transplantation* 1985;40:177–183.
26. Shiobara S, Witherspoon RP, Lum LG, et al. Immunoglobulin synthesis after HLA-identical marrow grafting. V. The role of peripheral blood monocytes in the regulation of in vitro immunoglobulin secretion stimulated by pokeweed mitogen. *J Immunol* 1984;132:2850–2856.
27. Brkic S, Tsoi MS, Mori T, et al. Cellular interactions in marrow-grafted patients. III. Normal interleukin 1 and defective interleukin 2 production in short-term patients and in those with chronic graft-versus-host disease. *Transplantation* 1985;39:30–35.
28. Castenskiold EC, Kelsey SM, Collins PW, et al. Functional hyperactivity of monocytes after bone marrow transplantation: possible relevance for the development of post-transplant complications or relapse. *Bone Marrow Transplant* 1995;15:879–884.
29. Storek J, Espino G, Dawson MA, et al. Low B-cell and monocyte counts on day 80 are associated with high infection rates between days 100 and 365 after allogeneic marrow transplantation. *Blood* 2000;96:3290–3293.
30. Shenoy S, Mohanakumar T, Todd G, et al. Immune reconstitution following allogeneic peripheral blood stem cell transplants. *Bone Marrow Transplant* 1999;23:335–346.
31. Volpi I, Perruccio K, Tosti A, et al. Postgrafting administration of granulocyte colony-stimulating factor impairs functional immune recovery in recipients of human leukocyte antigen haplotype-mismatched hematopoietic transplants. *Blood* 2001;97:2514–2521.
32. Stroncek DF, Confer DL, Leitman SF. Peripheral blood progenitor cells for HPC transplants involving unrelated donors. *Transfusion* 2000;40:731–741.
33. Mielcarek M, Graf L, Johnson G, et al. Production of interleukin-10 by granulocyte colony-stimulating factor-mobilized blood products: a mechanism for monocyte-mediated suppression of T-cell proliferation. *Blood* 1998;92:215–222.
34. Robertson MJ, Ritz J. Biology and clinical relevance of human natural killer cells. *Blood* 1990;76:2421–2438.
35. Brenner MK, Reittie JE, Grob J-P, et al. The contribution of large granular lymphocytes to B cell activation and differentiation after T-cell depleted allogeneic bone marrow transplantation. *Transplantation* 1986;42:257–261.
36. Klingemann H. Relevance and potential of natural killer cells in stem cell transplantation. *Biol Blood Marrow Transplant* 2000;6:90–99.
37. Ruggeri L, Capanni M, Casucci M, et al. Role of natural killer cell alloreactivity in HLA-mismatched hematopoietic stem cell transplantation. *Blood* 1999;94:333–339.
38. Ruggeri L, Capanni M, Urbani E, et al. Effectiveness of donor natural killer cell alloreactivity in mismatched hematopoietic transplants. *Science* 2002;295:2097–2100.
39. Livnat S, Seigneuret M, Storb R, et al. Analysis of cytotoxic effector cell function in patients with leukemia or aplastic anemia before and after marrow transplantation. *J Immunol* 1980;124:481–490.
40. Ault KA, Antin JH, Ginsburg D, et al. Phenotype of recovering lymphoid cell populations after marrow transplantation. *J Exp Med* 1985;161:1483.
41. Rooney CM, Wimperis JZ, Brenner MK, et al. Natural killer cell activity following T-cell depleted allogeneic bone marrow transplantation. *Br J Haematol* 1986;62:413–420.
42. Keever CA, Small TN, Flomenberg N, et al. Immune reconstitution following bone marrow transplantation: comparison of recipients of T-cell depleted marrow with recipients of conventional marrow grafts. *Blood* 1989;73:1340–1350.
43. Roberts MM, To LB, Gillis D, et al. Immune reconstitution following peripheral blood stem cell transplantation, autologous bone marrow transplantation and allogeneic bone marrow transplantation. *Bone Marrow Transplant* 1993;12:469–475.
44. Lowdell MW, Craston R, Ray N, et al. The effect of T cell depletion with Campath-1M on immune reconstitution after chemotherapy and allogeneic bone marrow transplant as treatment for leukaemia. *Bone Marrow Transplant* 1998;21:679–686.
45. Beelen DW, Peceny R, Elmaagacli A, et al. Transplantation of highly purified HLA-identical sibling donor peripheral blood $CD34^+$ cells without prophylactic post-transplant immunosuppression in adult patients with first chronic phase chronic myeloid leukemia: results of a phase II study. *Bone Marrow Transplant* 2000;26:823–829.
46. Giraud P, Thuret I, Reviron D, et al. Immune reconstitution and outcome after unrelated cord blood transplantation: a single paediatric institution experience. *Bone Marrow Transplant* 2000;25:53–57.

47. Morecki S, Nabet C, Ackerstein A, et al. The effect of in vitro T lymphocyte depletion on generation of IL2-activated cytotoxic cells. *Bone Marrow Transplant* 1991;7:269–273.
48. Drobyski WR, Klein J, Flomenberg N, et al. Superior survival associated with transplantation of matched unrelated versus one-antigen-mismatched unrelated or highly human leukocyte antigen-disparate haploidentical family donor marrow grafts for the treatment of hematologic malignancies: establishing a treatment algorithm for recipients of alternative donor grafts. *Blood* 2002;99:806–814.
49. Reittie JE, Gottlieb D, Heslop HE, et al. Endogenously generated activated killer cells circulate after autologous and allogeneic marrow transplantation but not after chemotherapy. *Blood* 1989;73:1351–1358.
50. Dokhelar MC, Wiels J, Lipinski M, et al. Natural killer cell activity in human bone marrow recipents. Early reappearance of peripheral natural killer activity in graft-versus-host disease. *Transplantation* 1981;31:61–65.
51. Gratama JW, Lipovich-Oosterveer MA, Ronteltap C, et al. Natural immunity and graft-versus-host disease. *Transplantation* 1985;40:256–260.
52. Keever CA, Klein J, Leong N, et al. Effect of GVHD on the recovery of NK cell activity and LAK precursors following BMT. *Bone Marrow Transplant* 1993;12:289–298.
53. Keever CA, Welte K, Small T, et al. Interleukin 2-activated killer cells in patients following transplants of soybean lectin-separated and E rosette-depleted bone marrow. *Blood* 1987;70:1893–1903.
54. Rhoades JL, Cibull ML, Thompson JS, et al. Role of natural killer cells in the pathogenesis of human acute graft-versus-host disease. *Transplantation* 1993;56:113–120.
55. Xun C, Brown SA, Jennings CD, et al. Acute graft-versus-host-like disease induced by transplantation of human activated natural killer cells into SCID mice. *Transplantation* 1993;56:409–417.
56. Hauch M, Gazzola MV, Small T, et al. Anti-leukemia potential of interleukin-2 activated natural killer cells after bone marrow transplantation for chronic myelogenous leukemia. *Blood* 1990;75:2250–2262.
57. MacKinnon S, Howes JM, Goldman JM. Induction of in vitro graft-versus-leukemia activity following bone marrow transplantation for chronic myeloid leukemia. *Blood* 1990;76:2037–2045.
58. Gottschalk LR, Bray RA, Kaizer H, et al. Two populations of CD56 (Leu-a9)$^+$/CD16$^+$ cells in bone marrow transplant recipients. *Bone Marrow Transplant* 1990;5:259–264.
59. Jacobs R, Stoll M, Stratmamm G, et al. CD16–CD56$^+$ natural killer cells after bone marrow transplantation. *Blood* 1992;79:3239–3244.
60. Ottinger HD, Beelen DW, Scheulen B, et al. Improved immune reconstitution after allotransplantation of peripheral blood stem cells instead of bone marrow. *Blood* 1996;88:2775–2779.
61. Beelen DW, Ottinger HD, Elmaagacli A, et al. Transplantation of filgrastim-mobilized peripheral blood stem cells from HLA-identical sibling or alternative family donors in patients with hematologic malignancies: a prospective comparison on clinical outcome, immune reconstitution, and hematopoietic chimerism. *Blood* 1997;90:4725–4735.
62. Miller JS, Prosper F, McCullar V. Natural killer (NK) cells are functionally abnormal and NK cell progenitors are diminished in granulocyte colony-stimulating factor-mobilized peripheral blood progenitor cell collections. *Blood* 1997;90:3098–3105.
63. Keever CA, Abu-Hajir M, Graf W, et al. Characterization of the alloreactivity and anti-leukemia reactivity of cord blood mononuclear cells. *Bone Marrow Transplant* 1995;15:407–419.
64. Thomson BG, Robertson KA, Gowan D, et al. Analysis of engraftment, graft-versus-host disease, and immune recovery following unrelated donor cord blood transplantation. *Blood* 2000;96:2703–2711.
65. Moretta A, Maccario R, Fagioli F, et al. Analysis of immune reconstitution in children undergoing cord blood transplantation. *Exp Hematol* 2001;29:371–379.
66. Niehues T, Rocha V, Filipovich AH, et al. Factors affecting lymphocyte subset reconstitution after either related or unrelated cord blood transplantation in children—a Eurocord analysis. *Br J Haematol* 2001;114:42–48.
67. Richard C, Baro J, Bello-Fernandez C, et al. Recombinant human granulocyte–macrophage colony stimulating factor (rhGM-CSF) administration after autologous bone marrow transplantation for acute myeloblastic leukemia enhances activated killer cell function and may diminish leukemic relapse. *Bone Marrow Transplant* 1995;15:721–726.
68. Spits H, Lanier LL, Philips JH. Development of human T and natural killer cells. *Blood* 1995;85:2654–2670.
69. Haynes BF, Markert ML, Sempowski GD, et al. The role of the thymus in immune reconstitution in aging, bone marrow transplantation, and HIV-1 infection. *Annu Rev Immunol* 2000;18:529–560.
70. Muller-Hermelink HK, Sale GE, Borisch B, et al. Pathology of the thymus after allogeneic bone marrow transplantation in man. A histologic immunohistochemical study of 36 patients. *Am J Pathol* 1987;129:242–256.

71. Fukushi N, Arase H, Wang B, et al. Thymus: a direct target tissue in graft-versus-host reaction after allogeneic bone marrow transplantation that results in abrogation of induction of self-tolerance. *Proc Natl Acad Sci USA* 1990;87:6301–6305.
72. Kook H, Goldman F, Padley D, et al. Reconstruction of the immune system after unrelated or partially matched T-cell-depleted bone marrow transplantation in children: immunophenotypic analysis and factors affecting the speed of recovery. *Blood* 1996;88:1089–1097.
73. Small TN, Avigan D, Dupont B, et al. Immune reconstitution following T-cell depleted bone marrow transplantation: effect of age and post-transplant graft rejection prophylaxis. *Biol Blood Marrow Transplant* 1997;3:65–75.
74. Small TN, Papadopoulos EB, Boulad F, et al. Comparison of immune reconstitution after unrelated and related T-cell-depleted bone marrow transplantation: effect of patient age and donor leukocyte infusions. *Blood* 1999;93:467–480.
75. Davison GM, Novitzky N, Kline A, et al. Immune reconstitution after allogeneic bone marrow transplantation depleted of T cells. *Transplantation* 2000;69:1341–1347.
76. Soiffer RJ, Bosserman L, Murray C, et al. Reconstitution of T-cell function after CD6-depleted allogeneic bone marrow transplantation. *Blood* 1990;75:2076–2084.
77. Mackall CL, Fleisher TA, Brown MR, et al. Age, thymopoiesis, and CD4+ T-lymphocyte regeneration after intensive chemotherapy. *N Engl J Med* 1995;332:143–149.
78. Fujimaki K, Maruta A, Yoshida M, et al. Immune reconstitution assessed during five years after allogeneic bone marrow transplantation. *Bone Marrow Transplant* 2001;27:1275–1281.
79. Storek J, Joseph A, Espino G, et al. Immunity of patients surviving 20 to 30 years after allogeneic or syngeneic bone marrow transplantation. *Blood* 2001;98:3505–3512.
80. Atkinson K, Farewell V, Storb R, et al. Analysis of late infections after human bone marrow transplantation: role of genotypic nonidentity between marrow donor and recipient and of nonspecific suppressor cells in patients with chronic graft-versus-host disease. *Blood* 1982;60:714–720.
81. Storek J, Dawson MA, Storer B, et al. Immune reconstitution after allogeneic marrow transplantation compared with blood stem cell transplantation. *Blood* 2001;97:3380–3389.
82. Handgretinger R, Schumm M, Lang P, et al. Transplantation of megadoses of purified haploidentical stem cells. *Ann NY Acad Sci* 1999;872:351–352.
83. Handgretinger R, Lang P, Schumm M, et al. Immunological aspects of haploidentical stem cell transplantation in children. *Ann NY Acad Sci* 2001;938:340–357.
84. Eyrich M, Lang P, Lal S, et al. A prospective analysis of the pattern of immune reconstitution in a paediatric cohort following transplantation of positively selected human leucocyte antigen-disparate haematopoietic stem cells from parental donors. *Br J Haematol* 2001;114:422–432.
85. Handgretinger R, Klingebiel T, Lang P, et al. Megadose transplantation of purified peripheral blood CD34+ progenitor cells from HLA-mismatched parental donors in children. *Bone Marrow Transplant* 2001;27:777–783.
86. Chakraverty R, Robinson S, Peggs K, et al. Excessive T cell depletion of peripheral blood stem cells has an adverse effect upon outcome following allogeneic stem cell transplantation. *Bone Marrow Transplant* 2001;28:827–834.
87. Mavroudis DA, Read EJ, Molldrem J, et al. T cell-depleted granulocyte colony-stimulating factor (G-CSF) modified allogenic bone marrow transplantation for hematological malignancy improves graft CD34+ cell content but is associated with delayed pancytopenia. *Bone Marrow Transplant* 1998;21:431–440.
88. Martinez C, Urbano-Ispizua A, Rozman C, et al. Immune reconstitution following allogeneic peripheral blood progenitor cell transplantation: comparison of recipients of positive CD34+ selected grafts with recipients of unmanipulated grafts. *Exp Hematol* 1999;27:561–568.
89. Urbano-Ispizua A, Carreras E, Marin P, et al. Allogeneic transplantation of CD34+ selected cells from peripheral blood from human leukocyte antigen-identical siblings: detrimental effect of a high number of donor CD34+ cells? *Blood* 2001;98:2352–2357.
90. Gorski J, Yassai M, Zhu X, et al. Circulating T cell repertoire complexity in normal individuals and bone marrow recipients analyzed by CDR3 size spectratyping. Correlation with immune status. *J Immunol* 1994;152:5109–5119.
91. Gorski J, Yassai M, Keever C, et al. Analysis of reconstituting T cell receptor repertoires in bone marrow transplant recipients. *Arch Immunol Ther Exp* 1995;43:93–97.
92. Roux E, Helg C, Chapuis B, et al. T-cell repertoire complexity after allogeneic bone marrow transplantation. *Hum Immunol* 1996;48:135–138.

93. Godthelp BC, van Tol MJ, Vossen JM, et al. T-Cell immune reconstitution in pediatric leukemia patients after allogeneic bone marrow transplantation with T-cell-depleted or unmanipulated grafts: evaluation of overall and antigen-specific T-cell repertoires. *Blood* 1999;94:4358–4369.
94. Hirokawa M, Horiuchi T, Kitabayashi A, et al. Delayed recovery of CDR3 complexity of the T-cell receptor-beta chain in recipients of allogeneic bone marrow transplants who had virus- associated interstitial pneumonia: monitor of T-cell function by CDR3 spectratyping. *J Allergy Clin Immunol* 2000;106:S32–S39.
95. Dumont-Girard F, Roux E, van Lier RA, et al. Reconstitution of the T-cell compartment after bone marrow transplantation: restoration of the repertoire by thymic emigrants. *Blood* 1998;92:4464–4471.
96. Verfuerth S, Peggs K, Vyas P, et al. Longitudinal monitoring of immune reconstitution by CDR3 size spectratyping after T-cell-depleted allogeneic bone marrow transplant and the effect of donor lymphocyte infusions on T-cell repertoire. *Blood* 2000;95:3990–3995.
97. Donnenberg AD, Margolick JB, Beltz LA, et al. Apoptosis parallels lymphopoiesis in bone marrow transplantation and HIV disease. *Res Immunol* 1995;146:11–21.
98. Hebib NC, Deas O, Rouleau M, et al. Peripheral blood T cells generated after allogeneic bone marrow transplantation: lower levels of bcl-2 protein and enhanced sensitivity to spontaneous and CD95-mediated apoptosis in vitro. Abrogation of the apoptotic phenotype coincides with the recovery of normal naive/primed T-cell profiles. *Blood* 1999;94:1803–1813.
99. Lin MT, Tseng LH, Frangoul H, et al. Increased apoptosis of peripheral blood T cells following allogeneic hematopoietic cell transplantation. *Blood* 2000;95:3832–3839.
100. Schroff RW, Gale RP, Fahey JL. Regeneration of T cell subpopulations after bone marrow transplantation: cytomegalovirus infection and lymphoid subset imbalance. *J Immunol* 1982;129:1926–1930.
101. Autran B, Leblond V, Sadat-Sowti B, et al. A soluble factor released by $CD8^{+}CD57^{+}$ lymphocytes from bone marrow transplanted patients inhibits cell-mediated cytolysis. *Blood* 1991;77:2237–2241.
102. Sadat-Sowti B, Debre P, Mollet L, et al. An inhibitor of cytotoxic functions produced by $CD8^{+}CD57^{+}$ T lymphocytes from patients suffering from AIDS and immunosuppressed bone marrow recipients. *Eur J Immunol* 1994;24:2882–2888.
103. Gorochov G, Debre P, Leblond V, et al. Oligoclonal expansion of $CD8^{+}$ $CD57^{+}$ T cells with restricted T-cell receptor beta chain variability after bone marrow transplantation. *Blood* 1994;83:587–595.
104. Morley JK, Batliwalla FM, Hingorani R, et al. Oligoclonal $CD8^{+}$ T cells are preferentially expanded in the $CD57^{+}$ subset. *J Immunol* 1995;154:6182–6190.
105. Weekes MP, Wills MR, Mynard K, et al. Large clonal expansions of human virus-specific memory cytotoxic T lymphocytes within the $CD57^{+}$ $CD28^{-}$ $CD8^{+}$ T-cell population. *Immunology* 1999;98:443–449.
106. Kern F, Khatamzas E, Surel I, et al. Distribution of human CMV-specific memory T cells among the CD8pos. subsets defined by CD57, CD27, and CD45 isoforms. *Eur J Immunol* 1999;29:2908–2915.
107. Hoshino T, Yamada A, Honda J, et al. Tissue-specific distribution and age-dependent increase of human $CD11B^{+}$ T cells. *J Immunol* 1993;151:2237–2246.
108. Klingemann HG, Lum LG, Storb R. Phenotypical and functional studies on a subtype of suppressor cells ($CD8^{+}/CD11^{+}$) in patients after bone marrow transplantation. *Transplantation* 1987;44:381–386.
109. Gebel HM, Kaizer H, Landay AL. Characterization of circulating suppressor T lymphocytes in bone marrow transplant recipients. *Transplantation* 1987;43:258–263.
110. Gottschalk LR, Kaizer H, Gebel HM. Characterization of peripheral blood CD8/11 cells in bone marrow transplant recipients. II. Two distinct populations of CD8/11 cells. *Transplantation* 1988;45:890–894.
111. Velardi A, Varese P, Terenzi A, et al. Lymphokine production by T-cell clones after human bone marrow transplantation. *Blood* 1989;74:1665–1672.
112. Lebeck LK, Kaizer H, Gebel HM. Characterization of peripheral blood CD8/11b cells in bone marrow transplant recipients. III. Subsets of CD8/11b cells differentially regulate immunoglobulin production. *Bone Marrow Transplant* 1992;9:35–39.
113. Bierer BE, Burakoff SJ, Smith BR. A large proportion of T lymphocytes lack CD5 expression after bone marrow transplantation. *Blood* 1989;73:1359–1366.
114. Douek DC, Vescio RA, Betts MR, et al. Assessment of thymic output in adults after haematopoietic stem-cell transplantation and prediction of T-cell reconstitution. *Lancet* 2000;355:1875–1881.
115. Heitger A, Neu N, Kern H, et al. Essential role of the thymus to reconstitute naive (CD45RA+) T-helper cells after human allogeneic bone marrow transplantation. *Blood* 1997;90:850–857.
116. Lamb LS, Abhyankar SA, Hazlett L, et al. Expression of CD134 (0X-40) on T cells during the first 100 days following allogeneic bone marrow transplantation as a marker for lymphocyte activation and therapy-resistant graft-versus-host disease. *Cytometry* 1999;38:238–243.

117. Atkinson K. T Cell subpopulations defined by monoclonal antibodies after HLA-identical sibling marrow transplantation. II. Activated and functional subsets of helper-inducer and cytotoxic-suppressor subpopulations defined by two-colour fluorescence flow cytometry. *Bone Marrow Transplant*1986;1:121–132.
118. Talvensaari K, Clave E, Douay C, et al. A broad T-cell repertoire diversity and an efficient thymic function indicate a favorable long-term immune reconstitution after cord blood stem cell transplantation. *Blood* 2002;99:1458–1464.
119. Carding SR, Egan PJ. The importance of gamma delta T cells in the resolution of pathogen- induced inflammatory immune responses. *Immunol Rev* 2000;173:98–108.
120. Ferrarini M, Ferrero E, Dagna L, et al. Human gammadelta T cells: a nonredundant system in the immune-surveillance against cancer. *Trends Immunol* 2002;23:14–18.
121. Norton J, al-Saffar N, Sloane JP. An immunohistological study of gamma/delta lymphocytes in human cutaneous graft-versus-host disease. *Bone Marrow Transplant* 1991;7:205–208.
122. Norton J, al-Saffar N, Sloane JP. Immunohistological study of distribution of g/d lymphocytes after allogeneic bone marrow transplantation. *J Clin Pathol* 1992;45:1027–1028.
123. Kawanishi Y, Passweg J, Drobyski WR, et al. Effect of T cell subset dose on outcome of T cell-depleted bone marrow transplantation. *Bone Marrow Transplant* 1997;19:1069–1077.
124. Drobyski WR, Majewski D, Hanson G. Graft-facilitating doses of ex vivo activated gammadelta T cells do not cause lethal murine graft-vs-host disease. *Biol Blood Marrow Transplant* 1999;5:222–230.
125. Gratama JW, Fibbe WE, Visser JW, et al. CD3+, 4-, 8- T cells and $CD3^+$, -4, -8 T cells repopulate at different rates after allogeneic bone marrow transplantation. *Bone Marrow Transplant* 1989;4:291–296.
126. Dechanet J, Merville P, Lim A, et al. Implication of gamma delta T cells in the human immune response to cytomegalovirus. *J Clin Invest* 1999;103:1437–1449.
127. Cela ME, Holladay MS, Rooney CM, et al. Gamma delta T lymphocyte regeneration after T lymphocyte-depleted bone marrow transplantation from mismatched family members or matched unrelated donors. *Bone Marrow Transplant* 1996;17:243–247.
128. Vilmer E, Guglielmi P, David V, et al. Predominant expression of circulating $CD3^+$ lymphocytes bearing gamma T cell receptor in a prolonged immunodeficiency after allogeneic bone marrow transplantation. *J Clin Invest* 1988;82:755–761.
129. Vilmer E, Triebel F, David V, et al. Prominent expansion of circulating lymphocytes bearing γ T-cell receptors, with preferential expression of variable γ genes after allogeneic bone marrow transplantation. *Blood* 1988;72:841–849.
130. van der Harst D, Brand A, van Luxemburg-Heijs SA, et al. Selective outgrowth of $CD45RO^+$ V gamma 9^+/V delta 2^+ T-cell receptor gamma/delta T cells early after bone marrow transplantation. *Blood* 1991;78:1875–1881.
131. Lamb LS, Henslee-Downey PJ, Parrish RS, et al. Increased frequency of TCR gamma delta + T cells in disease-free survivors following T cell-depleted, partially mismatched, related donor bone marrow transplantation for leukemia. *J Hematother* 1996;5:503–509.
132. Lamb LS, Gee AP, Hazlett LJ, et al. Influence of T cell depletion method on circulating γδ T cell reconstitution and potential role in the graft-versus-leukemia effect. *Cytotherapy* 1999;1:7–19.
133. Reusser P, Riddell SR, Meyers JD, et al. Cytotoxic T-lymphocyte response to cytomegalovirus after human allogeneic bone marrow transplantation: pattern of recovery and correlation with cytomegalovirus infection and disease. *Blood* 1991;78:1373–1380.
134. Drobyski WR, Dunne WM, Burd EM, et al. Human herpesvirus-6 (HHV-6) infection in allogeneic bone marrow transplant recipients: evidence of a marrow-suppressive role for HHV-6 in vivo. *J Infect Dis* 1993;167:735–739.
135. Wang FZ, Linde A, Dahl H, Ljungman P. Human herpesvirus 6 infection inhibits specific lymphocyte proliferation responses and is related to lymphocytopenia after allogeneic stem cell transplantation. *Bone Marrow Transplant* 1999;24:1201–1206.
136. Wagner H-J, Rooney C, Heslop H. Diagnosis and treatment of posttransplantation lymphoproliferative disease after hematopoietic stem cell transplantation. *Biol Blood Marrow Transplant* 2002;8:1–8.
137. Gratama JW, Verdonck LF, van der Linden JA, et al. Cellular immunity to vaccinations and herpesvirus infections after bone marrow transplantation. *Transplantation* 1986;41:719–724.
138. Atkinson K. Reconstruction of the haemopoietic and immune systems after marrow transplantation. *Bone Marrow Transplant* 1990;5:209–226.

139. Noel DR, Witherspoon RP, Storb R, et al. Does graft-versus-host disease influence the tempo of immunologic recovery after allogeneic human marrow transplantation? An observation on 56 long-term survivors. *Blood* 1978;51:1087–1105.
140. Kameoka J, Sato T, Torimoto Y, et al. Differential CD26-mediated activation of the CD3 and CD2 pathways after CD6-depleted allogeneic bone marrow transplantation. *Blood* 1995;85:1132–1137.
141. Meyers JD, Flournoy N, Thomas ED. Cell-mediated immunity to varicella-zoster virus after allogeneic marrow transplant. *J Infect Dis* 1980;141:479–487.
142. Meyers JD, Flournoy N, Thomas ED. Infection with herpes simplex virus and cell-mediated immunity after marrow transplant. *J Infect Dis* 1980;142:338–346.
143. Wade JC, Day LM, Crowley JJ, et al. Recurrent infection with herpes simplex virus after marrow transplantation: role of the specific immune response and acyclovir treatment. *J Infect Dis* 1984;149:750–756.
144. Walter E, Greenberg P, Gilbert M, et al. Reconstitution of cellular immunity against cytomegalovirus in recipients of allogeneic bone marrow by transfer of T-cell clones from the donor. *N Engl J Med* 1995;333:1038–1044.
145. Lopez-Botet M, De Landazuri MO, Izquierdo M, et al. Defective interleukin 2 receptor expression is associated with the T cell disfunction subsequent to bone marrow transplantation. *Eur J Immunol* 1987;17:1167–1174.
146. Yamagami M, McFadden PW, Koethe SM, et al. Failure of T cell receptor-anti-CD3 monoclonal antibody interaction in T cells from marrow recipients to induce increases in intracellular ionized calcium. *J Clin Invest* 1990;86:1347–1351.
147. Mori T, Tsoi MS, Gillis S, et al. Cellular interactions in marrow-grafted patients. I. Impairment of cell-mediated lympholysis associated with graft-vs-host disease and the effect of interleukin 2. *J Immunol* 1983;130:712–716.
148. Hebart H, Daginik S, Stevanovic S, et al. Sensitive detection of human cytomegalovirus peptide-specific cytotoxic T-lymphocyte responses by interferon-gamma-enzyme-linked immunospot assay and flow cytometry in healthy individuals and in patients after allogeneic stem cell transplantation. *Blood* 2002;99:3830–3837.
149. Emanuel D, Cunningham I, Jules-Elysee K, et al. Cytomegalovirus pneumonia after bone marrow transplantation successfully treated with the combination of ganciclovir and high-dose intravenous immune globulin. *Ann Intern Med* 1988;109:777–782.
150. Li CR, Greenberg PD, Gilbert MJ, et al. Recovery of HLA-restricted cytomegalovirus (CMV)-specific T-cell responses after allogeneic bone marrow transplant: correlation with CMV disease and effect of ganciclovir prophylaxis. *Blood* 1994;83:1971–1979.
151. Nguyen Q, Champlin R, Giralt S, et al. Late cytomegalovirus pneumonia in adult allogeneic blood and marrow transplant recipients. *Clin Infect Dis* 1999;28:618–623.
152. Broers AE, van Der Holt R, van Esser JW, et al. Increased transplant-related morbidity and mortality in CMV-seropositive patients despite highly effective prevention of CMV disease after allogeneic T-cell-depleted stem cell transplantation. *Blood* 2000;95:2240–2245.
153. Kern F, Faulhaber N, Khatamzas E, et al. Measurement of anti-human cytomegalovirus T cell reactivity in transplant recipients and its potential clinical use: a mini-review. *Intervirology* 1999;42:322–324.
154. Cwynarski K, Ainsworth J, Cobbold M, et al. Direct visualization of cytomegalovirus-specific T-cell reconstitution after allogeneic stem cell transplantation. *Blood* 2001;97:1232–12140.
155. Gratama JW, van Esser JW, Lamers CH, et al. Tetramer-based quantification of cytomegalovirus (CMV)-specific CD8$^+$ T lymphocytes in T-cell-depleted stem cell grafts and after transplantation may identify patients at risk for progressive CMV infection. *Blood* 2001;98:1358–1364.
156. Junghanss C, Boeckh M, Carter RA, et al. Incidence and outcome of cytomegalovirus infections following nonmyeloablative compared with myeloablative allogeneic stem cell transplantation, a matched control study. *Blood* 2002;99:1978–1985.
157. Duncombe AS, Grundy JE, Oblakowski P, et al. Bone marrow transplant recipients have defective MHC-unrestricted cytotoxic responses against cytomegalovirus in comparison with Epstein–Barr virus: the importance of target cell expression of lymphocyte function-associated antigen 1 (LFA1). *Blood* 1992;79:3059–3066.
158. Gross TG, Steinbuch M, DeFor T, et al. B Cell lymphoproliferative disorders following hematopoietic stem cell transplantation: risk factors, treatment and outcome. *Bone Marrow Transplant* 1999;23:251–258.

159. Meijer E, Slaper-Cortenbach IC, Thijsen SF, et al. Increased incidence of EBV-associated lymphoproliferative disorders after allogeneic stem cell transplantation from matched unrelated donors due to a change of T cell depletion technique. *Bone Marrow Transplant* 2002;29:335–339.
160. Lucas KG, Small TN, Heller G, et al. The development of cellular immunity to Epstein–Barr virus after allogeneic bone marrow transplantation. *Blood* 1996;87:2594–2603.
161. Warren HS, Atkinson K, Pembrey RG, et al. Human bone marrow allograft recipients: production of, and responsiveness to, interleukin 2. *J Immunol* 1983;131:1771–1775.
162. Azogui O, Gluckman E, Fradelizi D. Inhibition of IL 2 production after human allogeneic bone marrow transplantation. *J Immunol* 1983;131:1205–1208.
163. Welte K, Ciobanu N, Moore MA, et al. Defective interleukin 2 production in patients after bone marrow transplantation and in vitro restoration of defective T lymphocyte proliferation by highly purified interleukin 2. *Blood* 1984;64:380–385.
164. Welte K, Keever CA, Levick J, et al. Interleukin-2 production and response to interleukin-2 by peripheral blood mononuclear cells from patients after bone marrow transplantation. II. Patients receiving soybean lectin-separated and T cell-depleted bone marrow. *Blood* 1987;70:1595–1603.
165. Cooley MA, McLachlan K, Atkinson K. Cytokine activity after human bone marrow transplantation. III. Defect in IL2 production by peripheral blood mononuclear cells is not corrected by stimulation with Ca^{++} ionophore plus phorbol ester. *Br J Haematol* 1989;73:341–347.
166. Cooley MA. Cytokine activity after human bone marrow transplantation. Production of interferons by peripheral blood mononuclear cells from recipients of HLA-identical sibling bone marrow transplants. *J Immunol* 1987;138:3742–3745.
167. Lum LG, Joshi ID, Smith MR, et al. Constitutive and mitogen-stimulated cytokine mRNA expression by peripheral blood mononuclear cells from most autologous and allogeneic bone marrow transplant recipients is intact. *Bone Marrow Transplant* 1994;13:187–195.
168. Tanaka J, Imamura M, Kasai M, et al. Cytokine gene expression by concanavalin A-stimulated peripheral mononuclear cells after bone marrow transplantation: an indicator of immunological abnormality due to chronic graft-versus-host disease. *Bone Marrow Transplant* 1994;14:695–701.
169. Mitra DK, Singh HP, Singh M, et al. Reconstitution of naive T cells and type 1 function after autologous peripheral stem cell transplantation: impact on the relapse of original cancer. *Transplantation* 2002;73:1336–1339.
170. Small TN, Keever CA, Weiner-Fedus S, et al. B-Cell differentiation following autologous, conventional or T-cell depleted bone marrow transplantation: a recapitulation of normal B-cell ontogeny. *Blood* 1990;76:1647–1656.
171. Storek J, Ferrara S, Ku N, et al. B Cell reconstitution after human bone marrow transplantation: recapitulation of ontogeny? *Bone Marrow Transplant* 1993;12:387–398.
172. D'Costa S, Slobod KS, Benaim E, et al. Effect of extended immunosuppressive drug treatment on B cell vs T cell reconstitution in pediatric bone marrow transplant recipients. *Bone Marrow Transplant* 2001;28:573–580.
173. Lum LG, Seigneuret MC, Storb RF, et al. In vitro regulation of immunoglobulin synthesis after marrow transplantation. I. T-Cell and B-cell deficiencies in patients with and without chronic graft-versus-host disease. *Blood* 1981;58:431–439.
174. Witherspoon RP, Goehle S, Kretschmer M, et al. Regulation of immunoglobulin production after human marrow grafting. The role of helper and suppressor T cells in acute graft-versus-host disease. *Transplantation* 1986;41:328–335.
175. Storek J, Saxon A. Reconstitution of B cell immunity following bone marrow transplantation. *Bone Marrow Transplant* 1992;9:395–408.
176. Lortan JE, Vellodi A, Jurges ES, et al. Class- and subclass-specific pneumococcal antibody levels and response to immunization after bone marrow transplantation. *Clin Exp Immunol* 1992;88:512–519.
177. Fumoux F, Guigou V, Blaise D, et al. Reconstitution of human immunoglobulin VH repertoire after bone marrow transplantation mimics B-cell ontogeny. *Blood* 1993;81:3153–3157.
178. Storek J, King L, Ferrara S, et al. Abundance of a restricted fetal B cell repertoire in marrow transplant recipients. *Bone Marrow Transplant* 1994;14:783–790.
179. Gokmen E, Raaphorst FM, Boldt DH, et al. Ig heavy chain third complementarity determining regions (H CDR3s) after stem cell transplantation do not resemble the developing human fetal H CDR3s in size distribution and Ig gene utilization. *Blood* 1998;92:2802–2814.

180. Suzuki I, Milner EC, Glas AM, et al. Immunoglobulin heavy chain variable region gene usage in bone marrow transplant recipients: lack of somatic mutation indicates a maturational arrest. *Blood* 1996;87:1873–1880.
181. Kelsey SM, Lowdell MW, Newland AC. IgG subclass levels and immune reconstitution after T cell-depleted allogeneic bone marrow transplantation. *Clin Exp Immunol* 1990;80:409–412.
182. Sheridan JF, Tutschka PJ, Sedmak DD, et al. Immunoglobulin G subclass deficiency and pneumococcal infection after allogeneic bone marrow transplantation. *Blood* 1990;75:1583–1586.
183. Izutsu KT, Sullivan KM, Schubert MM, et al. Disordered salivary immunoglobulin secretion and sodium transport in human chronic graft-versus-host disease. *Transplantation* 1983;35:441–446.
184. Abedi MR, Hammarstrom L, Ringden O, et al. Development of IgA deficiency after bone marrow transplantation. The influence of acute and chronic graft-versus-host disease. *Transplantation* 1990;50:415–421.
185. Storek J, Witherspoon RP, Luthy D, et al. Low IgG production by mononuclear cells from marrow transplant survivors and from normal neonates is due to a defect of B cells. *Bone Marrow Transplant* 1995;15:679–684.
186. Saryan JA, Rappeport J, Leung DY, et al. Regulation of human immunoglobulin E synthesis in acute graft versus host disease. *J Clin Invest* 1983;71:556–564.
187. Walker SA, Rogers TR, Perry D, et al. Increased serum IgE concentrations during infection and graft versus host disease after bone marrow transplantation. *J Clin Pathol* 1984;37:460–462.
188. Lum LG, Munn NA, Schanfield MS, et al. The detection of specific antibody formation to recall antigens after human bone marrow transplantation. *Blood* 1986;67:582–587.
189. Lum LG, Noges JE, Beatty P, et al. Transfer of specific immunity in marrow recipients given HLA-mismatched, T cell-depleted, or HLA-identical grafts. *Bone Marrow Transplant* 1988;3:399–406.
190. Wahren B, Gahrton G, Linde A, et al. Transfer and persistence of viral antibody-producing cells in bone marrow transplantation. *J Infect Dis* 1984;150:358–365.
191. Saxon A, Mitsuyasu R, Stevens R, et al. Designed transfer of specific immune responses with bone marrow transplantation. *J Clin Invest* 1986;78:959–967.
192. Wimperis JZ, Brenner MK, Prentice HG, et al. Transfer of a functioning humoral immune system in transplantation of T-lymphocyte-depleted bone marrow. *Lancet* 1986;1:339–343.
193. Shiobara S, Lum LG, Witherspoon RP, et al. Antigen-specific antibody responses of lymphocytes to tetanus toxoid after human marrow transplantation. *Transplantation* 1986;41:587–592.
194. Vavassori M, Maccario R, Moretta A, et al. Restricted TCR repertoire and long-term persistence of donor-derived antigen-experienced CD4$^+$ T cells in allogeneic bone marrow transplantation recipients. *J Immunol* 1996;157:5739–5747.
195. Chaushu S, Chaushu G, Garfunkel AA, et al. Salivary immunoglobulins in recipients of bone marrow grafts. I. A longitudinal follow-up. *Bone Marrow Transplant* 1994;14:871–876.
196. Chaushu S, Chaushu G, Garfunkel A, et al. Salivary immunoglobulins in recipients of bone marrow grafts. II. Transient secretion of donor-derived salivary IgA following transplantation of T cell-depleted bone marrow. *Bone Marrow Transplant* 1994;14:925–928.
197. Wimperis JZ, Brenner MK, Prentice HG, et al. B Cell development and regulation after T cell-depleted marrow transplantation. *J Immunol* 1987;138:2445–2450.
198. Ljungman P, Lewensohn-Fuchs I, Hammarstrom V, et al. Long-term immunity to measles, mumps, and rubella after allogeneic bone marrow transplantation. *Blood* 1994;84:657–663.
199. Witherspoon RP, Storb R, Ochs HD, et al. Recovery of antibody production in human allogeneic marrow graft recipients: influence of time posttransplantation, the presence or absence of chronic graft-versus-host disease, and antithymocyte globulin treatment. *Blood* 1981;58:360–368.
200. Guinan EC, Molrine DC, Antin JH, et al. Polysaccharide conjugate vaccine responses in bone marrow transplant patients. *Transplantation* 1994;57:677–684.
201. King SM, Saunders EF, Petric M, et al. Response to measles, mumps and rubella vaccine in paediatric bone marrow transplant recipients. *Bone Marrow Transplant* 1996;17:633–636.
202. Gerritsen EJ, Van Tol MJ, Van't Veer MB, et al. Clonal dysregulation of the antibody response to tetanus-toxoid after bone marrow transplantation. *Blood* 1994;84:4374–4382.
203. Engelhard D, Nagler A, Hardan I, et al. Antibody response to a two-dose regimen of influenza vaccine in allogeneic T cell-depleted and autologous BMT recipients. *Bone Marrow Transplant* 1993;11:1–5.
204. Engelhard D, Handsher R, Naparstek E, et al. Immune response to polio vaccination in bone marrow transplant recipients. *Bone Marrow Transplant* 1991;8:295–300.
205. Ljungman P, Duraj V, Magnius L. Response to immunization against polio after allogeneic marrow transplantation. *Bone Marrow Transplant* 1991;7:89–93.

206. Perreault C, Pelletier M, Landry D, et al. Study of Langerhans cells after allogeneic bone marrow transplantation. *Blood* 1984;63:807–811.
207. Atkinson K, Munro V, Vasak E, et al. Mononuclear cell subpopulations in the skin defined by monoclonal antibodies after HLA-identical sibling marrow transplantation. *Br J Dermatol* 1986;114:145–160.
208. Witherspoon RP, Matthews D, Storb R, et al. Recovery of in vivo cellular immunity after human marrow grafting. Influence of time postgrafting and acute graft-versus-host disease. *Transplantation* 1984;37:145–150.
209. Auffermann-Gretzinger S, Lossos IS, Vayntrub TA, et al. Rapid establishment of dendritic cell chimerism in allogeneic hematopoietic cell transplant recipients. *Blood* 2002;99:1442–1448.
210. Shlomchik WD, Couzens MS, Tang CB, et al. Prevention of graft versus host disease by inactivation of host antigen- presenting cells. *Science* 1999;285:412–415.
211. Klangsinsirikul P, Carter GI, Byrne JL, et al. Campath-1G causes rapid depletion of circulating host dendritic cells (DCs) before allogeneic transplantation but does not delay donor DC reconstitution. *Blood* 2002;99:2586–2591.
212. Hale G, Jacobs P, Wood L, et al. CD52 antibodies for prevention of graft-versus-host disease and graft rejection following transplantation of allogeneic peripheral blood stem cells. *Bone Marrow Transplant* 2000;26:69–76.
213. Przepiorka D, Anderlini P, Saliba R, et al. Chronic graft-versus-host disease after allogeneic blood stem cell transplantation. *Blood* 2001;98:1695–1700.
214. Morecki S, Gelfand Y, Nagler A, et al. Immune reconstitution following allogeneic stem cell transplantation in recipients conditioned by low intensity vs myeloablative regimen. *Bone Marrow Transplant* 2001;28:243–249.
215. Powles R, Smith C, Milan S, et al. Human recombinant GM-CSF in allogeneic bone-marrow transplantation for leukaemia: double-blind, placebo-controlled trial. *Lancet* 1990;336:1417–1420.
216. Nemunaitis J, Rosenfeld CS, Ash R, et al. Phase III randomized, double-blind placebo-controlled trial of rhGM-CSF following allogeneic bone marrow transplantation. *Bone Marrow Transplant* 1995;15:949–954.
217. Lazarus HM, Rowe JM. Clinical use of hematopoietic growth factors in allogeneic bone marrow transplantation. *Blood Rev* 1994;8:169–178.
218. Soiffer R, Murray C, Cochran K, et al. Clinical and immunologic effects of prolonged infusion of low-dose recombinant interleukin-2 after autologous and T-cell-depleted allogeneic bone marrow transplantation. *Blood* 1992;79:517–526.
219. Soiffer R, Murray C, Gonin R, Ritz J. Effect of low-dose interleukin-2 on disease relapse after T-cell-depleted allogeneic bone marrow transplantation. *Blood* 1994;84:964–971.
220. Robinson N, Sanders JE, Benyunes MC, et al. Phase I trial of interleukin-2 after unmodified HLA-matched sibling bone marrow transplantation for children with acute leukemia. *Blood* 1996;87:1249–1254.
221. Fry TJ, Mackall CL. Interleukin-7: from bench to clinic. *Blood* 2002;99:3892–3904.
222. Bolotin E, Smogorzewska M, Smith S, et al. Enhancement of thymopoiesis after bone marrow transplant by in vivo interleukin-7. *Blood* 1996;88:1887–1894.
223. Abdul-Hai A, Or R, Slavin S, et al. Stimulation of immune reconstitution by interleukin-7 after syngeneic bone marrow transplantation in mice. *Exp Hematol* 1996;24:1416–1422.
224. Geiselhart LA, Humphries CA, Gregorio TA, et al. IL-7 administration alters the CD4 : CD8 ratio, increases T cell numbers, and increases T cell function in the absence of activation. *J Immunol* 2001;166:3019–3027.
225. Mackall CL, Fry TJ, Bare C, et al. IL-7 increases both thymic-dependent and thymic-independent T-cell regeneration after bone marrow transplantation. *Blood* 2001;97:1491–1497.
226. Alpdogan O, Schmaltz C, Muriglan SJ, et al. Administration of interleukin-7 after allogeneic bone marrow transplantation improves immune reconstitution without aggravating graft-versus-host disease. *Blood* 2001;98:2256–2265.
227. Fry TJ, Christensen BL, Komschlies KL, et al. Interleukin-7 restores immunity in athymic T-cell-depleted hosts. *Blood* 2001;97:1525–1533.
228. Woody MA, Welniak LA, Richards S, et al. Use of neuroendocrine hormones to promote reconstitution after bone marrow transplantation. *Neuroimmunomodulation* 1999;6:69–80.
229. Savino W, Postel Vinay MC, Smaniotto S, et al. The thymus gland: a target organ for growth hormone. *Scand J Immunol* 2002;55:442–452.
230. Murphy WJ, Durum SK, Longo DL. Role of neuroendocrine hormones in murine T cell development. Growth hormone exerts thymopoietic effects in vivo. *J Immunol* 1992;149:3851–3857.

231. De Mello-Coelho V, Savino W, Postel-Vinay MC, et al. Role of prolactin and growth hormone on thymus physiology. *Dev Immunol* 1998;6:317–323.
232. Savino W, Smaniotto S, De Mello-Coelho V, et al. Is there a role for growth hormone upon intrathymic T-cell migration? *Ann NY Acad Sci* 2000;917:748–754.
233. Tian ZG, Woody MA, Sun R, et al. Recombinant human growth hormone promotes hematopoietic reconstitution after syngeneic bone marrow transplantation in mice. *Stem Cells* 1998;16:193–199.
234. Savino W, de Mello-Coelho V, Dardenne M. Control of the thymic microenvironment by growth hormone/insulin-like growth factor-I-mediated circuits. *Neuroimmunomodulation* 1995;2:313–318.
235. Jardieu P, Clark R, Mortensen D, et al. In vivo administration of insulin-like growth factor-I stimulates primary B lymphopoiesis and enhances lymphocyte recovery after bone marrow transplantation. *J Immunol* 1994;152:4320–4327.
236. Robbins K, McCabe S, Scheiner T, et al. Immunological effects of insulin-like growth factor-I—enhancement of immunoglobulin synthesis. *Clin Exp Immunol* 1994;95:337–342.
237. de Mello-Coelho V, Gagnerault MC, et al. Growth hormone and its receptor are expressed in human thymic cells. *Endocrinology* 1998;139:3837–3842.
238. de Mello Coelho V, Villa-Verde DM, Farias-De-Oliveira DA, et al. Functional insulin-like growth factor-1/insulin-like growth factor-1 receptor-mediated circuit in human and murine thymic epithelial cells. *Neuroendocrinology* 2002;75:139–150.
239. Storb R, Doney KC, Thomas ED, et al. Marrow transplantation with or without donor buffy coat cells for 65 transfused aplastic anemia patients. *Blood* 1982;59:236–246.
240. Mackinnon S, Papadopoulos EB, Carabasi MH, et al. Adoptive immunotherapy using donor leukocytes following bone marrow transplantation for chronic myeloid leukemia: is T cell dose important in determining biological response? *Bone Marrow Transplant* 1995;15:591–594.
241. Papadopoulos EB, Ladanyi M, Emanuel D, et al. Infusions of donor leukocytes to treat Epstein–Barr virus-associated lymphoproliferative disorders after allogeneic bone marrow transplantation. *N Engl J Med* 1994;330:1185–1191.
242. Tiberghien P, Ferrand C, Lioure B, et al. Administration of herpes simplex–thymidine kinase-expressing donor T cells with a T-cell-depleted allogeneic marrow graft. *Blood* 2001;97:63–72.
243. Giralt S, Hester J, Huh Y, et al. CD8-depleted donor lymphocyte infusion as treatment for relapsed chronic myelogenous leukemia after allogeneic bone marrow transplantation. *Blood* 86(11):4337–4343.
244. Alyea EP, Soiffer RJ, Canning C, et al. Toxicity and efficacy of defined doses of $CD4^+$ donor lymphocytes for treatment of relapse after allogeneic bone marrow transplant. *Blood* 1998;91:3671–3680.
245. Alyea E, Weller E, Schlossman R, et al. T-Cell-depleted allogeneic bone marrow transplantation followed by donor lymphocyte infusion in patients with multiple myeloma: induction of graft-versus-myeloma effect. *Blood* 2001;98:934–939.
246. Thiele DL, Lipsky PE. Mechanism of L-leucyl-L-leucine methyl ester-mediated killing of cytotoxic lymphocytes: dependence on a lysosomal thiol protease, dipeptidyl peptidase I, that is enriched in these cells. *Proc Natl Acad Sci USA* 1990;87:83–87.
247. Thiele DL, Lipsky PE. The action of leucyl-leucine methyl ester on cytotoxic lymphocytes requires uptake by a novel dipeptide-specific facilitated transport system and dipeptidyl peptidase I-mediated conversion to membranolytic products. *J Exp Med* 1990;172:183–194.
248. Thiele DL, Lipsky PE. Apoptosis is induced in cells with cytolytic potential by L-leucyl-L-leucine methyl ester. *J Immunol* 1992;148:3950–3957.
249. Charley M, Thiele DL, Bennett M, et al. Prevention of lethal murine graft versus host disease by treatment of donor cells with L-leucyl-L-leucine methyl ester. *J Clin Invest* 1986;78:1415–1420.
250. Pecora AL, Bordignon C, Fumagalli L, et al. Characterization of the in vitro sensitivity of human lymphoid and hematopoietic progenitors to L-leucyl-L-leucine methyl ester. *Transplantation* 1991;51:524–531.
251. Rosenfeld CS, Thiele DL, Shadduck RK, et al. Ex vivo purging of allogeneic marrow with L-leucyl-L-leucine methyl ester. A phase I study. *Transplantation* 1995;60:678–683.
252. Greenberg PD, Reusser P, Goodrich JM, et al. Development of a treatment regimen for human cytomegalovirus (CMV) infection in bone marrow transplantation recipients by adoptive transfer of donor-derived CMV-specific T cell clones expanded in vitro. *Ann NY Acad Sci* 1991;636:184–195.

253. Riddell S, Walter B, Gilbert M, et al. Selective reconstitution of CD8+ cytotoxic T lymphocyte responses in immunodeficient bone marrow transplant recipients by the adoptive transfer of T cell clones. *Bone Marrow Transplant* 1994;14:78–84.
254. Sun Q, Pollok KE, Burton RL, et al. Simultaneous ex vivo expansion of cytomegalovirus and Epstein–Barr virus-specific cytotoxic T lymphocytes using B-lymphoblastoid cell lines expressing cytomegalovirus pp65. *Blood* 1999;94:3242–3250.
255. Peggs K, Verfuerth S, Mackinnon S. Induction of cytomegalovirus (CMV)-specific T-cell responses using dendritic cells pulsed with CMV antigen: a novel culture system free of live CMV virions. *Blood* 2001;97:994–1000.
256. Peggs KS, Mackinnon S. Clinical trials with CMV-specific T cells. *Cytotherapy* 2002;4:21–28.
257. Einsele H, Roosnek E, Rufer N, et al. Infusion of cytomegalovirus (CMV)-specific T cells for the treatment of CMV infection not responding to antiviral chemotherapy. *Blood* 2002;99:3916–3922.
258. Heslop HE, Ng CYC, Li C, et al. Long-term restoration of immunity against Epstein–Barr virus infection by adoptive transfer of gene-modified virus-specific T lymphocytes. *Nature Med* 1996;2:551–555.
259. Rooney CM, Smith CA, Ng CY, et al. Infusion of cytotoxic T cells for the prevention and treatment of Epstein–Barr virus-induced lymphoma in allogeneic transplant recipients. *Blood* 1998;92:1549–1555.
260. Regn S, Raffegerst S, Chen X, et al. Ex vivo generation of cytotoxic T lymphocytes specific for one or two distinct viruses for the prophylaxis of patients receiving an allogeneic bone marrow transplant. *Bone Marrow Transplant* 2001;27:53–64.
261. Flomenberg P, Babbitt J, Drobyski WR, et al. Increasing incidence of adenovirus disease in bone marrow transplant recipients. *J Infect Dis* 1994;169:775–781.
262. Williamson EC, Millar MR, Steward CG, et al. Infections in adults undergoing unrelated donor bone marrow transplantation. *Br J Haematol* 1999;104:560–568.
263. Mullighan CG, Heatley S, Doherty K, et al. Mannose-binding lectin gene polymorphisms are associated with major infection following allogeneic hemopoietic stem cell transplantation. *Blood* 2002;99:3524–3529.

10 Infection in the Hematopoietic Stem Cell Transplant Recipient

Lindsey Baden, MD
and Robert H. Rubin, MD, FACP, FCCP

CONTENTS

1. INTRODUCTION

Successful hematopoietic stem cell transplantation (HSCT) requires the accomplishment of several tasks: the application of a conditioning regimen that eliminates to the greatest possible extent the patient's malignant cell burden; the suppression of the patient's immunity in order to prevent rejection of the transplanted cells; and the creation of "space" for the donor cells within the bone marrow. A variety of conditioning regimens are being utilized, with irradiation and chemotherapy (most commonly, cyclophosphamide) being the mainstays of most conditioning regimens. In addition, nonmyeloablative chemotherapy regimens, without irradiation, are being explored as well. These may be supplemented with other chemotherapeutic agents, anti-T-cell antibodies to suppress recipient immunity, and a variety of cytokines and cytokine antagonists. From an infectious disease point of view, the possible consequences of the conditioning regimen are several: mucositis severe enough to affect nutrition and hydration, provide a portal of entry for bacteria and yeast to invade, and prevent the reliable absorption of medications; persistent pancytopenia; and impaired cell-mediated immunity, thus predisposing to viral-induced, especially cytomegalovirus (CMV) infection, as well as Epstein–Barr virus (EBV) posttransplant lymphoproliferative disease *(1,2)*. The importance of granulocytopenia in the pathogenesis of significant infection in patients undergoing treatment for cancer was first defined by Bodey in 1966 *(3)* and confirmed many times since then. He reported that

From: *Stem Cell Transplantation for Hematologic Malignancies*
Edited by: R. J. Soiffer © Humana Press Inc., Totowa, NJ

the incidence of infection was 14% if the absolute neutrophil count (ANC) fell below 500/mm^3, rising to 24–60% if it fell to less than 100/mm^3. The longer the duration of the granulocytopenia and the more rapid the fall in the ANC, the greater the risk of infection. Granulocytopenia of more than 5 wk duration has an incidence of infection that approaches 100% *(3–5)*.

A variety of sources for donor cells can be utilized for HSCT: autologous bone marrow or stem cells that may be purged of contaminating malignant cells (by in vitro chemotherapy or specific antitumor antibody treatment or by positive selection of stem cells by the use of antibodies against the CD34 antigen that these cells bear); syngeneic bone marrow or stem cells from an identical twin; and allogeneic bone marrow or stem cells from major histocompatibility complex (MHC)-defined donors (MHC-identical siblings, MHC-identical unrelated individuals, MHC haplotype-matched donors, both related and unrelated, and MHC-mismatched donors). In vitro treatment of bone marrow to eliminate T cells is often undertaken to limit the extent of graft-vs-host disease (GVHD), but with a resulting decrease in immune responses to microbes. Each of these has a unique profile in terms of the effects on the recipient: incidence and severity of GVHD, rejection of the transplant, and the rate of recovery of bone marrow and immunologic function. These, in turn, dictate the profile of infections that occur posttransplant *(1,2,4–6)*.

A number of factors interact to determine the risk of infection following HSCT: the underlying disease that led to the transplantation effort; the conditioning regimen employed; the source of the stem cells and the manipulation of them prior to infusion into the recipient; the degree of histocompatibility mismatch between donor and recipient; the presence of such metabolic abnormalities as protein-calorie malnutrition, uremia, and, probably, hyperglycemia; the severity of GVHD that develops and the nature of the immunosuppressive program needed to control the GVHD; and the environmental exposures to which the recipient is subjected *(1,3,6,7)*.

Environmental exposures of importance include both those experienced in the community and those encountered within the hospital (*see* Table 1). Of particular concern are hospital exposures to opportunistic mold infection (not only *Aspergillus* species, but also such newly emerging molds as *Fusarium* and *Scedosporium*), *Legionella* species, and resistant Gram-negative bacilli such as *Pseudomonas aeruginosa*. Hospital exposures are further divided into domiciliary and nondomiciliary. Domiciliary exposures are those that occur in the room or on the ward where the patient is housed within the hospital—often there is clustering of cases in time and space. Table 2 delineates the steps that should be taken to prevent the occurrence of opportunistic infection within the hospital environment *(6–8)*.

Nondomiciliary, nosocomial exposures occur when patients are taken to other sites in the hospital environment for essential procedures and are exposed to contaminated air and/or potable water at this time. Nondomiciliary exposures are more difficult to detect because of the lack of clear-cut clustering of cases, but they are actually more common than domiciliary exposures, particularly with the widespread use of HEPA filters on transplant wards. Avoidance of exposures as the patient travels through the hospital must be aggressively pursued. In addition, HSCT recipients are at risk for person-to-person spread of such organisms as methicillin-resistant *Staphylococcus aureus*, vancomycin-resistant enterococci, β-lactamase-producing Gram-negative bacilli, and azole-resistant yeast on the hands of medical personnel. Finally, as will be discussed subsequently, person-to-person spread of respiratory virus infection (e.g., influenza, respiratory syncythial virus, parainfluenza, and others) can have a major effect on HSCT patients *(7,9)*.

Table 1
Infections in HSCT Patients Resulting From Excessive Environmental Hazards

Infections related to excessive nosocomial hazard
Aspergillus species
Legionella species
Pseudomonas aeruginosa and other Gram-negative bacilli
Nocardia asteroides
Infections related to particular exposures within the community
Systemic mycotic infections in certain geographic areas
Histoplasma capsulatum
Coccidioides immitis
Blastomyces dermatidis
Strongyloides stercoralis
Community-acquired opportunistic infection resulting from ubiquitous saphrophytes in the environment
Cryptococcus neoformans
Aspergillus species
Nocardia asteroides
Pneumocystis carinii
Respiratory infections circulating in the community
Mycobacterium tuberculosis
Influenza
Adenoviruses
Parainfluenza
Respiratory syncytial virus
Infections acquired by the ingestion of contaminated food/water
Salmonella species
Listeria monocytogenes

2. TEMPORAL COURSE OF INFECTION POST-HSCT

The rate at which immune and bone marrow (BM) reconstitution occurs following transplantation is the major factor in determining which infections occur at different time-points posttransplant. The first issue is the duration of severe granulocytopenia (the impact of which is compounded by the effects of the conditioning regimen on the barrier function of the oral and gut mucosa). The duration of severe granulocytopenia varies with the source of stem cells utilized: 20–25 d following the infusion of BM cells, 10–20 d for peripheral blood stem cells (PBDCs), and 25–35 d for umbilical cord blood transplants. Both granulocyte colony-stimulating factor (G-CSF) and granulocyte-macrophage colony-stimulating factor (GM-CSF) administration can be useful in shortening these time periods in some patients. After an aggressive myeloablative conditioning regimen, both B- and T-cell deficiencies may be present for months to years, as are the number of dendritic cells. In addition, functional deficits of both B and T cells may persist for months after a return to adequate numbers. Manipulations of the stem cells after harvest and before infusion into the recipient may further delay normalization of cell number and function. For example, CD34 selection and other types of T-cell depletion (TCD) of stem cells results in a significant delay in the recovery of lymphocytes and monocytes

Table 2
Infection Control Guidelines

AI Recommendations[a]

1. All personals should wash their hands before entering and after leaving the rooms of HSCT recipients and candidates undergoing conditioning therapy, or before any direct contact with patients regardless of whether they were soiled from the patient, environment, or objects.
2. All health care workers with diseases transmissible by air, droplet, and direct contact (e.g., varicella zoster virus, infectious gastroenteritis, herpes simplex lesions of lips or fingers, and upper respiratory tract infections) should be restricted from patient contact and temporarily reassigned to other duties.
3. When a case of laboratory-confirmed legionellosis is identified in a person who was in the inpatient HSCT center during all or part of the 2–10 d before illness onset or if two or more cases of laboratory-confirmed Legionnaire's disease occur among patients who had visited an outpatient HSCT center, hospital personnel in consultation with the hospital infection control team should perform a thorough epidemiologic and environmental investigation or determine the likely environmental source(s) of *Legionella* species (e.g., showers, tap water faucets, cooling towers, and hot water tanks).
4. To control VRE exposure, strict adherence to standard infection control measures is necessary, as outlined in the text.
5. All HCWs who anticipate contact with a *Clostridium difficile*-infected patient or patient's environment or possessions should put on gloves before entering the patient's room and before handling the patient's secretions and excretions.
6. HSCT candidates with a recently positive tuberculin skin test or a history of a positive skin test and no prior preventive therapy should be administered a chest radiograph and evaluated for active TB.

AII Recommendations[a]

1. HCST centers should prevent birds from gaining access to hospital air-intake ducts.
2. Appropriate gloves should be used by all persons when handling potentially contaminated biological materials.
3. Work exclusion policies should be designed to encourage HCWs to report their illnesses or exposures.
4. Visitors who might have communicable infectious disease (e.g., upper respiratory tract infections, flulike illnesses, recent exposure to communicable disease, an active shingles rash whether covered or not, a VZV-like rash within 6 wk of receiving a live attenuated varicella vaccine, or a history of receiving an oral polio vaccine within the previous 3–6 wk) should not be allowed in the HSCT center or have direct contact with HSCT recipients or candidates undergoing conditioning therapy.
5. If *Legionella* species are detected in the water supplying an HSCT center, the water supply should be decontaminated and eradication of *Legionella* should be verified.
6. HSCT centers should follow basic infection control practices for control of MRSA infection and colonization, including hand washing between patients and use of barrier precautions, including wearing gloves whenever entering the MRSA-infected or MRSA-colonized patient's room.
7. HSCT personnel should institute prudent use of all antibiotics, particularly vancomycin, to prevent the emergence of staphylococci with reduced susceptibility to vancomycin.
8. Use of intravenous vancomycin is associated with the emergence of VRE; vancomycin and all other antibiotics, particularly antiagaerobic agents, should be used judiciously.
9. All patients with *Clostridium difficile* disease should be placed under contact precautions for the duration of the illness.
10. When caring for an HCST recipient or candidate undergoing conditioning therapy with upper or lower respiratory tract infection, HCWs and visitors should change gloves and wash hands in circumstances outlined in the text.
11. Visitors and HCWs with infectious conjunctivitis should be restricted from direct patient contact until the drainage resolves and the ophthalmology consultant concurs that the infection and inflammation have resolved to avoid possible transmission of adenovirus to HSCT recipients.
12. For patients with suspected or proven pulmonary or laryngeal TB, HSCT personnel should follow guidelines regarding the control of TB in health care facilities.

[a]*Abbreviations*: HSCT, hematopoietic stem cell transplantation; TB, tuberculosis; VRE, vancomycin-resistant enterococci; HCWs, health care workers; VZV, varicella-zoster virus; MRSA, methicillin-resistant *Staphylococcus aurea*; AI = obligatory recommendations; AII = recommendations that should be followed in the majority of situations.

Source: Modified from ref. *7*.

and an increased risk of cytomegalovirus (CMV) disease and, presumably, other herpes group viruses *(1,2)*.

From this brief description, it is clear that the temporal course of infection following HSCT can be divided into three time periods (*see* Fig. 1) *(1,2,6,7)*.

1. **Phase I**: the period of profound granulocytopenia, which lasts from the administration of the conditioning regimen until engraftment has occurred. On average, this period lasts approx 30 d. The combination of profound granulocytopenia and mucositis makes the patient particularly vulnerable to bacterial and candidal infection. In addition, infection present in the transplant recipient pretransplant may be amplified by the granulocytopenic state and deficiencies of T- and B-cell numbers and function. Thus, control of pretransplant infection is needed prior to the initiation of the conditioning regimen. Prior to engraftment (both with autologous and allogeneic transplants), approx 50% of patients will have fever of unknown origin, with bloodstream infection in approx 12.5% and pneumonia in approx 10%.
2. **Phase II**: the period between engraftment and posttransplant d 100. During this time period, viral infections, particularly CMV and the other herpes group viruses, and invasive mold infections are the major concerns. If antimicrobial prophylaxis against these organisms is administered during this time period, the occurrence of these infections may be delayed into the late period more than 100 d posttransplant. Patients who fail to engraft, and thus have even more prolonged periods of granulocytopenia, are at particular risk for invasive fungal infection by both yeast and mold organisms. A not uncommon clinical problem during phase II is the occurrence of the idiopathic pneumonia syndrome, a diffuse, interstitial form of pneumonia (with radiologic findings similar to those observed with CMV or *Pneumocystis carinii*) of noninfectious etiology.
3. **Phase III**: the late period more than 100 d posttransplant. The major determinant of infection in the latter half of phase II and in phase III is the presence or absence of GVHD. In the absence of GVHD, the incidence of infection has decreased significantly, with varicella-zoster virus (VZV) and pneumococcal infection being the classical problems of this time period. In addition, late or relapsing CMV infection may be manifest during this time period. If GVHD is present, it will be treated with such powerful immunosuppressive drugs as cyclosporine (or tacrolimus), high-dose corticosteroids, mycophenolate, and even monoclonal antibodies. Patients in this last category (GVHD under treatment) are at particular risk for invasive mold infection, viruses, *P. carinii*, and other opportunistic pathogens.

3. PRINCIPLES OF ANTIMICROBIAL THERAPY IN THE HSCT RECIPIENT

There are four modes in which antimicrobial therapy can be administered to the HSCT patient *(7)*:

1. A **therapeutic** mode, in which antimicrobial therapy is prescribed for the treatment and eradication of microbes causing clinical illness.
2. A **prophylactic** mode, in which antimicrobial therapy is prescribed to an entire population before an event to prevent clinically important infection. For such a strategy to be successful, the infection(s) being targeted must be important enough to justify the intervention and the antimicrobial therapy prescribed must be nontoxic enough and inexpensive enough to justify the intervention. By far the most effective antimicrobial prophylactic strategy is low-dose trimethoprim-sulfamethoxazole, which has virtually eliminated the occurrence of *P. carinii*, *Listeria monocytogenes*, *Nocardia asteroides*, and *Toxoplasma gondii* in patients compliant with the regimen. Other prophylactic strategies commonly utilized in HSCT patients include

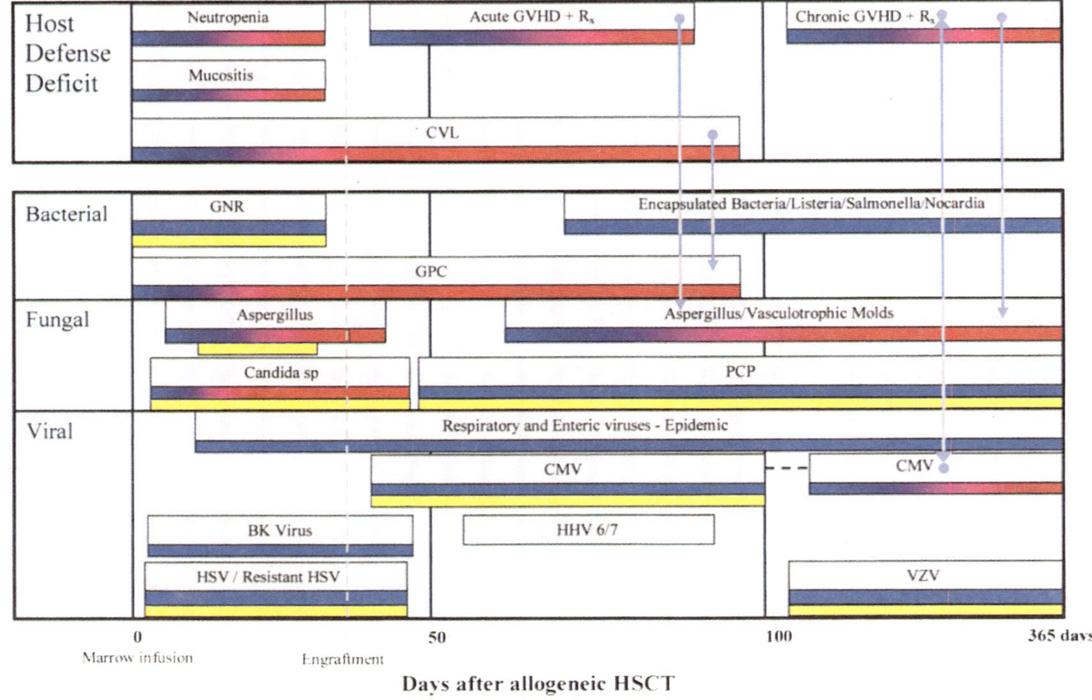

Fig. 1. Timetable of infection for allogeneic HSCT patients receiving antimicrobial prophylaxis. This figure outlines the time period of the major host deficits and infections, which occur during allogeneic HSCT in relation to when targeted pathogen-specific prophylactic, pre-emptive, and empiric therapies are deployed. Risk for infectious complications are temporally dependent and are significantly decreased in the setting of prophylactic, pre-emptive, or empiric therapy. The risk of certain infections after transplantation is highly associated with ongoing immunologic manipulation as seen with the therapy for GVHD (linkages noted by vertical arrows). CVL = central venous line, GVHD = graft-vs-host disease, GNR = Gram-negative rods, GPC = Gram-positive cocci, PCP = *Pneumocystis carnii* pneumonia, CMV = cytomegalovirus, HHV- 6/7 = human herpes virus 6/7, HSV = herpes simplex virus, and VZV = varicella-zoster virus. Standard prophylactic considerations in this context include the following: GNR= fluoroquinolone or trimethoprim/sulfamethoxazole; *Candida* sp. = fluconazole; PCP = trimethoprim/sulfamethoxazole, atovaquone, dapsone, or pentamidine; and HSV/VZV = acyclovir. Standard emipiric therapeutic considerations in this setting include the following: GNR = ceftazidime, piperacillin/gentamicin, or imipenem; aspergillus/molds/candida = amphotericin preparations or extended spectrum azoles; and CMV = iv ganciclovir, valganciclovir, or pre-emptive monitoring (by antigenemia or polymerase chain reaction).

fluoroquinolones *(5)* to prevent Gram-negative sepsis, fluconazole to prevent yeast infection, and anti-CMV prophylaxis.

3. An **empiric** mode, in which antimicrobial therapy is administered in response to a symptom complex. In this context, empiric antimicrobial therapy is initiated during the period of profound granulocytopenia in response to fever ± rigors or subtle signs of sepsis (unexplained hypotension, tachypnea, an ongoing volume requirement, or acidosis). In the patient deemed not to be a therapeutic emergency, initial therapy is usually aimed at aerobic Gram-negative bacilli (e.g., the Enterobacteriaceae or *Pseudomonas aeruginosa*). A variety of drugs have been utilized for this purpose, depending in part on the nature of particular problem organisms found at a given medical center. Advanced-spectrum β-lactams (e.g., ceftazadime or imipenem), either alone or together with an aminoglycoside or a fluoroquinolone, are the mainstays of this approach. In the setting of severe illness, vancomycin may be started cocontemperaneously with the diagnostic evaluation. If 2–5 d of such broad-spectrum therapy is unsuccessful, then empiric antifungal therapy with amphotericin B deoxycholate, a lipid-associated amphotericin preparation, intravenous itraconazole, or possibly voriconazole should be initiated. Thus, empiric therapy is based on an algorithm rather than on microbiologic or other studies.
4. A **pre-emptive** mode, in which antimicrobial therapy is prescribed to a small percentage of patients deemed to be at particularly high risk because of clinical/epidemiologic information or the isolation of microbial pathogens. This approach is being particularly evaluated for the prevention of CMV disease. Pre-emptive therapy is meant to prevent symptomatic infection by targeting individuals at particularly high risk as determined by objective information as opposed to an algorithm. Examples of pre-emptive therapy being used at many transplant centers include the following: control of CMV infection by monitoring patients for evidence of preclinical viremia (by antigenemia or polymerase chain reaction [PCR] assays), with initiation of antiviral therapy immediately on demonstration of viremia; initiation of antifungal therapy (with an amphotericin preparation or voriconazole) upon the demonstration of respiratory tract colonization by *Aspergillus* species, *Fusarium*, or *Scedosporium*. Such colonization in the case of *Aspergillus* (and by analogy the other two invasive molds) carries a greater than 50% risk of subsequent invasive disease; serial measurements of galactomannan, a cell wall antigen of *Aspergillus*, or a PCR assay for fungal nucleic acid appears to have potential as an "early warning system" for the presence of early invasive disease, which could then leadto pre-emptive therapy.

One other aspect of antimicrobial therapy in the HSCT patient bears emphasis here: the possibility of drug interactions between antimicrobial drugs and the calcineurin inhibitors (cyclosporine and tacrolimus), which are mainstays of the immunosuppressive regimens prescribed to prevent and treat GVHD. There are basically three categories of interaction, two of which are related to the major route of drug metabolism for the calcineurin inhibitors, hepatic cytochrome P450 enzymatic metabolism. These possible interactions are as follows: (1) Certain antimicrobial agents (most notably rifampin, rifabutin, nafcillin, and isoniazid) upregulate the metabolism of the calcineurin inhibitors, leading to a fall in blood levels and an increased risk of GVHD. (2) Certain antimicrobial agents (most notably the macrolides, erythromycin > clarithromycin > azithromycin, and the azoles, ketoconazole > itraconazole > voriconazole > fluconazole) will downregulate the metabolism of the calcineurin inhibitors, resulting in elevated blood levels of active drug, an increased risk of nephrotoxicity, as well as overimmunosuppression and an increased incidence of opportunistic infection. (3) Therapeutic blood levels of the calcineurin inhibitors, when combined with such drugs as amphotericin B, aminoglycosides, and vancomycin can cause significant renal toxicity. There are three forms of toxicity that can be observed in this situation: accelerated nephrotoxicity, in which renal dysfunction occurs at an accelerated rate (e.g., creatinine elevations occurring after only a few doses of amphotericin); idiosyncratic nephrotoxicity, in which single doses of amphotericin, gentamicin, or intravenous trimethoprim–sulfamethoxazole in the face of therapeutic blood levels of the calcineurin inhibitor precipitated oliguric renal failure; and dose-related nephrotoxicity such that prophylactic doses of trimethoprim–sulfamethoxazole (e.g., one single-strength tablet once or twice daily) are well tolerated, whereas *Pneumocystis* treatment doses are not; similarly, 250 mg of ciprofloxacin twice daily is without adverse effect, whereas 500 mg twice daily may produce nephrotoxicity *(7,10)*.

These issues related to antimicrobial therapy lead to the following policies. Particular emphasis is placed on the prevention of infection (usually via prophylactic or pre-emptive strategies, but with empiric intervention if necessary). Antimicrobial choices usually include advanced-spectrum β-lactams, fluoroquinolones, and azoles, whereas aminoglycosides and amphotericin must be used with great care. The effects of these drugs on calcineurin inhibitor metabolism should dictate close monitoring of blood levels of these drugs, with dosage adjustment as needed, both with the initiation of the antimicrobial agent in question and after its termination.

4. INFECTIONS OF PARTICULAR IMPORTANCE IN THE HSCT RECIPIENT

4.1. Bloodstream Infection

Given the nature, duration, and severity of host defense defects present in HSCT patients, it is not surprising that bloodstream infection is a regular feature of the posttransplant course. The greatest number of bloodstream infections occurs during the period prior to engraftment when a variety of factors interact with the severe granulocytopenia that is characteristic of the pre-engraftment period. These factors include mucositis, permitting the translocation of bacteria and *Candida species* from the oral cavity and gut into the circulation and the presence of vascular access devices that traverse the skin and serve as direct conduits into the systemic circulation. Thus, the primary mucocutaneous barriers to infection are compromised, and the absence of granulocytes only amplifies the susceptibility of the patient *(1,2,7)*.

Whereas Gram-negative bacteremia was the major cause of bloodstream infection 15–30 yr ago, today Gram-positive organisms are the most frequent cause of positive blood cultures. The possible reasons for this shift are many: the widespread use of fluoroquinolones, with their potent activity against Gram-negative bacteria, as prophylaxis during this period; the presence of indwelling central venous catheters for prolonged periods; and the widespread use of systemic anti-Gram-negative therapy—all of these contribute to the Gram-positive predominance. The bacteria isolated during the pre-engraftment period, then, include staphylococci (especially coagulase negative staphylococci), viridans streptococci, enterococci, and corynebacteria, with fewer isolates of Enterobacteriaceae or *P. aeruginosa* being identified. An increasing problem in the HSCT population is antibiotic-resistant organisms, particularly vancomycin-resistant enterococci, methicillin-resistant *Staphylococcus aureus*, and resistant Gram-negative bacilli (such as hyper-β-lactamase producing *Klebsiella* and chromosomal-inducible β-lactamase producing *Enterobacter* species) *(1,2,7,9,11–15)*.

The standard of care at present for the severely granulocytopenic patient is the initiation of empiric antibacterial therapy in response to an unexplained fever or other signs of sepsis. What remains controversial is what the regimen should be. Because of the rapidity with which clinical deterioration can occur with untreated Gram-negative sepsis in the granulocytopenic patient, anti-Gram-negative therapy is always employed. How best to accomplish this is an important issue. The traditional approach of a β-lactam plus an aminoglycoside is still favored by many experts, although nephrotoxicity from the aminoglycoside has led to the trial of other approaches: the substitution of a fluoroquinolone for the aminoglycoside (although if a fluoroquinolone is being used for prophylaxis, it is less attractive as part of a therapeutic regimen) or the prescription of a single advanced-spectrum drug such as imipenem, ceftazadime, or cefepime. An intermediate strategy is to combine an advanced-spectrum β-lactam with an aminoglycoside for 72 h and then continue with the β-lactam alone, thus allowing for early control of infection with a minimum incidence of toxicity. The second area of controversy is whether empiric Gram-positive coverage should be initiated at the same time, given the preponderance of Gram-positive infection. As there is typically time to evaluate culture data and deploy targeted Gram-positive antimicrobial therapy rather than empiricism, vancomycin is rarely required empirically. Indications for the immediate initiation of vancomycin as part of the empiric therapy regimen include the following *(5,9,11–15)*:

1. Line sepsis is likely because of evidence of infection at the insertion site (or within the tunnel).
2. Severe illness such as shock and/or respiratory distress are present.
3. The patient is at particular risk for seeding of a prosthetic device (e.g., a prosthetic valve, a hip prosthesis, etc.).
4. The empiric Gram-negative coverage exclusively covers aerobic Gram-negative rods, such as the combination of aztreonam and gentamicin.

The empiric approach taken should be based on a determination of how acutely ill the patient is. If it is deemed a therapeutic emergency with ongoing deterioration and shock, then the antibacterial regimen utilized should be imipenem or ceftazadime and gentamicin plus vancomycin, with appropriate revision once culture information becomes available. If the patient is stable, then any one of the following regimens would be reasonable: piperacillin plus gentamicin, ceftazadime alone, or imipenem alone. Vancomycin should be added if there is evidence for a Gram-positive infection such as a skin source or positive culture results. If the patient responds to the empiric regimen, then it is usually continued until the granulocytopenia resolves. Cessation of therapy after the patient has made a clinical response with resolution of fever and negative cultures but remains neutropenic has been shown to be associated with a high risk of clinical deterioration and should be avoided in most situations *(16)*.

Although patients with indwelling central venous catheters are at risk for bloodstream infection at any time, there is another specific situation in which the patient post HSCT is at risk. Patients with chronic GVHD are at risk for invasive infection from encapsulated organisms, particularly *S. pneumoniae*, *Haemophilus influenzae*, and *Neisseria meningitidis*. It is postulated that the combination of B-lymphocyte dysfunction secondary to the conditioning regimen and the effects of GVHD and its treatment have resulted in the loss and failure to develop opsonizing antibody to these organisms, particularly *S. pneumoniae* (with recurrent pneumococcal bacteremia being not uncommon in patients with chronic GVHD). In addition, for 1–2 yr posttransplant, HSCT patients have an inadequate response to pneumococcal vaccine. IgG levels should be monitored as well, with intravenous IgG being used when IgG level falls below 500 mg/mL *(17,18)*. For each of these reasons, antimicrobial prophylaxis is advocated. Before the widespread occurrence of penicillin-resistant pneumococci, penicillin was the treatment of choice. Presently, long-term, low-dose trimethoprim–sulfamethoxazole (one single-strength tablet daily) appears to be the prophylaxis of choice for this problem *(1,6)*.

Candidemia is the other major cause of bloodstream infection in phase I HSCT patients (pre-engraftment). Although there is the possibility that the portal of entry can be vascular access catheters, it is believed that translocation of *Candida* species across gut mucosa damaged by the pretransplant conditioning regimen is the major route of access to the bloodstream in the granulocytopenic patient. In the past, *C. albicans* and *C. tropicalis* accounted for virtually all of the *Candida* bloodstream infections. The incidence of candidemia was approx 11–16% (with a median time of onset of 2 wk posttransplant), resulting in a high rate of tissue invasion and an attributable mortality of nearly 40%. With the introduction of fluconazole prophylaxis (400 mg/d) during the pre-engraftment period and upon the diagnosis of GVHD, the incidence of candidemia has been halved (11% to 5%), *C. albicans* and *C. tropicalis* have been virtually eliminated, hepatosplenic candidiasis has become quite rare, and the attributable mortality has been significantly decreased (with maintenance of the mortality benefit over a period of several years). *Candida krusei* and *C. glabrata* have become not uncommon causes of candidemia in HSCT patients, as have the other non-*albicans Candida* species. The attributable mortality as a result of invasive candidiasis has been reported to range from 15% to 38%. In addition, late complications of candidemia may occur; these include endophthalmitis and chronic disseminated (hepatosplenic) candidiasis. These typically occur weeks to months after the episode of candidemia and are the reason that all cases of candidemia must trigger the use of systemic antifungal therapy for 2–4 wk even if the patient becomes asymptomatic just with the removal of the vascular access device *(1,4,7,19–24)*.

It is also important to recognize that other species of yeast (e.g., *Trichosporon* species) can cause clinical syndromes identical to those observed with invasive candidiasis (bloodstream infection, infection metastatic to the skin and subcutaneous tissues as well as other sites, including hepatosplenic disease identical to that caused by *Candida* species). Because organisms such as *Trichosporon* are often resistant to conventional antifungal drugs, (but with apparent susceptibility to the extended spectrum triazoles, such as newly licensed voriconazole), definitive diagnosis should be sought, even if tissue biopsy is required *(1,7,19)*.

4.2. Intravascular-Catheter-Related Infection

The surgical placement of tunneled multilumen central venous catheters for long-term use has become the standard of care for HSCT patients. The incidence of infection with these devices is significantly less than for short-term, nontunneled, single-lumen or multilumen central venous catheters (<1% vs 3–5%). Table 3 delineates the recommendations of the Healthcare Infection Control Practices Advisory Committee for the prevention of intravenous-access-device-related infection *(7,25–28)*.

Intravascular catheter infection should be considered in the febrile, granulocytopenic patient under the following circumstances: the presence of inflammation or gross purulence at the site of insertion; the absence of other sites of infection; abrupt onset of symptoms, including evidence of hypotension; positive blood cultures with microbial flora commonly found on the skin: *S. aureus*, coagulase-negative staphylococci, *Corynebacterium* spp., *Bacillus* spp., and *Candida* spp. The key question in patients with intravascular-catheter-related infection is whether or not effective therapy can be accomplished with the catheter remaining in place. Short-term, nontunneled catheters should be removed, with placement of a new catheter percutaneously at a new site *(26)*.

Table 3
Healthcare Infection Control Practices Advisory Committee (HICPAC) Recommendations for the Prevention of Intravenous-Device-Related Bloodstream Infections (IVDR BSI)

- General Measures
  - Education of all healthcare workers involved with vascular access regarding indications for use, proper insertion technique, and maintenance of IVDs
  - Surveillance
    - Institutional rates of IVDR BSI monitored routinely
    - Rates of central venous catheter (CVC)-related BSI using standardized definitions and denominators, expressed per 1000 CVC-d
- At Insertion
  - Aseptic technique
    - Hand washing before inserting or manipulation of any IVD
    - Clean or sterile gloves during insertion or manipulation of noncentral IVD
    - Maximal barrier precautions (mask, cap, long-sleeved sterile gown, sterile gloves, and sterile sheet-drape) during insertion of CVCs
  - Dedicated iv teams strongly recommended
  - Cutaneous antisepsis: chlorhexidine preferred; however, an iodophor, such as 10% povidone–iodine, tincture of iodine, or 70% alcohol also acceptable
  - Sterile gauze or a sterile semipermeable polyurethane film dressing
  - Systemic antibiotics at insertion strongly discouraged
- Maintenance
  - Remove IVDs as soon as their use is no longer essential
  - Monitor the IVD site on regular basis, ideally daily
  - Change dressing of CVC insertion site at least weekly
  - Topical antibiotic ointments not recommended
    - Systemic anticoagulation with low-dose warfarin (1 mg daily) for patients with long-term IVDs and no contraindication.
    - Replace PIVCs every 72 h
    - Replace administration sets every 72 h unless lipid-containing admixture or blood products given, then every 24 h
- Technology
  - Consider use of chlorhexidine-impregnated sponge dressing with adolescent and adult patients with noncuffed central venous or arterial catheters expected to remain in plance for 4 d or more.
  - *If* after consistent application of basic infection control precautions, the institutional rate of IVDR BSI is yet high with short-term CVCs (3.3 BSIs per 1000 IVD-days), consider the use of an anti-infective coated CVC (chlorhexidine–silver sulfadiazine or minocycline–rifampin).
  - *In individual patients* with long-term IVDs who have had recurrent IVDR BSIs despite consistent application of infection control practices, consider the use of a prophylactic antibiotic lock solution (i.e., heparin with vancomycin (25 μg/mL), with or without ciprofloxacin (2 μg/mL).

Source: Adapted from the draft of the Healthcare Infection Control Practices Advisory Committee (HICPAC) guideline for the prevention of intravascular-catheter-related infections *(10)*.

In contrast, salvage of a long-term, surgically placed (tunneled) catheter is possible under certain circumstances. First, there is an absolute requirement for bactericidal therapy if this salvage effort is to be made. The greatest success in this endeavor is when the infecting organisms are coagulase-negative staphylococci, with a success rate of approx 75% with 2–3 wk of therapy through the infected line. In addition, some authorities advocate the placement of a highly concentrated solution of the antimicrobial being used (e.g., vancomycin) locked into the catheter while systemic therapy is being administered, claiming 90% success with this combination approach. On the other hand, if infection is caused by *S. aureus*, *Bacillus* spp., *Corynebacterium JK*, *Stenotrophomonas* spp., *B. cepacia*, all *Pseudomonas* spp., fungi, or mycobacterial species, the catheter should be removed early in the treatment program *(1,2,4,7)*.

4.3. Viral Infections in HSCT Recipients

There are two classes of viral infection of particular importance in the HSCT recipient: those resulting from herpes group viruses (cytomegalovirus [CMV], Epstein–Barr virus [EBV], herpes simplex virus [HSV], varicella-zoster virus [VZV], and human herpesvirus-6, -7, and -8 [HHV-6, -7, -8]) and those resulting from respiratory viruses (e.g., influenza, respiratory syncytial virus [RSV], parainfluenza, adenoviruses, and others). The human herpes group viruses share a number of characteristics that make them particularly effective pathogens in HSCT recipients *(1,7,10)*:

1. **Latency**. Once infected with a herpes group virus, one is infected for life, with circulating antibody (seropositivity) in the absence of active viral replication being the marker for latent infection. The mechanisms by which latent virus is reactivated have been best studied with CMV where the major pathway for reactivation is triggered by tumor necrosis factor (TNF), with the catecholamines epinephrine and norepinephrine and pro-inflammatory prostaglandins also playing a role. Thus, virus is reactivated by such processes as sepsis, GVHD, and allogeneic reactions. Of interest, although OKT3 and antilymphocyte globulin are potent reactivators of CMV and presumably the other herpes viruses, cyclosporine, tacrolimus, and steroids play no role in reactivating these viruses. However, once a replicating virus is present, these agents, particularly cyclosporine and tacrolimus, amplify the extent of this replication (indeed, we refer to these agents as "in vivo PCRs for these viruses").
2. **Cell association**. These viruses are highly cell associated, meaning that transmission is through intimate person to person contact, transfusion, or transplantation of latently or actively replicating cells from a seropositive donor. Humoral immunity is hence less important than cell-mediated immunity. Indeed, the key host defense is accomplished by MHC-restricted, virus-specific, cytotoxic T cells—just that component of host defense most affected by GVHD and its treatment.
3. **Oncogenesis**. There are at least two mechanisms by which herpes group viruses can play a role in oncogenesis: EBV and HHV-8 are directly oncogenic, causing the posttransplant lymphoproliferative disease and Kaposi's sarcoma, respectively. In addition, it is highly likely that cytokines, chemokines, and growth factors produced by the transplant recipient in response to replication by these viruses can modulate the oncogenic potential in given patients. For example, among solid-organ transplant patients, symptomatic CMV disease increases the incidence of EBV-associated posttransplant lymphoproliferative disease approx 10-fold.
4. **Indirect effects**. In addition to the direct causation of infectious disease syndromes, human herpes viruses, particularly CMV, have indirect effects that are clinically important. It is believed that cytokines, chemokines, and growth factors produced in response to viral replication are responsible for these effects. These include, in addition to the modulation of oncogenesis, increasing the net state of immunosuppression so that the risk of opportunistic infection is increased and playing a role in the occurrence of GVHD. This last point is particularly important, as a variety of experiments have shown that GVHD and infection are closely linked

by the production of these mediators; that is, there is a bidirectional trafficking of mediators between the two processes that determines the clinical fate of the patient.

4.3.1. Cytomegalovirus

Manifestations of CMV post-HSCT are many, reflecting the fact that endothelial cell replication is an important part of the pathogenesis of CMV; this virus produces a "viral vasculitis" affecting multiple organs. The clinically most important direct effects of CMV in the HSCT recipient are pneumonia and gastrointestinal disease. CMV as a cause of fever is common, and other effects (hepatitis, BM dysfunction, retinitis, and encephalitis) may occur. The risk of CMV is greatest in the seropositive recipient, although the virus clearly can be transmitted via transfusion or transplantation. The risk of CMV is greater in allogeneic than autologous transplants, although if CD34 stem cell selection is employed, the incidence will increase. A traditionally important source of CMV has been viable leukocyte-containing transfusions; it is important to provide either CMV seronegative blood products or utilize effective leukocyte removal filters in order to prevent acquisition of the virus by this route. If an individual is CMV seronegative and is sexually active, then safe sex practices are urged, particularly the use of condoms *(1,7)*.

The most effective therapy for clinical CMV is ganciclovir, which can be administered either intravenously or orally in the form of a prodrug, valganciclovir, with an acceptable bioavailability profile (approx 50%). Typically, the parenteral form is administered until viremia has cleared (approx 3 wk) followed by approx 3 mo of the oral agent. In the case of serious illness, particularly pneumonia, anti-CMV hyperimmune globulin is usually administered as well. The mortality from CMV pneumonia despite these efforts remains at an unacceptable level of greater than 50%. The major toxicity of ganciclovir is BM toxicity, so that great effort is placed in monitoring these patients closely and adjusting doses appropriately *(1,7)*.

There is a form of pneumonia that closely resembles CMV pneumonia (peak incidence approx 6 wk posttransplant, interstitial infiltrates on X-ray, subacute onset) that is of unknown etiology. There are currently two theories of pathogenesis: The first is that the pneumonia the result of radiation and chemotherapy toxicity; others have suggested that HHV-6 is involved. Optimal therapy for this process is unknown, although most centers usually end up using corticosteroids *(1,7)*.

Emphasis is placed as well in preventing CMV disease, with two preventative strategies used. The first is prophylaxis with a ganciclovir preparation from the time of engraftment until at least d 100 posttransplant *(29,30)*. Alternatively, a pre-emptive strategy is employed in which patients are monitored for viremia weekly through either a PCR assay for CMV DNA or an antigenemia assay. Typically, these assays turn positive several days to weeks prior to the onset of clinical disease, permitting the use of effective pre-emptive therapy (3 wk or more of ganciclovir treatment, with continuing close follow-up for viremia posttreatment) *(1,7,31–35)*.

In the preganciclovir era, CMV disease occurred primarily approx 6 wk posttransplant. Increasingly, with the widespread use of a prophylactic or pre-emptive antiviral strategy, breakthrough occurs much later, 170 or more days posttransplant. Risk factors for late CMV disease include chronic GVHD, low CD4– T-cell counts, and CMV infection before d 100. Relapsing disease also can occur, particularly in the face of high viral loads and inadequate courses of ganciclovir. In that case, combination therapy with foscarnet and ganciclovir or with foscarnet alone becomes necessary. Foscarnet and the third-choice drug cidofovir are both associated with significant nephrotoxicity and are to be avoided if possible, being utilized only in the setting of antiviral resistance *(1,7)*.

4.3.2. Epstein–Barr Virus

The major recognizable clinical effect of EBV in the HSCT patient is in the pathogenesis of posttransplant lymphoproliferative disease (PTLD). Following the recovery from primary EBV infection (>95% of the adult population), ongoing lytic infection of B cells occurs in the oropharynx, with latent infection of B cells being seen in the peripheral blood and lymphoid tissues. These latently infected cells are transformed and immortalized, resulting in polyclonal proliferation. In the normal seropositive individual, these cells are kept in check by a specific cytotoxic T-cell response. In the presence of immunosuppressive therapy, this surveillance system is inhibited in a dose-related fashion, thus permitting continued B-cell proliferation. Such ongoing proliferation results in particular clones being favored and the potential for the development of cytogenetic abnormalities, which leads to the development of a truly malignant process—PTLD *(1,7,10,36)*.

The spectrum of clinical disease seen with PTLD is quite broad, ranging from a polyclonal mononucleosislike process that usually responds to decreasing immunosuppressive therapy to a monoclonal, highly malignant B-cell lymphoma. The mononucleosislike process is seen particularly in children with primary EBV infection. The clinical presentation is one of fever, sore throat, cervical adenopathy, and tonsillar hypertrophy and inflammation. Unlike B-cell lymphoma in the normal host, in the transplant patient, particularly the adult, the process can be totally extranodal. Thus, presentations include central nervous system (CNS) invasion (from involvement of the meninges to focal cerebral lesions) and liver, lung, and BM disease. Not uncommonly, involvement of the gut (particularly the small bowel) may lead to recognition of the PTLD, with a clinical presentation of small bowel obstruction, perforation, or occult gastrointestinal bleeding. Disseminated, multiorgan disease is quite common in the HSCT patient *(1,7,10,36)*.

Risk factors for the development of PTLD include the following: (1) primary EBV infection in association with high-dose immunosuppression; (2) such interventions as T-cell depletion, myeloablative conditioning regimens, and the systemic administration of antithymocyte globulin or OKT3 increase the risk significantly; (3) mismatched BM and the accompanying GVHD appear to increase the risk of PTLD, with a postulated mechanism that chronic MHC antigenic stimulation results in increased numbers of B cells that become immortalized, providing a rich background for the development of PTLD; (4) Intensive immunosuppression that results in suppression of the key host defense against EBV transformed cells (MHC-restricted, EBV-specific, cytotoxic T cells) significantly increases the risk of PTLD. In addition to the host characteristics mentioned, high EBV viral loads correlate with an increased risk of PTLD. It has been suggested that EBV viral load surveillance in the oropharynx and/or peripheral blood be carried out in high-risk patients (those with primary EBV infection, anti-T-cell antibody therapy for GVHD, non-MHC-identical, T-cell-depleted HSCT recipients), with decreased immunosuppression ± antiviral therapy (acyclovir or ganciclovir) carried out in the setting of high viral loads *(1,7,10,36)*.

Treatment of PTLD remains controversial. All patients with diagnosed PTLD should have greater than 50% decrease in immunosuppressive drugs, particularly cyclosporine and tacrolimus. Most centers also prescribe antiviral therapy. Patients not responding to these measures are usually then treated with an anti-B-cell monoclonal antibody (rituximab, an anti-CD20 monoclonal antibody) *(37,38)*. After that, therapies have ranged from antilymphoma chemotherapy to IFN-α and intravenous γ-globulin. Two interesting new approaches include the infusion of lymphocytes from the stem cell donor and treatment with a monoclonal antibody to interleukin (IL)-6 *(39,40)*. The response of patients to the antibody to IL-6 re-emphasizes the importance of the cytokine milieu in the pathogenesis of this and other processes in HSCT patients.

4.3.3. Herpes Simplex Virus

Herpes simplex virus infection prior to the introduction of acyclovir was a major problem in the HSCT recipient. Occurring in the pre-engraftment period, HSV infection greatly exacerbated the severity of mucositis. Not only were ulcers observed in the oral cavity and anogenital areas, ulcerations of the esophagus, stomach, and intestine were observed. HSV pneumonia was also noted, with rare cases of cutaneous dissemination and encephalitis noted. The standard of care now is to test all candidates for HSCT for antibody to HSV, with seropositive individuals then placed on antiviral prophylaxis, beginning 1 wk before HSCT and continuing for 1 mo. Effective agents include the following: acyclovir (intravenous or oral), valacyclovir, or famciclovir. Recurrence of HSV may occur later in the course and should again be treated with an acyclovir regimen, with repeated episodes justifying long-term prophylaxis. Acyclovir resistance is uncommon in this situation, but can occur, and it requires treatment with foscarnet *(1,7)*.

4.3.4. Varicella-Zoster Virus

All patients prior to transplant should have serologic testing for VZV. If possible, VZV vaccine (a live, attenuated vaccine) should be administered prior to immunosuppression. Seronegative individuals post-transplant should avoid exposures to VZV, but when such occurs varicella-zoster immune globulin (VZIG), and valacyclovir should be promptly initiated. An estimated 40% of HSCT patients may develop active VZV, with a median time of onset being approx 5 mo posttransplant. The great majority of these patients have zoster, but approx 20% will have a more generalized process resembling primary varicella. Without prompt antiviral therapy, at least one-third of these patients will die. VZV is more common and severe in patients with allogeneic transplants, particularly those with chronic GVHD. If CD34 selection is utilized, then autologous patients parallel the allogeneic patients in incidence and severity. The big fear is visceral involvement in the setting of disseminated disease. Early treatment is mandatory, with high-dose intravenous acyclovir for 3–7 d, followed by oral valacyclovir. Relapsing infection can occur and sustained treatment is indicated if this occurs. VZV vaccine post-HSCT is contraindicated for at least 2 yr posttransplant, and unless a research study or close follow-up is involved, it should be omitted indefinitely posttransplant *(1,41–43)*.

4.3.5. Human Herpesvirus-6

Herpesvirus-6 is a β-herpesvirus (as is CMV), whose role is just now being defined. In the great majority of instances, HHV-6 primary infection occurs in the first year of life, with a seroprevalence rate of 90% at 1 yr and close to 100% at 3 yr. The clinical effects associated with primary HHV-6 infection include a febrile exanthem called exanthem subitum and a form of encephalitis. It has also been suggested that HHV-6 plays a role in the pathogenesis of multiple sclerosis. In HSCT patients, BM suppression, especially delayed platelet engraftment, has been associated with this virus. In addition, interstitial pneumonia and encephalitis have been linked, but not definitively shown, to this virus. HHV-6 is associated with CMV much of the time, and the suggestion has been made that the combination of these viruses is clinically more potent than either virus by itself. Diagnosis of HHV-6 infection is best accomplished by PCR assay of plasma. Ganciclovir is the treatment of choice for this virus. It is clearly possible that anti-CMV preventative strategies with ganciclovir are also having a beneficial effect on this virus as well *(1)*.

4.3.6. Respiratory Viruses

Hematopoeitic SCT recipients are at significant risk for infection with respiratory viruses circulating in the community. These infections can occur at any time in the posttransplant course and can be acquired in the community or during hospitalization from infected staff, family, and friends. Overall, an estimated 10–20% of HSCT patients will become infected in the first year posttransplant, with the potential for this figure to rise significantly in the setting of a communitywide outbreak. The dilemma for the clinician is how to prevent these infections, as there is a far higher rate of progression to pneumonia (viral and/or bacterial or fungal superinfection), which carries a far higher morbidity and mortality than what is observed in the general population. In addition, antiviral therapy for these agents is in its infancy, and although influenza vaccine can be administered as a killed viral vaccine, its efficacy is greatly attenuated by the immunosuppressed state present in HSCT patients. Thus, at the present time, avoidance of exposure to infected individuals is the best preventative strategy available *(44–47)*.

4.3.7. Respiratory Syncytial Virus

Although RSV can be acquired through inhalation of an aerosol, direct contact with infected secretions is the usual mode of spread between individuals. In the HSCT patient, both adult and pediatric, RSV is a cause of significant morbidity and mortality. The illness begins with the signs and symptoms of a viral upper-respiratory-tract infection (rhinorrhea, sinus congestion, sore throat, and/or otitis media), with progression to pneumonia being common, especially if the virus is acquired in the pre-engraftment phase. The advent of rapid RSV diagnosis by antigen detection in nasopharyngeal swabs has resulted in the recognition that RSV is a significant pathogen for both adults and children, particularly in immunosuppressed patients. Optimal antiviral management, however, remains unclear. There are reports that aerosolized ribavirin ± anti-RSV polyclonal or monoclonal antibody has therapeutic benefit, but this remains unproven. The data currently available suggest that therapy is most effective if instituted prior to progression to pneumonia—a preemptive strategy. There is also interest in prophylaxis with an anti-RSV antibody, although there have been no trials in HSCT patients *(44–47)*.

4.3.8. Influenza

As with RSV, the incidence of influenza infection in HSCT patients reflects the level of influenza activity in the community. Thus, there is considerable variation in incidence; the best estimate is that 10–30% of patients requiring hospitalization for acute respiratory complaints have influenza. The impact of this virus when HSCT recipients are infected are demonstrated by the following statistics: approx 60% of the patients with influenza developed pneumonia and approx 25% of patients with influenza die of progressive respiratory failure. Therapy of influenza in this patient population is in its infancy; therefore, prevention is of great importance. Vaccination each year is recommended, but its benefit is attenuated; indeed, it is probably fair to say that maximal benefit from vaccination occurs when the vaccine is administered to healthcare workers, family, friends, and other contacts of the patient. Prevention with amantadine, rimantadine, or the new neuraminidase inhibitors has not yet been accomplished, so, at present, this cannot be recommended outside a research environment. When an infection is diagnosed, early treatment should be considered *(47)*.

4.3.9. Other Respiratory Viruses

Parainfluenza, adenoviruses, rhinoviruses, and coronaviruses are all capable of causing lower respiratory tract infection in HSCT recipients. Again, therapy is not available, emphasizing infection-control strategies in the hospital setting and avoidance of individuals with respiratory tract complaints at home. When upper-respiratory-tract complaints occur in HSCT patients, they should have a diagnosis made, utilizing rapid diagnostic techniques (e.g., antigen-detection assays), pre-emptive therapy, when available, should be initiated, immunosuppressive therapy should be diminished, and isolation from other HSCT patients should be accomplished.

4.4. Fungal Infections in the HSCT Recipient

There are three categories of fungal infection that can invade the HSCT patient: (1) the opportunistic fungi, which cause greater than 90% of the fungal infections that occur in the HSCT patient (*Candida*, *Aspergillus*, and *Cryptococcus* being the most important of these infections); (2) the geographically restricted systemic mycoses (*Blastomyces dermatitidis*, *Coccidioides immitis*, and *Histoplasma capsulatum*); and (3) invasive infection as a result of the so-called "newly emerging fungi" (*Fusarium*, *Paecilomyces*, the zygomycetes, and such dematiaceous fungi as *Scedosporium*, *Scopulariopsis*, and *Dactylaria*) *(7)*.

There are three major routes by which invasive fungal infections occur in this patient population: inhalation of the fungi that have been aerosolized by some factor; direct delivery of endogenous organisms to damaged skin and intraperitoneal anatomic abnormalities; direct inoculation of fungal species, often fluconazole resistant because of previous exposure to the drug. Because of the aerosol problem, HSCT patients should be instructed in avoiding circumstances in which aerosols of fungal spores might be encountered: areas of high dust exposure, urban renewal and other construction projects, chicken coops, bat caves, avocational (e.g., gardening) and vocational activities that require digging up soil, marijuana smoking, and the preparation and handling of foods that contain molds (e.g., blue cheese). Similarly, HSCT recipients should avoid exposures to naturopathic medicines, which can be contaminated by mold *(1,7)*.

Although *Candida* spp., as previously discussed, are the most common cause of invasive fungal infection in the HSCT patients, the most feared are those caused by *Aspergillus* spp., with *A. fumigatus*, *A. flavus*, *A. terreus*, and *A. niger* being the most common causes of invasive aspergillosis. The portal of entry for 90% of cases of invasive aspergillosis is the lungs, with the nasal sinuses and the skin accounting for virtually all of the remaining cases. There are two major host defenses that are mobilized in response to inhalation of the *Aspergillus* spores—granulocytes and cell-mediated immunity, specifically cytotoxic T cells. The importance of both of these mechanisms is demonstrated by the clustering of cases of invasive aspergillosis at two time-points in the posttransplant course: pre-engraftment when profound granulocytopenia is present, with the incidence of invasive aspergillosis increasing steadily as the period of granulocytopenia is extended; the second time that invasive aspergillosis is a major problem is after the diagnosis of GVHD and the treatment of this adverse event. Indeed, these late cases of invasive aspergillosis have become more common than the pre-engraftment cases. Mortality rates are high in patients who developed invasive aspergillosis in either time period *(1,7,48,49)*.

The clinical syndromes caused by *Aspergillus* invasion reflect the pathologic consequences of the vasculotropic nature of this mold, with there being three major consequences of the vascular invasion that characterizes *Aspergillus* invasion: hemorrhage, infarction, and metastases. Initial clinical complaints include fever, chest pain, tachypnea, hypoxemia, and hemoptysis, as well as symptoms related to metastases. In 50% or more of patients disseminated infection is present at the time of first diagnosis, accounting for the more than 80% mortality observed in allogeneic HSCT recipients. A particular problem is infection in the CNS, where mortality approaches 100%. Metastases can be to any site, but particularly important is the skin, as innocent appearing skin lesions can lead to early recognition of the disease and should be aggressively biopsied *(7)*.

Diagnosis is usually accomplished by biopsy of a site of abnormality. Early diagnosis is the key to effective therapy. The isolation of *Aspergillus* spp. from respiratory secretions in an asymptomatic HSCT patient carries a 50% risk of subsequent invasive disease and should be treated pre-emptively, with amphotericin or, possibly, voriconazole. Unfortunately, not all cases of invasive aspergillosis provide such a useful "early warning signal." Therefore, considerable effort has been made to find another technology that will lead to an early diagnosis. For example, monitoring the serum or plasma of a patient who is deemed to be at high risk for the shedding of galactomannan antigen (from the cell wall of *Aspergillus*) or the detection of circulating fungal DNA in the blood by PCR. Finally, a particular chest computed tomography (CT) finding, the halo sign (*see* Fig.2) is highly suggestive in this setting of invasive aspergillosis (although other pathogens can cause the same radiologic finding: *Fusarium* and other vasculotrophic molds and *Nocardia asteroids* being examples of this). European groups have been advocating protocol serial chest CT scans to find such pathology as a guide to early diagnosis. Suffice it to say that if prevention fails, then early diagnosis is the key to the patient's survival *(7,48,49)*.

Given the limitations of current diagnostic techniques and the significant morbidity associated with invasive fungal infection, two strategies of antimicrobial use are commonly deployed in the HSCT patient. The first is prophylactic fluconazole during the transplant period, which has been shown to decrease fungal infections *(50)* in one study and overall mortality *(51)* in another, when given starting at d 0, until engraftment *(50)* or d +75 *(51)*. It is important to note that a high background rate of *Candida* infections was noted in both of these reports. The second common strategy is empiric antifungal therapy in neutropenic patients with persistent fever without a source, despite broad-spectrum antimicrobial therapy for more than 96 h. In this setting, the primary concern is invasive mold infection, especially *Aspergillus (3)*. The traditional antifungal therapy utilized as empiric therapy is an amphotericin product *(52)*. However, recent data suggest a potential role for itraconazole *(53)* and, possibly, voriconazole *(54)*. Caspofungin is currently under active investigation for use in this setting.

When treating invasive aspergillosis, several approaches should be considered simultaneously: (1) antifungal therapy, (2) reverse the host defect (decrease corticosteroids, increase WBC; consider GM-CSF), (3) control permissive viral infections (e.g., CMV), and (4) consider surgical excision, if possible. Antifungal therapy has been revolutionized by the recent head-to-head comparison of voriconazole to amphotericin, with voriconazole demonstrating improved efficacy with decreased toxicity. Voriconazole has become a cornerstone of therapy for invasive mold infections *(55)*. The recent licensure of the first echinocandin, caspofungin, suggests the possibility of combination therapy; how to combine these classes (polyenes,

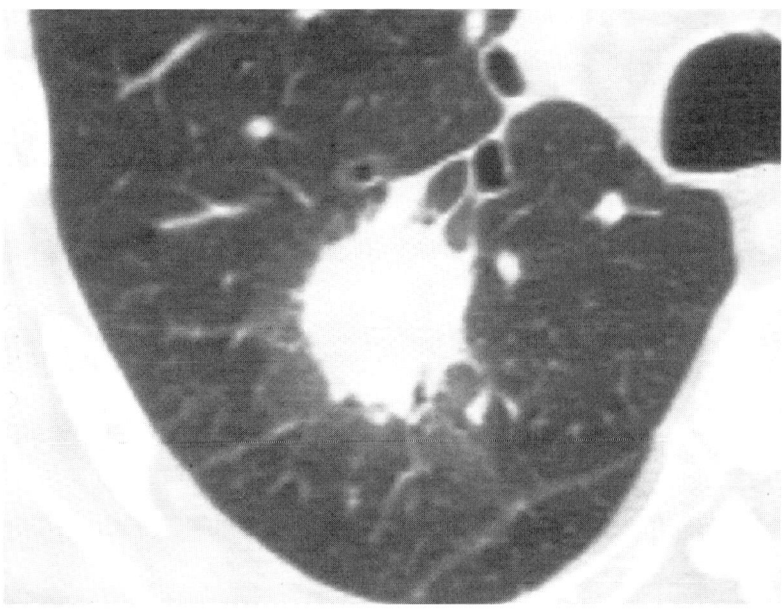

Fig. 2. Computerized tomographic scan of the chest in a patient with a "halo sign" as a result of invacine aspergillosis. Note that halo signs most commonly occur in granulocytopenic HSCT recipients with invasive aspergillosis. However, it must be emphasized that a halo sign is occasionally seen in patients with *Nocardia*, *Scedosporium*, *Fusarium*, and other forms of pneumonia.

azoles, and echinocandins) of antifungal agents for optimal therapeutic benefit has yet to be determined.

Therapy for the new and emerging fungi, *Fusarium* and *Scedosporium*, should be guided by in vitro sensitivity testing (if available), but voriconazole use should be considered early. When therapy for the endemic mycoses is indicated, initial therapy (induction therapy) is with an amphotericin preparation, followed by a prolonged course of consolidative therapy with itraconazole. Cryptococcal disease should be treated with an amphotericin preparation plus fluorocytosine to gain rapid control, followed by a prolonged course of fluconazole.

5. SUMMARY AND CONCLUSIONS

Hematopoietic SCT has become one of the great success stories of modern medicine. It is the therapy of choice for an increasing number of conditions, including a variety of cancers, BM failure states, congenital immunodeficiencies, metabolic disorders, and even as a means for introducing new genes. The major hurdle in most of these attempts, however, remains infection. Bacterial and fungal sepsis as well as herpes group viral infection and community acquired respiratory virus infection threaten the well-being of these patients. There are two phases of the posttransplant course when the patient is at particular risk: pre-engraftment with profound granulocytopenia and mucositis, and postengraftment when GVHD and its therapy render the patient vulnerable to both fungal and viral infection. New preventative strategies are being formulated involving both prophylaxis and pre-emptive therapy. Similarly, new nonculture diagnostic approaches are being developed that rely on antigen detection or PCR detection of microbial DNA. These should prompt much more effective prevention and therapeutic strategies. New therapies, both antiviral and antifungal, have emerged. Thus, there is much ferment in the study and management of the infections that afflict HSCT patients; much has been accomplished and there is much to be accomplished.

REFERENCES

1. Boeckh M, Marr KA. Infection in hematopoietic stem cell transplantation. In: Rubin RH, Young LS, eds. *Clinical Approach to Infection in the Compromised Host*, 4th ed. New York: Kluwer Academic/Plenum, 2002:527–571.
2. Deeg HC, Bowden RA. Introduction to marrow and blood stem cell transplantation. In: Bowden RA, Ljungman P, Paya CV, eds. *Transplant Infections*. Philadelphia: Lippencott–Raven, 1998:1–12.
3. Bodey GP, Buckley M, Sathe YS, et al. Quantitative relationships between circulating leukocytes and infection in patients with acute leukemia. *Ann Intern Med* 1966;64:328–340.
4. Donowitz GR, Maki DG, Crnich CJ, et al. Infections in the neutropenic patient—new views of an old problem. *Hematology (Am Soc Hematol Educ Program)* 2001:113–139.
5. Hughes WT, Armstrong D, Bodey GP, et al. 2002 Guidelines for the use of antimicrobial agents in neutropenic patients with cancer. *Clin Infect Dis* 2002;34:730–751.
6. Anon. Guidelines for preventing opportunistic infections among hematopoietic stem cell transplant recipients. MMWR Recomm Rep 2000;49:1–125, 1–7.
7. Sullivan KM, Dykewicz CA, Longworth DL, et al. Preventing opportunistic infections after hematopoietic stem cell transplantation: the Centers for Disease Control and Prevention, Infectious Diseases Society of America, and American Society for Blood and Marrow Transplantation Practice Guidelines and beyond. *Hematology (Am Soc Hematol Educ Program)* 2001:392–421.
8. Hopkins CC, Weber DJ, Rubin RH. Invasive aspergillus infection: possible non-ward common source within the hospital environment. *J Hosp Infect* 1989;13:19–25.
9. Elting LS, Bodey GP, Keefe BH. Septicemia and shock syndrome due to viridans streptococci: a case-control study of predisposing factors. *Clin Infect Dis* 1992;14:1201–1207.
10. Rubin RH, Ikonen T, Gummert JF, et al. The therapeutic prescription for the organ transplant recipient: the linkage of immunosuppression and antimicrobial strategies. *Transplant Infect Dis* 1999;1:29–39.
11. Zinner SH. Changing epidemiology of infections in patients with neutropenia and cancer: emphasis on gram-positive and resistant bacteria. *Clin Infect Dis* 1999;29:490–494.
12. Elting LS, Rubenstein EB, Rolston KV, et al. Outcomes of bacteremia in patients with cancer and neutropenia: observations from two decades of epidemiological and clinical trials. *Clin Infect Dis* 1997;25:247–259.
13. Cometta A, Calandra T, Bille J, et al. Escherichia coli resistant to fluoroquinolones in patients with cancer and neutropenia. *N Engl J Med* 1994;330:1240–1241.
14. EORTC International Antimicrobial Therapy Cooperative Group. Ceftazidime combined with short or long course of amikacin for empirical therapy of gram-negative bacteremia in cancer patients with granulocytopenia. *N Engl J Med* 1997:317:1692–1698.
15. Rubin M, Hathorn JW, Marshall D, et al. Gram-positive infections and the use of vancomycin in 550 episodes of fever and neutropenia. *Ann Intern Med* 1988;108:30–35.
16. Pizzo PA, Robichaud KJ, Gill FA, et al. Duration of empiric antibiotic therapy in granulocytopenic patients with cancer. *Am J Med* 1979;67:194–200.
17. Buckley RH, Schiff RI. The use of intravenous immune globulin in immunodeficiency diseases. *N Engl J Med* 1991;325:110–117.
18. Sullivan KM, Storek J, Kopecky KJ, et al. A controlled trial of long-term administration of intravenous immunoglobulin to prevent late infection and chronic graft-vs.-host disease after marrow transplantation: clinical outcome and effect on subsequent immune recovery. *Biol Blood Marrow Transplant* 1996;2:44–53.
19. Walsh TJ, Pizzo PA. Fungal infections in granulocytopenic patients: current approaches to classifications, diagnosis. In: Holmberg K, Meyer R, eds. *Diagnosis and Therapy of Systemic Fungal Infections*. New York: Raven, 1989:47–70.
20. Meunier F, Aoun M, Bitar N. Candidemia in immunocompromised patients. *Clin Infect Dis* 1992;14(suppl 1):S120–S125.

21. Wingard JR. Infections due to resistant *Candida* species in patients with cancer who are receiving chemotherapy. *Clin Infect Dis* 1994;19(Suppl 1):S49–S53.
22. Brooks RG. Prospective study of *Candida* endophthalmitis in hospitalized patients with candidemia. *Arch Intern Med* 1989;149:2226–2228.
23. Chubachi A, Miura I, Ohshima A, et al. Risk factors for hepatosplenic abscesses in patients with acute leukemia receiving empiric azole treatment. *Am J Med Sci* 1994;308:309–312.
24. Rex JH, Walsh TJ, Sobel JD, et al. Practice guidelines for the treatment of candidiasis. Infectious Diseases Society of America. *Clin Infect Dis* 2000;30:662–678.
25. Maki D, Mermel L. Infections due to infusion therapy. In: Bennett JV, Brachman PS, eds. *Hospital Infections*, 4th ed. Philadelphia: Lippincott–Raven, 1998:689–724.
26. Maki DG, Crnich CJ. Line sepsis in the granulocytopenic patient: precaution, diagnosis and management. *Hematology* 2001:228–139.
27. Kluger D, Maki D. The relative risk of intravascular device-related bloodstream infections with different types of intravascular devices in adults. A meta-analysis of 206 published studies. Fourth Decennial International Conference on Nosocomial and Healthcare Associated Infections, 2000; submitted for publication, 2001.
28. Grohskopf LA, Maki DG, Sohn AH, et al. Reality check: should we use vancomycin for the prophylaxis of intravascular catheter-associated infections? *Infect Control Hosp Epidemiol* 2001;22:176–179.
29. Goodrich JM, Mori M, Gleaves CA, et al. Early treatment with ganciclovir to prevent cytomegalovirus disease after allogeneic bone marrow transplantation. *N Engl J Med* 1991;325:1601–1607.
30. Goodrich JM, Bowden RA, Fisher L, et al. Ganciclovir prophylaxis to prevent cytomegalovirus disease after allogeneic marrow transplant. *Ann Intern Med* 1993;118:173–178.
31. Boeckh M, Gooley TA, Myerson D, et al. Cytomegalovirus pp65 antigenemia-guided early treatment with ganciclovir versus ganciclovir at engraftments after allogeneic marrow transplantation: a randomized double-blind study. *Blood* 1996;88:4063.
32. Einsele H, Ehninger G, Hebart H, et al. Polymerase chain reaction monitoring reduces the incidence of cytomegalovirus disease and the duration and side effects of antiviral therapy after bone marrow transplantation. *Blood* 1995;86:2815.
33. Boeckh M, Bowden RA, Gooley T, et al. Successful modification of a pp65 antigenemia-based early treatment strategy for prevention of cytomegalovirus disease in allogeneic marrow transplant recipients. *Blood* 1999;93:1781–1782.
34. Einsele H, Hebart H, Kauffmann-Schneider C, et al. Risk factors for treatment failures in patients receiving PCR-based preemptive therapy for CMV infection. *Bone Marrow Transplant* 2000;25:757–763.
35. Rubin RH. Preemptive therapy in immunocompromised hosts. *N Engl J Med* 1991;324:1057–1059.
36. Preiksaitis JK, Cockfield SM. Epstein–Barr virus and lymphoproliferatic disorders after transplantation. In: Bowden RA, Ljungman P, Paya CV, eds. *Transplant Infections*. Philadelphia: Lippincott–Raven, 1998:245–263.
37. Kuehnle I, Huls MH, Liu Z, et al. CD20 monoclonal antibody (rituximab) for therapy of Epstein–Barr virus lymphoma after hemopoietic stem-cell transplantation. *Blood* 2000;95:1502–1505.
38. Fischer A, Blanche S, Le Bidois J, et al. Anti-B-cell monoclonal antibodies in the treatment of severe B-cell lymphoproliferative syndrome following bone marrow and organ transplantation. *N Engl J Med* 1991;324:1451–1456.
39. Bollard CM, Rooney CM, Huls MH, et al. Long term follow-up of patients who received EBV specific CTLs for the prevention or treatment of EBV lymphoma. *Blood* 2000:96(suppl):478a (Abstract 2057).
40. Durandy A. Anti-B cell and anti-cytokine therapy for the treatment of post-transplant lymphoproliferative disorder: past, present, and future. *Transplant Infect Dis* 2001;3:104–107.
41. Bowden RA, Rogers KS, Meyers JD. Oral acyclovir for the long-term suppression of varicella zoster virus infection after marrow transplantation. 29th Interscience Conference on Antimicrobial Agents and Chemotherapy, 1989:Abstract 62.
42. Vazquez M, LaRussa PS, Gershon AA, et al. The effectiveness of the varicella vaccine in clinical practice. *N Engl J Med* 2001;344:955–960.
43. Asano Y, Yoshikawa T, Suga S, et al. Postexposure prophylaxis of varicella in family contact by oral acyclovir. *Pediatrics* 1993;92:219–222.
44. Boeckh M, Berrey MM, Bowden RA, et al. Phase 1 evaluation of the respiratory syncytial virus-specific monoclonal antibody palivizumab in recipients of hematopoietic stem cell transplants. *J Infect Dis* 2001;184:350–354.

45. Boeckh M, Hayden F, Corey K, et al. Detection of rhinovirus RNA in bronchoalveolar lavage in hematopoietic stem cell transplant recipients with pneumonia. 40th Interscience Conference on Antimicrobial Agents and Chemotherapy, 2000:262 (Abstract 190).
46. Ghosh S, Champlin R, Couch R, et al. Rhinovirus infections in myelosuppressed adult blood and marrow transplant recipients. *Clin Infect Dis* 1999;29:528–532.
47. Whimbey EE, Englan JA. Community respiratory virus infections in transplant recipients. In: Bowden RA, Ljungman P, Paya CV, eds. *Transplant Infections*. Philadelphia: Lippincott–Raven, 1998:309–324.
48. Marr KA, Seidel K, White TC, et al. Candidemia in allogeneic blood and marrow transplant recipients: evolution of risk factors after the adoption of prophylactic fluconazole. *J Infect Dis* 2000;181:309–316.
49. Wald A, Leisenring W, van Burik JA, et al. Epidemiology of *Aspergillus* infections in a large cohort of patients undergoing bone marrow transplantation. *J Infect Dis* 1997;175:1459–1466.
50. Goodman JL, Winston DJ, Greenfield RA, et al. A controlled trial of fluconazole to prevent fungal infections in patients undergoing bone marrow transplantation. *N Engl J Med* 1992;326:845–851.
51. Slavin MA, Osborne B, Adams R, et al. Efficacy and safety of fluconazole prophylaxis for fungal infections after marrow transplantation—a prospective, randomized, double-blind study. *J Infect Dis* 1995;171:1545–1552.
52. Walsh TJ, Finberg RW, Arndt C, et al. Liposomal amphotericin B for empirical therapy in patients with persistent fever and neutropenia. National Institute of Allergy and Infectious Diseases Mycoses Study Group. *N Engl J Med* 1999;340:764–771.
53. Boogaerts M, Winston DJ, Bow EJ, et al. Intravenous and oral itraconazole versus intravenous amphotericin B deoxycholate as empirical antifungal therapy for persistent fever in neutropenic patients with cancer who are receiving broad-spectrum antibacterial therapy. A randomized, controlled trial. *Ann Intern Med* 2001;135:412–422.
54. Walsh TJ, Pappas P, Winston DJ, et al. Voriconazole compared with liposomal amphotericin B for empirical antifungal therapy in patients with neutropenia and persistent fever. *N Engl J Med* 2002;346:225–234.
55. Herbrecht R, Denning DW, Patterson TF, et al. Voriconazole versus amphotericin B for primary therapy of invasive aspergillosis. *N Engl J Med* 2002;347:408–415.

11 EBV Lymphoproliferative Disease After Transplantation

Stephen Gottschalk, MD, *Cliona M. Rooney,* PhD, *and Helen E. Heslop,* MD

Contents

1. INTRODUCTION

Epstein–Barr virus (EBV) associated posttransplant lymphoproliferative disease (PTLD) is a serious, life-threatening complication after hematopoietic stem cell transplantation (HSCT). Major risk factors include the use of unrelated or human leukocyte antigen (HLA)-mismatched related donors, T-cell depletion of the graft, the use of T-cell antibodies for the prophylaxis and therapy of graft-vs-host disease (GVHD), and an underlying diagnosis of primary immunodeficiency *(1–4)*. Over the last decade, effective immunotherapies have been developed either reconstituting EBV-specific T-cell responses *(5,6)* or targeting PTLD with anti-B-cell monoclonal antibodies like rituximab *(7,8)*. In addition to careful clinical monitoring of high-risk patients, serial measurement of EBV–DNA load in peripheral blood samples by polymerase chain reaction (PCR)-based methods has proven to assist in the identification of high-risk patients *(9,10)*. However, the indication for pre-emptive therapy remains a major challenge because not all HSCT recipients with elevated EBV–DNA develop PTLD.

2. EBV-ASSOCIATED DISEASES

Epstein–Barr virus was the first human virus implicated in oncogenesis and its original description has since been linked to a heterogeneous group of nonmalignant and malignant

From: *Stem Cell Transplantation for Hematologic Malignancies*
Edited by: R. J. Soiffer © Humana Press Inc., Totowa, NJ

diseases *(11)*. EBV is a latent herpes virus that infects more than 90% of all human population worldwide. Primary EBV infection usually occurs through the oropharynx, where mucosal epithelial cells and/or B cells become primarily infected *(12)*. The virus produced in these cells may then infect neighboring epithelial cells and B cells circulating through the mucosa-associated lymphoid tissues. Primary infection results in a self-limiting illness characterized by fever, lymphadenopathy, and pharyngitis that are followed by lifelong virus latency in B cells. In healthy, seropositive individuals, EBV latency is tightly controlled by the cellular immune system. The importance of CD8-positive EBV-specific T cells in the control of primary EBV infection and latency has been well documented *(13,14)* and, recently, the potential role of CD4-positive EBV-specific T cells has also been highlighted *(15,16)*.

All EBV-associated malignancies are associated with the virus' latent cycle. Four patterns of EBV latent gene expression have been described, termed type 0, I, II, and III, and types I–III are found in malignancies *(11)*. In all types of latency, the EBV-derived polyadenylated viral RNAs, being EBERs 1 and 2, are expressed; however, the pattern of latent viral protein expressing varies. Type 0 latency characterizes EBV latency after primary infection in healthy individuals; the virus persists episomally in resting memory B cells, and of the almost 100 viral proteins, only LMP2 is expressed *(17)*. In type I latency, only EBNA-1 and BARFO are expressed and it is associated with EBV-positive Burkitt's lymphoma and gastric adenocarcinoma. Type II latency, characterized by EBNA-1, BARFO, LMP1, and LMP2 expression, is found in EBV-positive Hodgkin's disease, nasopharyngeal carcinoma, and peripheral T/natural-killer (NK)-cell lymphomas. Whereas malignancies associated with type I and II latency occur in individuals with minimal or no immune dysfunction, type III latency is associated with malignancies in severely immunocompromised patients. It is characterized by the expression of the entire array of nine EBV latency proteins (EBNAs 1, 2, 3A, 3B, 3C, LP, BARFO, LMP1 and LMP2) and this pattern of gene expression is found in PTLD after solid-organ transplant (SOT) or HSCT and in EBV-associated lymphomas occurring in patients with congenital immunodeficiency or human immunodeficiency virus (HIV) infections. In addition, type III latency is found in lymphoblastoid cell lines (LCLs), which (1) can be readily prepared by infecting B cells in vitro with EBV and (2) were instrumental in the generation of EBV-specific cytotoxic T lymphocytes (CTL) for the prophylaxis and therapy of PTLD after HSCT (*see* Subheading 1.7.2.).

3. PATHOGENESIS OF PTLD

In EBV-seropositive individuals with compromised T-cell function, the control of EBV-infected B cells is impaired, leading to an increase in the number of EBV-infected B cells. The expansion of latent EBV-infected B cells occurs without significant reactivation from latency into the lytic cycle, explaining why antiviral agents, like acyclovir, that prevent productive viral replication are of limited therapeutic value *(18)*. The importance of T-cell dysfunction in the pathogenesis of PTLD in HSCT recipients is highlighted by the fact that the majority of PTLD cases occur within the first 6 mo posttransplant when the T-cell deficiency is most profound *(2)*. In addition, as discussed in Subheading 1.4., therapies that selectively deplete T cells or impair their function increase the incidence of PTLD. Because not all patients with similar T-cell dysfunction develop PTLD, other contributing risk factors may play a role in the outgrowth of EBV-transformed B cells, like the local concentrations of cytokines or chemokines, which could potentially promote B-cell proliferation.

Table 1
Risk Factors for PTLD After HSCT

Risk factor	*Relative risk*		
	Bhatia et al. (1)	*Curtis et al. (2)*	*Socie et al. (3)*
HLA-Mismatched transplant	8.9	3.7	7.5
T-Cell depletion	11.9	9.1	4.8
ATG as prophylaxis or therapy for GVHD	5.9	5.5	3.1
Immunodeficiency as primary diagnosis	2.5	NR[a]	NR[a]

[a]NR, not reported.

4. INCIDENCE AND RISK FACTORS

The overall prevalence of PTLD after allogeneic HSCT (alloHSCT) is approx 1%, with the majority of cases developing in the first 6 mo after transplantation. However, the incidence is significantly increased by risk factors including (1) the use of HLA-mismatched family members, (2) closely unrelated donors, (3) T-cell depletion of donor cells, (4) intensive immunosuppression with T-cell antibodies for the prophylaxis and therapy of graft-vs-host disease (GVHD), and (5) an underlying diagnosis of primary immunodeficiency (*see* Table 1) *(1–3,19)*. The incidence is much lower when T and B cells are depleted simultaneously, indicating that the incidence of PTLD may depend on the balance between EBV-infected B cells and EBV-specific T-cell precursors. In a large review of HSCT recipients treated with the Campath-1 antibody, which removes mature T and B cells *(20)*, the incidence of PTLD was less than 2%. Other methods of B-cell depletion, like elutriation, which removes over 90% of B cells from the donor graft *(21)*, or the addition of monoclonal antibodies for B-cell depletion to the T-cell-depletion regimen, have also proven to be effective. The use of anti-CD19, anti-CD20, or a combination of anti-CD19 and anti-CD20 monoclonal antibodies for the depletion of B cells in stem cell products prevented the development of PTLD and acute GVHD without a reduction in the engraftment rate, as compared with historical controls *(22,23)*.

Only a few cases of PTLD have been described after autologous HSCT (autoHSCT) and most have involved patients who had previously received long-standing intensive immunosuppressive therapy or received a CD34-selected product that may delay immune reconstitution *(24)*. The incidence of PTLD after allogeneic umbilical cord blood transplant (UCBT) is low, and in a recent review, only 5 of 272 transplanted patients (2%) developed PTLD *(25)*. PTLD occurred 4–14 mo after UCBT, with four out of five patients being treated for GVHD grade II–IV, indicating that, as for alloHSCT, recipient T-cell suppressive therapy is an important risk factor.

5. CLINICAL PRESENTATION AND PATHOLOGY

In HSCT recipients, PTLD may present with a diverse spectrum of clinical symptoms and signs, underscoring the need for a high index of suspicion in making the diagnosis. Symptoms and signs include fever, sweats, generalized malaise, enlarged tonsils, and cervical lymphadenopathy, not unlike that seen in primary EBV infection *(12)*. EBV-associated B-cell proliferation may involve other organs, including lung, liver, spleen, kidneys, small intestine, bone marrow, or the central nervous system. Often, diffuse disease is only diagnosed at autopsy in patients thought to have severe GVHD or fulminant sepsis *(26)*. The pathology ranges from polymorphic B-cell lymphomas to immunoblastic lymphomas *(27)*. They are usually oligoclonal or monoclonal, almost always of donor origin, and in some cases, mutations in oncogene or tumor suppressor genes have been found *(28)*.

6. LABORATORY TEST

Because the presenting clinical symptoms of PTLD are not specific, there has been a great interest in developing tests that would predict the development of PTLD. The usefulness of PCR-based methods to monitor EBV–DNA load has been well documented and EBV–DNA load monitoring is now routinely available in large transplant centers *(9,10,19)*. In addition, functional assays to monitor EBV-specific T-cell responses are being developed that may play an important role in the future laboratory assessment of HSCT recipients at risk for PTLD *(29,30)*.

6.1. Monitoring of EBV–DNA Load in HSCT Patients

The onset of PTLD in the majority of cases is preceded by a large increase in EBV load and several investigators have shown that frequent monitoring of EBV–DNA load in peripheral blood by PCR is a valuable diagnostic test for early detection of PTLD after both SOT and HSCT *(9,31,32)*. The threshold levels of EBV–DNA suggestive of impending PTLD vary according to sample (plasma, serum, peripheral blood mononuclear cells, or whole blood) and PCR method of quantifying viral DNA. We and others currently favor real-time quantitative (RQ) PCR *(33)* as a detection method because it has several advantages in comparison to conventional PCR methods: It is (1) fast and safe, requiring minimal specimen handling, (2) flexible, allowing the detection of DNA from different specimen material, (3) highly sensitive, (4) reproducible, and (5) precise. Initial studies in recipients of T-cell-depleted grafts suggested that a high EBV–DNA level has a strong prognostic value for the development of lymphoma *(6,9,32)*. However, over the past few years, it has become clear that although EBV reactivation is a frequent event after both T-cell-depleted and unmanipulated transplant, high EBV loads only have a high correlation with the development of EBV lymphoma after T-cell-depleted transplants *(34,35)*. In patients with high EBV–DNA load after solid-organ transplant, recent studies indicate several distinct pattern of EBV latent gene expression in memory B cells, with type III latency conferring the highest risk for PLTD development *(36)*. Thus, an elevated EBV–DNA load can lead to early diagnosis of PTLD, although other factors such a clinical symptoms and signs and results of diagnostic imagining studies must be taken into account before therapy is initiated.

6.2. Monitoring EBV-Specific CTL Responses

In contrast to monitoring EBV–DNA load in peripheral blood, measurement of EBV-specific T-cell responses by (1) interferon (IFN)-γ secretion assays using intracellular cytokine staining or Elispot assays or (2) major histocompatibility class (MHC) I–peptide tetrameric complexes for enumerating EBV-specific CTLs are not routinely available. Yang et al. *(29)* used IFN-γ Elispot assays successfully in two SOT patients to monitor EBV-specific immune reconstitution after adoptive immunotherapy with EBV-specific CTL. Using tetramer analysis and IFN-γ secretion assays in HIV patients, van Baarle et al. *(30)* demonstrated dysfunctional EBV-specific CD8-positive T cells prior to the development of EBV-associated non-Hodgkin's lymphomas (NHLs). These studies indicate that functional analysis of EBV-specific T-cell responses is feasible and may be useful in assessing the risk of PTLD development in the HSCT recipient with increased EBV–DNA load.

7. TREATMENT

Treatment of PTLD has largely focused on strategies to boost the immune response to EBV *(37)*. In SOT recipients, withdrawing immunosuppressive therapy has proven effective, but it carries a high risk of graft rejection *(38)*. Because HSCT patients receive high-dose chemotherapy and/or radiation to completely ablate their immune system, withdrawal of immune suppression posttransplant in the majority cases is ineffective; therefore, more active immunotherapeutic strategies have been pursued. Therapy with IFN-α and intravenous immune globulin has been used in SOT recipients and in a small number of HSCT patients with some responses *(39)*. Active immunization is not feasible because of the patients' severe immunosuppression, and the most successful modalities of therapy have been the adoptive immunotherapy of donor T cells or donor-derived EBV-specific CTL and the infusion of monoclonal antibodies against B cells.

7.1. Treatment With Donor T Cells

Adoptive immunotherapy with donor T cells for PTLD was originally reported by Papadopoulos et al. *(40)*. All five patients had therapeutic responses, but three developed GVHD and two died from respiratory insufficiency. In an update of their experience, 17 of 19 patients responded positively to donor T cells (*see* Table 2) *(41)*. Other investigators have also documented success with this approach *(32,42,43)* but emphasize the risk of GVHD and, in some instances, a lower response rate to donor leukocyte infusions (DLIs) than originally reported. In a series of 13 patients after T-cell-depleted alloHSCT, only 4 (31%) responded to DLIs *(32)*, 1 of whom died from acute GVHD and another from aspergillosis. Of the two surviving patients who had complete remission, one also received EBV-specific CTLs. Five of the nine patients with disease progression died within 10 d of receiving donor leukocytes, most likely because of advanced PTLD at the time of treatment, prompting the authors to advocate earlier diagnosis and initiation of therapy. In three smaller series, none of five patients responded to DLIs *(39,44,45)*. Reasons for the discrepancies in response rates to DLIs are unclear but may reflect different types of disease or better outcome with early diagnosis and treatment. To reduce the risk of GVHD, several groups have transduced T cells with the herpes simplex virus thymidine kinase gene, which renders transduced cells sensitive to the cytotoxic effects of ganciclovir *(46)*. Although there are reports that this strategy can be effective when GVHD occurs, two concerns are that the transgene may be immunogenic and that the ex vivo activation necessary for retroviral transduction may inhibit virus-reactive cells *(47)*.

7.2. Treatment With EBV-Specific CTLs

One strategy to reduce the potential risk of GVHD after donor T-cell infusions is the administration of in vitro-expanded antigen-specific CTLs, which was pioneered by Riddell et al. in Seattle for prophylaxis of CMV disease in HSCT recipients *(48,49)*. The CMV-specific CD8-positive CTL clones reconstituted CMV-specific immune responses without adverse effects, and none of the patients developed CMV disease. However, the CTL did not persist long term except in patients who either endogenously recovered CMV-specific CD4-positive T helper cells or were coinfused with CMV-specific CD4-positive T-cell clones, underscoring the need for such cells in the maintenance of CD8-positive CTL populations *(50)*.

Table 2
Treatment and Prophylaxis of PTLD With Donor T Cells or EBV-Specific CTL After HSCT

	Indication for therapy				
Study	*Prophylaxis*	*Therapeutic*	*Cell product*	*Response*	*GVHD*
Gustafsson et al. *(6)*	+		EBV-specific CTL	1/6 developed PTLD	1/6
Rooney et al. *(5)*	+		EBV-specific CTL	0/39 developed PTLD	1/39
Gross et al. *(39)*		+	Donor T cells	0/3	NR[a]
Heslop et al. *(43)*		+	Donor T cells	1/1	1/1
Lucas et al. *(32)*		+	Donor T cells	4/13[b]	4/13
Nagafuji et al. *(44)*		+	Donor T cells	0/1	0/1
O'Reilly et al. *(41)*		+	Donor T cells	17/19	3 acute, 8 chronic
Rooney et al. *(5)*		+	EBV-specific CTL	2/3	0/3
Sasahara et al. *(42)*		+	Donor T cells, EBV-specific CTL	0/1	0/1

[a]NR, not reported.
[b]One responding patient received EBV-specific CTL.

In the majority of PTLD cases that occur in HSCT recipients, the transformed B cells are of donor origin and express all latent cycle virus-associated antigens, providing excellent targets for virus-specific T cells. EBV-transformed LCLs also express all latent cycle virus-associated antigens and several costimulatory molecules that facilitate CTL generation. They can be readily prepared from any donor and provide a source of antigen-presenting cells that endogenously expresses the appropriate antigens for presentation of HLA class I-restricted epitopes. Most likely, HLA class II-restricted EBV epitopes are presented through phagocytosis of dead cells *(41,51)*. The generation of EBV-specific CTLs from seropositive, healthy donors takes 8–12 wk, of which 4–6 wk are needed to generate sufficient numbers of LCLs for CTL stimulation. The resultant EBV-specific CTLs are polyclonal and contain both CD4- and CD8-positive EBV-specific T cells, which is considered advantageous because the presence of antigen-specific CD4 helper T cells is important for in vivo survival of cytotoxic CD8-positive T-cell populations *(49)*.

We have infused 60 recipients of allogeneic T-cell-depleted graft products with donor-derived EBV-specific CTL. As prophylaxis, infusions were well tolerated with minimal side effects and no development of acute GVHD. More importantly, none of the CTL recipients developed PTLD, in comparison to 11.5% of untreated historic controls from our institution *(5)*. The trial was initially designed as a dose-escalation study and the first 12 patients received either 4×10^7 cells/m^2 (n=6) or 1.8×10^7 cells/m^2 (n=6) over 4 wk. At both dose levels, efficacy was noted and subsequent dose de-escalation showed that a single dose of 2×10^7 cells/m^2 was effective with no change in outcome. In nine patients with high EBV–DNA load, CTL infusion resulted in a 2–3 log decline of DNA levels, indicating that the infused CTL had antiviral effects and reconstituted cellular immunity to EBV. A subset of patients received EBV-specific CTLs, which were gene marked with the neomycin-resistant gene *(52)*. Gene-marked CTL persisted for up to 7 yr, and in one patient, a transient increase in EBV–DNA load was mirrored by an increase in gene-marked CTLs, followed by a subsequent decline of both values, demonstrating the intricate balance between EBV latency and EBV-specific CTLs. Other investigators also showed the safety and efficacy of EBV-specific CTLs in reducing high

EBV–DNA load post-HSCT *(6)*. The infused cell dose was similar to our study (1×10^7 cells/$m^2 \times 4$); however, one out of six patients developed fatal PTLD. In vitro testing of the infused CTL line of this patient showed only a weak EBV-specific component, which might explain this case of immunotherapy failure.

In our study, three patients with overt PTLD received EBV-specific CTLs, of whom two had a complete response. One of the responders experienced a potential complication of CTL therapy: An increase in tumor size as a result of infiltrating T cells caused airway compromise at a nasopharyngeal tumor site requiring intubation and mucosal ulceration at other tumor sites in the soft palate and intestine *(5)*. All lesions resolved and the patient is in remission more than 5 yr after therapy. The nonresponder died 24 days after CTL therapy and a limited autopsy showed progressive PTLD. Molecular analysis revealed that the patient harbored two genetically distinct viruses prior to CTL infusion, one of which carried a deletion of two immunodominant CTL epitopes *(53)*. After CTL infusion, the epitope deleted virus persisted, causing progressive, fatal PTLD. Because CTL mutants have been recently described in other diseases *(54,55)*, they may present a problem even when polyclonal CTL lines with a fixed epitope repertoire are used for immunotherapy. The incidence of both observed complications of CTL therapy (morbidity secondary to T-cell infiltration and occurrence of CTL escape mutants) is most likely to be higher in patients with high tumor burden, arguing to infuse patients with EBV-specific CTL as prophylaxis or with minimal disease.

Although therapy with EBV-specific CTLs has proved to be effective, the process of generating such lines is labor intensive and takes 10–12 wk. Koehne et al. have recently described methodology for selecting virus-specific cells early in culture by their susceptibility to transduction with a retroviral vector *(56)* that may allow a more rapid CTL generation. An additional issue is that recipients are only protected from one of the many viruses that may cause morbidity and mortality during the period of immunosuppression posttransplant. Several groups have investigated approaches for modifying antigen-presenting cells to generate multispecific CTLs. Transduction of LCLs with a retroviral vector encoding the CMV protein pp65 has allowed the generation of CTLs specific for both CMV and EBV *(57)*, whereas infection of LCLs with adenovirus results in the generation of CTL specific for both adenovirus and EBV *(58)*. An alternative strategy to generate broad antiviral immunity is to culture donor mononuclear cells with recipient cells and then deplete populations expressing activation markers such as CD25, which should contain alloreactive cells *(59)*. The residual allodepleted T-cell product will contain CTLs specific for multiple viruses and potentially residual tumor cells.

Other cellular therapies, like the infusion of interleukin (IL)-2-activated killer cells, have been tested in small numbers of SOT recipients with PTLD *(60)*. However, the initial promising result have not been repeated.

7.3. Treatment With Monoclonal Antibodies

In addition to cellular immunotherapy, monoclonal antibodies have been used for the treatment of PTLD after HSCT (*see* Table 3). In a European multicenter study, 58 patients were treated with anti-CD21 and anti-CD24 murine monoclonal antibodies and 35 (61%) entered complete remission *(61)*. However, these antibodies are no longer available and, in addition, murine monoclonal antibodies may cause anaphylaxis and the production of neutralizing human anti-mouse antibodies (HAMA). To reduce the incidence of HAMA, chimeric murine/human monoclonal antibodies have been developed and one of the most successful examples is rituximab (Rituxan; Genentech and IDEC Pharmaceuticals Corp.), an anti-CD20 mono-

Table 3
Treatment of PTLD After HSCT With Rituximab

Study	*Indication for Therapy*		*Response*
	Pre-emptive	*Therapeutic*	
Faye et al. *(8)*	+		4/4
Faye et al. *(70)*		+	1/1
Faye et al. *(8)*		+	4/8
Gruhn et al. *(71)*	+		3/3
Kuehnle et al. *(7)*	+		3/3
Milpied et al. *(65)*	+ (4)	+ (2)	4/6[a]
Wagner et al. *(34)*	+		2/2

[a]Responders not specified.

clonal antibody *(62–67)*. It has been used in the treatment of CD20-positive B-cell NHL as a single agent or in combination with conventional therapy and also is an effective agent for the treatment of PTLD. In a multicenter retrospective analysis of 32 patients with PTLD after SOT or HSCT, rituximab was well tolerated and the overall response rate was 69%, with 20 complete responses and two partial responses *(65)*. So far, we have treated nine patients with rituximab for PTLD after SOT (three liver and one kidney) or HSCT (n=5) *(7)*, with all patients having a complete remission. One patient, who had received high-dose steroids and antithymocyte globulin (ATG) for GVHD prior to rituximab therapy, died of aspergillosis. Three of the five HSCT recipients have now been followed for more almost 2 yr after rituximab infusion, with no evidence of PTLD recurrence. Faye et al. *(8)* reported 12 patients with PTLD after HSCT treated with rituximab. Eight patients had a complete remission and seven are alive with a median follow-up of almost 2 yr. Of the eight patients, two received DLI after rituximab and one patient died of staphylococcal sepsis. The four nonresponders had more extensive disease, with mediastinal involvement and a lower CD4 T-cell count. Other smaller cases series describing the use of rituximab for PTLD have been reported, and although no major complications were noted, the outcome varied in between studies. As for T-cell therapies, this most likely reflects better outcome with early diagnosis and treatment.

Rituximab has also been used prophylactically in patients with high EBV viral load. In a study evaluating a humanized anti-CD3 monoclonal antibody in the treatment of GVHD, elevated EBV viral load and lymphoproliferative disease developed in two of the first seven patients. Five of the next 10 patients were therefore given rituximab when their EBV viral load increased and all had a virological response with none developing lymphoma *(66)*. However, the use of rituximab as pre-emptive therapy for PTLD should be confined to such clinical scenarios where there is a strong association with the development of lymphoma because of its known side effects. The profound B-cell depletion induced by rituximab for 6–8 mo may exacerbate the immunodeficiency in transplant recipients, and a lack of EBV-infected B cells could potentially delay recovery of EBV-specific immunity, increasing the risk of PTLD late in the posttransplant period. Neither complication was observed in our transplant patients treated with rituximab, but long-term follow-up is necessary to adequately assess these risk factors. It is also possible that monoclonal antibody therapy may result in the selection of B cells negative for the targeted antigen, as reported in some lymphoma patients after anti-CD20 therapy *(67)* and recently for a patient with PTLD after lung transplant *(68)*.

In addition to B-cell antibodies, anti-IL-6 monoclonal antibodies have been used to treat PTLD *(69)*. In multicenter phase I and II clinical trials, 12 patients were treated with anti-IL-6 antibodies after SOT, with 5 achieving complete remission and three partial remissions. The treatment was well tolerated and further studies are needed to define the role of anti-IL-6 antibodies in therapy for PTLD.

8. CONCLUSIONS

Combined B- and T-cell depletion has lowered the incidence of PTLD; however, it remains a serious and life-threatening complication post-HSCT. Over the last decade, effective immunotherapies for PTLD have been developed, including donor-derived EBV-specific CTLs and monoclonal antibodies like rituximab. In contrast to EBV-specific CTLs, rituximab is readily available and pre-emptive therapy of imminent PTLD is becoming a clinical reality. Currently, it is advisable to consider pre-emptive therapy in patients with a high EBV–DNA load and risk factors such as T-cell depletion of the donor graft, infusion of anti-T-cell antibodies for GVHD therapy, or an underlying diagnosis of primary immunodeficiency. In patients with high EBV–DNA levels without risk factors and no clinical symptoms and signs of PTLD, possible side effects of therapy must be balanced against the risk of developing PTLD. In the future, in addition to EBV–DNA load monitoring by PCR, a laboratory test assessing EBV-specific T-cell function may become available to assist in the management of HCST patients who are at high-risk of developing PTLD. Because therapy failures have been reported with monoclonal antibodies as well as cellular immunotherapies, one of the major challenges for the future remains how to combine these treatment modalities. For such an approach, identification of patients at high risk for PTLD is a prerequisite because EBV-specific CTLs cannot be generated for every patient as prophylaxis. Patients with imminent PTLD could then receive as pre-emptive therapy, rituximab alone or in combination with other monoclonal antibodies, like anti-IL6, which would allow for the time required to expand EBV-specific CTLs. Such integrative immunotherapeutic approach may ultimately reduce current failure rates and improve long-term outcome of patients with PTLD.

ACKNOWLEDGMENTS

This work was supported by National Institutes of Health grants RO1 CA61384 and RO1 CA74126 and the GCRC at Baylor College of Medicine (NIH-RR00188). SG is the recipient of a Doris Duke clinical scientist development award. HEH is the recipient of a Doris Duke distinguished clinical scientist award.

REFERENCES

1. Bhatia S, Ramsay NK, Steinbuch M, et al. Malignant neoplasms following bone marrow transplantation. *Blood* 1996;87(9):3633–3639.
2. Curtis RE, Travis LB, Rowlings PA, et al. Risk of lymphoproliferative disorders after bone marrow transplantation: a multi-institutional study. *Blood* 1999;94(7):2208–2216.
3. Socie G, Curtis RE, Deeg HJ, et al. New malignant diseases after allogeneic marrow transplantation for childhood acute leukemia. *J Clin Oncol* 2000;18(2):348–357.
4. Gerritsen EJ, Stam ED, Hermans J, et al. Risk factors for developing EBV-related B cell lymphoproliferative disorders (BLPD) after non-HLA-identical BMT in children. *Bone Marrow Transplant* 1996;18(2):377–382.
5. Rooney CM, Smith CA, Ng CYC, et al. Infusion of cytotoxic T cells for the prevention and treatment of Epstein–Barr virus-induced lymphoma in allogeneic transplant recipients. *Blood* 1998;92(5):1549–1555.

6. Gustafsson A, Levitsky V, Zou JZ, et al. Epstein–Barr virus (EBV) load in bone marrow transplant recipients at risk to develop posttransplant lymphoproliferative disease: prophylactic infusion of EBV-specific cytotoxic T cells. *Blood* 2000;95(3):807–814.
7. Kuehnle I, Huls MH, Liu Z, et al. CD20 monoclonal antibody (rituximab) for therapy of Epstein–Barr virus lymphoma after hemopoietic stem-cell transplantation. *Blood* 2000;95(4):1502–1505.
8. Faye A, Quartier P, Reguerre Y, et al. Chimaeric anti-CD20 monoclonal antibody (rituximab) in post-transplant B-lymphoproliferative disorder following stem cell transplantation in children. *Br J Haematol* 2001;115(1):112–118.
9. Rooney CM, Loftin SK, Holladay MS, et al. Early identification of Epstein–Barr virus-associated post-transplant lymphoproliferative disease. *Br J Haematol* 1995;89:98–103.
10. Stevens SJ, Verschuuren EA, Pronk I, et al. Frequent monitoring of Epstein–Barr virus DNA load in unfractionated whole blood is essential for early detection of posttransplant lymphoproliferative disease in high-risk patients. *Blood* 2001;97(5):1165–1171.
11. Hsu JL, Glaser SL. Epstein–Barr virus-associated malignancies: epidemiologic patterns and etiologic implications. *Crit Rev Oncol Hematol* 2000;34(1):27–53.
12. Cohen JI. Epstein–Barr virus infection. *N Engl J Med* 2000;343(7):481–492.
13. Rickinson AB, Moss DJ. Human cytotoxic T lymphocyte responses to Epstein–Barr virus infection. *Annu Rev Immunol* 1997;15:405–431.
14. Callan MF, Tan L, Annels N, et al. Direct visualization of antigen-specific CD8+ T cells during the primary immune response to Epstein–Barr virus In vivo. *J Exp Med* 1998;187(9):1395–1402.
15. Munz C, Bickham KL, Subklewe M, et al. Human CD4(+) T lymphocytes consistently respond to the latent Epstein–Barr virus nuclear antigen EBNA1. *J Exp Med* 2000;191(10):1649–1660.
16. Nikiforow S, Bottomly K, Miller G. CD4+ T-cell effectors inhibit Epstein–Barr virus-induced B-cell proliferation. *J Virol* 2001;75(8):3740–3752.
17. Thorley-Lawson DA, Babcock GJ. A model for persistent infection with Epstein–Barr virus: the stealth virus of human B cells. *Life Sci* 1999;65(14):1433–1453.
18. Yao QY, Ogan P, Rowe M, et al. Epstein–Barr virus-infected B cells persist in the circulation of acyclovir-treated virus carriers. *Int J Cancer* 1989;43:67–71.
19. Hoshino Y, Kimura H, Tanaka N, et al. Prospective monitoring of the Epstein–Barr virus DNA by a real-time quantitative polymerase chain reaction after allogenic stem cell transplantation. *Br J Haematol* 2001;115(1):105–111.
20. Hale G, Waldmann H, for CAMPATH Users. Risks of developing Epstein–Barr virus-related lymphoproliferative disorders after T-cell-depleted marrow transplants. *Blood* 1998;91:3079–3083.
21. Gross TG, Hinrichs SH, Davis JR, et al. Depletion of EBV-infected cells in donor marrow by counterflow elutriation. *Exp Hematol* 1998;26(5):395–399.
22. Cavazzana-Calvo M, Bensoussan D, Jabado N, et al. Prevention of EBV-induced B-lymphoproliferative disorder by ex vivo marrow B-cell depletion in HLA-phenoidentical or non-identical T-depleted bone marrow transplantation. *Br J Haematol* 1998;103(2):543–551.
23. Liu Z, Wilson JM, Jones MC, et al. Addition of B cell depletion of donor marrow with anti-CD20 antibody to a T cell depletion regimen for prevention of EBV lymphoma after bone marrow transplant. *Blood* 1999;94(10, suppl 1):638a.
24. Hauke RJ, Greiner TC, Smir BN, et al. Epstein–Barr virus-associated lymphoproliferative disorder after autolgous bone marrow transplantation: report of two cases. *Bone Marrow Transplant* 1998;21(12):1271–1274.
25. Barker JN, Martin PL, Coad JE, et al. Low incidence of Epstein–Barr virus-associated posttransplantation lymphoproliferative disorders in 272 unrelated-donor umbilical cord blood transplant recipients. *Biol Blood Marrow Transplant* 2001;7(7):395–399.
26. Deeg HJ, Socie G. Malignancies after hemopoietic stem cell transplantation: many questions, some answers. *Blood* 1998;91(6):1833–1844.
27. Orazi A, Hromas RA, Neiman RS, et al. Posttransplantation lymphoproliferative disorders in bone marrow transplant recipients are aggressive diseases with a high incidence of adverse histologic and immunobiologic features. *Am J Clin Pathol* 1997;107(4):419–429.
28. Knowles DM, Cesarman E, Chadburn A, et al. Correlative morphologic and molecular genetic analysis demonstrates three distinct categories of posttransplantation lymphoproliferative disorders. *Blood* 1995;85(2):552–565.
29. Yang J, Tao Q, Flinn IW, et al. Characterization of Epstein–Barr virus-infected B cells in patients with posttransplantation lymphoproliferative disease: disappearance after rituximab therapy does not predict clinical response. *Blood* 2000;96(13):4055–4063.

30. van Baarle D, Hovenkamp E, Callan MF, et al. Dysfunctional Epstein–Barr virus (EBV)-specific CD8(+) T lymphocytes and increased EBV load in HIV-1 infected individuals progressing to AIDS-related non-Hodgkin lymphoma. *Blood* 2001;98(1):146–155.
31. Kimura H, Morita M, Yabuta Y, et al. Quantitative analysis of Epstein–Barr virus load by using a real-time PCR assay. *J Clin Microbiol* 1999;37(1):132–136.
32. Lucas KG, Burton RL, Zimmerman SE, et al. Semiquantitative Epstein–Barr virus (EBV) polymerase chain reaction for the determination of patients at risk for EBV-induced lymphoproliferative disease after stem cell transplantation. *Blood* 1998;91(10):3654–3661.
33. Niesters HG, van Esser J, Fries E, et al. Development of a real-time quantitative assay for detection of Epstein–Barr virus. *J Clin Microbiol* 2000;38(2):712–715.
34. Wagner HJ, Cheng YC, Liu Z, et al. Monitoring of transplanted patients at risk of Epstein–Barr virus (EBV)-induced lymphoproliferative disorder (LPD) by real time PCR quantification of EBV DNA in peripheral blood. *Blood* 2001;98(11, suppl 1):480a.
35. van Esser JW, van der HB, Meijer E, et al. Epstein–Barr virus (EBV) reactivation is a frequent event after allogeneic stem cell transplantation (SCT) and quantitatively predicts EBV-lymphoproliferative disease following T-cell—depleted SCT. *Blood* 2001;98(4):972–978.
36. Rose C, Green M, Webber S, et al. Pediatric solid-organ transplant recipients carry chronic loads of Epstein–Barr virus exclusively in the immunoglobulin d-negative B-cell compartment. *J Clin Microbiol* 2001;39(4):1407–1415.
37. Gottschalk S, Heslop HE, Rooney CM. Treatment of Epstein–Barr virus-associated malignancies with specific T cells. *Adv Cancer Res* 2002;84:175–201.
38. Swinnen LJ. Treatment of organ transplant-related lymphoma. *Hematol Oncol Clin North Am* 1998;11(5):963–973.
39. Gross TG, Steinbuch M, DeFor T, et al. B cell lymphoproliferative disorders following hematopoietic stem cell transplantation: risk factors, treatment and outcome. *Bone Marrow Transplant* 1999;23:251–258.
40. Papadopoulos EB, Ladanyi M, Emanuel D, et al. Infusions of donor leukocytes to treat Epstein–Barr virus-associated lymphoproliferative disorders after allogeneic bone marrow transplantation. *N Engl J Med* 1994;330:1185–1191.
41. O'Reilly RJ, Small TN, Papadopoulos E, et al. Biology and adoptive cell therapy of Epstein–Barr virus-associated lymphoproliferative disorders in recipients of marrow allografts. *Immunol Rev* 1997;157:195–216.
42. Sasahara Y, Kawai S, Itano M, et al. Epstein–Barr virus-associated lymphoproliferative disorder after unrelated bone marrow transplantation in a young child with Wiskott-Aldrich syndrome. *Pediatr Hematol Oncol* 1998;15(4):347–352.
43. Heslop HE, Brenner MK, Rooney CM. Donor T cells to treat EBV-associated lymphoma. *N Engl J Med* 1994;331:679–680.
44. Nagafuji K, Eto T, Hayashi S, et al. Donor lymphocyte transfusion for the treatment of Epstein–Barr virus-associated lymphoproliferative disorder of the brain. *Bone Marrow Transplant* 1998;21(11):1155–1158.
45. Imashuku S, Goto T, Matsumura T, et al. Unsuccessful CTL transfusion in a case of post-BMT Epstein–Barr virus-associated lymphoproliferative disorder (EBV-LPD). *Bone Marrow Transplant* 1998;20(4):337–340.
46. Tiberghien P. Use of suicide gene-expressing donor T-cells to control alloreactivity after haematopoietic stem cell transplantation. *J Intern Med* 2001;249(4):369–377.
47. Sauce D, Bodinier M, Garin M, et al. Retrovirus-mediated gene transfer in primary T lymphocytes impairs their anti-Epstein–Barr virus potential through both culture-dependent and selection process-dependent mechanisms. *Blood* 2002;99(4):1165–1173.
48. Riddell SR, Watanabe KS, Goodrich JM, et al. Restoration of viral immunity in immunodeficient humans by the adoptive transfer of T cell clones. *Science* 1992;257:238–241.
49. Riddell SR, Greenberg PD. T-Cell therapy of cytomegalovirus and human immunodeficiency virus infection. *J Antimicrob Chemother* 2000;45(suppl T3):35–43.
50. Walter EA, Greenberg PD, Gilbert MJ, et al. Reconstitution of cellular immunity against cytomegalovirus in recipients of allogeneic bone marrow by transfer of T-cell clones from the donor. *N Engl J Med* 1995;333(16):1038–1044.
51. Heslop HE, Rooney CM. Adoptive Immunotherapy of EBV lymphoproliferative diseases. *Immunol Rev* 1997;157:217–222.
52. Heslop HE, Ng CYC, Li C, et al. Long-term restoration of immunity against Epstein–Barr virus infection by adoptive transfer of gene-modified virus-specific T lymphocytes. *Nature Med* 1996;2:551–555.

53. Gottschalk S, Ng CYC, Smith CA, et al. An Epstein–Barr virus deletion mutant that causes fatal lymphoproliferative disease unresponsive to virus-specific T cell therapy. *Blood* 2001;97(4):835–843.
54. Goulder PJ, Brander C, Tang Y, et al. Evolution and transmission of stable CTL escape mutations in HIV infection. *Nature* 2001;412(6844):334–338.
55. Furukawa Y, Kubota R, Tara M, et al. Existence of escape mutant in HTLV-I tax during the development of adult T-cell leukemia. *Blood* 2001;97(4):987–993.
56. Koehne G, Gallardo HF, Sadelain M, et al. Rapid selection of antigen-specific T lymphocytes by retroviral transduction. *Blood* 2000;96(1):109–117.
57. Sun Q, Pollok KE, Burton RL, et al. Simultaneous ex vivo expansion of cytomegalovirus and Epstein–Barr virus-specific cytotoxic T lymphocytes using B-lymphoblastoid cell lines expressing cytomegalovirus pp65. *Blood* 1999;94(9):3242–3250.
58. Regn S, Raffegerst S, Chen X, et al. Ex vivo generation of cytotoxic T lymphocytes specific for one or two distinct viruses for the prophylaxis of patients receiving an allogeneic bone marrow transplant. *Bone Marrow Transplant* 2001;27(1):53–64.
59. Montagna D, Yvon E, Calcaterra V, et al. Depletion of alloreactive T cells by a specific anti-interleukin-2 receptor p55 chain immunotoxin does not impair in vitro antileukemia and antiviral activity. *Blood* 1999;93(10):3550–3557.
60. Nalesnik MA, Rao AS, Furukawa H, et al. Autologous lymphokine-activated killer cell therapy of Epstein–Barr virus-positive and -negative lymphoproliferative disorders arising in organ transplant recipients. *Transplantation* 1998;63:1200–1205.
61. Fischer A, Blanche S, LeBidois J, et al. Anti-B-cell monoclonal antibodies in the treatment of severe B-cell lymphoproliferative syndrome following bone marrow and organ transplantation. *N Engl J Med* 1991;324:1451–1456.
62. Levy R. A perspective on monoclonal antibody therapy: where we have been and where we are going. *Semin Hematol* 2000;37(4, suppl 7):43–46.
63. Maloney DG, Grillo-Lopez AJ, White CA, et al. IDEC-C2B8 (rituximab) anti-CD20 monoclonal antibody therapy in patients with relapsed low-grade non-Hodgkin's lymphoma. *Blood* 1997;90(6):2188–2195.
64. Maloney GD. Monoclonal antibodies in lymphoid neoplasia: principles for optimal combined therapy. *Semin Hematol* 2000;37(4, suppl 7):17–26.
65. Milpied N, Vasseur B, Parquet N, et al. Humanized anti-CD20 monoclonal antibody (Rituximab) in post transplant B-lymphoproliferative disorder: a retrospective analysis on 32 patients. *Ann Oncol* 2000;11(suppl 1):113–116.
66. Carpenter PA, Appelbaum FR, Corey L, et al. A humanized non-FcR-binding anti-CD3 antibody, visilizumab, for treatment of steroid-refractory acute graft-versus-host disease. *Blood* 2002;99(8):2712–2719.
67. Davis TA, Czerwinski DK, Levy R. Therapy of B-cell lymphoma with anti-CD20 antibodies can result in the loss of CD20 antigen expression. *Clin Cancer Res* 1999;5(3):611–615.
68. Verschuuren EA, Stevens SJ, van Imhoff GW, et al. Treatment of posttransplant lymphoproliferative disease with rituximab: the remission, the relapse, and the complication. *Transplantation* 2002;73(1):100–104.
69. Haddad E, Paczesny S, Leblond V, et al. Treatment of B-lymphoproliferative disorder with a monoclonal anti-interleukin-6 antibody in 12 patients: a multicenter phase 1–2 clinical trial. *Blood* 2001;97(6):1590–1597.
70. Faye A, Van Den Abeele T, Peuchmaur M, et al. Anti-CD20 monoclonal antibody for post-transplant lymphoproliferative disorders. *Lancet* 1998;352:1285.
71. Gruhn B, Meerbach A, Haefer R, et al. Early diagnosis and pre-emptive therapy of Epstein–Barr virus-associated lymphoproliferative disease following hematopoietic stem cell transplantation. *Blood* 2001;98(11, suppl 1):393a.

12 Pathophysiology of Lung Injury After Hematopoietic Stem Cell Transplantation

Kenneth R. Cooke, MD

Contents

1. INTRODUCTION

Over the last several decades, hematopoietic stem cell transplantation (SCT) has emerged as an important therapeutic option for a number of malignant and nonmalignant conditions. Unfortunately, the utility of this treatment strategy is limited by several side effects, the most serious of which include the development of graft-vs-host disease (GVHD) and pulmonary toxicity. Pulmonary dysfunction, specifically diffuse lung injury, is a major complication of SCT; it occurs in 25–55% of SCT recipients and can account for approximately 50% of transplant-related mortality *(1–6)*. Diffuse lung injury is described as either acute or chronic with respect to both the time of onset after SCT and the tempo of disease progression once the diagnosis has been established. Approximately 50% of the time, an infectious etiology is uncovered, whereas in the remaining 50% of cases, no microbial organisms are identified in the lungs of affected patients *(7)*. In recent years, the judicious use of broad-spectrum antimicrobial prophylaxis has tipped the balance of pulmonary complications after SCT from infectious to noninfectious. In this context, two types of pulmonary dysfunction have been recognized: acute noninfectious lung injury (termed idiopathic pneumonia syndrome [IPS]) and subacute or chronic noninfectious lung injury. Two forms of subacute/chronic lung injury are common in patients over 100 d posttransplant: airflow obstruction and restrictive lung injury *(8–16)*. Each form of noninfectious lung injury is associated with significant morbidity and mortality and, unfortunately, clinical responses to standard therapeutic approaches are limited. This chapter will be devoted to noninfectious lung injury occurring both early and late

From: *Stem Cell Transplantation for Hematologic Malignancies*
Edited by: R. J. Soiffer © Humana Press Inc., Totowa, NJ

after allogeneic SCT (alloSCT), with the goal of providing a better understanding of the definition, risk factors, and pathogenesis of these important transplant-related complications.

2. ACUTE LUNG INJURY: IDIOPATHIC PNEUMONIA SYNDROME

2.1. Overview

Idiopathic pneumonia syndrome refers to diffuse, noninfectious lung injury that occurs early in the time-course of SCT. In 1993, a panel convened by the National Institutes of Health (NIH) proposed a broad working definition of IPS to include widespread alveolar injury in the absence of active lower-respiratory-tract infection following SCT *(7)*. The NIH panel was careful to stress that they considered this definition to be that of a clinical *syndrome*, with variable histopathologic correlates and several potential etiologies *(7)*. Diagnostic criteria of IPS include signs and symptoms of pneumonia, evidence for nonlobar radiographic infiltrates, abnormal pulmonary function, and the absence of infectious organisms in the lower respiratory tract as determined by broncho-alveolar lavage (BAL) or lung biopsy *(2,7)*. A variety of histopathologic findings have been associated with IPS, including hyaline membranes, bronchiolitis obliterans organizing pneumonia (BOOP), and lymphocytic bronchitis; however, the most frequently reported pattern is interstitial pneumonitis, a term historically used interchangeably with IPS *(17)*. The median time of onset for IPS was initially described to be 6–7 wk after SCT, with a range from 14 to 90 d after the infusion of donor stem cells *(7)*. Perhaps the most striking feature of IPS is its impact on overall survival; mortality rates of 50–80% have been reported, with survival being less than 5% for patients requiring mechanical ventilation *(2,3,5–7,18,19)*. Although a more recent retrospective study from the Seattle group showed a lower incidence and earlier onset of IPS than previously reported, the typical clinical course involving the rapid onset of respiratory failure leading to death remained unchanged *(6)*. A retrospective review performed at the University of Michigan Medical Center demonstrated that the frequency of IPS after alloSCT ranged from 5% to 25% depending on donor source and the degree of antigenic mismatch. Consistent with the Seattle report, the median time for development of IPS was 18 days after transplant in unrelated donor (URD) recipients, and 13 d in the allogeneic peripheral blood stem cell (PBSC) group. Strikingly, the overall d 100 mortality in patients with IPS was 90% and the median time to death from onset of IPS was 13 days, despite high-dose steroids and broad-spectrum antimicrobial therapy *(20)*. As noted, these findings are consistent with published reports and underscore the critical nature of this transplant-related problem.

Potential risk factors for IPS are several and include SCT conditioning with total-body irradiation (TBI), acute graph-vs-host disease (GVHD), older recipient age, SCT for malignancies other than leukemia, and methotrexate (MTX) for GVHD prophylaxis *(5,21–23)*. Furthermore, the likelihood of developing IPS increases with the number of identified risk factors *(3)*. Whereas the effects of MTX and recipient age on IPS have been disputed, the correlation of TBI use or the development of acute GVHD with IPS has been observed in several reports *(2,5,6,23–25)*. The definition of IPS encompasses numerous descriptive forms of pulmonary toxicity as well, including diffuse alveolar hemorrhage (DAH), peri-engraftment respiratory distress syndrome (PERDS), and delayed pulmonary toxicity syndrome (DPTS) *(19)*. DAH generally develops in the immediate post-SCT period and is characterized by progressive shortness of breath, cough, and hypoxemia with or without fever *(19,26–28)*. Although hemoptysis is rare, BAL showing progressively bloodier aliquots of lavage return has traditionally diagnosed DAH *(26)*. Mortality has been reported in up to three-quarters of affected patients despite high-dose (250 mg/kg to 2 g/kg) steroids, with death occurring within 3 wk of diagnosis *(27)*. Peri-engraftment syndrome and DPTS typically occur after autologous SCT (autoSCT) *(19)*. Each is characterized by fever, dyspnea, and hypoxemia and tends to have a more favorable response to corticosteroids and overall prognosis *(29–31)*. By definition, PERDS occurs within 5 d of engraftment, whereas the onset of DPTS may be delayed for months and commonly occurs following high-dose chemotherapy (HDC) containing cyclophosphamide, cisplatin, and bischloroethylinitrosurea (BCNU) and stem cell rescue for breast cancer *(31)*.

2.2. Pathogenesis of Idiopathic Pneumonia Syndrome: The Lung As a Potential Target of the GVH Response

Potential etiologies for IPS are several and include direct toxic effects of SCT conditioning regimens, occult pulmonary infections, and inflammatory cytokines that have been implicated in other forms of pulmonary injury *(32–36)*. In addition, immunologic factors may be important. Support for the latter can be found in several large series in which IPS was associated with allogeneic (vs autologous or syngeneic) SCT and severe GVHD (vs mild or absent) *(2,3,5,6,18,19)*. In many instances, acute GVHD often precedes IPS, suggesting a possible causal relationship between the two entities *(5,21,37,38)*. Although the lung is not recognized as a classic target organ of GVHD, the clinical association between lung injury and GVHD and the demonstration of pathologic lung changes in rodents with acute GVHD make this possibility intriguing *(2,3,5,6,39–43)*. The pathophysiology of GVHD is complex and is now known to involve donor T-cell responses to host antigens, inflammatory cytokine effectors such as tumor necrosis factor-α (TNF-α) and interleukin-1 (IL-1), and endotoxin *(16,44–48)*. Endotoxin or lipopolysaccharide (LPS) is a component of endogenous bowel flora and is a potent enhancer of inflammatory cytokine release. Translocation of LPS across a gut mucosa damaged early in the posttransplant period by the effects of conditioning regimens and GVHD has been demonstrated after both experimental and clinical SCT *(49–52)*. When LPS reaches the systemic circulation, it induces the release of inflammatory cytokines, which, together with cellular effectors, contribute to GVHD target organ damage and dysfunction *(44,53,54)*.

The role of GVHD and specifically alloreactive donor lymphocytes in the pathogenesis of IPS remains a topic of considerable debate. Although acute pulmonary dysfunction has been associated with the development of systemic GVHD, IPS has also been reported after allogeneic T-cell-depleted SCT and when signs and symptoms of GVHD are limited or absent *(55–58)*, making a causal relationship between the two entities difficult to establish. The principal objection to the identification of the lung as a target of the GVH reaction is that epithelial apoptosis, a finding classically attributed to selective T-cell-mediated injury and considered pathognomonic for acute GVHD in other target tissue, has not been consistently identified in the lungs of patients with IPS *(38,59–61)*. In 1978, Beschorner and colleagues reported an association between the severity of clinical GVHD and a histologic pattern consistent with lymphocytic bronchitis found on postmortem exams. This finding was not seen in patients who received auto SCT or in untransplanted controls *(38)*. Although initially considered a potential histopathologic correlate for GVHD of the lung, the association between lymphocytic bronchitis and the development of systemic GVHD was not consistently identified in subsequent reports *(59–61)*.

The heterogeneity of pulmonary histopathology after clinical SCT is complicated further by the nonspecific changes that occur after mechanical ventilation and by the risks associated with lung biopsy procedures that can significantly limit the quality and quantity of pathology specimens obtained. Despite the lack of classic GVHD histopathology, it is not unreasonable to suggest that pulmonary epithelial and endothelial cells can be potential targets for activated donor T cells after allo SCT. First, the lung is a rich source of major and minor histocompatibility (HC) antigens and professional antigen-presenting cells *(62,63)* and is the site of complex immunologic networks, the proper balance of which allows for infectious surveillance and maintenance of structural integrity, whereas dysregulation of such networks can result in tissue injury and scarring *(64)*. Furthermore, the inflammatory mediators TNF-α and LPS, which are believed to play a part in GVHD *(52,54,65)*, have also been implicated as contributors to pulmonary dysfunction in several experimental systems and clinical syndromes, including adult respiratory distress syndrome (ARDS), lung allograft rejection, and pneumonitis after toxin exposure *(32–36,39,66–69)*. The role of T lymphocytes in immune-mediated pulmonary inflammation has recently been confirmed by several groups and is thought to involve dendritic cells, macrophages, and the secretion of cytokines *(70,71)*. Enhanced lymphocyte activation has been reported in the lungs of patients after BMT and during lung allograft rejection as well *(55,56,72)*.

Second, as discussed in detail later in this chapter, the association of chronic GVHD with obstructive lung disease after alloSCT is well accepted *(8,9,73–76)*. Although a causal link between these two entities has yet to be definitively established, the striking similarities between the consistent histopathologic features of bronchiolitis obliterans seen after SCT and that observed during lung transplant rejection, along with reports of improvement in lung function with immunosuppressive agents, strongly suggest an immunologic component to this pulmonary process *(9,74–76)*. Third, epithelial cell apoptosis is not a requirement of GVHD pathology; the thymus is a known target of GVHD and displays extensive cytolytic damage early in the course of this process, but epithelial cell apoptosis is not a prominent histologic feature *(77)*. Finally, recent studies have demonstrated that GVHD target organs vary with respect to their susceptibility to injury by inflammatory effectors such as cytotoxic T lymphocytes (CTLs), TNF-α, and FasL *(48,78)*. If the mechanisms of GVHD related tissue injury can differ between individual target organs, it is possible that the histopathologic manifestation of this injury may also vary.

2.3. Murine Models of IPS After Allogeneic BMT

2.3.1. Overview

Using well-established rodent SCT models, several investigators have recently explored the relationship between alloreactivity and IPS and have consistently shown that animals with systemic GVHD develop lung injury *(39,42,79,80)*. Importantly, these studies have uncovered potential roles for both inflammatory mediators and cellular effectors in the evolution of IPS and support the hypothesis that the lung may, indeed, be vulnerable to a "two-pronged" immunologic attack after allo SCT. Advantages of these systems include the unlimited availability of tissue for pathologic analysis, tight control over SCT parameters (including HC differences between donor and host, SCT conditioning regimens, and T-cell dose) and the ability to analyze the development of tissue injury without the confounding influences of immunosuppressive chemoprophylaxis, underlying disease, or prior treatment. Surprisingly, even under controlled experimental conditions, several patterns of lung injury have been identified. For example, using a B10 → (CBA × B10)F1 murine SCT model, Piguet and co-workers observed both an acute hemorrhagic alveolitis and a late-onset interstitial pneumonitis (IP) after infusion of B10 parental lymphocytes, whereas induction of GVHD with T cells from CBA donors led to IP only *(39)*. In addition, the development of interstitial pneumonitis along with a lymphocytic bronchiolitis/bronchitis comparable to the histopathology seen in lung allograft rejection was noted in an unirradiated rat GVHD model *(79)*. Similar pulmonary pathology has been reported in several mouse SCT systems that model a variety of HC antigenic mismatches between donor and host *(40–43,80,81)*.

In studies completed by Cooke and colleagues, B10.BR donor stem cells and T lymphocytes were transplanted into CBA recipients. This donor/recipient strain combination is matched at the loci but differs at multiple minor HC antigens and therefore most closely models a SCT from a matched unrelated donor. At 6 wk after SCT, lungs of mice receiving syngeneic transplants maintained virtually normal histology. By contrast, two major abnormalities were apparent in the allogeneic group: a dense mononuclear cell infiltrate around both pulmonary vessels and bronchioles and an acute pneumonitis involving the interstitium and alveolar spaces *(42)*. The alveolar infiltrate was composed of macrophages, lymphocytes, epithelial cells, and scattered polymorphonuclear cells within a fibrin matrix *(42)*. Both of these histopathologic patterns closely resemble the microscopic features of the nonspecific, diffuse interstitial pneumonias seen in allo SCT recipients *(7,17,38,59)*. As noted earlier, similar histopathology has been observed using other strain combinations where the GVH reaction is induced across (1) other minor antigens, (2) class I or class II antigens only, and (3) major and minor HC antigenic differences, whereas findings of diffuse alveolar injury, including alveolar hemorrhage, edema, or hyaline membranes, were not seen *(82–84)*. Pulmonary function has been measured in live transplanted mice in order to assess the physiologic consequences of lung pathology present after SCT *(43,80)*. Mice with GVHD showed significant reductions in both dynamic compliance and airway conductance compared with syngeneic controls consistent with both the interstitial and peribronchial infiltrates seen microscopically *(43)*. Of note, no differences in pulmonary function or lung histopathology were observed between animals with mild and moderate GVHD. Thus, initial studies suggested that the development of IPS after allo SCT correlated with the presence, but not the severity, of systemic GVHD. The nonlinear relationship between lung injury and the severity of acute GVHD was consistent with clinical reports of IPS in patients whose signs and symptoms of GVHD were mild or absent *(8,9,57,73,74)*. Physiologically significant lung injury has also been reported in a fully major HC mismatched system within the first 2 wk of SCT *(80)*, suggesting that increasing antigenic disparity between donor and host may directly correlate with the time of onset of IPS in these mouse BMT systems.

2.3.2. Inflammatory Effectors TNF-α and LPS and the Development of IPS

Experimental models have also provided insight into the possible pathophysiologic mechanisms responsible for acute noninfectious lung injury occurring after SCT. Consistent with the mixed inflammatory alveolar infiltrates observed on histopathology, lung injury in recipients of allo SCT has been shown to be associated with a significant increase in the number of BAL lymphocytes, macrophages, and neutrophils *(42)*. Furthermore, increased expression of TNF-α mRNA and protein has been detected in the lungs and BAL fluid of animals with GVHD *(40–42,45,81)*. The correlation between increased BAL fluid TNF-α levels, neutrophil content, and pulmonary pathology in the absence of infection suggests that endotoxin (LPS) might also play an important role in the observed damage. Not only are increased levels of LPS noted in the BAL fluid of mice with IPS, but LPS may also be a "trigger" for the release of inflammatory cytokines that directly contribute to lung damage; LPS injection 6 wk after SCT increased the total number of neutrophils in the BAL fluid and significantly amplified the severity of lung injury in animals with advanced GVHD *(42)*. These pathologic changes were associated with large increases in BAL fluid levels of TNF-α and LPS and with the development of alveolar hemorrhage *(42,81)*. The role of TNF-α in the development of experimental IPS has been examined further by using strategies that neutralize the effects of this inflammatory cytokine *(45,81,82)*. Recently, the effects of a soluble, dimeric, TNF-binding protein (rhTNFR:Fc; Immunex Corp. Seattle, WA) on lung injury were studied after allo SCT. Administration of rhTNFR:Fc around the time of LPS challenge effectively reduced mortality and prevented increases in pulmonary pathology, BAL fluid cellularity and endotoxin content, confirming that TNF-α is central to LPS-mediated systemic and pulmonary toxicity in this setting *(81)*. Furthermore, TNF-α neutralization from wk 4 to wk 6 after SCT significantly reduced the severity of lung injury and prevented the progression of systemic and hepatic GVHD seen in the control group during the treatment period *(81)*.

TNF-α is likely to contribute to the development of IPS through both direct and indirect mechanisms. TNF-α increases MHC expression, modulates leukocyte migration, facilitates cell-mediated cytotoxicity, and is itself cytotoxic *(45,85)*. It is also possible that the protective effects seen in the lung are secondary to a systemic anti-inflammatory response *(86)* because TNF-α blockade also attenuates the progression systemic and hepatic GVHD *(81)*. The partial reduction in lung injury provided by TNF-α neutralization is consistent with reports from many groups *(39,45,51,52,78,87,88)* and suggests that other inflammatory mediators and cellular mechanisms that are involved in acute GVHD may also contribute to the development of IPS *(47,48,78)*. Specifically, interleukin (IL)-1β, transforming growth factor-β (TGF-β), and nitrating species including nitric oxide and peroxynitrite have been implicated in the generation of early lung toxicity after allo SCT, particularly when cyclophosphamide is included in the conditioning regimen *(80,89,90)*.

The results of endotoxin challenge experiments confirm that TNF-α mediates systemic and pulmonary toxicity caused by LPS *(91–93)*. The reduction in BAL fluid LPS after TNF-α neutralization was intriguing however and strongly suggested that in addition to directly neutralizing TNF-α in the alveolar space, treatment with rhTNFR:Fc altered the systemic inflammatory response to LPS "upstream" from the lung *(86)*. From this perspective, the structural and functional integrity of the liver is likely to be critical. The liver is pivotally located between the intestinal reservoir of Gram-negative bacteria and their toxic byproducts and the rich capillary network in the lung. Kupffer cells in the liver detoxify and subsequently clear endotoxin from the systemic circulation *(94)* and protect the lung in experimental models of sepsis and ARDS *(95,96)*. Inflammation engendered during the normal clearance of endotoxin remains contained within the reticulo-endothelial system of the liver *(94)*. If, however, the capacity of the liver to clear an endotoxin challenge is exceeded, both inflammatory cytokines and unprocessed LPS can traverse into the systemic circulation and cause acute end-organ damage. Several experimental studies have shown that pre-existing injury decreases the ability of the liver to neutralize endotoxin effectively *(97–100)*. In the setting of acute GVHD, an endotoxin surge can arise from increased leakage of LPS across damaged intestinal mucosa. In this scenario, underlying hepatic damage as a consequence of direct target organ injury could then serve to decrease the liver's capacity for LPS uptake and clearance. Animals with mild or no GVHD effectively detoxify exogenous endotoxin and protect their lungs from further damage, whereas mice with extensive disease are unable to do so and ultimately develop severe pulmonary toxicity, including alveolar hemorrhage *(42)*. In the studies noted earlier using rhTNFR:Fc, all animals had advanced GVHD at the time of analysis. As expected, administration of LPS to animals treated with control IgG overwhelmed the liver's capacity to clear circulating endotoxin and caused enhanced hepatic injury and the propagation of systemic and pulmonary disease. By contrast, systemic neutralization of TNF-α protected the liver from endotoxin-induced inflammation and resulted in decreased mortality and a reduction of BAL fluid LPS levels and pulmonary inflammation *(81)*.

These data demonstrate that the inflammatory mediators TNF-α and LPS both contribute to experimental IPS. Moreover, they support the hypothesis that a "gut–liver–lung" axis of inflammation may play a role in IPS pathophysiology and suggest that any process or combination of events that eventually results in large amounts of endotoxin and/or TNF-α into the pulmonary circulation could contribute to the development of lung injury. This hypothesis is supported by the clinical observation of increased levels of TNF-α in the serum of patients that develop IPS *(101)*. A role for hepatic dysfunction in pulmonary toxicity after SCT is also consistent with clinical reports of acute noninfectious pulmonary toxicity associated with severe GVHD and veno-occlusive disease (VOD) *(2,102)*. Furthermore, evidence for cytokine activation and LPS amplification in the broncho-alveolar compartment, which has been noted during ARDS *(103)*, has recently been demonstrated in patients with IPS after SCT as well *(1)*. Clark and colleagues found increased pulmonary vascular permeability and BAL fluid levels of IL-1, IL-12, IL-6, and TNF-α and components of the LPS amplification system (LPB and CD14) in patients with IPS *(1)*. The investigators conclude that pro-inflammatory cytokine activation contributes to IPS and suggest that patients with this complication may be at increased risk for LPS-mediated lung injury.

2.3.3. Cellular Effectors and the Development of IPS

2.3.3.1. The Role of Neutrophil/Polymorphonuclear Cells

As demonstrated earlier, the presence of neutrophils, in the absence of infection, is a major component of the inflammatory infiltrate seen in animals with IPS *(42)*. A role for neutrophils in noninfectious lung injury has been observed in both the acute and chronic setting; neutrophilia is a prominent finding in acute respiratory distress syndrome (ARDS) and in the early and late stages of bronchiolitis obliterans (BO) that develops during lung allograft rejection *(104–109)*. Polymorphonuclear (PMN) products are abundant in the BAL fluid of patients with ARDS and are believed to significantly contribute to endothelial and epithelial damage that occurs in this setting *(104)*, whereas similar increases in PMN activation markers may be early indicators of BO after lung transplant *(106)*. Neutrophils are likely to play a role in lung injury after SCT as well; more that 60% of patients diagnosed with IPS at the University of Michigan developed signs and symptoms of pulmonary dysfunction within 7 d of neutrophil engraftment *(20)*. Furthermore, a significant neutrophilic influx has also been observed in the BAL fluid and biopsy specimens of SCT recipients with BO *(110,111)*. In mouse IPS models, the influx of neutrophils is most prominent between wk 4 and 6 after SCT and is associated with the presence of TNF-α and LPS in the BAL fluid *(42,81)*. The relationship among neutrophils, TNF-α, and LPS is underscored by the outcome of LPS challenge and TNF-α neutralization experiments; administration of rhTNFR:Fc completely abrogated the robust influx of PMN cells resulting from LPS administration *(81)*. Importantly, this finding directly correlated with protection from enhanced pulmonary histopathology (including hemorrhage) and the preservation of pulmonary function *(81)*. Furthermore, reduction in lung injury resulting from neutralizing TNF from wk 4 to 6 was also accompanied by a significant decrease in neutrophils in BAL fluid. Taken together, these data support a role for neutrophils in the injury incurred during IPS and suggest that aspects of the innate immune response may also contribute to this process.

2.3.3.2. Role of Donor Accessory Cells in the Development of IPS

The relationship among LPS, TNF-α, and donor leukocytes in the pathophysiology IPS has been examined further by determining whether the responsiveness of donor cells to LPS stimulation would influence the development of lung injury after allo SCT. To test this hypothesis, two related substrains of mice, C3H/Hej and C3Heb/Fej, that differ in their response to the lethal effects of LPS *(112)* were used as SCT donors. C3Heb/Fej animals exhibit normal murine sensitivity to LPS challenge (LPS-s), whereas a genetic mutation in the Toll-like receptor 4 (Tlr 4) gene of C3H/Hej mice has made this strain resistant to LPS (LPS-r) *(112–115)*. Initial experiments demonstrated that transplantation of cells from LPS-r donors resulted in a significant decrease in systemic GVHD. Specifically, LPS-r SCT reduced early intestinal injury mediated by TNF-α, a finding that was independent of donor T-cell response to host antigens *(52)*. In subsequent experiments, recipients of LPS-r SCT were also found to develop significantly less lung toxicity as measured by pathology, function, and BAL fluid cellularity *(82)*. This protective effect was associated with decreased TNF-α secretion in vivo and in vitro; BAL fluid TNF-α levels were lower after LPS-r SCT and BAL cells harvested from LPS-r recipients produced approx 30-fold less TNF-α to LPS stimulation compared to cells collected from recipients of LPS-s SCT *(82)*. This finding correlated with the naïve phenotype of C3H/Hej and C3Heb/Fej BAL cells, respectively, and was consistent with the observation that more than 98% of BAL cells are of donor origin by wk 4 after transplant. BAL LPS concentrations were also decreased after LPS-r SCT and correlated with a reduction in intestinal toxicity and serum LPS levels at wk 1 and with decreased intestinal and hepatic injury at wk 5 *(52,82)*. Similar reductions in systemic GVHD and lung injury have also been observed when animals deficient in CD14, a cell surface receptor critical to the innate immune response and an important receptor for LPS, were used as SCT donors in a second P → F1 SCT model *(116)*. These data demonstrate that resistance of donor accessory cells to LPS stimulation reduces the severity of lung injury after allo SCT. Importantly, these findings also reveal a significant role for donor-derived macrophages in IPS and support an etiologic link between gut and lung damage that occurs after alloSCT.

2.3.3.3. Role of Donor-Derived T-Cell Effectors

Although the induction of GVHD fundamentally depends on interactions between donor T cells and host antigen-presenting cells *(117)*, the role of alloreactive donor T cells in the pathogenesis of IPS has been a topic of considerable debate. The importance of lymphocytes to lung injury after experimental SCT has, however, been suggested by several groups *(40,80,118,119)*. Donor T cells are critical to the early pro-inflammatory events associated with lung toxicity that develops within the first week of SCT across MHC antigens, whereas in a minor HC antigen mismatch system, donor lymphocytes have been shown to persistently respond to host antigens and contribute to physiologically significant lung histopathology at later time-points after SCT *(43,80)*. Furthermore, donor T-cell clones that recognize CD45 polymorphisms result in a rapidly progressive pulmonary vasculitis within the first 3 d after their injection into nonirradiated recipients *(40,119)*. Finally, Gartner and colleagues showed that pulmonary natural killer (NK)-cell activity remained increased over an extended period of time during GVHD in contrast to the transient and mild increase in splenic NK activity that occurred during the same interval *(120)*. These experimental data support clinical observations suggesting that alveolar lymphocytosis associated with interstitial pneumonitis after allo BMT could represent a pulmonary manifestation of chronic GVHD *(121)*.

Additional experiments have been completed to determine whether donor cytotoxic T lymphocyte (CTL) effectors contribute to lung injury via cell–cell-mediated killing. Two primary cytolytic pathways have been identified: the perforin–granzyme pathway and the Fas–Fas ligand (FasL) pathway. Both perforin and Fas pathways contribute to cytolysis mediated by CTLs and lymphokine-activated killer (LAK) cells *(122–125)*. The Fas pathway is primarily used by CD4+ cells *(126)*, whereas perforin-mediated killing has been shown to involve both CD4+ and CD8+ T-cell populations *(48,127)*. Furthermore, each cytolytic pathway has been shown to play a role in the development of GVHD and lung injury in non-SCT settings *(128–131)*. Using a parent → F1 model, significant CTL activity has been observed in the lungs of allo SCT recipients; alloantigen-specific killing using both perforin and Fas/FasL pathways was present as early as wk 2 after BMT and persisted over time as lung injury developed *(83)*. The relative contribution of each cytolytic pathway to the development of IPS was determined by using wild-type mice or animals deficient in either perforin (*pfp*) or FasL (*gld*) as SCT donors. Recipients of *gld*, but not *pfp–/–* SCT developed significantly less lung injury compared to allogeneic controls, a finding that was associated with reductions in BAL fluid cellularity, donor CD4+ and CD8+ T cells, and TNF-α levels *(83)*.

As mentioned earlier however, noninfectious lung injury has been reported in patients in whom systemic GVHD is mild or absent, making a causal relationship between alloreactive T cells and IPS difficult to establish *(8,9,57,73,74)*. Of interest, T-cell depletion (TCD) at the time of SCT using the B10.BR → CBA system reduced, but did not abrogate, lymphocyte responses in the lungs even though the number of T cells in the donor stem cell inoculum was insufficient to cause clinical or histologic GVHD. The observation that host reactive donor lymphocytes were present in the BAL fluid but not the spleens of animals after TCD SCT was intriguing and suggested that the lung may be particularly sensitive to the effects of these cells even when systemic tolerance has been established. Clinically, BAL fluid lymphocytosis has been described after TCD SCT in association with pneumonitis that resulted from a local immune response; pulmonary T cells appeared to be activated despite systemic immune suppression *(55)*. Collectively, these data support a role for cellular effector mechanisms in IPS pathophysiology. Donor-derived T cells can contribute to lung injury after SCT, even when systemic GVHD is mild or absent. In addition, CTL activity is present in the lungs of mice with IPS, and Fas–FasL but not perforin-mediated killing significantly contributes to the development of lung injury in an experimental system.

2.3.4. Role of Host Antigen-Presenting Cells in the Development of IPS

Although several groups have generated data to support a role for alloreactive donor T cells in the evolution of lung injury after SCT, the precise mechanisms by which these cells interact with host antigens and cause injury remain unresolved. This process is likely to be complex and to ultimately involve the interaction of donor lymphocytes with pulmonary antigen-presenting cells (APCs). It is conceivable that pulmonary dendritic cells, which are potent stimulators of primary T-cell responses, are intimately involved with this process *(132,133)*. These cells are thought to play a critical role in the initiation and regulation of immune responses in the lung, and recent data suggest that they are important to both acute and chronic rejection after lung transplantation *(134–137)*. Furthermore, the Th1 cytokines IL-2, and interferon-γ (IFN-γ), which are critical to the development of GVHD *(138)* are felt to be involved in the activation and recruitment of dendritic cells to sites of inflammation *(139,140)*. The specific requirement of host APCs for the generation of acute GVHD was recently reported in a CD8+ T-cell-driven GVHD model in which chimeric animals that did not express alloantigen (MHC class I) on their APCs were used as SCT recipients *(117)*. These results were recently extended by the work of Teshima and colleagues, who showed that alloantigen expression on host epithelial cells is not required for the development of acute GVHD; rather, recognition of alloantigen on host APCs is necessary and sufficient to induce a GVH reaction in which early cytotoxic damage to GVHD target organs is driven by inflammatory cytokines *(65)*. It is possible that radio-resistant, pulmonary APCs in the host persist longer than those in other organs, thus allowing sustained presentation of host antigens in the lung (but not in other visceral sites) to small numbers of donor T cells trapped within the pulmonary microvascular circulation. This hypothesis could account for the apparent "sanctuary" status of the lung with respect to donor T cells and may have important implications with regard to the evaluation and treatment of pulmonary dysfunction after SCT even when clinical GVHD is absent.

2.3.5. Mechanisms of Leukocyte Recruitment to the Lung After Allo SCT

Although cellular effectors likely play a significant role in development of IPS, the mechanisms by which white blood cells (WBCs) traffic to the lung and cause inflammation have yet to be determined. WBC trafficking to sites of inflammation is a complex process involving interactions between leukocytes and endothelial cells that are facilitated by adhesion molecules, chemokines, and their receptors *(141)*. Chemokines are a large family of 8- to 10-kDa polypeptide molecules that have well-defined roles in directing cell movements of lymphocytes, monocytes, and neutrophils during immune responses and do so both directly via their chemoattractant properties (i.e., by providing "directional clues") and indirectly via integrin activation *(142,143)*. The 50+ chemokines that have been identified to date are classified structurally into 4 main groups according to the configuration of cysteine residues near the NH2-terminus (CC, CXC, C, and CX_3C) *(143)*. Actions of chemokines are mediated through a large family of seven-transmembrane-spanning, serpentine, G_i-protein-coupled receptors that have ligand specificity and a restricted expression on subclasses of leukocytes. However, ligand specificities can overlap; some chemokines bind to several receptors and some receptors bind multiple ligands *(144)*. Chemokines and their receptors can be functionally divided into two broad categories: "inducible" or "inflammatory" chemokines that are regulated by proinflammatory stimuli, help orchestrate innate and adaptive immunity, and recruit leukocytes to sites of inflammation in response to physiologic stress and "constitutive" or "homeostatic" chemokines responsible for basal leukocyte migration during immune surveillance and formation of the architectural framework of secondary lymphoid organs. "Inducible" or "inflammatory" chemokines are produced by a variety of cell types and are induced to high levels of expression by inflammatory stimuli such as LPS, IL-1 and TNF-α *(141)*. The corresponding "inflammatory" chemokine receptors tend to have more promiscuous or redundant ligand-binding interactions compared to "homeostatic" receptors and tend to be expressed on cells with an "effector" phenotype *(145)*.

Although chemokines have been shown to facilitate the recruitment of leukocytes to the lung in a variety of inflammatory states, including asthma, ARDS, infectious pneumonia, pulmonary fibrosis, and lung allograft rejection *(145,146)*, investigators have just begun to explore their role in IPS. In each scenario, the composition of the accompanying leukocytic infiltrate is determined by the pattern of chemokine expression in the inflamed lung. The mixed pulmonary infiltrate observed in mice after allo SCT suggests, therefore, that chemokines responsible for the recruitment of monocytes, lymphocytes, and neutrophils may be upregulated during the development of IPS. This hypothesis is supported by the work of Panoskaltsis-Mortari and co-workers, who noted that enhanced expression of monocyte- and T-cell-attracting chemokines in the lungs correlated with lung injury that developed within the first 2 wk after SCT *(147)*. Work by the same group specifically demonstrated that T-lymphocyte production of MIP-1α is critical to the recruitment of CD8+ T cells to GVHD target organs, including the lung at later time-points after SCT *(148)*. These findings are supported by the observation that specific interactions between MIP-1α and CCR5+ CD8+ T cells also contribute to the pathogenesis of liver GVHD *(149)*. Studies are ongoing to more specifically determine the role of inflammatory chemokines in leukocyte recruitment during the development of IPS.

2.3.6. Summary

Extensive preclinical and clinical data suggest that both inflammatory and cellular effectors participate in the development of IPS after alloSCT; TNF-α and LPS appear to be significant, albeit not exclusive, contributors to IPS, and cells of both myeloid and lymphoid origin also play a direct role in lung injury that occurs in this setting. In particular, the contribution of donor accessory cells appears to be tightly linked to the relationship between LPS and TNF-α as it exists along a "gut–liver–lung" axis of inflammation, whereas donor-derived T-cell effectors can home to the lung and cause damage even when systemic GVHD is mild or absent. These findings have led to the development of a schema of IPS pathophysiology wherein it is hypothesized that the lung is susceptible to two distinct but interrelated pathways of injury involving aspects of both the adaptive and innate immune response (*see* Fig. 1). These studies are significant because they support a paradigm shift away from the current understanding of acute lung injury after SCT as an idiopathic clinical syndrome to a process in which the lung is the target of an alloantigen-specific, immune-mediated attack. It is anticipated that mechanistic insights gained using experimental models will form the basis for translational research protocols with the specific intent of treating or preventing IPS after SCT.

2.4. Treatment Strategies for IPS After AlloSCT

Currently, standard treatment regimens for IPS include supportive care measures in conjunction with broad-spectrum antimicrobial agents with or without intravenous corticosteroids *(6,20)*. Although reports of anecdotal responses to standard therapy are available, these responses are limited; despite such measures, the mortality of patients diagnosed with IPS remains unacceptably high *(19)*. Furthermore, prospective studies addressing the treatment of IPS and specifically the use of steroids are lacking in the literature. In the light of the poor response rate to standard treatment and preclinical and clinical data that suggest a potential role for TNF-α in the development of IPS, etanercept (Enbrel, Immunex, Seattle, WA) a soluble, dimeric TNF-α binding protein, was administered to three consecutive pediatric patients at the University of Michigan SCT program who met criteria for IPS *(20)*. All three patients underwent bronchoscopy with BAL 24–48 h prior to etanercept administration, and in each case, BAL fluid analysis was negative for infection. Pulmonary edema from fluid overload and cardiogenic etiologic factors were also ruled out in all cases. Each patient received empiric broad-spectrum antimicrobial therapy and methylprednisolone (2 mg/kg/d) prior to and during etanercept therapy. The administration of etanercept in combination with standard immunosuppressive therapy was well tolerated and associated with significant improvements in pulmonary function within the

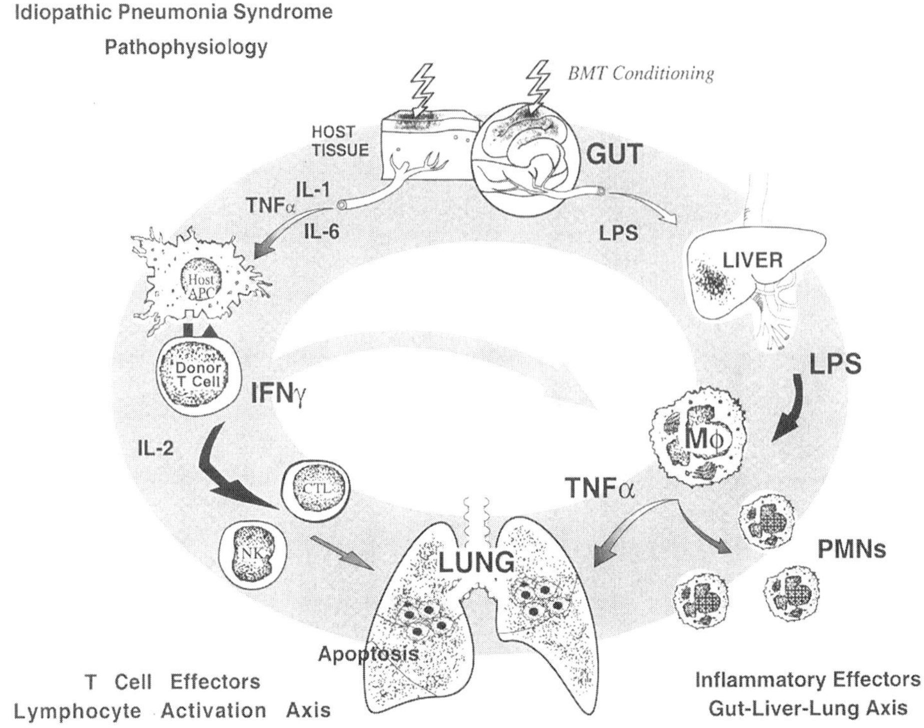

Fig. 1. Pathophysiology of noninfectious lung injury. Data generated using murine SCT models have been incorporated into a working hypothesis of IPS physiology. This schema postulates that the lung is susceptible to two distinct but interrelated pathways of immune-mediated injury that occur along a T-lymphocyte activation axis and a "gut–liver–lung" axis of inflammation. The lymphocyte-activation axis fundamentally depends on interactions between donor T cells and host APCs. Chemo-radiotherapy of SCT conditioning causes TNF-α and IL-1 release that enhances the ability of host APC to present alloantigens to mature donor T cells present in the BM inoculum *(16,182)*. Once engaged, donor T cells become activated and secrete a number of cytokines, including IFN-γ, which is a critical cytokine for the priming of pulmonary macrophages (Mϕ) and monocytes *(183–185)*, and IL-2, which facilitates T-cell activation, and proliferation and generation of both CTL and NK cells. Donor-derived, host reactive T cells and CTLs are present in the lung after alloSCT and contribute to pulmonary toxicity via Fas–FasL-mediated cell killing. The inflammatory axis focuses on the relationship between the cellular activating effects of LPS and the downstream production of TNF-α as it occurs along a gut–liver–lung axis of inflammation. During GVHD, the production of IFN-γ by allogeneic donor T cells is both necessary and sufficient to prime macrophages in those animals to secrete lethal amounts of TNF-α *(44)*. These primed macrophages are triggered to secrete inflammatory cytokines by doses of exogenous endotoxin too small to stimulate normal cells. Endotoxin enters the systemic circulation through gaps in the intestinal mucosa *(44,49–52)*. The ability of systemic endotoxin to reach the alveolar space is related to the consequences of GVHD in other target organs, particularly the liver, which is pivotally located immediately downstream (via the splanchnic circulation) of the intestinal reservoir of Gram-negative bacteria and their toxic byproducts. When confronted with a sudden endotoxin surge from increased LPS crossing a damaged intestinal mucosa, liver macrophages secrete inflammatory cytokines. If the endotoxin load surpasses the hepatic capacity for its clearance, both inflammatory cytokines (TNF-α) and unprocessed LPS spill over into the systemic circulation *(96,97,100)*. Underlying liver damage from hepatic GVHD decreases the liver's capacity for LPS uptake and clearance; thus, LPS remains in the systemic circulation for prolonged periods. Once in the alveolar space, LPS triggers pulmonary macrophage populations to secrete additional TNF-α, which results in the recruitment of neutrophils to the lung and enhances tissue damage.

first week of therapy. These data suggest that etanercept may represent a safe, noncrossreactive, therapeutic option for patients with IPS, and clinical trials studying etanercept for this indication are ongoing *(20)*.

3. SUBACUTE PULMONARY TOXICITY AFTER SCT: OBSTRUCTIVE LUNG DISEASE AND RESTRICTIVE LUNG DISEASE

3.1. Overview

Two forms of subacute pulmonary toxicity are common in patients over 100 d posttransplant: obstructive lung disease and restrictive lung injury *(8,9,14,74,150,151)*. Obstructive lung disease involves enhanced resistance to airflow on expiration and reflects conditions in the smaller airways and bronchioles. Obstructive defects are demonstrated by decreases in forced expiratory volumes at 1 s (FEV_1) and specifically by reductions in the forced expiratory ratio FEV_1/FVC (defined below) as measured by standard pulmonary function testing (PFT) *(150,152)*. By contrast, restrictive lung disease is classically associated with reductions in forced vital capacity (FVC), total lung capacity (TLC) and diffusion capacity of the lung for carbon monoxide (DLCO) with the FEV_1/FVC ratio maintained near 100% *(10,14,19,74,150)*. The reported incidence of both airflow obstruction and restrictive lung disease in alloSCT survivors ranges from 20% to 50% depending on donor source and time interval post SCT *(8,15,57,150)*.

3.2. Obstructive Lung Disease After SCT

Obstructive lung disease (OLD) is a well-recognized cause of morbidity following alloSCT *(8,74,151–154)*. Obstructive defects as defined by a FEV1.0/FVC < 70% on pulmonary function testing have been observed in approx 15–25% of allogeneic transplant recipients by d 100 and can persist for years after SCT *(10,57,74,150)*. Airflow obstruction may be a sequelae of extensive restrictive changes in small airways or may be related to small-airway destruction *(155)*. Lung biopsies from patients with OLD have shown a variety of histologic patterns, including lymphocytic bronchitis, chronic and acute interstitial pneumonitis, and varying degrees of bronchiolar inflammation, including BO *(8,57,76,111,153)*. This variation in histopathology is complicated further by the methods used to procure lung tissue; specifically, transbronchial lung biopsies rarely include an adequate sampling of distal bronchiolar structures and, therefore, are frequently considered nondiagnostic.

Despite these limitations, BO remains the most common form of histopathology associated with OLD and has been used historically to describe "GVHD of the lung" and interchangeably with OLD after SCT *(8,57,76,111,153)*. As the name implies, BO describes the histopathologic pattern of small-airway inflammation with fibrinous obliteration of the bronchiolar lumen that is classically associated with a fixed obstructive defect on PFT *(8,9,12,57,155)*. Airflow obstruction may, however, exist without BO, and BO may be present on biopsy without evidence for significant pulmonary dysfunction *(156)*. Furthermore, OLD is diagnosed by the appropriate clinical and PFT findings without histopathologic confirmation in the majority of cases. In this context, two phrases have been used to identify affected patients. The term "obstructive bronchiolitis" has been used to describe patients with airflow obstruction noted on PFT that have signs and symptoms consistent with bronchiolar inflammation *(151)*. Second, the phrase "bronchiolitis obliterates syndrome" or "BOS" has been developed to define the constellation of clinical, functional, and pathologic findings that accompany rejection after lung transplantation *(157)*. BOS is specifically defined as an irreversible decline in FEV1 of at least 20% from baseline and is graded using the international heart and lung transplantation criteria: BOS stage 0 = FEV1 80% baseline; stage 1 = FEV1 from 66% to 79%; stage 2 = FEV1 from 51% to 65%; stage 3 = FEV1 50% of baseline value *(157)*.

The lack of consistent terminology and variability in diagnostic criteria used to define OLD has contributed to the wide variation in the reported incidence of this form of lung injury after SCT. A review by Afessa and colleagues found that OLD was reported in 8.3% of 2152 allo SCT patients included in 9 studies and that the incidence varied between 6% and 20% in long-term survivors with chronic GVHD *(19)*. When compared to IPS, the onset of airflow obstruction tends to be later (ranging from 3 to 18 mo after SCT) and more insidious. However, the rate of progression of disease once symptoms are established is variable, with rapid deterioration in FEV1 being associated with a poor outcome *(8,9,73,152)*. Symptoms may include cough, dyspnea, and wheezing; however, many patients remain asymptomatic despite having evidence of moderate to severe airway obstruction on PFTs *(8,74)*. Chest radiographs may show patchy, diffuse infiltrates but are frequently unrevealing except for hyperinflation and flattening of the diaphragm *(8,57,73)*. Likewise, findings on chest computed tomography (CT) can range from essentially normal early in the course of disease to demonstrating extensive peribronchial inflammation, bronchiectasis, significant air trapping, and diffuse parenchymal hypoattenuation *(9,158,159)*.

The clinical course of OLD varies from mild, with slow deterioration, to diffuse, necrotizing, fatal bronchiolitis of the small airways. Mortality rates of 25–50% have been reported in association with the latter form of lung injury *(11–13,152)*. Response to bronchodilator therapy is usually marginal because airflow obstruction tends to be "fixed" rather than "reversible." Furthermore, response to immunosuppressive therapy, including steroids alone or in combination with cyclosporine, or azathioprine, is limited and typically results in preservation (rather than significant improvement) of existing lung function, suggesting that early detection of disease is important *(8,9,13,152)*. In this light, two studies have suggested that analysis of maximum mid-expiratory flow rates (MMFR) may be used as an earlier indicator of impending airflow obstruction than FEV_1 *(13,73)*. Because enhanced immunosuppression significantly increases the risk of infection, the utility of such therapy is questionable when a clinical response is not seen within the first months of treatment or when pulmonary dysfunction is long standing.

As with IPS, the etiology of airflow obstruction after SCT is likely to be multifactorial and may include the effects of pretransplant conditioning regimens, concomitant infections, chronic aspiration, and the occurrence of GVHD targeting the lung. Significant airflow obstruction has been reported in association with older donor age, use of methotrexate for GVHD prophylaxis, lower levels of serum immunoglobulins, the presence of esophageal dysfunction (with aspiration), mismatched stem cell grafts, and busulfan (rather than TBI)-containing SCT conditioning regimens *(8,9,13,74,151,152,160)*. From an infectious disease perspective, donor and recipient baseline cytomegalovirus (CMV) status have not been shown to impact on the development of OLD. However, a history of both respiratory syncytial virus (RSV) and adenoviral infections has been suggested as possible etiologies for the higher incidence of OLD in the pediatric population *(9)*. From an immunologic standpoint, the development of OLD is strongly associated with cGVHD, particularly in patients with low serum IgG levels *(8,152)* and chronic hepatic GVHD *(9)*. Furthermore, recipients of mismatched related donor or matched unrelated donor grafts have a much higher incidence of OLD than patients receiving matched related donor transplants (40% vs 13%) *(9)*. Collectively, these data suggest that immunologic mechanisms that are responsible for systemic GVHD may also contribute to OLD after alloSCT.

3.3. Restrictive Lung Disease After SCT

Reductions in lung volume (FVC, TLC) and diffusion capacity (DLCO) are common during the posttransplant period *(10,14,74,150)*. By 100 d posttransplant, significant decreases in FVC or TLC have been reported in as many as 25–45% of allogeneic transplant recipients and occur with greater frequency than obstructive abnormalities at this time *(10,14,15,150)*. An increase in nonrelapse mortality has been associated with the presence of a decline in TLC or FVC at 100 d posttransplant, even if the absolute values for each were within the normal range *(10)*. The presence of restrictive lung disease (RLD) at 1 yr or more posttransplant has likewise correlated with increased nonrelapse mortality *(14)*. Increasing recipient age, underlying diagnosis, total-body irradiation (TBI) containing conditioning regimens and the presence of acute GVHD have been associated with lower lung capacities and higher mortality rates *(10,14,15,161–163)*. In contrast to airflow obstruction, RLD posttransplant has not been consistently associated with chronic GVHD *(10)*. In one pediatric study, the incidence of RLD was less common than in adult patients, but the incidence of these defects increased with increasing patient age *(15)*. A more recent report revealed that a large proportion of children receiving SCT in the 1990s were at risk for significant pulmonary dysfunction despite the absence of symptoms *(150)*. This risk was greatest for patients with more advanced disease at the time of SCT.

3.4. Pathogenesis of Subacute Pulmonary Toxicity After SCT

3.4.1. Obstructive Lung Disease/Bronchiolitis Obliterans Syndrome

In comparison to IPS, the pathophysiology of subacute lung injury after SCT is less well defined. This limitation stems from the lack of correlative data obtained from afflicted SCT recipients and the paucity of suitable SCT animal models for either form of injury. The development of OLD is characterized by bronchiolar leukocyte recruitment leading to fibro-obliteration of the airway. The mechanism of injury likely involves an initial insult to the small airway epithelium followed by an ongoing inflammatory response. The duration of the inciting stimulus determines the ultimate outcome of the ensuing inflammatory response: A static insult may result in wound healing with resolution and repair, whereas a persistent stimulus can lead to an overexuberant reparative response resulting in a more destructive and less reversible state characterized by airway obliteration and airflow obstruction. The normal repair mechanism is predicated on the proper balance between pro-inflammatory and anti-inflammatory "mediators" and changes in this balance can significantly influence the ultimate outcome of the immune response.

Most of what is known about the pathogenesis of OLD has been formulated from clinical investigation of lung allograft recipients and from murine heterotopic tracheal transplant models. The absence of an initial inflammatory response from BMT conditioning regimens and the presence of a "host vs graft" rather than "graft vs host" reaction are just two of the issues that limit the extrapolation of data obtained from these systems to that which occurs after SCT. However, clinical and experimental pulmonary allograft rejection are characterized by exuberant alloantigen-driven, immune-mediated injury to the bronchial structures of the lung. This response most certainly involves antigen presentation, T-cell activation, leukocyte recruitment, and enhanced expression of various mediators of inflammation, suggesting therefore that mechanisms of lung injury may be similar in each scenario. Data generated from humans and mice support the hypothesis that the development of OLD or BO involves the interactions among cytokine, chemokine, and cellular effectors. Compared to healthy transplant recipients, analysis of BAL fluid obtained from patients with BO has revealed elevations in IL-1ra, TGF-β, IL-8, and MCP-1, all of which have been implicated in other fibro-proliferative processes *(106,164–166)*. Elevations of TGF-β and MCP-1 have also been observed in murine models of BO *(164,167)*. TNF-α is also known to play a critical role in the development of interstitial lung disease and fibrosis *(168,169)*. Although marked elevations of TNF-α have been reported during the development of murine BO, similar increases have not been observed in the BAL fluid of lung allograft recipients with BO *(165)*.

Because IL-8 is a potent chemoattractant for neutrophils, elevations of this chemokine during the development of BO is consistent with the reproducible finding of BAL neutrophilia that accompanies this process *(109,170)*. Clinical data also support a role for the interaction between pulmonary APCs and lymphocytes in the development of BO because effector T cells and dendritic cells expressing the costimulatory molecules CD80 and CD86 are present in the lungs of patients with BOS *(171,172)*. These observations have been extended by animal models; BO developing in heterotopic tracheal allografts requires donor-type rather than host-type APCs and can occur in the absence of either MHC class I or II antigens on donor tissue. These findings suggest that direct allorecognition by either CD8+ or CD4+ cells is important to this form of airway injury *(173)*. Additional studies have shown that CD28–B7 interactions are critical to this response because blocking this pathway using CTLA4IgG abrogates the development of BO *(174)*.

3.4.2. Restrictive Lung Injury

Similar to that which occurs during the development of BO, the pathogenesis of restrictive lung injury involves a chronic inflammatory process and the interplay between immune effector cells (that have been recruited to the lung) with the resident cellular constituents of the pulmonary vascular endothelium and interstitial space. In the setting of BMT, expression of class II MHC antigens on pulmonary epithelium, APCs, and vascular endothelium could promote alloantigen recognition and immune activation. The resulting inflammatory response would likely include secretion of pro-inflammatory cytokines, including TNF-α, IL-1β, IL-6, and TGF-β along with chemokines like IL-8, MCP-1, and MIP-1-α, all of which are known to stimulate fibroblast proliferation and promote collagen synthesis and deposition or leukocyte recruitment to inflamed tissue *(175,176)*. As chronic inflammation proceeds, fibroblasts increase dramatically in number within the lung leading to the loss of type I epithelial cells, proliferation of type II cells, the recruitment and proliferation of endothelial cells, and enhanced collagen deposition *(176)*. Ultimately, this process would result in interstitial thickening, loss of alveolar architecture, and end-stage fibrosis leading to significant loss of lung volume and severely impaired gas exchange.

Within this conceptual framework, Shankar and colleagues have suggested a biphasic model of noninfectious lung injury involving the interplay of ionizing irradiation and alloreactive donor T cells. This irradiated murine SCT model is characterized by early pro-inflammatory cytokine release and the promotion of lymphocyte influx, followed by a shift to a pro-fibrotic environment and the persistent secretion of TNF-α and IL-12 *(175)*. As noted earlier, TNF-α is one of several mediators that is known to promote chemotaxis, activation and proliferation of fibroblasts, and stimulation of collagen synthesis in vitro *(176)*. TNF-α gene expression has been shown to rise after administration of agents that cause pulmonary fibrosis in rats *(168)*. A causal role for TNF-α in the development of interstitial lung disease and fibrosis has been shown using various methods to block the effects of TNF-α. Neutralization of TNF-α results in reduction of lung fibrosis in murine models by decreasing the cellularity of the lung parenchyma, attenuating destruction of the alveolar architecture, and reducing total lung hydroxyproline content *(168,169)*. In addition, mutant mice deficient in both TNF receptors (p55 and p75 knockout mice) are protected from injury after silica and bleomycin exposure *(177)*. Perhaps the most compelling evidence for a role of TNF-α in interstitial lung injury stems from a study in which targeted overexpression of TNF-α in the lungs of transgenic mice resulted in the development of lymphocytic and fibrosing alveolitis *(178)*. Although early lung histopathology observed in the TNF transgenic mice was not dissimilar to that seen in experimental IPS models *(42)*, the histologic changes associated with more chronic exposure to TNF-α resembled those seen in interstitial lung disease *(175)*.

3.5 Treatment of Subacute Lung Injury After SCT

Evaluation of treatment strategies for subacute lung injury after SCT is again hampered by the absence of controlled clinical trials addressing this problem. Furthermore, most reports focus on patients treated for OLD rather than RLD. Although the etiology of airflow obstruction after SCT is likely to be multifactorial, the undoubted association of OLD and chronic GVHD has resulted in a general acceptance that immunologic damage contributes to this process. Thus, "standard" therapy has historically employed enhanced immunosuppression in conjunction with supportive care, including supplemental oxygen therapy and broad-spectrum antimicrobial prophylaxis. Unfortunately, the response to agents, including steroids, cyclosporine, tacrolimus, and azathioprine, is limited, and when present, it tends to occur early in the course of treatment *(8,13,57,73,152)*. Patients with more severe disease at the start of treatment have a poor prognosis and high mortality rates, suggesting that recognition of OLD at a more reversible stage may be important *(13,73,152)*. Although no agent or combination of agents has been proven superior with respect to treating OLD, a study by Payne and colleagues showed that when compared to historical controls receiving prednisone and methotrexate for GVHD prophylaxis, the use of cyclosporine and methotrexate was protective against the development of OLD *(179)*. Unfortunately, results of prospective, randomized trials studying the impact of current GVHD prophylaxis regimens on the incidence and severity of OLD, have yet to be reported. However, a recent clinical trial examining the effectiveness of inhaled steroids in addition to standard systemic immunosuppression to prevent BOS after lung transplant was completed and found no benefit to such treatment when compared to placebo controls *(180)*. The poor response to standard therapy and the unacceptable morbidity and mortality associated with subacute lung injury after SCT is underscored by the recent report of a successful lung transplant in a SCT recipient with BO *(181)*. Collectively, these findings necessitate the development of prospective trials that will 1) enhance our understanding of the immunologic mechanisms responsible for OLD and RLD after SCT, 2) determine the most appropriate therapeutic approach, and 3) test new agents in this clinical setting.

4. SUMMARY

Diffuse noninfectious lung injury remains a significant problem following allo SCT both in the immediate posttransplant period and in the months to years that follow. Along with the development of GVHD, pulmonary toxicity limits the broader application of SCT and can have significant implications with respect to the quality of life of SCT survivors. Although it is plausible that noninfectious lung injury and GVHD are connected mechanistically, a causal relationship between these two entities has yet to be definitively determined. Our understanding of the immunologic mechanisms involved with lung injury is limited by the absence of controlled clinical and the resultant paucity of clinical data, but these limitations have been overcome in part by observations made using animal SCT models; significant preclinical data suggest that the lung may be vulnerable to a two-pronged immunologic attack involving both inflammatory cytokine/chemokine and cellular effectors. As animal models for acute lung injury after SCT are explored further and those for subacute lung injury are developed, it is hoped that insights gained from each will improve our understanding of these disease processes and ultimately lead to the development of successful therapeutic strategies designed to diagnose, treat, or prevent noninfectious pulmonary toxicity in our SCT recipients.

REFERENCES

1. Clark J, Madtes D, Martin T, et al. Idiopathic pneumonia after bone marrow transplantation: cytokine activation and lipopolysaccharide amplification in the bronchoalveolar compartment. *Crit Care Med* 1999;27:1800.
2. Crawford S, Hackman R. Clinical course of idiopathic pneumonia after bone marrow transplantation. *Am Rev Respir Dis* 1993;147:1393.
3. Weiner RS, Mortimer MB, Gale RP, et al. Interstitial pneumonitis after bone marrow transplantation. *Ann Intern Med* 1986;104:168–175.
4. Quabeck K. The lung as a critical organ in marrow transplantation. *Bone Marrow Transplant* 1994;14:S19–S28.
5. Crawford S, Longton G, Storb R. Acute graft versus host disease and the risks for idiopathic pneumonia after marrow transplantation for severe aplastic anemia. *Bone Marrow Transplant* 1993;12:225.
6. Kantrow SP, Hackman RC, Boeckh M, et al. Idiopathic pneumonia syndrome: changing spectrum of lung injury after marrow transplantation. *Transplantation* 1997;63:1079–1086.
7. Clark J, Hansen J, Hertz M, et al. Idiopathic pneumonia syndrome after bone marrow transplantation. *Am Rev Respir Dis* 1993;147:1601–1606.
8. Holland HK, Wingard JR, Beschorner WE, et al. Bronchiolitis obliterans in bone marrow transplantation and its relationship to chronic graft-versus-host disease and low serum IgG. *Blood* 1988;72:621–627.
9. Schultz KR, Green GJ, Wensley D, et al. Obstructive lung disease in children after allogeneic bone marrow transplantation. *Blood* 1994;84:3212–3220.
10. Crawford SW, Pepe M, Lin D, et al. Abnormalities of pulmonary function tests after marrow transplantation predict nonrelapse mortality. *Am J Respir Crit Care Med* 1995;152:690–695.
11. Sullivan K, Mori M, Sanders J, et al. Late complications of allogeneic and autologous bone marrow transplantation. *Bone Marrow Transplant* 1992;10:127–134.
12. Wiesendanger P, Archimbaud E, Mornex J, et al. Post transplant obstructive lung disease ("broncliolitis obliterans"). *Eur Respir J* 1995;8:551–558.
13. Sanchez J, Torres A, Serrano J, et al. Long term follow up of immunosuppressive treatment for obstructive airway disease after allogeneic bone marrow transplantation. *Bone Marrow Transplant* 1997;20:403–408.
14. Badier M, Guillot C, Delpierre S, et al. Pulmonary function changes 100 days and one year after bone marrow transplantation. *Bone Marrow Transplant* 1993;12:457–461.
15. Quigley P, Yeager A, Loughlin G. The effects of bone marrow transplantation on pulmonary function in children. *Pediatr Pulmonary* 1994;18:361–367.
16. Abhyankar S, Gilliland DG, Ferrara JLM. Interleukin 1 is a critical effector molecule during cytokine dysregulation in graft-versus-host disease to minor histocompatibility antigens. *Transplantation* 1993;56:1518–1523.
17. Yousem SA. The histological spectrum of pulmonary graft-versus-host disease in bone marrow transplant recipients. *Hum Pathol* 1995;26:668–675.
18. Neiman P, Wasserman PB, Wentworth BB, et al. Interstitial pneumonia and cytomegalovirus infection as complications of human marrow transplantation. *Transplantation* 1973;15:478–485.
19. Afessa B, Litzow MR, Tefferi A. Bronchiolitis obliterans and other late onset non-infectious pulmonary complications in hematopoietic stem cell transplantation. *Bone Marrow Transplant* 2001;28:425–434.

20. Yanik G, Hellerstedt B, Custer J, et al. Etanercept as a novel therapy for idiopathic pneumonia syndrome after allogenic bone marrow transplantation. *Biol Blood Marrow Transplant* 2002; 8:395–400.
21. Wingard JR, Mellits ED, Sostrin MB, et al. Interstitial pneumonitis after allogeneic bone marrow transplantation. Nine-year experience at a single institution. *Medicine* 1988;67:175–186.
22. Weiner RS, Horowitz MM, Gale RP, et al. Risk factors for interstitial pneumonitis following bone marrow transplantation for severe aplastic anemia. *Br J Haematol* 1989;71:535.
23. Meyers JD, Flournoy N, Thomas ED. Nonbacterial pneumonia after allogeneic marrow transplantation: a review of ten years' experience. *Rev Infect Dis* 1982;4:1119–1132.
24. Atkinson K, Turner J, Biggs JC, et al. An acute pulmonary syndrome possibly representing acute graft-versus-host disease involving the lung interstitium. *Bone Marrow Transplant* 1991;8:231.
25. Della Volpe A, Ferreri AJ, Annaloro C, et al. Lethal pulmonary complications significantly correlate with individually assessed mean lung dose in patients with hematologic malignancies treated with total body irradiation. *Int J Radiat Oncol Biol Phys* 2002;52:483–488.
26. Robbins RA, Linder J, Stahl MG, et al. Diffuse alveolar hemorrhage in autologous bone marrow transplant recipients. *Am J Med* 1989;87:511–518.
27. Lewis ID, DeFor T, Weisdorf DJ. Increasing incidence of diffuse alveolar hemorrhage following allogeneic bone marrow transplantation: cryptic etiology and uncertain therapy. *Bone Marrow Transplant* 2000;26:539–543.
28. Metcalf JP, Rennard SI, Reed EC, et al. Corticosteroids as adjunctive therapy for diffuse alveolar hemorrhage associated with bone marrow transplantation. University of Nebraska Medical Center Bone Marrow Transplant Group. *Am J Med* 1994;96:327–334.
29. Capizzi SA, Kumar S, Huneke NE, et al. Peri-engraftment respiratory distress syndrome during autologous hematopoietic stem cell transplantation. *Bone Marrow Transplant* 2001;27:1299–1303.
30. Wilczynski SW, Erasmus JJ, Petros WP, et al. Delayed pulmonary toxicity syndrome following high-dose chemotherapy and bone marrow transplantation for breast cancer. *Am J Respir Crit Care Med* 1998;157:565–573.
31. Bhalla KS, Wilczynski SW, Abushamaa AM, et al. Pulmonary toxicity of induction chemotherapy prior to standard or high-dose chemotherapy with autologous hematopoietic support. *Am J Respir Crit Care Med* 2000;161:17–25.
32. Kelley J. Cytokines of the lung. *Am Rev Respir Dis* 1990;141:765–788.
33. Piguet P, Collart M, Grau G, et al. Requirement of tumour necrosis factor for development of silica-induced pulmonary fibrosis. *Nature* 1990;344:245–247.
34. Schmidt J, Pliver CN, Lepe-Zuniga JL, et al. Silica-stimulated monocytes release fibroblast proliferation factors identical to interleukin-1. A potential role for interleukin-1 in the pathogenesis of silicosis. *J Clin Invest* 1984;73:1462–1472.
35. Suter P, Suter S, Girardin E, et al. High bronchoalveolar levels of tumor necrosis factor and its inhibitors, interleukin-1, interferon, and elastase, in patients with adult respiratory distress syndrome after trauma, shock or sepsis. *Am Rev Resp Dis* 1992;145:1016.
36. Hyers T, Tricomi S, Dettenmier P, et al. Tumor necrosis factor levels in serum and bronchoalveolar lavage fluid of patients with the adult respiratory distress syndrome. *Am Rev Respir Dis* 1991;144:268.
37. Bortin M, Ringden O, Horowitz M, et al. Temporal relationships between the major complications of bone marrow transplantation for leukemia. *Bone Marrow Transplant* 1989;4:339.
38. Beschorner W, Saral R, Hutchins G, et al. Lymphocytic bronchitis associated with graft versus host disease in recipients of bone marrow transplants. *N Engl J Med* 1978;299:1030–1036.
39. Piguet PF, Grau GE, Collart MA, et al. Pneumopathies of the graft-versus-host reaction. Alveolitis associated with an increased level of tumor necrosis factor MRNA and chronic interstitial pneumonitis. *Lab Invest* 1989;61:37–45.
40. Clark JG, Madtes DK, Hackman RC, et al. Lung injury induced by alloreactive Th1 cells is characterized by host-derived mononuclear cell inflammation and activation of alveolar macrophages. *J Immunol* 1998;161:1913–1920.
41. Shankar G, Bryson J, Jennings C, et al. Idiopathic pneumonia syndrome in mice after allogeneic bone marrow transplantation. *Am J Respir Cell Mol Biol* 1998;18:235–242.
42. Cooke KR, Kobzik L, Martin TR, et al. An experimental model of idiopathic pneumonia syndrome after bone marrow transplantation. I. The roles of minor H antigens and endotoxin. *Blood* 1996;8:3230–3239.
43. Cooke KR, Krenger W, Hill GR, et al. Host reactive donor T cells are associated with lung injury after experimental allogeneic bone marrow transplantation. *Blood* 1998;92:2571–2580.

44. Nestel FP, Price KS, Seemayer TA, et al. Macrophage priming and lipopolysaccharide-triggered release of tumor necrosis factor alpha during graft-versus-host disease. *J Exp Med* 1992;175:405–413.
45. Piguet PF, Grau GE, Allet B, et al. Tumor necrosis factor/cachectin is an effector of skin and gut lesions of the acute phase of graft-versus-host disease. *J Exp Med* 1987;166:1280–1289.
46. Antin JH, Ferrara JLM. Cytokine dysregulation and acute graft-versus-host disease. *Blood* 1992;80:2964–2968.
47. Braun YM, Lowin B, French L, et al. Cytotoxic T cells deficient in both functional Fas ligand and perforin show residual cytolytic activity yet lose their capacity to induce lethal acute graft-versus-host disease. *J Exp Med* 1996;183:657–661.
48. Baker MB, Altman NH, Podack ER, et al. The role of cell-mediated cytotoxicity in acute GVHD after MHC-matched allogeneic bone marrow transplantation in mice. *J Exp Med* 1996;183:2645–2656.
49. Fegan C, Poynton C, Whittaker J. The gut mucosal barrier in bone marrow transplantation. *Bone Marrow Transplant* 1990;5:373–377.
50. Jackson SK, Parton J, Barnes RA, et al. Effect of IgM-enriched intravenous immunoglobulin (Pentaglobulin) on endotoxaemia and anti-endotoxin antibodies in bone marrow transplantation. *Eur J Clin Invest* 1993;23:540–545.
51. Hill GR, Crawford JM, Cooke KJ, et al. Total body irradiation effects on acute graft versus host disease. The role of gastrointestinal damage and inflammatory cytokines. *Blood* 1997;90 pp. 3204–3213.
52. Cooke K, Hill G, Crawford J, et al. Tumor necrosis factor-α production to lipopolysaccharide stimulation by donor cells predicts the severity of experimental acute graft versus host disease. *J Clin Invest* 1998;102:1882–1891.
53. Hill GR, Teshima T, Rebel VI, et al. The p55 TNF-alpha receptor plays a critical role in T cell alloreactivity. *J Immunol* 2000;164:656–663.
54. Cooke K, Gerbitz A, Hill G, et al. LPS Antagonism reduces graft-versus-host disease and preserves graft-versus-leukemia activity after experimental bone marrow transplantation. *J Clin Invest* 2001;7:1581–1589.
55. Milburn HJ, Poulter LW, Prentice HG, et al. Pulmonary cell populations in recipients of bone marrow transplants with interstitial pneumonitis. *Thorax* 1989;44:570.
56. Milburn HJ, Du Bois RM, Prentice HG, et al. Pneumonitis in bone marrow transplant recipients results from a local immune response. *Clin Exp Immunol* 1990;81:232.
57. Schwarer AP, Hughes JMB, Trotman-Dickenson B, et al. A chronic pulmonary syndrome associated with graft-versus-host disease after allogeneic marrow transplantation. *Transplantation* 1992;54:1002–1008.
58. Sutedja TG, Apperley JF, Hughes JMB, et al. Pulmonary function after bone marrow transplantation for chronic myeloid leukemia. *Thorax* 1988;43:163–169.
59. Sloane J, Depledge M, Powles R, et al. Histopathology of the lung after bone marrow transplantation. *J Clin Pathol* 1983;36:546–554.
60. Hackman RC, Sale GE. Large airway inflammation as a possible manifestation of a pulmonary graft-versus-host reaction in bone marrow allograft recipients. *Lab Invest* 1981;44:26A.
61. Connor R, Ramsay N, McGlave P, et al. Pulmonary pathology in bone marrow transplant recipients. *Lab Invest* 1982;46:3.
62. Madtes DK, Crawford SW. Lung injuries associated with graft-versus-host reactions. In: Ferrara JLM, Deeg HJ, Burakoff SJ, eds. *Graft-vs.-Host Disease*. New York: Marcel Dekker, 1997:425.
63. Beaumont F, Schilizzi BM, Kallenberg CG, et al. Expression of class II-MHC antigens on alveolar and bronchiolar epithelial cells in fibrosing alveolitis. *Chest* 1986;89:136.
64. Kunkel SL, Strieter RM. Cytokine networking in lung inflammation. *Hosp Prac* 1990:63–76 Vol 10 pp. 63–66, 69 73–76..
65. Teshima T, Ordemann R, Reddy P, et al. Acute graft-versus-host disease does not require alloantigen expression on host epithelium. *Nature Med* 2002;8:575–581.
66. Jordana M, Richards C, Irving LB, et al. Spontaneous in vitro release of alveolar-macrophage cytokines after the intratracheal instillation of bleomycin in rats. *Am Rev Respir Dis* 1988;137:1135–1140.
67. Fattal-German M, Le Roy Ladurie F, et al. Expression of ICAM-1 and TNF alpha in human alveolar macrophages from lung-transplant recipients. *Ann NY Acad Sci* 1996;796:138–148.
68. Sumitomo M, Sakiyama S, Tanida N, et al. Difference in cytokine production in acute and chronic rejection of rat lung allografts. *Transplant Int* 1996;9:S223–S225.
69. Stephens KE, Ishizaka A, Larrick JW, et al. Tumor necrosis factor causes increased pulmonary permeability and edema. Comparison to septic acute lung injury. *Am Rev Respir Dis* 1988;137:1364–1370.

70. Curtis JL, Byrd PK, Warnock ML, et al. Requirement of CD4-positive T cells for cellular recruitment to the lungs of mice in response to a particulate intratracheal antigen. *J Clin Invest* 1991;88:1244.
71. Toews GB. Pulmonary dendritic cells: sentinels of lung associated lymphoid tissues. *Am J Respir Cell Mol Biol* 1991;4:204.
72. Rabinowich H, Zeevi A, Paradis IL, et al. Proliferative responses of bronchoalveolar lavage lymphocytes from heart-lung transplant patients. *Transplantation* 1990;49:115.
73. Curtis DJ, Smale A, THien F, et al. Chronic airflow obstruction in long-term survivors of allogeneic bone marrow transplantation. *Bone Marrow Transplant* 1995;16:169–173.
74. Clark JG, Schwartz DA, Flournoy N, et al. Risk factors for air-flow obstruction in recipients of bone marrow transplants. *Ann Intern Med* 1987;107:648–656.
75. Urbanski SJ, Kossakowska AE, Curtis J, et al. Idiopathic small airways pathology in patients with graft-versus-host disease following allogeneic bone marrow transplantation. *Am J Surg Pathol* 1987;11:965.
76. Wyatt SE, Nunn P, Hows JM, et al. Airways obstruction associated with graft-versus-host disease after bone marrow transplantation. *Thorax* 1984;39:887.
77. Hakim FT, Mackall CL. The immune system: effector and target of graft-versus-host disease. In: Ferrara JLM, Deeg HJ, Burakoff SJ, eds. *Graft-vs.-Host Disease*. New York: Marcel Dekker, 1997:257.
78. Hattori K, Hirano T, Miyajima H, et al. Differential effects of anti-fas ligand and anti-tumor necrosis factor a antibodies on acute graft-versus-host disease pathologies. *Blood* 1998;91:4051–4055.
79. Workman D, Clancy JJ. Interstitial pneumonitis and lymphocytic bronchiolitis/bronchitis as a direct result of acute lethal graft-versus-host disease duplicate the histopathology of lung allograft rejection. *Transplantation* 1994;58:207.
80. Panoskaltsis-Mortari A, Taylor PA, Yaegar TM, et al. The critical early proinflammatory events associated with idiopathic pneumonia syndrome in irradiated murine allogenic recipients are due to donor T cell infusion and potentiated by cyclophoshamide. *J Clin Invest* 1997;100:1015–1027.
81. Cooke K, Hill G, Gerbitz A, et al. TNFα neutralization reduces lung injury after experimental allogeneic bone marrow transplantation. *Transplantation* 2000;70:272–279.
82. Cooke K, Hill G, Gerbitz A, et al. Hyporesponsiveness of donor cells to LPS stimulation reduces the severity of experimental idiopathic pneumonia syndrome: potential role for a gut–lung axis of inflammation. *J Immunol* 2000;165:6612–6619.
83. Cooke K, Kobzik L, Teshima T, et al. A role for Fas–Fas ligand but not perforin mediated cytolysis in the development of experimental idiopathic pneumonia syndrome. *Blood* 2000;96:768a.
84. Gerbitz A, Wilke A, Eissner G, et al. Critical role for CD54 (ICAM-1) in the development of experimental indiopathic pneumonia syndrome. *Blood* 2000;96:768a.
85. Jasinski M, Wieckiewicz J, Ruggiero I, et al. Isotype-specific regulation of MHC Class II gene expression in human monocytes by exogenous and endogenous tumor necrosis factor. *J Clin Immunol* 1995;15:185.
86. Smith S, Skerrett S, Chi E, et al. The locus of tumor necrosis factor-α action in lung inflammation. *Am J Respir Cell Mol Biol* 1998;19:881.
87. Vallera DA, Taylor PA, Vannice JL, et al. Interleukin-1 or tumor necrosis factor-alpha antagonists do not inhibit graft-versus-host disease induced across the major histocompatibility barrier in mice. *Transplantation* 1995;60:1371–1374.
88. Clark JG, Mandac JB, Dixon AE, et al. Neutralization of tumor necrosis factor-alpha action delays but does not prevent lung injury induced by alloreactive T helper 1 cells. *Transplantation* 2000;70:39–43.
89. Haddad I, Ingbar D, Panoskaltsis-Mortari A, et al. Activated alveolar macrophage-derived nitric oxide predicts the development of lung damage after marrow transplantation in mice. *Chest* 1999;116:37S.
90. Haddad I, Panoskaltsis-Mortari A, Ingbar D, et al. High levels of peroxynitrite are generated in the lungs of irradiated mice given cyclophosphamide and allogeneic T cells: a potential mechanism of injury after marrow transplantation. *Am J Respir Cell Mol Biol* 1999;20:1125.
91. Christ W, Asano O, Robidoux A, et al. E5531, a pure endotoxin antagonist of high potency. *Science* 1995;268:80–83.
92. Garbrecht B, Di Silvio M, Demetris A, et al. Tumor necrosis factor-a regulates in vivo nitric oxide synthesis and induces liver injury during endotoxemia. *Hepatology* 1994;20:1055.
93. Freudenberg M, Galanos C. Tumor necrosis factor alpha mediates lethal activity of killed gram-negative and gram-positive bacteria in D-galactosamine treated mice. *Infect Immun* 1991;59:2110.

94. Crawford J. Cellular and molecular biology of the inflamed liver. *Curr Opin Gastroenterol* 1997;13:175.
95. Matuschak G, Pinksy M, Klein E, et al. Effects of D-galactosamine induced acute liver injury on mortality and pulmonary responses to Escherichia coli lipopolysaccharide. *Am Rev Respir Dis* 1990;141:1296.
96. Matuschak GM, Mattingly ME, Tredway TL, et al. Liver–lung interactions during *E. coli* endotoxemia. *Am J Respir Crit Care Med* 1994;149:41–49.
97. Nakao A, Taki S, Yasui M, et al. The fate of intravenously injected endotoxin in normal rats and in rats with liver failure. *Hepatology* 1994;19:1251.
98. Lehmann V, Freudenberg M, Galanos C. Lethal toxicity of lipopolysaccharide and tumor necrosis factor in normal and D-galactosamine treated mice. *J Exp Med* 1987;165:657.
99. Galanos C, Freudenber M, Reutter W. Galactosamine induced sensitization to the lethal effects of endotoxin. *Proc Natl Acad Sci USA* 1987;76:5939.
100. Katz M, Grosfeld J, Gross K. Impaired bacterial clearance and trapping in obstructive jaundice. *Am J Surg* 1984;199 Vol 199 pp. 14–20.
101. Holler E, Kolb HJ, Moller A, et al. Increased serum levels of tumor necrosis factor alpha precede major complications of bone marrow transplantation. *Blood* 1990;75:1011–1016.
102. Borin M, Ringden O, Horowitz M, et al. Temporal relationship between the major complications of bone marrow transplantation for leukemia. *Bone Marrow Transplant* 1989;4:339.
103. Martin T, Rubenfeld G, Ruzinski J. Relationship between soluble CD14, lipopolysaccharide binding protein, and the alveolar inflammatory response in patients with acute respiratory distress syndrome. *Am J Respir Crit Care Med* 1997;155:937.
104. Martin T, Goodman R. The role of chemokines in the pathophysiology of the acute respiratory distress syndrome (ARDS). In: Hebert C, ed. *Chemokines in Disease*. Totowa, NJ: Humana, 1999:81–110.
105. DiGiovine B, Lynch J, Martinez F, et al. Bronchoalveolar lavage neutrophilia is associated with obliterative bronchiolitis after lung transplantation: role of IL-8. *J Immunol* 1996;157:4194–5202.
106. Riise GC, Andersson BA, Kjellstrom C, et al. Persistent high BAL fluid granulocyte activation marker levels as early indicators of bronchiolitis obliterans after lung transplant. *Eur Respir J* 1999;14:1123–1130.
107. Zheng L, Walters EH, Ward C, et al. Airway neutrophilia in stable and bronchiolitis obliterans syndrome patients following lung transplantation. *Thorax* 2000;55:53–59.
108. Reynaud-Gaubert M, Thomas P, Badier M, et al. Early detection of airway involvement in obliterative bronchiolitis after lung transplantation. Functional and bronchoalveolar lavage cell findings. *Am J Respir Crit Care Med* 2000;161:1924–1929.
109. Elssner A, Vogelmeier C. The role of neutrophils in the pathogenesis of obliterative bronchiolitis after lung transplantation. *Transplant Infect Dis* 2001;3:168–176.
110. St John RC, Gadek JE, Tutschka PJ, et al. Analysis of airflow obstruction by bronchoalveolar lavage following bone marrow transplantation. Implications for pathogenesis and treatment. *Chest* 1990;98:600–607.
111. Urbanski SJ, Kossakowska AE, Curtis J, et al. Idiopathic small airways pathology in patients with graft-versus-host disease following allogeneic bone marrow transplantation. *Am J Surg Pathol* 1987;11:965–971.
112. Glode LM, Rosenstreich DL. Genetic control of B cell activation by bacterial lipopolysaccaride is mediated by multiple distinct genes or alleles. *J Immunol* 1976;117:2061–2066.
113. Poltorak A, Ziaolong H, Smirnova I, et al. Defective LPS signaling in C3H/HeJ and C57BL/20ScCr mice: mutations in Tlr4 gene. *Science* 1998;282:2085.
114. Watson J, Kelly K, Largen M, et al. The genetic mapping of a defective LPS response gene in C3H/Hej mice. *J Immunol* 1978;120:422–424.
115. Sultzer BM, Castagna R, Bandeakar J, et al. Lipopolysaccharide nonresponder cells: the C3H/HeJ defect. *Immunobiology* 1993;187:257–271.
116. Cooke K, Olkiewicz K, Clouthier S, et al. Critical role for CD14 and the innate immune response in the induction of experimental acute graft-versus-host disease. *Blood* 2001;98:776a.
117. Shlomchik W, Couzens M, Tang C, et al. Prevention of graft versus host disease by inactivation of host antigen-presenting cells. *Science* 1999;285:412–415.
118. Watanabe T, Kawamura T, Kawamura H, et al. Intermediate TCR cells in mouse lung. Their effector function to induce pneumonitis in mice with autoimmune-like graft-versus-host disease. *J Immunol* 1997;158:5805.
119. Chen W, Chatta K, Rubin W, et al. Polymorphic segments of CD45 can serve as targets for GVHD and GVL responses. *Blood* 1995;86(suppl):158a.
120. Gartner JG, Merry AC, Smith CI. An analysis of pulmonary natural killer cell activity in F1-hybrid mice with acute graft-versus-host reactions. *Transplantation* 1988;46:879–886.

121. Leblond V, Zouabi H, Sutton L, et al. Late CD8+ lymphocytic alveolitis after allogeneic bone marrow transplantation and chronic graft-versus-host disease. *Am J Crit Care Med* 1994;150:1056.
122. Trauth BC, Klas C, Peters AM, et al. Monoclonal antibody-mediated tumor regression by induction of apoptosis. *Science* 1989;245:301–305.
123. Itoh N, Yonehara S, Ishii A, et al. The polypeptide encoded by the cDNA for human cell surface antigen Fas can mediate apoptosis. *Cell* 1991;66:233–243.
124. Lowin B, Hahne M, Mattmann C, et al. Cytolytic T-cell cytotoxicity is mediated through perforin and Fas lytic pathways. *Nature (London)* 1994;370:650–652.
125. Lee RK, Spielman J, Zhao DY. Perforin fas ligand and tumor necrosis factor are the major cytotoxic molecules used by lymphokine-activated killer cells. *J Immunol* 1996;157:1919–1925.
126. Teshima T, Hill G, Pan L, et al. IL-11 separates graft-versus-leukemia effects from graft-versus-host disease after bone marrow transplantation. *J Clin Invest* 1999;104:317–325.
127. Blazar B, Taylor P, Vallera D. CD4+ and CD8+ T cells each can utilize a perforin-dependent pathway to mediate lethal graft versus host disease in major histocompatibility complex-disparate recipients. *Transplantation* 1997;64:571–576.
128. Rafi AQ, Zeytun A, Bradley M, et al. Evidence for the Involvement of Fas ligand and perforin in the induction of vascular leak syndrome. *J Immunol* 1998;161:3077–3086.
129. Matute-Bello G, Liles WC, Steinberg KP, et al. Soluble Fas ligand induces epithelial cell apoptosis in humans with acute lung injury (ARDS). *J Immunol* 1999;163:2217–2225.
130. Hiroyasu S, Shiraishi M, Koji T, et al. Analysis of Fas system in pulmonary injury of graft-versus-host disease after rat intestinal transplantation. *Transplantation* 1999;68:933–938.
131. Hashimoto S, Kobayashi A, Kooguchi K, et al. Upregulation of two death pathways of perforin/granzyme and FasL/Fas in septic acute respiratory distress syndrome. *Am J Respir Crit Care Med* 2000;161:237–243.
132. Massard G, Tongiio MW, Wihlm JM, et al. The dendritic cell lineage: an ubiquitous antigen-presenting organization. *Ann Thorac Surg* 1996;61:252.
133. Armstrong LR, Christensen PJ, Paine R, et al. Regulation of the immunostimulatory activity of rat pulmonary interstitial dendritic cells by cell–cell interactions and cytokines. *Am J Repir Cell Mol Biol* 1994;11:682.
134. Dupuis M, McDonald DM. Dendritic-cell regulation of lung immunity. *Am J Respir Cell Mol Biol* 1997;17:284.
135. Christensen PJ, Armstrong LR, Fak JJ, et al. Regulation of rat pulmonary dendritic cell immunostimulatory activity by alveolar epithelial cell-derived granulocyte macrophage colony-stimulating factor. *Am J Respir Cell Mol Biol* 1995;13:426.
136. van Haarst JM, de Wit HJ, Drexhage HA, et al. Distribution and immunophenotype of mononuclear and dendritic cells in the human lung. *Am J Respir Cell Mol Biol* 1994;10:487.
137. Yousem SA, Ray L, Paradis IL, et al. Potential role of dendritic cells in bronchiolitis obliterans in heart-lung transplantation. *Ann Thorac Surg* 1990;49:424.
138. Ferrara JLM, Deeg HJ. Graft versus host disease. *N Engl J Med* 1991;324:667–674.
139. Kradin RL, Xia W, Pike M, et al. Interleukin-2 promotes the motility of dendritic cells and their accumulation in lung and skin. *Pathobiology* 1996;64:180.
140. Suda T, Callahan RJ, Wilkerson RA, et al. Interferon-gamma reduces Ia+ dendritic cells traffic to the lung. *J Leukocyte Biol* 1996;60:519.
141. Mackay CR. Chemokines: immunology's high impact factors. *Nature Immunol* 2001;2:95–101.
142. Luster AD. Chemokines—chemotactic cytokines that mediate inflammation. *N Engl J Med* 1998;338:436–445.
143. Rollins BJ. Chemokines. *Blood* 1997;90:909–928.
144. Nelson PJ, Krensky AM. Chemokines, chemokine receptors, and allograft rejection. *Immunity* 2001;14:377–386.
145. Gerard C, Rollins BJ. Chemokines and disease. *Nature Immunol* 2001;2:108–115.
146. Luster AD. The role of chemokines in linking innate and adaptive immunity. *Curr Opin Immunol* 2002;14:129–135.
147. Panoskaltsis-Mortari A, Strieter RM, Hermanson JR, et al. Induction of monocyte- and T-cell-attracting chemokines in the lung during the generation of idiopathic pneumonia syndrome following allogeneic murine bone marrow transplantation. *Blood* 2000;96:834–839.
148. Serody JS, Burkett SE, Panoskaltsis-Mortari A, et al. T-Lymphocyte production of macrophage inflammatory protein-1alpha is critical to the recruitment of CD8(+) T cells to the liver, lung, and spleen during graft-versus-host disease. *Blood* 2000;96:2973–2980.
149. Murai M, Yoneyama H, Harada A, et al. Active participation of CCR5(+)CD8(+) T lymphocytes in the pathogenesis of liver injury in graft-versus-host disease. *J Clin Invest* 1999;104:49–57.
150. Cerveri I, Fulgoni P, Giorgiani G, et al. Lung function abnormalities after bone marrow transplantation in children: has the trend recently changed? *Chest* 2001;120:1900–1906.

151. Ringden O, Remberger M, Ruutu T, et al. Increased risk of chronic graft-versus-host disease, obstructive bronchiolitis, and alopecia with busulfan versus total body irradiation: long-term results of a randomized trial in allogeneic marrow recipients with leukemia. *Blood* 1999;93:2196–2201.
152. Clark JG, Crawford SW, Madtes DK, et al. Obstructive lung disease after allogeneic marrow transplantation. Clinical presentation and course. *Ann Intern Med* 1989;111:368–376.
153. Ralph DD, Springmeyer SC, Sullivan KM, et al. Rapidly progressive air-flow obstruction in marrow transplant recipients. Possible association between obliterative bronchiolitis and chronic graft-versus-host disease. *Am Rev Respir Dis* 1984;129:641–644.
154. Sullivan KM, Agura E, Anasetti C, et al. Chronic graft-versus-host disease and other late complications of bone marrow transplantation. *Semin Hematol* 1991;28:250–259.
155. King TE Jr. Overview of bronchiolitis. *Clin Chest Med* 1993;14:607–610.
156. Crawford SW, Clark JG. Bronchiolitis associated with bone marrow transplantation. *Clin Chest Med* 1993;14:741–749.
157. Cooper JD, Billingham M, Egan T, et al. A working formulation for the standardization of nomenclature and for clinical staging of chronic dysfunction in lung allografts. International Society for Heart and Lung Transplantation. *J Heart Lung Transplant* 1993;12:713–716.
158. Ooi GC, Peh WC, Ip M. High-resolution computed tomography of bronchiolitis obliterans syndrome after bone marrow transplantation. *Respiration* 1998;65:187–191.
159. Bankier AA, Van Muylem A, Knoop C, et al. Bronchiolitis obliterans syndrome in heart-lung transplant recipients: diagnosis with expiratory CT. *Radiology* 2001;218:533–539.
160. Beinert T, Dull T, Wolf K, et al. Late pulmonary impairment following allogeneic bone marrow transplantation. *Eur J Med Res* 1996;1:343–348.
161. Depledge MH, Barrett A, Powles RL. Lung function after bone marrow grafting. *Int J Radiat Oncol Biol Phys* 1983;9:145–151.
162. Gore EM, Lawton CA, Ash RC, et al. Pulmonary function changes in long-term survivors of bone marrow transplantation. *Int J Radiat Oncol Biol Phys* 1996;36:67–75.
163. Tait RC, Burnett AK, Robertson AG, et al. Subclinical pulmonary function defects following autologous and allogeneic bone marrow transplantation: relationship to total body irradiation and graft-versus-host disease. *Int J Radiat Oncol Biol Phys* 1991;20:1219–1227.
164. Belperio JA, Keane MP, Burdick MD, et al. Critical role for the chemokine MCP-1/CCR2 in the pathogenesis of bronchiolitis obliterans syndrome. *J Clin Invest* 2001;108:547–556.
165. Belperio JA, DiGiovine B, Keane MP, et al. Interleukin-1 receptor antagonist as a biomarker for bronchiolitis obliterans syndrome in lung transplant recipients. *Transplantation* 2002;73:591–599.
166. Elssner A, Jaumann F, Dobmann S, et al. Elevated levels of interleukin-8 and transforming growth factor-beta in bronchoalveolar lavage fluid from patients with bronchiolitis obliterans syndrome: proinflammatory role of bronchial epithelial cells. Munich Lung Transplant Group. *Transplantation* 2000;70:362–367.
167. El-Gamel A, Sim E, Hasleton P, et al. Transforming growth factor beta (TGF-beta) and obliterative bronchiolitis following pulmonary transplantation. *J Heart Lung Transplant* 1999;18:828–837.
168. Piguet P, Collart M, Grau G, et al. Tumor necrosis factor/cachectin plays a key role in bleomycin-induced pneumopathy and fibrosis. *J Exp Med* 1989;170:655–663.
169. Piguet P, Vesin C. Treatment by human recombinant soluble TNF receptor of pulmonary fibrosis induced by bleomycin or silica in mice. *Eur Respir J* 1994;7:515–518.
170. Reynaud-Gaubert M, Thomas P, Gregoire R, et al. Clinical utility of bronchoalveolar lavage cell phenotype analyses in the postoperative monitoring of lung transplant recipients. *Eur J Cardiothorac Surg* 2002;21:60–66.
171. Leonard CT, Soccal PM, Singer L, et al. Dendritic cells and macrophages in lung allografts: a role in chronic rejection? *Am J Respir Crit Care Med* 2000;161:1349–1354.
172. Ward C, Whitford H, Snell G, et al. Bronchoalveolar lavage macrophage and lymphocyte phenotypes in lung transplant recipients. *J Heart Lung Transplant* 2001;20:1064–1074.
173. Szeto WY, Krasinskas AM, Kreisel D, et al. Donor antigen-presenting cells are important in the development of obliterative airway disease. *J Thorac Cardiovasc Surg* 2000;120:1070–1077.
174. Yamada A, Konishi K, Cruz GL, et al. Blocking the CD28-B7 T-cell costimulatory pathway abrogates the development of obliterative bronchiolitis in a murine heterotopic airway model. *Transplantation* 2000;69:743–749.

175. Shankar G, Cohen DA. Idiopathic pneumonia syndrome after bone marrow transplantation: the role of pre-transplant radiation conditioning and local cytokine dysregulation in promoting lung inflammation and fibrosis. *Int J Exp Pathol* 2001;82:101–113.
176. Coker R, Laurent G. Pulmonary fibrosis: cytokines in the balance. *Eur Respir J* 1998;11:1218–1221.
177. Ortiz L, Lasky J, Lungarella G, et al. Upregulation of the p75 but not the p55 TNFα receptor mRNA after silica and bleomycin exposure and protectin from lung injury in double receptor knockout mice. *Am J Respir Cell Mol Biol* 1999;20:825–833.
178. Miyazaki Y, Araki K, Vesin C, et al. Expression of a tumor necrosis factor-α transgene in murine lung causes lymphocytic and fibrosing alveolitis. *J Clin Invest* 1995;96:250–259.
179. Payne L, Chan CK, Fyles G, et al. Cyclosporine as possible prophylaxis for obstructive airways disease after allogeneic bone marrow transplantation. *Chest* 1993;104:114–118.
180. Whitford H, Walters EH, Levvey B, et al. Addition of inhaled corticosteroids to systemic immunosuppression after lung transplantation: a double-blind, placebo-controlled trial. *Transplantation* 2002;73:1793–1799.
181. Rabitsch W, Deviatko E, Keil F, et al. Successful lung transplantation for bronchiolitis obliterans after allogeneic marrow transplantation. *Transplantation* 2001;71:1341–1343.
182. Xun CQ, Thompson JS, Jennings CD, et al. Effect of total body irradiation, busulfan–cyclophosphamide, or cyclophosphamide conditioning on inflammatory cytokine release and development of acute and chronic graft-versus-host disease in H-2-incompatible transplanted SCID mice. *Blood* 1994;83:2360–2367.
183. O'Garra A, Murphy K. Role of cytokines in determining T-lymphocyte function. *Curr Opin Immunol* 1994;6:458–466.
184. Swain SL, Weinberg AD, English M, et al. IL-4 directs the development of Th2-like helper effectors. *J Immunol* 1990;145:3796–3806.
185. Swain SL, Bradley LM, Croft M, et al. Helper T-cell subsets: phenotype, function and the role of lymphokines in regulating their development. *Immunol Rev* 1991;123:115–144.

13 Hepatic Veno-Occlusive Disease

Paul G. Richardson, MD

Contents

1. INTRODUCTION

The clinical syndrome of hepatic veno-occlusive disease (VOD) after hematopoietic stem cell transplantation (HSCT) is characterized by liver enlargement and pain, fluid retention, weight gain, and jaundice *(1–3)*. Its onset is typically by d +30 after stem cell transplantation (SCT), although later onset has been described *(4)*. As the diagnosis is based on clinical criteria, the incidence reported and severity seen is variable, ranging from 10% to 60%, and may be influenced by differences in conditioning regimens and patient characteristics *(5,6)*. Prognosis is also variable. Mild disease is defined by no apparent adverse effect from liver dysfunction with complete resolution of symptoms and signs. Moderate disease is characterized by adverse effects of liver dysfunction requiring therapy such as diuresis for fluid retention and analgesia for right upper-quadrant pain but with eventual complete resolution. The majority of patients fall into the mild to moderate category, but a significant fraction of VOD is severe, and although occasional patients may recover, most are essentially incurable, with a fatality rate approaching 100% *(5,7)*. VOD is considered to be part of the spectrum of nonmyeloid organ injury syndromes that can occur after high-dose therapy and SCT, which include idiopathic pneumonitis, diffuse alveolar hemorrhage, thrombotic microangiopathy, and capillary-leak syndrome. There is a growing body of evidence indicating that early injury to vascular endothelium

From: *Stem Cell Transplantation for Hematologic Malignancies*
Edited by: R. J. Soiffer © Humana Press Inc., Totowa, NJ

either directly by the conditioning regimen or indirectly through the production of certain cytokines is a common denominator of these events *(8–10)*. This may explain why VOD is more common in allogeneic SCT (alloSCT), where there is a greater degree of cytokine dysregulation and immune dysfunction, as compared to autologous SCT (autoSCT) *(5)*.

2. HISTOPATHOLOGY

Sinusoidal endothelium in the liver is notable for a cobblestone appearance with numerous small pores *(11)*. These fenestrations create a unique microvascular architecture within the surrounding extracellular matrix and tissues subserved by zone 3 of the hepatic acinus as they drain into the hepatic venules *(12,13)*. Hepatic venules manifest the first histologic change in VOD with subendothelial edema and endothelial cell damage with microthromboses, fibrin deposition, and the expression of factor VIII/ vWF within venular walls *(14)*. Dilatation of the sinusoids is also present, and hepatocyte necrosis follows with later features, including intense collagen deposition in the sinusoids, sclerosis of the venular walls, and the development of collagen deposition both within venular lumens and abluminally *(13)* (*see* Fig. 1A). This progresses to obliteration of the venule with further hepatocyte necrosis. Advanced veno-occlusion is similar to severe cirrhosis with widespread fibrous tissue replacement of normal liver *(13)*.

Gemtuzumab ozogamicin (Mylotarg)-related VOD, a newly observed complication of this anti-CD33 monoclonal antibody therapy for acute myelogenous leukemia (AML), is noteworthy for marked sinusoidal obstruction *(15)* and fibrosis (*see* Fig. 1B). Recently, the term "sinusoidal obstruction syndrome" (SOS) has been suggested as an alternate to the established terminology of VOD *(15)*. Whereas sinusoidal obstruction is clearly apparent in rat models of VOD *(16)* and is seen in human disease *(15)*, the first recognizable histologic change of liver toxicity in SCT patients is of widening of the subendothelial space between the basement membrane and the lumen of central veins *(13)*. Accompanying venular changes, dilation and engorgement of the sinusoids with extravasation of red cells, and frank necrosis of perivenular hepatocytes follow, which progress and become more widespread as the extent of venular injury advances *(13)*. Moreover, correlation of histologic findings in a cohort study of 76 consecutive necropsy patients post-SCT found the strongest statistical association between the severity of VOD and the extent of hepatocyte necrosis, sinusoidal fibrosis, thickening of the subendothelium, phlebosclerosis, and venular narrowing *(13)*. Until additional prospective studies show otherwise, a change in the term VOD in SCT patients to SOS would seem premature.

3. PATHOGENESIS

Injury to sinusoidal endothelial cells and hepatocytes in zone 3 of the liver acinus appear to be key initial events in VOD. Evidence for this include the observation that pyrrolizidine alkaloids cause denigration of hepatic venular endothelium in experimental animals *(17)*, and the ingestion of these compounds in contaminated grains and teas has been reported to result in VOD in humans *(18)*. Hepatocytes in zone 3 contain both a high concentration of cytochrome P450 enzymes, which metabolize many chemotherapeutic agents used in high-dose regimens, and glutathione-*S*-transferase enzymes, which catalyze the reaction of glutathione with electrophilic compounds *(19,20)*. Depletion of glutathione has been reported to result in hepatocyte necrosis, whereas glutathione mono-8-diester can selectively protect hepatocytes from high-dose alkylator injury *(21,22)*. It has been shown in a number of trials that higher

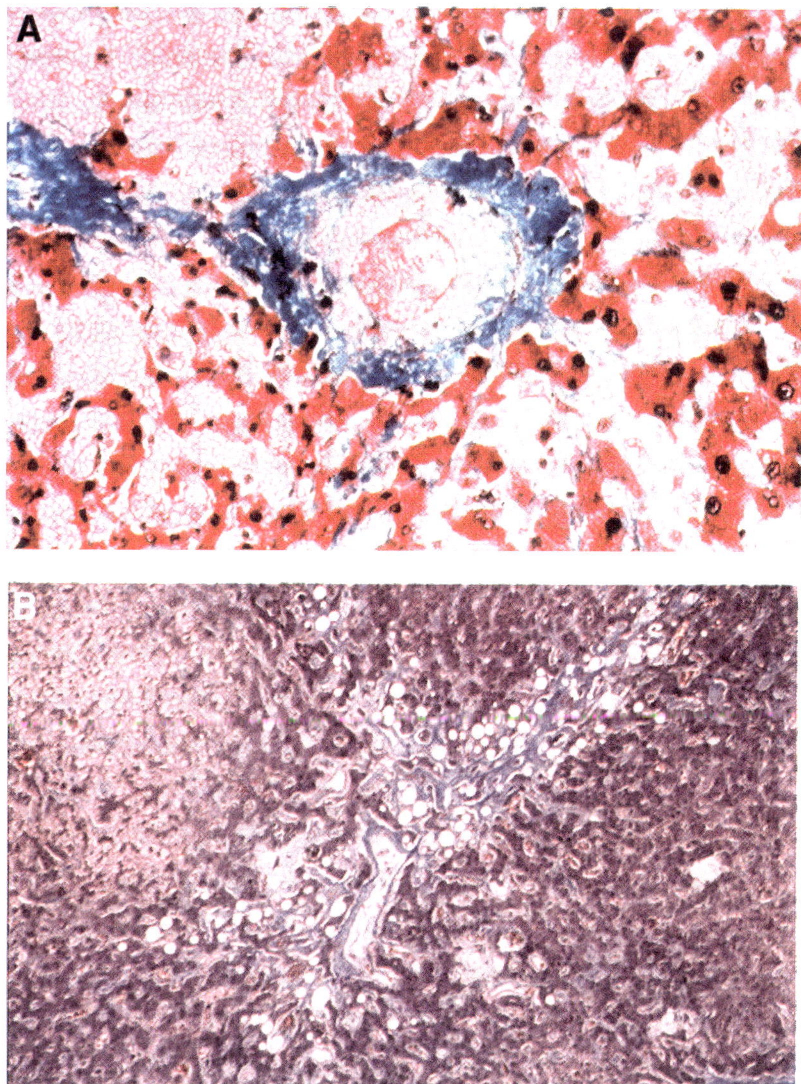

Fig. 1. (A) Liver biopsy showing characteristic dyes of VOD in a SCT patient with terminal venular fibrosis, fibrin deposition, subendothelial edema, and marked zone 3 hepatocellular damage. (B) Liver biopsy in a patient with prior Mylotarg exposure and severe VOD: Sinusoidal obstruction is prominent. (Photomicrographs courtesy of Howard Shulman, MD, with permission.)

plasma levels of cytotoxic drugs used in SCT such as busulfan or the metabolites of cyclophosphamide are associated with an increase risk of VOD *(18–21)*.

Commensurate with this, it has been observed that VOD is more common in patients whose area under the curve (AUC) of concentration vs time of busulfan is elevated *(23–25)*. Furthermore, when busulfan dosing is adjusted to reduce the AUC in patients whose AUC after first dose is elevated, the incidence of VOD has generally been shown to be significantly reduced *(23,26)*. More recently, the importance of busulfan in VOD pathogenesis has been re-evaluated by Slattery et al. who measured the pharmacokinetics of either busulfan and cyclophosphamide, or cyclophosphamide plus total-body irradiation (TBI) in patients prior to SCT *(27)*. These investigators reported that average plasma steady-state concentrations of busulfan correlated with exposure to cyclophosphamide. Subsequent studies have confirmed the importance of cyclophosphamide and its metabolites in sinusoidal endothelial cell and hepatocyte injury *(28)*. DeLeve et al. demonstrated that the direct exposure of sinusoidal endothelium to cyclophosphamide did not result in toxicity, but when sinusoidal endothelium was exposed to the metabolites acrolein or 4-hydroxy cyclophosphamide, a dose-dependent toxicity was observed *(16)*. In contrast, when sinusoidal endothelium and hepatocytes were cocultured in the presence of cyclophosphamide, marked toxicity to sinusoidal endothelium was apparent. This suggested that the increased injury to sinusoidal endothelium, which was greater than that seen to hepatocytes, was the result of acrolein generated by the metabolic activation of cyclophosphamide by hepatocytes. In the same study, DeLeve demonstrated that the effect was reversed by sustaining levels of hepatocyte glutathione with serine–methionine, and this protective effect was abolished by proparglyglycine, an inhibitor of glutathione synthesis *(16)*. These studies imply that increased exposure to the toxic metabolites of cyclophosphamide contribute to the development of VOD and that supporting levels of hepatic glutathione might prevent VOD, consistent with earlier experiments done by Teicher et al. *(22)*. Most recently, more evidence of the potential importance of glutathione in VOD was demonstrated by the abrogation of the effects of monocrotaline induced injury in a rat model with the targeted support of sinusoidal endothelial cell glutathione *(29)* and by a clinical report of the successful use of *N*-acetyl cysteine in the treatment of VOD *(30)*.

4. ENDOTHELIAL CELL INJURY

Several investigators have reported marked elevations in markers of endothelial injury in patients with VOD. Catani and colleagues measured plasma thrombomodulin (TM) and P-selectin levels prior to and after SCT prospectively in 25 patients, 2 of whom developed reversible VOD and 1 who developed fatal VOD. TM and P-selectin levels were normal in all but the one patient with severe VOD, where these endothelial stress products were found to be markedly elevated *(31)*. Salat et al. have measured plasma levels of plasminogen activator inhibitor I (PAI-1) in patients undergoing SCT. Levels of PAI-I were increased nearly fivefold in 4 patients with VOD compared to 28 patients without VOD *(32)*. They subsequently reported that levels of PAI-1 were significantly greater in VOD patients than those in other forms of liver injury after SCT and hypothesized a lipopolysaccharide (LPS)-based mechanism of sinusoidal endothelial injury and Kupffer cell activation, as illustrated in Fig. 2 *(33)*. Studies by other investigators have subsequently confirmed the elevation of PAI-1 levels in SCT-associated VOD and demonstrated elevation of tissue factor pathway inhibitor (TFPI), soluble tissue factor (sTF), TM, P-selectin, and E-selectin *(34–37)*. It is noteworthy that hepatic stellate cells (also known as Ito cells, lipocytes, or perisinusoidal cells) produce large amounts of PAI-1 when stressed, with recent evidence pointing to a key role for activated stellate cells in the pathogenesis of VOD through the production of extracellular matrix and the promotion of hepatic fibrosis *(38)* (*see* Fig. 2).

The role of cytokines has been an area of interest in the study of VOD pathogenesis (*see* Fig. 2). Tumor necrosis factor-α (TNF-α) levels in serum are low in established disease, but it has been postulated that high levels of TNF-α and interleukin (IL)-1β may contribute to initial endothelial damage *(39,40)*. More recent studies of IL-6, IL-8, as well as TNF-α and IL-1β levels in patients during SCT have suggested a possible relationship between IL-6 and IL-8 with jaundice, renal dysfunction, and pulmonary disease, but, in contrast, serum TNF-α and

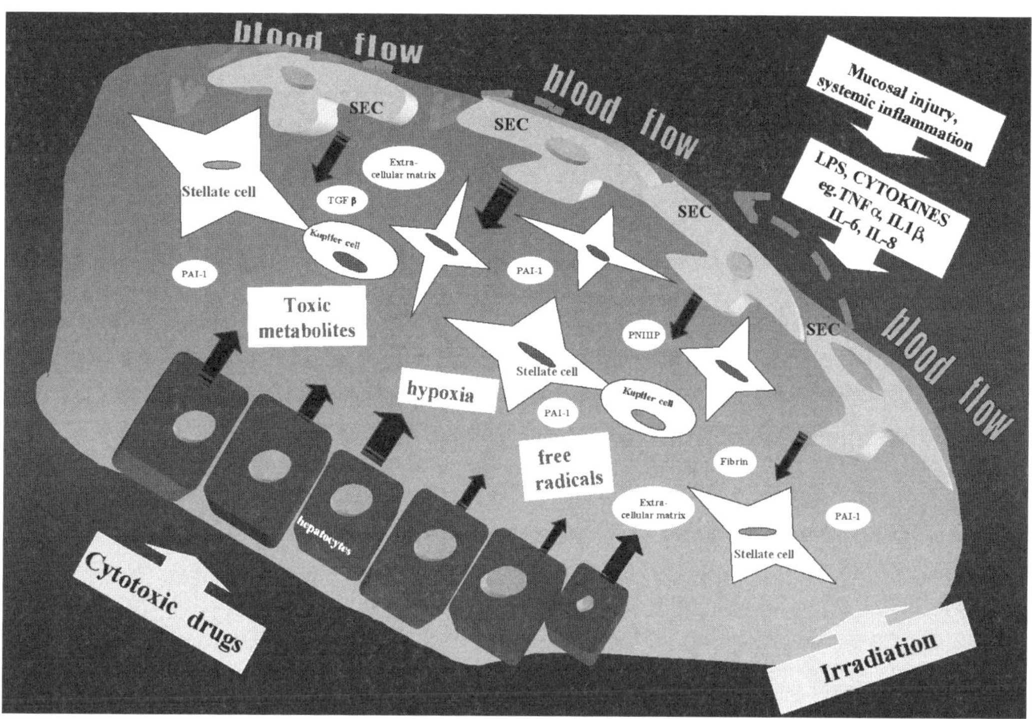

Fig. 2. Potential key cellular, biochemical, and cytokine events in VOD pathogenesis. SEC, sinusoidal endothelial cell. (From ref. *34* with permission.)

IL-Iβ concentrations were not predictive of SCT-related complications *(41)*. Data showing elevation of plasma levels of C-reactive protein in alloSCT patients with severe VOD, as compared to those without, support the possible role of IL-6 in the disease process *(42)*. Elevation of transforming growth factor-β (TGF-β), collagen propeptides, and hyaluronic acid have been observed in VOD *(43–45)*. Moreover, elevated serum levels of the immunopropeptide of type 3 procollagen (PIIINP) have been reported at the onset of clinically evident VOD in a study by Rio and colleagues *(46)*. Given that elevated levels of PIIINP have been associated with fibrotic liver disease, it has been speculated that serum levels of PIIINP are surrogates for the intrahepatic accumulation of type 3 collagen in VOD *(47,48)*.

Plasma levels of certain endothelial stress products increase after high-dose cytoreductive therapy, including von Willebrand factor (vWF) and serum angiotensin-converting enzyme *(40,49)*. Conversely, levels of anticoagulants fall shortly after high-dose cytoreductive therapy *(50,51)*. As an extension of these observations and the connection between endothelial damage and VOD, several studies have reported low baseline levels of naturally occurring anticoagulants in patients who subsequently developed VOD *(40,45,52)* compared to those who did not develop VOD. The same groups and others have also shown marked fluctuation in both the levels of various procoagulant proteins (including serum proteases and fibrinogen) and fibrinolytic parameters (such as D-dimer) *(40,49,52,53)*. However, a clear relationship between these levels and the development of VOD remains to be established and these data have been unable to distinguish whether the changes seen in coagulation parameters are directly involved in the pathogenesis of VOD or are epiphenomena of the disease process.

In patients with established VOD, profound thrombocytopenia and refractoriness to platelet transfusion is common. This may represent splenic sequestration as a result of portal hypertension or consumption through endothelial cell injury, and thrombopoietin levels are commensurately high *(45,54)*. Factor VII levels are usually low, but it is not known if this is specific to VOD, as a function of increased activation at the endothelial cell surface, or a result of global hepatic dysfunction *(40,49)*.

5. RISK FACTORS

Risk factors for developing VOD can be divided into pre-SCT and SCT-related factors *(5,7,55)*. Pre-SCT factors include elevation of liver transaminase levels (specifically AST), older age, poor performance status, female gender, advanced malignancy, prior abdominal radiation, the number of days on broad-spectrum antibiotics pre-SCT, prior exposure to amphotericin B, vancomycin, and/or acyclovir therapy, the number of days with fever pre-SCT, and the degree of histocompatibility in alloSCT *(2,5)*. Reduced pre-SCT diffusion capacity of the lung may be an independent risk factor for VOD *(56)*.

Norethisterone treatment, previously used in women to minimize menstrual bleeding during the thrombocytopenic period post-SCT, has been incriminated as a risk factor, possibly by causing microthrombotic injury in hepatic venules *(57)*. Some factors also appear to predict VOD severity—for example, a fourfold elevation of AST above normal and increasing histoincompatibility between donor and recipient being associated with severe VOD and high fatality *(7)*. Conversely, in nonrandomized studies, a low incidence of VOD has been found in patients receiving T-cell-depleted grafts *(58,59)*. SCT factors include TBI dose, dose rate, and dose of busulfan *(2,5)*. A randomized study showed a significantly higher incidence in patients receiving busulfan and cyclophosphamide compared to cyclophosphamide and TBI conditioning *(60)*. In a study of 350 patients treated with 16 mg/kg busulfan and 120 mg/kg cyclophosphamide, the overall incidence of VOD was 27% *(61)*. In an International Bone Marrow Transplant Registry (IBMTR) study of 1717 recipients of human leukocyte antigen (HLA)-identical sibling SCT for leukemia between 1988 and 1990, variables associated with an increased risk of VOD were conditioning with busulfan and cyclophosphamide compared to TBI *(62)*. Conversely, VOD also appears less frequent when peripheral blood progenitor SCT is used compared to bone marrow alone *(63)*. The reasons for this could be several, including more rapid engraftment resulting in less prolonged cytopenia, toxic injury, and cytokine disturbance. A more intriguing notion is that this may reflect superior endothelial re-engraftment from stem cells, a hypothesis that has been strengthened by the observation of donor endothelial cell engraftment in coronary vessels post-SCT *(64)*.

An important new risk factor for VOD is the administration of gemtuzumab ozogamicin (Mylotarg), an anti-CD33 monoclonal antibody linked to the potent toxin calicheamycin *(65,66)*. Sinusoidal endothelial cells and stellate cells in zone 3 of the hepatic sinus express CD33, and as a result, significant toxic liver injury has been reported both when this agent is given to AML patients prior to and after SCT, with resultant severe VOD and a high case fatality rate described *(66)*.

6. DIAGNOSIS

Ultrasound and computed tomography (CT) imaging can be useful in identifying hepatomegaly, confirming the presence of ascites and, together with Doppler studies, may be useful in determining whether or not there is attenuation or reversal of venous flow or portal vein thrombosis *(67)*. Both CT and ultrasound are useful in excluding pericardial effusion, constrictive pericarditis, extrahepatic venous obstruction, and mass lesions of the liver *(68,69)*. Doppler ultrasound has gained popularity in the assessment of VOD because it is noninvasive and can be performed at the bedside. However, pulsatile hepatic venous flow is a relatively nonspecific finding and reversal of portal flow is a late feature of VOD. More recently, Doppler measurement of hepatic arterial resistance has been studied prospectively in a limited number of patients with VOD as a means of providing earlier clues to diagnosis and prognosis *(70)*. Magnetic resonance imaging (MRI) has attracted interest, but its role remains to be established, other than as a means to exclude other causes of liver dysfunction *(71)*. Transvenous liver biopsy and wedged hepatic venous pressure gradient measurement (WHVPG) remain gold standards of diagnosis. In this setting, the transfemoral or transjugular method is generally preferred and percutaneous biopsy has little or no place in the evaluation of VOD given the high risk for bleeding *(72)*. As well as providing tissue, this technique permits measurement of WHVPG, with a gradient of greater than 10 mm of mercury having a 91% specificity and 86% positive predictive value, but more modest sensitivity at 52% *(73)*.

7. PROGNOSIS

In attempting to develop an aid to estimate prognosis, a Cox regression analysis was used by Bearman and colleagues to generate risk curves predictive of severe VOD based on a large cohort of patients from the Seattle Transplant Registry. In these patients, VOD occurrence was defined within the first 16 d post-SCT after preparation with one of three specific regimens: cyclophosphamide and TBI (Cy/TBI); busulfan and cyclophosphamide (Bu/Cy), or cyclophosphamide, BCNU, and VP-16 (CBV) *(74)*. Severe VOD in turn was associated with a case fatality rate of 98% by d +100 after SCT (*see* Fig. 3). Calculations were based on total serum bilirubin and percentage weight gain at various time points subsequent to SCT, up to d +16. Similar models have not been proposed for other temporal or therapeutic settings, and models based on possible surrogates, such as cytokines, endothelial stress products, or markers of fibrosis, have yet to be defined.

Regardless of time frame and conditioning, the rates of rise in bilirubin and weight gain are much higher in patients with severe VOD, and the mean maximum bilirubin and percent weight gain are significantly greater in patients with severe VOD compared to those with milder illness *(6)* (*see* Table 1). Other clinical features associated with worse outcome include the development of ascites, which occurs in fewer than 20% of patients with mild to moderate VOD compared to 48% or more patients with severe disease and is reflective of increased portal hypertension *(6)* (*see* Table 1). Commensurate with this, WHVPG values in patients with VOD beyond 20 mm of mercury are associated with a particularly poor prognosis *(73)*. A cardinal feature predicting high mortality in VOD is the presence of multiorgan failure (MOF). In fact, patients with severe VOD usually die of renal, pulmonary, and/or cardiac failure, rather than from hepatic insufficiency *per se (6)*.

8. PREVENTION

Given the lack of effective therapies, the prevention of fatal VOD is an obvious priority. Selection of particular conditioning regimens for patients at high risk is one approach, and this is perhaps best embodied by the emerging field of nonmyeloablative transplant, where the

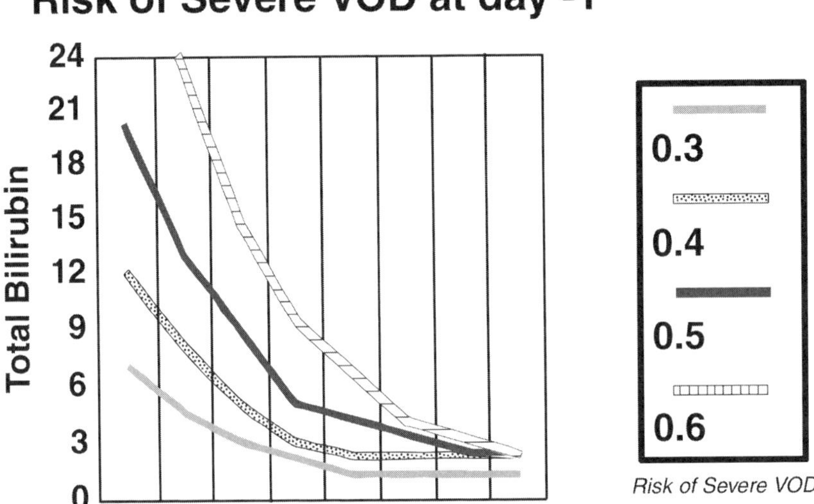

Fig. 3. Prognosis factors. (From ref. *74* with permission.)

Table 1
Clinical Features of Patients With VOD of the Liver According to Severity of Disease

	Mild	*Moderate*	*Severe*
Weight gain (% increase)	7.0 (± 3.5%)	10.1 (±5.3%)	15.5 (±9.2)
Maximum total serum bilirubin before d 20 (mg/dL)	4.73 (±2.9)	7.95 (±6.6)	26.15 (±15.3)
Percent of patients with peripheral edema	23%	70%	85%
Percent of patients with ascites	5%	16%	48%
Platelet transfusion requirements to d 20	53.8 (±27.6)	83.6 (±5.0)	118.3 (±51.8)
D 100 mortality (all causes) (%)	3	20	98

incidence of VOD is low *(75)*. However, depending on the underlying disease, this may or may not be an optimal therapeutic strategy *(75,76)*. Assessment of risk by virtue of genetic predisposition to VOD may be one possible avenue in the future. Preliminary studies of genetic polymorphisms in SCT patients have suggested a possible association between a mutation of glutathione-*S*-transferase synthesis and increased VOD risk *(77,78)*. Similarly, in a large, prospective study of allelic variants for TNF-α in SCT patients, a high incidence of MOF was seen in association with a specific allelic variant (TNF-d3), which causes increased TNF-α production in response to injury *(79)*. Therefore, the possibility of risk stratification pre-SCT for both the development and the sequelae of VOD exists, but, further, more comprehensive studies to better define such risk are needed. Moreover, the relationship of genetic risk, if able to be defined, to specific regimens and agents will also need to be established.

The most established practice in VOD prevention has been the use of pharmacokinetics to monitor drug levels with the intent of minimizing hepatic injury. This approach is currently best illustrated by the monitoring of busulfan levels *(17,23–26)*. The observed relationship between elevated busulfan levels and VOD may possibly be in part the result of busulfan-mediated depletion of hepatic glutathione, which, in turn, predisposes hepatocytes to additional injury from ensuing cyclophosphamide exposure. This argument is consistent with data suggesting that increased exposure to the toxic metabolites of cyclophosphamide may contribute to the development of VOD *(27)*. Moreover, the observation that ursodiol has important antioxidant properties within hepatocytes may explain why ursodiol's protective effect has been most apparent in patients receiving busulfan-based conditioning *(80)*.

The prophylactic administration of ursodeoxycholic acid, a hydrophilic water-soluble bile acid, has been studied in a number of randomized placebo-controlled prospective trials. Several have shown a statistically significant benefit in patients predicted to be at high risk of VOD *(80,81)*, although a recent large phase III study by the Nordic Bone Marrow Transplantation group did not demonstrate significant benefit *(82)*.

The supplement of hepatic gluthathione has been tested in experimental models *(22,28)* but this has been difficult to translate into patients because of concerns regarding tumor protection. The feasibility of restoring hepatic glutathione levels to concentrations that are truly effective in humans is also unclear. However, reports of a significant decline in gluthathione and other antioxidants after chemotherapy in SCT coupled with a recent report of *N*-acetyl cysteine supplementation in the successful treatment of VOD suggest that further evaluation of supportive nutrition, including antioxidants such as vitamin E, is warranted *(30,83,84)*.

Other approaches to VOD prevention, such as the role of steroids, have also attracted interest *(85)*. Given that inflammation does not appear to be a central component to the pathogenesis of VOD, it is difficult to understand why steroids should be of direct benefit. However, it is possible that they may abrogate other intercurrent or separate forms of liver injury. Modulating inflammation with pentoxifylline and TNF-α neutralization has been unsuccessful to date. Pentoxifylline administration in prospective randomized placebo-controlled trials has been either ineffective or associated with more VOD than placebo *(86,87)*.

Treatments targeted at preventing vascular injury have been more extensively examined. A small number of randomized trials have studied the effect of low-dose continuous intravenous heparin, but only one randomized study has demonstrated a beneficial effect of heparin prophylaxis *(88)*. However, this study was conducted mainly in low-risk patients, and other uncontrolled studies have suggested that heparin was ineffective and/or dangerous because of the increased risk of hemorrhage *(5,57,89,90)*. The use of antithrombin III (ATIII) concentrates has been shown to be of no protective value in a prospective study *(91)*. Low-molecular-weight heparins seem to be relatively safe and may have some effect in the prevention of VOD *(92,93)*, but well-designed, randomized studies are needed to confirm these preliminary results.

Prostaglandin E_1 (PGE_1) is a vasodilator with a cytoprotective effect on endothelium as well as platelet aggregation inhibitory and prothrombolytic activity *(94)*. In one trial, in which PGE_1 was given in combination with low-dose heparin, the incidence of VOD was 12.2% in the PGE_1-treated group compared to an incidence of 25.5% in historic controls, suggesting that prophylactic PGE_1 might decrease the incidence and severity of VOD *(95)*. A randomized trial performed in Buffalo, NY also showed that prophylactic PGE_1, heparin, and tissue plasminogen activator (tPA) treatment demonstrated an improved d +100 survival post-SCT compared to heparin and tPA alone *(96)*. However, a prospective study by the Seattle group using higher doses of PGE_1 in a phase I/II study, without concomitant heparin, could not demonstrate any beneficial effect of this drug, and PGE_1 administration was complicated by significant toxicity *(74)*.

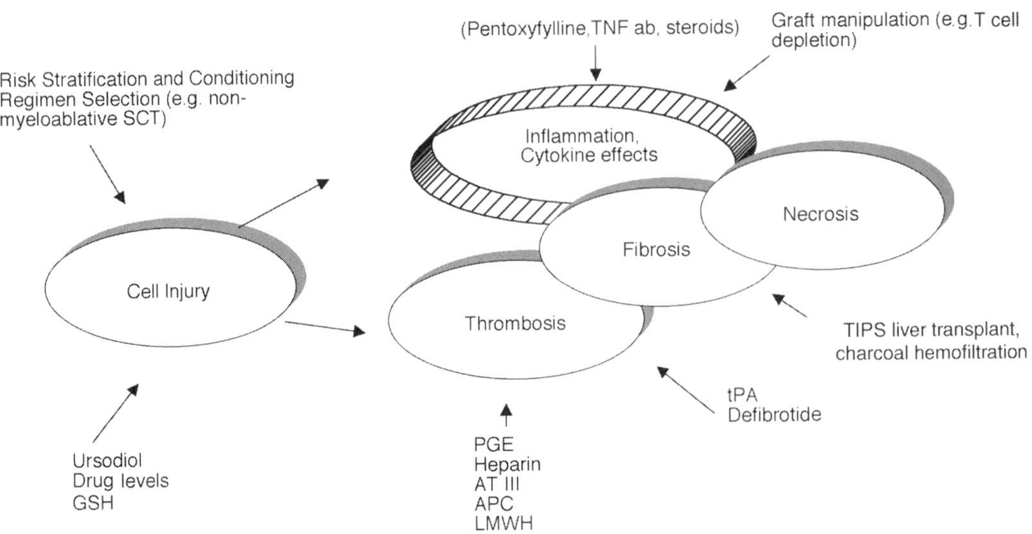

Fig. 4. Potential points for intervention in VOD. Whereas cell injury, microthrombosis, fibrosis and necrosis are established as events in VOD pathogenesis, the role of inflammation and cytokine-mediated injury remains to be defined. GSH, gluthathione; ATIII, antithrombin 3; LMWH, low-molecular-weight heparin; APC, activated protein C; TIPS, transjugular intrahepatic portosystemic shunt; TNF ab, tumor necrosis factor antibody. (Adapted with permission from ref. *34*.)

9. TREATMENT (SEE FIG. 4)

Based on the histologic observation of microthrombosis and fibrin deposition as well as intense factor VIII/vWF staining in VOD, strategies aimed at promoting fibrinolysis with or without concomitant anticoagulant therapy have been developed *(97,98)*. More than 100 patients have been reported in the literature to be treated to date with thrombolytic therapy with or without anticoagulation, but only a few series have included more than 10 patients (see Table 2). In the largest study published in patients with established VOD, 42 patients received treatment with tPA and concomitant heparin for severe disease. Twelve of 42 (29%) patients responded, with response defined as a reduction in pretreatment bilirubin by at least 50%. No patient with MOF defined as renal insufficiency and/or hypoxemia at the time of treatment responded and 10 (24%) developed severe secondary bleeding secondary to treatment, with a significant number experiencing fatal hemorrhage. The authors concluded that tPA/heparin should not be given to patients with MOF and treatment should be given early in the disease course or not at all *(99)*.

The administration of ATIII and activated protein C (APC) has not been shown to be effective in a number of studies *(100,101)*, although a trial in 10 patients using ATIII for the treatment of chemotherapy-induced organ dysfunction following SCT suggested some clinical benefit in 3 patients with VOD *(102)*. PGE_1 infusions for established VOD have been largely unsuccessful *(103)*.

Defibrotide (DF), a single-stranded polydeoxyribonucleotide with a molecular weight of 15–30 kDa *(104)*, has been identified as an agent that might be able to modulate endothelial cell injury without enhancing systemic bleeding and protect host hepatocytes and sinusoidal endothelium without compromising the antitumor effects of cytotoxic therapy *(105,106)*. DF

Table 2
tPA for the Treatment of VOD

Author	No. of patients (n)	Dose (mg/d)	Duration (d)	Heparin (Yes/No)	No. of Responses	No. of Life-threatening or serious hemorrhage
Baglin *(84)*	1	50	4	No	1	0
Bearman *(79)*	42	5.4–30	2–4	Yes	12	10
LaPorte *(85)*	1	50	4	No	1	0
Rosti *(86)*	1	50	4	No	1	0
Ringden *(87)*	1	50	4	No	0	1
Leahey *(78)*	9	5–10	2–4	Yes	5	0
Feldman *(88)*	3	15	4	No	3	0
Goldberg *(89)*	1	20	4	Yes	1	0
Higashigawa *(90)*	1	2–5	4	Yes[a]	1	0
Hagglund*(91)*	10	3–50	3–8	Yes[b]	4	4
Lee *(92)*	3	10–20	7–14	Yes	3	0
Yu *(93)*	8	0.25–0.5[c]	4	No	4	0
Schriber *(94)*	37	30–40	1–21	Yes	10[d]	13
Kulkarni *(95)*	17	10	1–12	Yes	6	0

[a]Patient also received PGE_1.
[b]Three patients received heparin; 7 patients did not.
[c]Dose reported as mg/kg.
[d]In patients who met established criteria for VOD. (From ref. *99* with permission.)

has specific aptameric binding sites on vascular endothelium, namely adenosine receptors A1 and A2, which are part of the growing family of nucleotide receptors involved in endothelial cell regulation and response to injury *(106)*. Studies have shown that DF increases prostacyclin (PGI_2), prostaglandin E_2, and thrombomodulin in vivo. DF also upregulates TFPI and tPA *(107–110)*. It decreases thrombin generation and also decreases circulating PAI-1 *(111)*. DF inhibits fibrin deposition and may modulate vitronectin and fibronectin release, which, as components of the extracellular matrix, are linked to collagen formation and fibrosis *(112–114)*. Clinical trials of DF have demonstrated activity in peripheral vascular disease, microvascular thrombotic states, ischemic organ injury, and chemotherapy-related hemolytic uremic syndrome (HUS) *(108,113,115,116)*. Recent preclinical studies of human-derived, LPS-exposed microvascular and macrovascular endothelium by Falanga et al. have shown selective and protective effects of DF in LPS-mediated microvascular injury through enhanced fibrinolysis and modulation of sTF and TFPI expression *(117,118)*. This differential activity of the drug on microvascular rather than macrovascular endothelium is particularly intriguing in the context of its application to diseases of the microvasculature such as VOD.

A pilot treatment plan was launched in the United States for patients with severe VOD, defined by a greater than 40% risk per the Bearman model or by the presence of MOF *(119)*. DF treatment was given intravenously, typically every 6 h and infused over 2 h with a dose range of 10–60 mg/kg/d. In the first cohort of 19 evaluable patients, complete remissions (defined as a bilirubin less than 2 mg/dL) were seen in 8/19 (42%), most of whom had resolution of MOF and survived to d +100 and beyond. Response was typically evident within the first 7 d and the active dose appeared to be approx 25 mg/kg/d. None of the nonresponders survived past d +100, with a median survival of only 36 d post-SCT (range: 15–89 d) *(119)*. Additional trials of DF administration to patients with severe VOD and MOF by other groups have produced similar results *(120–124)*. Although the natural history of more moderate VOD is less morbid, the complete remission rate in the European experience with DF therapy was higher in patients with moderate but significant VOD, suggesting that earlier intervention may be more effective *(124)*. A recent analysis of the expanded US experience has confirmed the favorable safety profile of DF when used in a multi-institutional setting following specific treatment guidelines *(125)*, where a complete remission rate of 36% and an overall survival of 35% was observed in a total of 88 SCT patients with severe VOD and MOF. Predictors of survival included younger age, autoSCT, and abnormal portal flow, whereas busulfan-based conditioning and encephalopathy predicted the worse outcome. Decreases in mean creatinine and PAI-1 levels during DF therapy also predicted better survival, suggesting that certain features associated with successful outcome could correlate with DF-related treatment effects, and further evaluation of DF therapy for severe VOD may, therefore, allow better definition of predictors of response or failure *(125)*. Prospective, multi-institutional trials of DF in the treatment of severe VOD are now underway in the United States and Europe *(126)*.

Liver transplant in those who have been able to undergo the procedure has resulted in clinical improvement in about 30%, as estimated from small cases series, but difficulties with this approach include finding a suitable liver graft, managing the effects of multisystem organ failure, and the prevention of liver graft rejection *(127)*. Transjugular intrahepatic portosystemic shunts (TIPS), which have been used successfully in patients with cirrhosis and bleeding esophageal varices, ascites, and Budd–Chiari syndrome, have also been tested to treat VOD after SCT *(128–130)*. This procedure involves the creation of a channel between the hepatic vein and the portal vein using a subcutaneously inserted catheter and the maintenance of the channel using a metal stent. Although the procedure has appeal because it does not require an open surgical procedure and any bleeding that results is intrahepatic, it probably has no value for patients whose VOD is not characterized by significant fluid retention and ascites. It is also limited in terms of long-term efficacy, as evidenced by the poor overall survival data in the patient series published to date. Another modality, charcoal hemofiltration, capable of adsorbing bilirubin and other factors from the circulation has been reported to be useful *(131)* and may be helpful as a supportive measure in selected patients.

10. CONCLUSIONS

Hepatic VOD is a manifestation of conditioning regimen-related toxicity in SCT (with a contribution from previous chemotherapy, including newer agents such as Mylotarg) and is most probably increased by allogeneic effects between donor cells, cytokine release, and recipient tissues. It is currently a major limiting factor for improving the efficacy of both autoSCT and alloSCT, and better methods of both prophylaxis and treatment are needed to overcome this much feared complication. Prevention is clearly a priority, and efforts designed to identify at-risk patients, utilize pharmacokinetics to better individualize chemotherapy administration, and prevent vascular and hepatocyte injury are ongoing. The treatment of severe VOD remains inadequate with a very high fatality rate. Current directions in the investigation of VOD therapy target endothelial injury. The use of rh-tPA in conjunction with heparin has been confounded by the risk of serious toxicity. An alternative agent, DF, has shown considerable potential with remarkably little toxicity, and the results of prospective trials will, hopefully, confirm this drug's current promise. TIPS, charcoal hemofiltration, and liver transplantation are other approaches currently under investigation in severe disease and may have adjunctive roles as better systemic approaches to treatment evolve.

ACKNOWLEDGMENTS

The author gratefully acknowledges the assistance of Parisa Momtaz in the preparation of this manuscript. The photomicrographs were kindly provided by Howard Shulman, MD.

REFERENCES

1. McDonald GB, Sharma P, Matthews DE, et al. Venocclusive disease of the liver after bone marrow transplantation: diagnosis, incidence, and predisposing factors. *Hepatology* 1984;4:116–122.
2. Bearman SI. The syndrome of hepatic veno-occlusive disease after marrow transplantation. *Blood* 1995;85:3005–3020.
3. Richardson PG, Guinan EC. The pathology, diagnosis and treatment of hepatic veno-occlusive disease: current status and novel approaches. *Br J Haematol* 1999;107:485–493.
4. Lee JL, Gooley T, Bensinger W, et al. Venocclusive disease of the liver after high-dose chemotherapy with alkylating agents: incidence, outcome and risk factors. *Hepatology* 1997;26(pt 2):149A.
5. Carreras E, Bertz H, Arcese W, et al. Incidence and outcome of hepatic veno-occlusive disease after blood or marrow transplantation: a prospective cohort study of the European Group for Blood and Marrow Transplantation. European Group for Blood and Marrow Transplantation Chronic Leukemia Working Party. *Blood* 1998;92:3599–3604.
6. McDonald GB. Venocclusive disease of the liver following marrow transplantation. *Marrow Transplant Rev* 1993;3:49–56.
7. McDonald GB, Hinds MS, Fisher LD, et al. Veno-occlusive disease of the liver and multiorgan failure after bone marrow transplantation: a cohort study of 355 patients. *Ann Intern Med* 1993;118:255–267.

8. Holler E, Kolbe HJ, Moller A, et al. Increased serum levels of TNFa precede major complications of bone marrow transplantation. *Blood* 1990;75:1011–1016.
9. Krenger W, Hill GR, Ferrara JLM. Cytokine cascades in acute graft-versus-host disease. *Transplantation* 1997;64:553–558.
10. Baglin TP. Veno-occlusive disease of the liver complicating bone marrow transplantation. *Bone Marrow Transplant* 1994;13:1–4.
11. Shirai M, Nagashima K, Iwasaki S, et al. A light and scanning electron microscopic study of hepatic veno-occlusive disease. *Acta Pathol Jpn* 1987;37:1961–1971.
12. Shulman HM, McDonald GB, Matthews D, et al. An analysis of hepatic venocclusive disease and centrilobular hepatic degeneration following bone marrow transplantation. *Gastroenterology* 1980;79:1178–1191.
13. Shulman HM, Fisher LB, Schoch HG, et al. Venoocclusive disease of the liver after marrow transplantation: histological correlates of clinical signs and symptoms. *Hepatology* 1994;19:1171–1180.
14. Shulman HM, Gown AM, Nugent DJ. Hepatic veno-occlusive disease after bone marrow transplantation. Immunohistochemical identification of the material within occluded central venules. *Am J Pathol* 1987;127:549–558.
15. DeLeve L, Shulman HM, McDonald GB. Toxic injury to hepatic sinusoids: sinusoidal obstruction syndrome (veno-occlusive disease). *Semin Liver Dis* 2002;22:27–42.
16. DeLeve LD. Cellular target of cyclophosphamide toxicity in the murine liver: role of glutathione and site of metabolic activation. *Hepatology* 1996;24:830–837.
17. Allen JR, Carstens LA, Katagiri GJ. Hepatic veins of monkeys with veno-occlusive disease. Sequential ultrastructural changes. *Arch Pathol* 1969;87:279–289.
18. Ridker PN, McDermont WV. Hepatotoxicity due to comfrey herb tea [letter; comment] [see comments]. *Am J Med* 1989;87:701.
19. Traber PG, Chianale J, Gumucio JJ. Physiologic significance and regulation of hepatocellular heterogeneity [see comments]. *Gastroenterology* 1988;95:1130–1143.
20. el Mouelhi M, Kauffman FC. Sublobular distribution of transferases and hydrolases associated with glucuronide, sulfate and glutathione conjugation in human liver. *Hepatology* 1986;6:450–456.
21. Deleve LD. Dacarbazine toxicity in murine liver cells: a model of hepatic endothelial injury and glutathione defense. *J Pharmacol Exp Ther* 1994;268:1261–1270.
22. Teicher BA, Crawford JM, Holden SA, et al. Glutathione monoethyl ester can selectively protect liver from high dose BCNU or cyclophosphamide. *Cancer* 1988;62:1275–1281.
23. Grochow LB. Busulfan disposition: the role of therapeutic monitoring in bone marrow transplantation induction regimens. *Semin Oncol* 1993;20:18–25.
24. Hassan M, Oberg G, Bekassy AN, et al. Pharmacokinetics of high-dose busulphan in relation to age and chronopharmacology. *Cancer Chemother Pharmacol* 1991;28:130–134.
25. Schuler U, Schroer S, Kuhnle A, et al. Busulfan pharmacokinetics in bone marrow transplant patients: is drug monitoring warranted? *Bone Marrow Transplant* 1994;14:759–765.
26. Yeager AM, Wagner JE Jr, Graham ML, et al. Optimization of busulfan dosage in children undergoing bone marrow transplantation: a pharmacokinetic study of dose escalation. *Blood* 1992;80:2425–2428.
27. Slattery JT, Kalhorn TF, McDonald GB, et al. Conditioning regimen-dependent disposition of cyclophosphamide and hydroxycyclophosphamide in human marrow transplantation patients. *J Clin Oncol* 1996;14:1484–1494.
28. DeLeve LD. Glutathione defense in non-parenchymal cells. *Semin Liver Dis* 1998;18:403–413.
29. Wang X, Kanel GC, DeLeve LD. Support of sinusoidal endothelial cell glutathione prevents hepatic veno-occlusive disease in the rat. *Hepatology* 2000;31:428–434.
30. Ringden O, Remberger M, Lehmann S, et al. *N*-Acetylcysteine for hepatic veno-occlusive disease after allogeneic stem cell transplantation. *Bone Marrow Transplant* 2000;25:993–996.
31. Catani L, Gugliotta L, Vianelli N, et al. Endothelium and bone marrow transplantation. *Bone Marrow Transplant* 1996;17:277–280.
32. Salat C, Holler E, Reinhardt B, et al. Parameters of the fibrinolytic system in patients undergoing BMT: elevation of PAI-1 in veno-occlusive disease. *Bone Marrow Transplant* 1994;14:747–750.
33. Salat C, Holler E, Kolbe HJ, et al. Plasminogen activator inhibitor-1 confirms the diagnosis of hepatic veno-occlusive disease in patients with hyperbilirubinemia after bone marrow transplant. *Blood* 1997;89:2184–2188.
34. Richardson P, Guinain E. Hepatic veno-occlusive disease following hematopoietic stem cell transplantation. *Acta Haematol* 2001;106:57–68.

35. Richardson P, Hoppensteadt D, Elias A, et al. Elevation of tissue factor pathway inhibitor [TFPI], thrombomodulin [TM] and plasminogen activator inhibitor-1 [PAI-1] levels in stem cell transplant [SCT]-associated veno-occlusive disease [VOD] and changes seen with the use of defibrotide [DF]. *Blood* 1997;90:219a.
36. Richardson PG, Hoppensteadt DA, Elias AD, et al. Elevation of endothelial stress products and trends seen in patients with severe veno-occlusive disease treated with defibrotide. *Thromb Haemost* 1999;3185(Suppl):628.
37. Nurnberger W, Michelmann I, Burdach S, et al. Endothelial dysfunction after bone marrow transplantation: increase of soluble thrombomodulin and PAI-1 in patients with multiple transplant-related complications. *Ann Hematol* 1998;76:61–65.
38. Sato Y, Asada Y, Hara S, et al. Hepatic stellate cells (Ito cells) in veno-occlusive disease of the liver after allogeneic bone marrow transplantation. *Histopathology* 1999;34:66–70.
39. Bianchi M, Tracey KJ. The role of TNF in complications of marrow transplantation. *Marrow Transplant Rev* 1993/94;3:57–61.
40. Scrobohaci ML, Drouet L, Monem-Mansi A, et al. Liver veno-occlusive disease after bone marrow transplantation changes in coagulation parameters and endothelial markers. *Thromb Res* 1991;63:509–519.
41. Ferra C, de Sanjose S, Gallardo D, et al. IL-6 and IL-8 levels in plasma during hematopoietic progenitor transplantation. *Haematologica* 1998;83:1082–1087.
42. Schots R, Kaufman L, Van Riet I, et al. Monitoring of C-reactive protein after allogeneic bone marrow transplantation identifies patients at risk of severe transplant-related complications and mortality. *Bone Marrow Transplant* 1998;22:79–85.
43. Anscher MS, Peters WP, Reisenbichler H, et al. Transforming growth factor beta as a predictor of liver and lung fibrosis after autologous bone marrow transplantation for advanced breast cancer. *N Engl J Med* 1993;328:1592–1598.
44. Eltumi M, Trivedi P, Hobbs J, et al. Monitoring of veno-occlusive disease after bone marrow transplantation by serum aminopropepide of type III procollagen. *Lancet* 1993;342:518–521.
45. Park YD, Yasui M, Yoshimoto T, et al. Changes in hemostatic parameters in hepatic veno-occlusive disease following bone marrow transplantation. *Bone Marrow Transplant* 1997;19:915–920.
46. Rio B, Bauduer F, Arrago JP, et al. *N*-Terminal peptide of type III procollagen: a marker for the development of hepatic veno-occlusive disease after BMT and a basis for determining the timing of prophylactic heparin. *Bone Marrow Transplant* 1993;11:471–472.
47. Eltumi M, Trivedi P, Hobbs JR, et al. Monitoring of veno-occlusive disease after bone marrow transplantation by serum aminopropeptide of type III procollagen [see comments]. *Lancet* 1993;342:518–521.
48. Heikinheimo M, Halila R, Fasth A. Serum procollagen type III is an early and sensitive marker for veno-occlusive disease of the liver in children undergoing bone marrow transplantation. *Blood* 1994;83:3036–3040.
49. Collins PW, Gutteridge CN, O'Driscoll A, et al. von Willebrand factor as a marker of endothelial cell activation following BMT. *Bone Marrow Transplant* 1992;10:499–506.
50. Harper PL, Jarvis J, Jennings I, et al. Changes in the natural anticoagulants following bone marrow transplantation. *Bone Marrow Transplant* 1990;5:39–42.
51. Haire WD, Ruby EI, Gordon BG, et al. Multiple organ dysfunction syndrome in bone marrow transplantation. *JAMA* 1995;274:1289–1295.
52. Faioni EM, Krachmalnicoff A, Bearman SI, et al. Naturally occuring anticoagulants and bone marrow transplantation: plasma protein C predicts the development of venocclusive disease of the liver. *Blood* 1993;81:3458–3462.
53. Sudhoff T, Heins M, Sohngen D, et al. Plasma levels of D-dimer and circulating endothelial adhesion molecules in veno-occlusive disease of the liver following allogeneic bone marrow transplantation. *Eur J Haematol* 1998;60:106–111.
54. Oh H, Tahara T, Bouvier M, et al. Plasma thrombopoietin levels in marrow transplant patients with veno-occlusive disease of the liver. *Bone Marrow Transplant* 1998;22:675–679.
55. Nevill TJ, Barnett MJ, Klingemann H-G, et al. Regimen-related toxicity of busulfan–cyclophosphamide conditioning regimen in 70 patients undergoing allogeneic bone marrow transplantation. *J Clin Oncol* 1991;9:1224–1232.
56. Matute-Bello G, McDonald GD, Hinds MS, et al. Association of pulmonary function testing abnormalities and severe veno-occlusive disease of the liver after marrow transplantation. *Bone Marrow Transplant* 1998;21:1125–1130.

57. Hagglund H, Remberger M, Klaesson S, et al. Norethisterone treatment, a major risk-factor for veno-occlusive disease in the liver after allogeneic bone marrow transplantation [see comments]. *Blood* 1998;92:4568–4572.
58. Soiffer R, Dear K, Rabinowe SN, et al. Hepatic dysfunction follwoing T-cell-depleted allogeneic bone marrow transplantation. *Transplantation* 1991;52:1014–1019.
59. Moscardo F, Sanz GF, De la Rubia J. Marked reduction in the incidence of hepatic veno-occlusive disease after allogeneic hematopoietic stem cell transplantation with CD34+ positive selection. *Bone Marrow Transplant* 2001;27:983–988.
60. Ringden O, Ruutu T, Remberger M, et al. A randomized trial comparing busulfan with total body irradiation as conditioning in allogeneic marrow transplant recipients with leukemia: a report from the Nordic Bone Marrow Transplantation Group. *Blood* 1994;83:2723–2730.
61. Styler MJ, Crilley P, Biggs J. Hepatic dysfunction following busulfan and cyclophosphamide myeloblation: a retrospective, multicenter analysis. *Bone Marrow Transplant* 1996;18:171–176.
62. Rozman C, Carreras E, Qian C, et al. Risk factors for hepatic veno-occlusive disease following HLA-identical sibling bone marrow transplants for leukemia. *Bone Marrow Transplant* 1996;17:75–80.
63. Fisher DC, Vredenburgh JJ, Petros WP, et al. Reduced mortality following bone marrow transplantation for breast cancer with the addition of peripheral blood progenitor cells is due to a marked reduction in veno-occlusive disease of the liver. *Bone Marrow Transplant* 1998;21:117–122.
64. Korbling M, Katz RL, Khanna A, et al. Hepatocytes and epithelial cells of donor origin in recipients of peripheral-blood stem cells. *N Engl J Med* 2002;346:738–746.
65. Tack DK, Letendre L, Kamath P, et al. Development of hepatic veno-occlusive disease after Mylotarg infusion for relapsed acute myeloid leukemia. *Bone Marrow Transplant* 2001;28:895–897.
66. McDonald GB. Management of hepatic sinusoidal obstruction syndrome following treatment with gemtuzmab ozogamicin (Mylotarg®). *Clin Lymphoma* 2002;2:S35–S39.
67. Brown BP, Abu-Yousef M, Farner R, et al. Doppler sonography: a noninvasive method for evaluation of hepatic venocclusive disease. *Am J Roentgenol* 1990;154:721–724.
68. Hosoki T, Kuroda C, Tokunaga K, et al. Hepatic venous outflow obstruction: evaluation with pulsed duplex sonography. *Radiology* 1989;170:733–737.
69. Nicolau C, Concepcio B, Carreras E, et al. Sonographic diagnosis and hemodynamic correlation in veno-occlusive disease of the liver. *J Ultrasound Med* 1993;12:437–440.
70. Sonneveld P, Lameris JS, Cornelissen J, et al. Color-flow imaging sonography of portal and hepatic vein flow to monitor fibrinolytic therapy with r-TPA for veno-occlusive disease following myeloablative treatment. *Bone Marrow Transplant* 1998;21:731–734.
71. van den Bosch MA, van Hoe L. MR imaging findings in two patients with hepatic veno-occlusive disease following bone marrow transplantation [in process citation]. *Eur Radiol* 2000;10:1290–1293.
72. Carreras E, Granena A, Navasa M, et al. Transjugular liver biopsy in BMT. *Bone Marrow Transplant* 1993;11:21–26.
73. Shulman HM, Gooley T, Dudley MD, et al. Utility of transvenous liver biopsies and wedged hepatic venous pressure measurements in sixty marrow transplant recipients. *Transplantation* 1995;59:1015–1022.
74. Bearman SI, Anderson GL, Mori M, et al. Venocclusive disease of the liver: Development of a model for predicting fatal outcome after marrow transplantation. *J Clin Oncol* 1993;11:1729–1736.
75. Barrett J, Childs R. Non-myeloblative stem cell transplants. *Br J Haematol* 2000;111:6–17.
76. Maris M, Sandmaier BM, Maloney DG, et al. Non-myeloblative hematopoietic stem cell transplantation. *Transfus Clin Biol* 2001;8:231–234.
77. Tse WT, Beyer W, Pendleton JD, et al. Genetic Polymorphisms in glutathione-*S*-transferase and plasminogen activator inhibitor and risk of veno-occlusive disease (VOD). in American Society of Hematology. 2000. San Francisco: The Journal of American Society of Hematology.
78. Poonkuzhali S, Vidya S, Shaji RV, et al. Glutathione *S*-transferase gene polymorphism and risk of major undergoing allogeneic bone marrow transplantation. *Blood* 2001;98:852a.
79. Haire WD, Cavet J, Pavletic SZ, et al. Tumor necrosis factor d3 allele predicts for organ dysfunction after allogeneic blood stem cell transplantation (ABSCT). in American Society of Hematology. 2000. San Francisco: Journal of the American Society of Hematology.
80. Ohashi K, Tanabe J, Watanabe R, et al. The Japanese multicenter open randomized trial of ursodeoxycholic acid prophylaxis for hepatic veno-occlusive disease after stem cell transplantation. *Am J Hematol* 2000;64:32–38.
81. Essell JH, Schroeder MT, Harman GS, et al. Ursodiol prophylaxis against hepatic complications of allogeneic bone marrow transplantation. A randomized, double-blind, placebo-controlled trial. *Ann Intern Med* 1998;128:975–981.

82. Ruutu T, Eriksson B, Remes K, et al. Ursodiol prevention of hepatic complications in allogeneic stem cell transplantation: results of a prospective, randomized, placebo-controlled trial. *Bone Marrow Transplant* 1999;23:756 [Abstract].
83. Jonas CR, Puckett AB, Jones DP, et al. Plasma antioxidant status after high-dose chemotherapy: a randomized trial of parenteral nutrition in bone marrow transplantation patients. *Am J Clin Nutr* 2000;72:181–189.
84. Goringe AP, Brown S, O'Callaghan U, et al. Glutamine and vitamin E in the treatment of hepatic veno-occlusive disease following high-dose chemotherapy. *Bone Marrow Transplant* 1998;21:829–832.
85. Khoury H, Adkins D, Trinkaus K, et al. Treatment of hepatic veno-occlusive disease with high dose corticosteroids: an update on 28 stem cell transplant recipients. *Blood* 1998;92:1132 [Abstract].
86. Ferra C, Sanjose S, Lastra CF, et al. Pentoxifylline, ciprofloxacin and prednisone failed to prevent transplant-related toxicities in bone marrow transplant recipients and were associated with an increased incidence of infectious complications. *Bone Marrow Transplant* 1997;20:1075–1080.
87. Clift RA, Bianco JA, Appelbaum FR, et al. A randomized controlled trial of pentoxifylline for the prevention of regimen-related toxicities in patients undergoing allogeneic marrow transplantation. *Blood* 1993;82:2025–2030.
88. Attal M, Huguet F, Rubie H. Prevention of hepatic veno-occlusive disease after bone marrow transplantation by continuous infusion of low-dose heparin: a prospective, randomized trial. *Blood* 1992;79:2834–2840.
89. Bearman SI, Hinds MS, Wolford JL. A pilot study of continuous infusion heparin for the prevention of hepatic veno-occlusive disease after bone marrow transplantation. *Bone Marrow Transplant* 1990;5:407–411.
90. Marsa-Vila L, Gorin NC, Laporte JP. Prophylactic heparin does not prevent liver veno-occlusive disease following autologous bone marrow transplantation. *Eur J Haematol* 1991;47:346–352.
91. Budinger MD, Bouvier M, Shah A, et al. Results of a phase 1 trial of anti-thrombin III as prophylaxis in bone marrow transplant patients at risk for venocclusive disease. *Blood* 1996;88:172a [Abstract].
92. Lee JH, Lee KH, Choi JS, et al. Veno-occlusive disease (VOD) of the liver in Korean patients following allogeneic bone marrow transplantation (BMT): efficacy of recombinant human tissue plasminogen activator (rt-PA) treatment. *J Korean Med Sci* 1996;11:118–126.
93. Or R, Nagler A, Shpilberg O, et al. Low molecular weight heparin for the prevention of veno-occlusive disease of the liver in bone marrow transplantation patients. *Transplantation* 1996;61:1067–1071.
94. Vaughan DE, Plavin SR, Schafer AI. PGE1 accelerates thrombolysis by tissue plasminogen activator. *Blood* 1989;73:1213–1217.
95. Gluckman E, Jolivet I, Scrobohaci ML. Use of prostaglandin E1 for prevention of liver veno-occlusive disease in leukaemic patients treated by allogeneic bone marrow transplantation. *Br J Haematol* 1990;74:277–281.
96. Schriber JR, Milk BJ, Baer MR. A randomized phase II trial comparing heparin (Hep) +/– prostaglandin E1 (PG) to prevent hepatotoxicity (HT) following bone marrow transplantation (BMT): preliminary results. *Blood* 1996;88:1642.
97. Bearman SI, Shuhart MC, Hinds MS, et al. Recombinant human tissue plasminogen activator for the treatment of established severe venocclusive disease of the liver after bone marrow transplantation. *Blood* 1992;80:2458–2462.
98. Leahey AM, Bunin NJ. Recombinant human tissue plasminogen activator for the treatment of severe hepatic veno-occlusive disease in pediatric bone marrow transplant patients. *Bone Marrow Transplant* 1996;17:1101–1104.
99. Richardson P, Bearman SI. Prevention and treatment of hepatic venocclusive disease after high-dose cytoreductive therapy. *Leuk Lymphoma* 1998;31;267–277.
100. Haire WD, Stephens LC, Ruby EI. Antithrombin III (AT3) treatment of organ dysfunction during bone marrow transplantation (BMT)—results of a pilot study. *Blood* 1996;88:458a [Abstract].
101. Strasser SI, McDonald GB. Gastrointestinal and hepatic complications. In: Forman SJ, Blume KG, Thomas ED, eds. *Hematopoietic Cell Transplantation* 2nd ed. Boston: Blackwell Scientific, 1998.
102. Morris JD, Harris RE, Hashmi R, et al. Antithrombin-III for the treatment of chemotherapy-induced organ dysfunction following bone marrow transplantation. *Bone Marrow Transplant* 1997;20:871–878.
103. Ibrahim A, Pico JL, Maraninchi D, et al. Hepatic veno-occlusive disease following bone marrow transplantation treated by prostaglandin E1. *Bone Marrow Transplant* 1991;7(suppl):53.
104. Bianchi G, Barone D, Lanzarotti E, et al. Defibrotide, a single-stranded polydeoxyribonucleotide acting as an adenosine receptor agonist. *Eur J Pharmacol* 1993;238:327–334.
105. Eissner G, Multhoff G, Gerbitz A, et al. Fludarabine induces apoptosis, activation, and allogenicity in human endothelial and epithelial cells: protective effect of defibrotide. *Blood* 2002;100:334–340.

106. Bracht F, Schror, K. Isolation and identification of aptamers from defibrotide that act as thrombin antagonists in vitro. *Biochem Biophys Res Commun* 1994;200:933–936.
107. Berti F, Rossoni G, Biasi G, et al. Defibrotide by enhancing prostacyclin generation prevents endothelin-I induced contraction in human saphenous veins. *Prostaglandins* 1990;40:337–350.
108. Coccheri S, Biagi G. Defibrotide. *Cardiovasc Drug Rev* 1991;9:172–196.
109. Fareed J. Modulation of endothelium by heparin and related polyelectrolytes. In: Nicolaides A, Novo S, eds. *Advances in Vascular Pathology 1997*. Amsterdam: Elsevier Science, 1997.
110. Zhou Q, Chu X, Ruan, C. Defibrotide stimulates expression of thrombomodulin in human endothelial cells. *Thromb Hemost* 1994;71:507–510.
111. Palmer KJ, Goa KL. Defibrotide: a review of its pharmacodynamic and pharmacokinetic properties, and therapeutic use in vascular disorders. *Drugs* 1993;45:259–294.
112. Coccheri S, Biagi G, Legnani C, et al. Acute effects of defibrotide, an experimental antithrombotic agent, on fibrinolysis and blood prostanoids in man. *Eur J Clin Pharmacol* 1988;35:151–156.
113. Ulutin ON. Antithrombotic effect and clinical potential of defibrotide. *Semin Thromb Hemost* 1993;19:186–191.
114. Jamieson A, Alcock P, Tuffin DP. The action of polyanionic agents defibrotide and pentosan sulphate on fibrinolytic activity in the laboratory rat. *Fibrinolysis* 1996;10:27–35.
115. Bonomini V, Vangelista A, Frasca GM. A new antithrombotic agent in the treatment of acute renal failure due to hemolytic-uremic syndrome and thrombotic thrombocytopenic purpura [letter]. *Nephron* 1984;37:144.
116. Viola F, Marubini S, Coccheri G, et al. Improvement of walking distance by defibrotide in patients with intermittent claudication: results of a randomized, placebo-controlled study (the DICLIS study). *Thromb Haemost* 2000;83:672–677.
117. Falanga A, Marchetti M, Vignoli A, et al. Defibrotide (DF) modulates tissue factor expression by microvascular endothelial cells. *Blood* 1999;94:146a.
118. Falanga A, Marchetti M, Vignoli A, et al. Impact of defibrotide on the fibrinolytic and procoagulant properties of endothelial cell macro- and micro-vessels. *Blood* 2000;96:53a.
119. Richardson PG, Elias AD, Krishnan A, et al. Treatment of severe veno-occlusive disease with defibrotide: compassionate use results in response without significant toxicity in a high-risk population. *Blood* 1998;92:737–744.
120. Abecasis M, Ferreira I, Guimaraes A, et al. Defibrotide as salvage therapy for hepatic veno-occlusive disease (VOD). *Bone Marrow Transplant* 1999;23:749 [Abstract].
121. Salat C, Pihusch R, Fries S, et al. Successful treatment of veno-occlsive disease with defibrotide—a report of two cases. *Bone Marrow Transplant* 1999;23:757 (Abstract).
122. Zinke W, Neumeister P, Linkesch W. Defibrotide—an approach in the treatment of severe veno-occlusive disease? *Bone Marrow Transplant* 1999;23:760 (Abstract).
123. Jenner MJ, Micallef IN, Rohatiner AZ, et al. Successful therapy of transplant-associated veno-occlusive disease with a combination of tissue plasminogen activator and defibrotide [in process citation]. *Med Oncol* 2000;17:333–336.
124. Chopra R, Eaton JD, Grassi A, et al. Defibrotide for the treatment of hepatic veno-occlusive disease: results of the European compassionate-use study. *Br J Haematol* 2000;100:4337–4343.
125. Richardson P, Murakami C, Jin Z, et al. Multi-institutional use of defibrotide in 88 patients post stem cell transplant with severe veno-occlusive disease and multi-system organ failure; response without significant toxicity in a high risk population and factors predictive of outcome. *Blood* 2002;100:4337–4343.
126. Richardson P, Warren D, Momtaz P, et al. Multi-institutional phase II randomized dose finding study of defibrotide (DF) in patients (pts) with severe veno-occlusive disease (VOD) and multi-system organ failure (MOF) post stem cell transplantation (SCT): promising response rate without significant toxicity in a high risk population. *Blood* 2001;98:853a.
127. Schlitt HJ, Tischler HJ, Ringe B, et al. Allogeneic liver transplantation for hepatic veno-occlusive disease after bone marrow transplantation—clinical and immunological considerations. *Bone Marrow Transplant* 1995;16:473–478.
128. Fried MW, Connaghan DG, Sharma S, et al. Trans jugular intrahepatic protosystemic shunt for the management of severe venocclusive disease following bone marrow transplantation. *Hepatology* 1996;24:588–591.
129. Smith FO, Johnson MS, Scherer LR, et al.Transjugular intrahepatic portosystemic shunting (TIPS) for the treatment of severe hepatic veno-occlusive disease. *Bone Marrow Transplant* 1996;18:643–646.
130. Alvarez R, Banares R, Casariego J, et al. Percutaneous intrahepatic portosystemic shunting in the treatment of veno-occlusive disease of the liver after bone marrow transplantation. *Gastroenterol Hepatol* 2000;23:177–180.
131. Tefferi A, Kumar S, Wolf R, et al. Charcoal hemofiltration for hepatic veno-occulsive disease after hematopoietic stem cell transplantation. *Bone Marrow Transplant* 2001;28:997–999.

14 Quality-of-Life Issues Posttransplantation

Stephanie J. Lee, MD, MPH

Contents

1. OVERVIEW

Quality of life (QOL) refers to every dimension of life except for its length, and it includes physical abilities, symptoms, social well-being, psychoemotional status, and spiritual/existential qualities. It reflects how well people feel, what they can accomplish, how satisfied they are with their lives, and whether their lives have meaning and purpose. Within this broad concept, health-related quality of life (HR-QOL) refers to aspects of QOL that are attributable to health, disease, or medical treatment. (In this chapter, the abbreviation QOL is used for simplicity.) Following hematopoietic stem cell transplantation (HSCT), QOL can range from perfect, with no physical, emotional, or social sequelae and a greater appreciation for life, to severely compromised, with physical disability, pain, and psychological despair. Of course, most patients who have undergone HSCT fall within this spectrum. The goal of this chapter is to provide an overview of concepts and published work rather than review individual studies exhaustively. Additional sections address how to evaluate QOL studies and use QOL data in the care of individual patients.

From: *Stem Cell Transplantation for Hematologic Malignancies*
Edited by: R. J. Soiffer © Humana Press Inc., Totowa, NJ

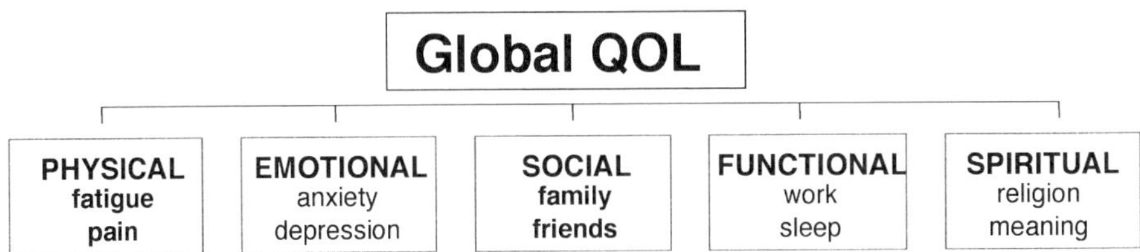

Fig. 1. Components of quality of life.

2. DEFINITIONS

Figure 1 shows the general taxonomy of QOL. Overall or global QOL is at the top of the pyramid and is the short answer to the question How are you doing today? Conceptually, global QOL is based on a composite of domains representing physical, emotional, social, functional, and spiritual/existential considerations. These domains are best assessed by familiar queries: Are you bothered by any symptoms? How are you holding up? These domains reflect specific issues (e.g., Do you have any mouth sores? Can you walk up a flight of stairs? Have you gone back to work yet? Are you sleeping all right? How are things at home?) The exact segregation of some QOL components varies according to the author. For example, sexual functioning has been grouped variably under the physical, functional and social domains.

By definition, QOL is multidimensional, individual, and subjective *(1)*. Studies of concurrent measures of patient- and surrogate-reported QOL show that physicians, nurses, spouses, and parents often think differently about patients' QOL than they do *(2)*. For example, nurses thought some specific problems would have a greater impact on QOL than patients reported *(3)*. These findings suggest that QOL is best assessed directly from patients and that surrogate assessments may be misleading.

Several qualitative studies have probed the meaning of QOL for HSCT patients. Ferrell analyzed survey responses to six open-ended questions about QOL from 119 HSCT survivors (63% response rate, transplanted 1976–1990). Content analysis suggested six themes about the meaning of QOL. These may be summarized into two overarching concepts: appreciating and cherishing what one has (family, relationships, life) and desire to regain pretransplant functioning (independence, health, return to work, normalcy). The impact of HSCT on QOL emphasized several losses (side effects, decreased strength and stamina, limited work and activities) and some positive effects (second chance, opportunity to improve QOL, increased spirituality and meaning, increased appreciation for life). When asked what physicians or nurses could do to improve QOL, patients responded with many practical suggestions (be accessible, provide support groups, provide education and coping strategies, increase patient participation in decision-making) *(4,5)*. Haberman studied 125 adult HSCT survivors (64% response rate, transplanted prior to 1983, 87% allogeneic recipients) more than 6 yr posttransplantation using an open-ended questionnaire. Many patients reported using cognitive and attitudinal strategies (acceptance, looking on the positive side) and behavior- and action-oriented strategies (staying active, setting goals, taking care of oneself) to cope with problems. Patients who believe HSCT improved their QOL focused on the lessons learned through the experience and improved health. Patients who reported poorer QOL after HSCT focused on physical and social limitations and increased life stress from finances and job *(6)*. Baker et al. *(7)* interviewed 84 survivors after their departure from the Johns Hopkins Oncology Center, and again at 6 mo and

1 yr (80–84% response rate, 42% allogeneic recipients). In addition to physical and psychological problems, respondents noted problems with resuming roles put on hold because of illness. Specifically, they reported issues with returning home, work, and social situations such as stigmatization, problems with family and children, and financial and job concerns *(7)*.

3. SPECIFIC ISSUES POSTTRANSPLANTATION

Survivors generally report high global QOL following HSCT, but also many specific symptoms *(1,8–13)* and limitations on their daily activities *(14)*. However, despite many problematic long-term complications, almost all patients indicate they would undergo the procedure again given similar circumstances *(12,15,17)*. For some problems, such as fatigue, sleep, and sexual functioning, documented dissatisfaction is high in the general population and also chemotherapy-treated patients too *(10,18)*. The following subsections briefly highlight the major themes reported in the literature.

3.1. Physical Functioning and Physical Symptoms

The physical domain encompasses strength, stamina, and symptoms. HSCT patients, particularly those suffering from chronic graft-vs-host disease (cGVHD) report lower physical functioning and poorer overall health than the general population *(13,19,20)*. HSCT can be associated with a variety of irreversible physical sequelae, including cataracts, premature menopause, infertility, and avascular necrosis of bone. Treatment-related pulmonary, cardiovascular, and renal complications occur. Many of the medications prescribed after HSCT have bothersome side effects.

Patients report many specific symptoms, particularly involving skin changes, fatigue, weakness, pain, stiff joints, headache, poor appetite, mouth sores, dry eyes and mouth, and frequent colds. Fatigue and lack of stamina may be overwhelming *(21)* (*see* Table 1).

3.2. Psychoemotional

The psychoemotional domain encompasses emotions (e.g., anxiety, depression, and fear) and cognition. Rates of true psychiatric diagnoses are high, including a 20–30% incidence of depression *(22,23)* and a 5% incidence of posttraumatic stress disorder *(24,25)*. Surprisingly, most studies find a similar rate of psychoemotional problems between autologous and allogeneic recipients *(26,27)*, and even better functioning in allogeneic recipients *(28,29)*. Patients continue to worry about relapse and whether they will recover to their pretransplant functioning *(7,19,30)*.

Post-HSCT neurobehavioral outcomes are strongly predicted by baseline cognitive and social functioning *(31)*. Frequent mild cognitive deficits are seen in 20% of patients even before HSCT, and early decline in cognitive function is observed during hospitalization *(32)*. One of the most common patient concerns is loss of memory and ability to concentrate, and, indeed, short-term memory problems do increase with time since HSCT *(31)*. A cross-sectional study of 66 HSCT patients with a mean of 34 mo postprocedure showed that 37% of allogeneic and 17% of autologous patients had abnormal neuropsychological exams with detectable deficits in orientation, memory, and reasoning. Concurrent magnetic resonance imaging (MRI) exams showed abnormalities in most of these patients *(33)*. In children, intelligence quotients are lower 1 yr after HSCT, although no further decline was seen at 3 yr *(34)*.

Table 1
Percentage of Autologous and Allogeneic Recipients Agreeing or Strongly Agreeing With Qualitative Statements About Recovery at 6, 12, and 24 mo Following Transplantation

Variable	*Autologous*			*Allogeneic*		
	6 mo	12 mo	24 mo	6 mo	12 mo	24 mo
No. of patients	93	69	35	112	79	45
Life has returned to normal	53%***	61%	63%	31%***	58%	68%
I feel back to my old self	42%	62%	60%	31%	56%	47%
I have been able to enjoy my normal activities since bone marrow transplantation (BMT)	42%**	62%	60%	21%**	48%	62%
I have been able to enjoy socializing with family and friends since BMT	75%***	87%	83%	52%***	77%	84%
I have been able to put my illness and BMT behind me and get on with life	55%***	68%	66%	33%***	59%	67%
I am satisfied with my physical appearance	76%***	72%	77%*	43%***	58%	56%*
I have recovered from my transplant	55%*	65%	65%	41%*	66%	71%
In general, my health is very good or excellent	37%	46%	46%	33%	39%	36%

Note: Asterisks refer to comparison of autologous and allogeneic patients at identical time-points: *$p<0.05$, **$p<0.01$, ***$p<0.001$.
Source: From ref. *40*, with permission.

3.3. Social

Social functioning is concerned with relationships, roles, and leisure activities. Social relationships are generally preserved or even enhanced posttransplant *(12)*. However, one study reports that a greater time since HSCT is associated with decrease in social support *(29)*. Dissatisfaction with appearance is common. Sexual problems are also very common, with women reporting more sexual difficulties than men. Estrogen and testosterone levels, whether endogenous or the result of replacement, seem to correlate with sexual satisfaction *(11,35–40)*.

3.4. Functional

Approximately 60–90% of HSCT survivors eventually return to work, with higher rates noted in office workers compared to people employed in physically demanding jobs *(20,29,41–47)*. Return to work is significantly associated with better QOL, but both may be attributable to physical and mental health *(42,48)*. Failure to return to work or school is common even in untransplanted patients with hematologic malignancies (26%) and, thus, may not be attributable to HSCT itself *(49,50)*. Concerns over finances *(40)* and obtaining health insurance are common after HSCT *(41)*, as they are for other cancer survivors. Sleep difficulties are also noted *(51)*.

3.5. Spiritual/Existential

The spiritual/existential domain refers to religion, spirituality, hope, and the meaning of life. Many patients experience a greater appreciation for life compared to patients not treated with HSCT *(4,9,10,21,47,52–54)*. A sense of global meaning, defined as the feeling that life has meaning and purpose, may facilitate adaptation *(55)*, as can the ability to find meaning in illness *(56)*. Looking at survival as a second chance for a different, perhaps more meaningful life can accentuate QOL, whereas struggling to regain a lifestyle and outlook similar to before HSCT may lead to dissatisfaction. Indeed, reordering priorities is a common theme for survivors *(29)*, and although gains in the spiritual/existential domain may greatly improve overall QOL, at least one author has suggested that full recovery is not complete until patients are no longer acutely aware and appreciative of being alive *(57)*.

4. PHASES OF TRANSPLANTATION

Hematopoietic SCT is a procedure with substantial risks of treatment-related morbidity and mortality. Beyond the early risks, survivors are faced with increased susceptibility to infections and restrictions on a normal lifestyle for months to years after the procedure. Patients are generally advised to wear protective masks and gloves and avoid crowded public areas until they have physically recovered. They are not allowed to return to work for 6–12 mo following HSCT, so for many patients, their roles as a worker, parent, and caregiver are threatened simultaneously *(42,48)*. In addition, there remains a persistent risk of relapse of the original disease, potential need for rehospitalization, and late complications that can interfere with complete recovery.

It is helpful to conceptualize the HSCT process into three broad phases that have particular implications for QOL *(1,58,59)*. The first phase begins when the decision is made to pursue HSCT and ends with commencement of the procedure. Researchers have focused on the psychoemotional distress associated with this period, including high levels of anxiety and depression as patients await transplantation *(60–64)*. The second phase encompasses the period of hospitalization for HSCT through early recovery. Quality of life during this time is compromised by physical discomfort, fatigue, social isolation, and fears of imminent death. However, most patients view this phase as temporary and not representative of long-term QOL. In fact, Zittoun et al. have reported that overall QOL is most influenced by depression and fatigue and not physical symptoms during this period *(65)*.

Whereas physical concerns and survival predominate early after HSCT, with time concerns shift towards integrating survivorship and moving on *(7,17)*. The third phase entails long-term readaptation and return to some form of normalcy *(10,16)*, although the transplant experience may inexorably alter an individual's perceptions of "normal" *(59)*. Reports on the trajectory of recovery vary. Continued improvement over time has been observed *(29,45,66,67)*, others report a plateau after 1–2 yr *(14,40)* (*see* Table 2). Yet another study suggests that problems vary over time, with physical recovery dominating early after transplantation then ebbing, and issues of reintegration, discrimination, and ability to attain long-range goals becoming increasingly important as time from transplantation increases *(17)*. Patients struggle to regain or redefine their roles as spouses, parents, caregivers, students, or workers within the context of their HSCT experience and any sequelae from the procedure.

5. SUMMARY OF LARGE HSCT SURVIVOR STUDIES

In 1999, it was estimated that there were more than 20,000 patients surviving longer than 5 yr post-HSCT *(68)*. Most studies report very good health and adaptation *(46)*, although up to 31% of survivors report serious functional limitations or poor QOL *(39,69,70)*. This section briefly summarizes six cohorts in which long-term or longitudinal QOL has been evaluated after HSCT.

Andrykowski et al. assembled a large cross-sectional cohort of more than 200 patients from 5 transplant centers. Approximately half had an allogeneic transplant procedure, and average time since HSCT was 3.5 yr. Patients were surveyed by mail using several validated instruments assessing mood, psychological adjustment to illness, self-esteem, positive and negative affect, impact of illness, perceived recovery and current health, sleep, and symptoms. A subset (n=172) was interviewed by phone at the time of enrollment and 137 returned a follow-up survey 18 mo later. The authors concluded that less than half of survivors report normal functional status in most domains. Fatigue and sleep disturbances were common for both autologous and allogeneic patients. Many specific physical symptoms and limitations persist, particularly for allogeneic recipients. Interestingly, discordance between pre-HSCT expectations for returning to normal and current health status was associated with the greatest psychological distress *(16,45,51)*.

Sutherland et al. mailed a self-administered questionnaire to 251 allogeneic recipients and achieved a response rate of 93% (n=231). Patients completed Short Form 36, (SF36) Satisfaction with Life Domains Scale, and a symptom scale at a median of 40 mo post-HSCT. The major finding was that patients within 3 yr from HSCT had significantly worse scores compared to the general population on all SF36 subscales except the mental health scale. In contrast, patients more than 3 yr post-HSCT displayed better functioning on the social, mental health, and vitality subscales, and equivalent functioning on the other SF36 scales compared to the general population. However, Kiss et al. reported 28 subjects from this same population who had survived at least 10 yr following allogeneic transplantation for chronic myelogenous leukemia (CML). In these very late survivors, they found poorer physical functioning, role

Table 2

Bothersome Symptoms Reported by Autologous and Allogeneic Recipients Reported at 6, 12, and 24 mo Following Transplantation; Patients Reported Being Bothered a Lot or Extremely Bothered

Variable	*Autologous*			*Allogeneic*		
	6 mo	12 mo	24 mo	6 mo	12 mo	24 mo
No. of patients	93	69	35	112	79	45
Fatigue	42%	30%	35%	44%	35%	33%
Anxiety	15%	7%	11%	13%	10%	18%
Depression	9%	9%	11%	8%	4%	16%
Pain	11%	7%	14%	12%	5%	11%
Difficulty concentrating	14%	13%	17%	9%	14%	13%
Feeling isolated	8%*	3%	3%	20%*	5%	11%
Mouth sores	2%	1%**	0%	2%	15%**	9%
Painful joints	17%	12%	11%	12%	14%	20%
Skin changes	9%	4%***	11%	18%	24%***	16%
Memory loss	13%	9%	17%	9%	13%	16%
Finances	23%	17%	11%	25%	27%	22%
Sexual difficulties	24%	29%	37%	21%	29%	36%

Note: Asterisks refer to comparison of autologous and allogeneic patients at identical time points: * $p<0.05$, ** $p<0.01$, *** $p<0.001$.
Source: From ref. *40*, with permission.

physical functioning, and general health than an age-adjusted normative US population. Several late medical complications adversely affected QOL including cGVHD, relapse, osteoporosis, and need for medications *(12,13)*.

Bush et al. measured QOL in autologous and allogeneic survivors within 4 yr of transplantation (*n*=415) or greater than 6 yr post-HSCT (*n*=125) via self-administered surveys with the QLQC30, a symptom scale, demands of bone marrow transplantation (BMT) recovery, Profile of Mood States, health perceptions survey, and a open-ended module. They found that overall QOL was good for most survivors and improved over the first 4 yr posttransplant, but many patients had residual deficits. Approximately 5% of very long-term survivors rated their health as poor *(11,29)*.

The Hopkins group reported a cohort of 135 patients (86% response rate, 71% allogeneic recipients) who were at least 6 mo posttransplant. Participants completed a battery of instruments measuring functional status (SF36), occupational information, self-esteem, coping, optimism, social ties, satisfaction, mood, and positive and negative affect. Approximately 70% reported good to excellent health, felt that social and physical functioning was normal or only slightly limited, and had returned to work. Many positive changes were seen in relationships and existential/psychological domains, and 75–90% of patients were to able to maintain their family, friend, and homemaker roles. However, 23% reported job discrimination, 39% had insurance problems, and 22% were dissatisfied with their sexual functioning *(9,35,41,48,52)*.

Broers et al. reported a prospective, longitudinal study of 125 patients (approx 50% allogeneic). Subjects completed surveys measuring QOL, functional limitations, psychological distress, anxiety and depression, self-esteem, and health locus of control prior to HSCT and 1 mo, 6 mo, 1 yr, and 3 yr afterward. Follow-up of survivors was 63–80% at each time-point. The authors report that 25% of patients still had severe functional limitations at 3 yr, although 90% reported overall good to excellent health *(70)*.

Lee et al. studied 320 patients (70% response rate, 63% allogeneic) by self-administered survey prior to transplantation, and at 6, 12, and 24 mo post-HSCT. Instruments included the SF36, two utility measurements, a symptom scale, and qualitative questions. Results showed that although autologous patients had fewer physical symptoms and better perceptions of recovery at 6 mo, by 12 mo autologous and allogeneic patients were indistinguishable and little further gains were made by 2 yr *(40)*.

6. PREDICTORS OF BETTER QOL POSTTRANSPLANTATION

Better post-HSCT adaptation and QOL are predicted by younger age, male sex, higher educational level, better QOL and social support at the time of HSCT, longer time since HSCT, and absence of late complications, including cGVHD *(11,20,30,39,45,66,71–73)*. Surprisingly, the type of HSCT procedure does not seem to be influential, as autologous and allogeneic recipients have remarkably similar QOL given the differences in the their risks of treatment-related mortality and late complications *(40,49,54,66,74)* (*see* Fig. 2). In autologous HSCT, use of peripheral blood stem cells (PBSCs) is associated with fewer physical symptoms within the first 3 mo than marrow, although overall QOL was similar in a randomized study of 91 patients (62 received peripheral blood, 29 received marrow) *(75)*. In allogeneic HSCT (alloHSCT), only one study has compared QOL associated with methods of acute GVHD prevention. No differences were seen in an observational study of 146 recipients of unrelated donor marrow whether T-cell depletion or a methotrexate-based regimen was used as prophy-

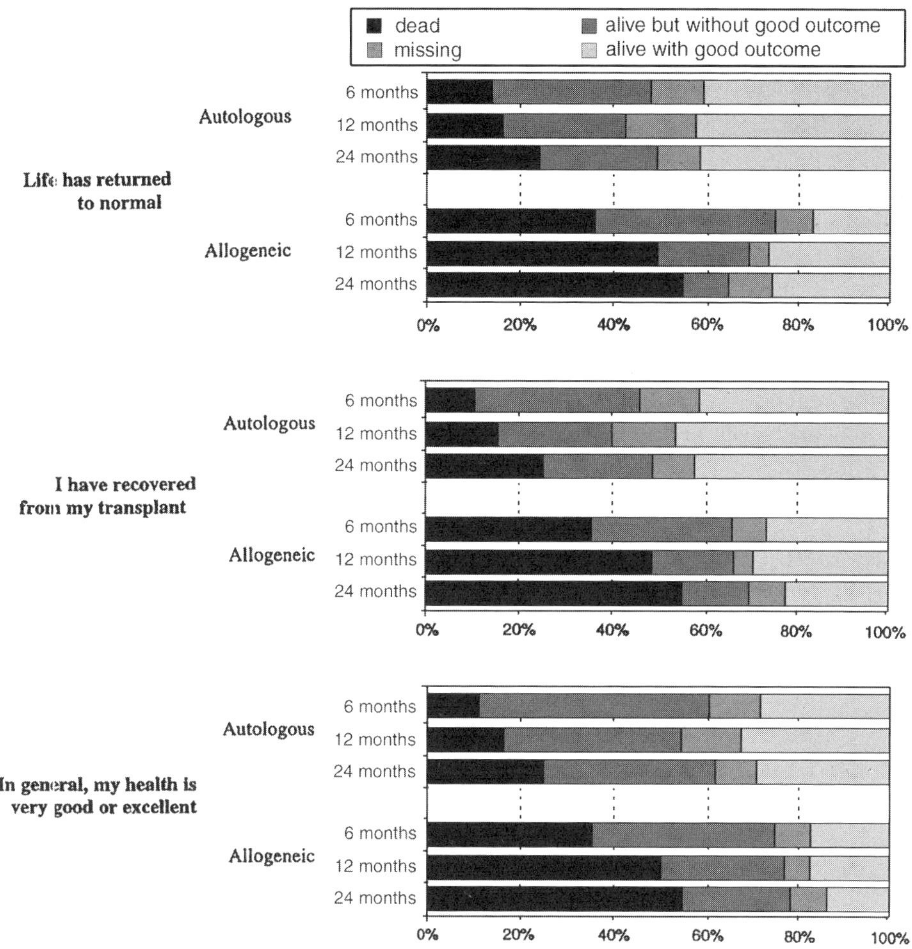

Fig. 2. Absolute proportions of patients at 6, 12, and 24 mo somewhat or strongly agreeing with the listed statements of indicating very good or excellent health. (From ref. *40*, reprinted, with permission.)

laxis *(76)*. Thus, with the exception of graft source for autologous patients, very few modifiable factors have been associated with post-HSCT QOL.

In solid-organ transplantation where donors are a limited resource, the concept that psychosocial profiles predict survival and success of the procedure is widely accepted and is part of the patient-selection process. In HSCT, studies of QOL and survival have focused more on depression and coping styles with contradictory results *(77–81)*. Several psychological assessment scales to identify HSCT patients at high risk for poor QOL and shortened survival posttransplant have been proposed, but they have either not been shown to predict outcome or are not widely applied *(82–86)*.

7. QOL FOLLOWING TRANSPLANTATION COMPARED TO OTHER MEDICAL PROCEDURES

Although HSCT patients appear to have poorer QOL relative to normal, healthy people, they appear remarkably similar to other patient populations. Comparison to patients with hematologic malignancies treated with chemotherapy alone *(8,18,19,87,88)* or recipients of solid-organ transplants *(23,71)* suggest more similarities than differences. When differences exist, there are usually greater physical problems in HSCT patients but better psychoemotional functioning than comparison groups *(49,75)*. However, most of these comparative studies included fewer than 100 patients total, and differences may have been missed. Molassiotis et al. used a cross-sectional design to study 91 long-term HSCT survivors and 73 matched controls treated with chemotherapy alone. Measures included psychosocial adjustment to illness, anxiety and depression, symptoms, social support and psychosexual functioning. They concluded that transplant patients were doing as well or better than chemotherapy patients *(49)*. Zittoun et al. reported a cross-sectional comparison of 98 patients participating in a multicenter study comparing alloHSCT (assigned to this arm if an human leukocyte antigen [HLA]-matched sibling was available, *n*=35), autoHSCT (*n*=29), or intensive chemotherapy (*n*=34) (randomized between these latter two options). Patients were surveyed a median of 4 yr after attaining complete remission using a multidimensional QOL instrument, a HSCT-specific symptom scale, and a measure of perceived changes in several domains. The authors concluded that alloHSCT survivors had poorer overall QOL and more physical problems than the other groups, but were similar in cognitive, emotional, and social outcomes *(18)*. Hjermstad et al. longitudinally assessed 177 (41 allogeneic recipients, 51 autologous patients, 85 chemotherapy recipients) with the EORTC QLQ C30, an anxiety and depression scale, and a symptom scale. They found that at 1 yr, all groups had lower physical, role, and social scores than a population sample. However, in the two transplanted groups, the rates of anxiety and depression and QOL was similar *(19,74,89)*.

8. CLINICAL USES FOR QOL DATA

8.1. Patient Counseling

Despite acknowledgment that QOL considerations may be paramount for some patients, studies suggest that for most patients, potential length of life is more important in choosing among treatment options *(90–93)*. This is supported by observations that many patients seem to have already made up their minds to pursue HSCT even before they are aware of what the procedure entails *(10,58,94,95)*. For many HSCT candidates, it may seem that there is "no choice," as transplantation offers the only realistic hope of cure *(96)*. Indeed, many physicians have observed that patients wish to avoid discussion of the specific risks and QOL issues surrounding HSCT once they have made the decision to proceed *(10,61,97)*.

However, even if QOL considerations do not influence treatment choice, knowledge of probable QOL outcomes may help patients and their families prepare for challenges they will face during and after the procedure *(40)*. Some authors hypothesize that realistic expectations facilitate better recovery, and overly optimistic expectations impede adaptation. However, given the wide range of possible outcomes and inability to predict individual problems accurately, it is difficult to know what expectations patients ought to have. Also, even on a population basis, concrete estimates of symptom prevalence after transplantation and reasonable expectations for recovery are rarely presented in the literature.

8.2. Designing Interventions to Improve QOL

Although observational data are useful descriptively and to help identify vulnerable patients at risk for poor QOL post-HSCT, for most researchers the ultimate goal is to improve the QOL of present or future patients. However, most interventions either have not been tested in clinical trials or have failed to show significant improvements over standard practice.

As noted earlier, one proposed approach to improving post-HSCT QOL is to align expectations with experiences. In theory, fostering realistic expectations may help adjustment following HSCT and actually improve perceptions of QOL *(16,22,61)*. However, operationalizing and scientifically testing this concept is difficult.

Another psychological strategy to improve QOL is to help patients retain as much personal control as possible during HSCT *(26)*. However, a fact sheet designed to empower patients by providing a list of common concerns and suggestions for where to obtain information actually increased feelings of helplessness and hopelessness, although patients were less anxious, better prepared, and reported fewer problems *(98)*.

A third approach advocates a systems approach to psychosocial complications and QOL issues. In theory, this would help establish a therapeutic relationship before it is needed, normalize the experience of distress to make it more acceptable, integrate psychosocial providers into the treating team, and allow routine screening for distress *(7,59,89)*. However, a randomized trial of psychosocial screening and disclosure to treating physicians failed to demonstrate a benefit of intervention during acute hospitalization (n=178) *(65)*.

A final approach to improving QOL is to institute procedures to counteract specific problems. For example, Dimeo and colleagues showed that aerobic exercise programs improve fatigue, physical performance, and psychological distress in HSCT patients. A larger randomized trial of aerobic exercise after autologous and allogeneic transplantation is being conducted in Germany *(99–101)*. A randomized controlled trial of a comprehensive coping program involving preparatory information, cognitive restructuring, and relaxation with guided imagery administered to patients undergoing autologous transplantation for breast cancer (n=110) demonstrated less nausea and anxiety in the intervention group within 7 d posttransplantation, but it did not affect pain or psychological distress *(102)*. Syrjala et al. performed a randomized controlled trial (n=94) with four different groups: standard care, therapist support, relaxation and imagery, and a package of cognitive-behavioral techniques that included relaxation and imagery. The two groups that were taught relaxation and imagery had significantly less pain. However, the addition of cognitive-behavioral techniques to one group did not improve pain control, and no intervention improved nausea *(103)*. Thus, although aerobic exercise and relaxation imagery have shown benefits in small studies, they have not been embraced by the HSCT community as part of routine care.

9. QOL ISSUES FOR SPECIAL POPULATIONS

9.1. Pediatrics

Studies of pediatric QOL in HSCT have been limited, but the bulk of evidence suggests better recovery in children than adults. Badell et al. interviewed 98 disease-free survivors more than 3 yr after pediatric HSCT (74% allogeneic recipients) and compared results with 58 healthy control subjects. Transplant survivors reported higher global QOL than the controls. They reported better sleep, family and friend relationships, and leisure possibilities, but they perceived more problems with physical appearance, school, and work possibilities than their peers. The authors concluded that pediatric survivors seem to value both their lives and their free time more highly *(54)*. Schmidt et al. interviewed 212 survivors (90% participation rate) at least 1 yr following allogeneic transplantation using the City of Hope/Stanford survivor index. Fifty subjects were pediatric survivors. Adults suffered from more cGVHD, frequent colds, and skin changes than pediatric survivors. Thirty-six percent of adults and 50% of children rated their overall QOL as a 10 out of a possible 10. The authors concluded that younger patients recover more fully from HSCT than adults *(43)*. Matthes-Martin et al. assessed 73 pediatric allogeneic survivors at least 1 yr posttransplantation. They reported that 75% of patients (or surrogates for patients less than 12 yr old) had excellent QOL and few had detectable organ impairments, although 27% had cGVHD *(104)*.

9.2. Family Members

There is little doubt that HSCT is a process that families go through together, and that QOL for all is probably impacted by the demands of the procedure. Dermatis and Lesko studied 61 parents prior to transplantation of their children and found very high levels of psychological distress, with mothers displaying more difficulties than fathers *(105)*.

Surprisingly, little is reported about the impact of HSCT on adult patients' families. Qualitative studies hint at the family distress instigated by HSCT *(5,7)*. Keogh et al. studied 28 patients and 25 relatives (not the donor) prior to transplant, and at 3, 6, and 12 mo after HSCT. The study design specified that if a patient died, the relative was no longer contacted. The authors concluded that relatives were quite stressed prior to transplant and at 3 mo, but most were no longer distressed by 12 mo. However, qualitative statements suggested that the support of others (not the patient) "kept them going" (68%) and that most expected the patient's life to resume and get back to normal by 3–6 mo. When this did not occur, they were surprised by the "reluctance" of patients to do so and by the patient's unhappiness and irritability. Forty-five percent reported tension and conflict around this issue and 64% expressed feelings of resentment and frustration at the continued dependence of the patient *(106)*. Preliminary reports from a large, cross-sectional, multicenter study of HSCT survivors, significant others, and controls suggest that spouses suffer considerably from social isolation (Wingard, personal communication, 2002).

Although many patients have dependent children, little is written in the HSCT literature about effects on children and ways to minimize adverse impacts on their development and parent–child relationships. Similarly, given that HSCT is a semielective procedure associated with extremely high mortality rates, little is written about approaches to manage family stress or family bereavement issues.

9.3. Donors

For every patient undergoing allogeneic transplantation, there is a donor somewhere whose QOL may be affected by the procedure. Although the absolute risk of severe or life-threatening complications is quite low *(107)*, marrow donors undergo painful procedures to provide stem cells. Although almost all recover and return to normal function, this may take a prolonged period of time and may not be complete for some patients. Studies suggest that unrelated donors, who provide anonymous stem cells for purely altruistic reasons, report less discomfort than related donors *(108)*. Certain techniques, such as use of long-acting local anesthetics after marrow donation, may decrease the pain further *(109)*. Even when marrow aspiration is avoided, as with peripheral cell donation, donors receive injections of growth factors and undergo leukapheresis to remove stem cells. Growth factor use in normal donors is commonly associated with a need for narcotic pain relief, particularly for severe back pain. There are rare reports of major complications (splenic rupture).

Two studies of the first 493 unrelated donors who participated in the National Marrow Donor Program suggest that the risk of acute complications is low (6%) and that most donors experience positive psychological benefits from marrow donation. At 1 yr, 87% felt donation was "very worthwhile" and 91% would donate again in the future. However, some donors did experience stress and inconvenience as a result of the donation, and longer collection times predicted poorer outcomes. At 1 wk postharvest, more than half still reported fatigue, pain at marrow collection sites, and low back pain. Mean recovery time was 15.8 d, but 10% took longer than 30 d to recover fully *(110,111)*. Qualitative interviews with 52 unrelated donors participating in the early years of the National Marrow Donor Program suggest that donors have high self-esteem and believe that marrow donation is consistent with their values and personal concepts. Interestingly, scores on the self-esteem scale 1 yr after donation correlated with whether the patient was still alive *(112)*. Another study of 565 unrelated Japanese marrow donors showed that physical functioning, role functioning, and pain were significantly affected 1 wk after harvest, but functioning returned to baseline after 3 mo. Prior to harvest, donors scored above the national average in all areas of functioning *(113)*.

10. RESEARCH ISSUES

10.1. Topics

Quality-of-life research seems poised to move to the next level and evolve from observation to intervention and influence. This will depend on the field's ability to (1) translate the observations of the past 20 yr into successful interventions that maintain or improve QOL for future patients *(59)*, (2) incorporate QOL end points alongside clinical trials to help present a balanced picture of outcomes *(10)*, and (3) translate findings of QOL studies into meaningful data accessible and influential to clinicians, patients, and policy-makers *(114)*. Several ongoing large, multicenter studies typify these goals, including (1) a randomized trial of T-cell depletion vs immunosuppressive medications for acute GVHD prophylaxis in which QOL is a secondary end point (sponsored by the National Heart, Lung and Blood Institute) and (2) a study organized through the International Bone Marrow Transplant Registry and the University of Florida concurrently studying long-term survivors, spouses, and controls.

10.2. Study Design Challenges

Because by definition QOL is individual, patients are the only reliable source of data. In addition, QOL data must be collected in real time, as patients do not accurately recall their past QOL *(115)* and data cannot be collected retrospectively from chart review. Missing data particularly pose analytic problems if data are missing informatively (because death, poor health, or even good health cause missing assessments). Counterbalancing these potential problems is the fact that QOL studies in HSCT survivors routinely enjoy very high response rates (70–90%) *(96)*. Methods to address the missing-data problem include rigorous attempts to collect complete data from surviving patients, depiction of results as absolute proportions (that take into account patients who die or fail to provide QOL data) *(40)*, and statistical models that combine QOL and survival data *(116,117)* (Fig. 2).

Readers evaluating the quality of QOL studies should consider how QOL was measured, how representative the study population is of the universe of patients, and whether appropriate analytic methods were used. When available, a pretransplant baseline and appropriate repeated measures techniques should be used because means can be deceptive, as some subjects improve while others worsen *(118)*. Comparison or control groups should be included whenever possible to acknowledge the variation in QOL and help place the results in context. Specific broad domains as well as symptoms should be measured because HSCT patients tend to report very high global QOL while suffering from multiple problems. Finally, readers should consider whether the reported outcomes are clinically meaningful and whether the authors have helped readers translate results into communicable concepts to patients.

11. FUTURE DIRECTIONS

Although most patients and health care providers acknowledge the importance of QOL, several factors in HSCT have conspired to limit the extent to which this concern is translated into practice and decision-making. First, QOL after HSCT is variable, to a large extent unpredictable, and, thus far, unmodifiable. It is difficult to factor QOL into treatment decisions when outcome varies so much. Second, most patients have diseases for which there is no other reasonable chance of cure. Thus, QOL concerns may be relegated to a more informational role. Third, most reports do not translate results of QOL studies back into language and concepts that are accessible to patients and practicing physicians. Finally, several authors have suggested that the field needs to move beyond small cross-sectional studies. Larger, longitudinal studies evaluating potential interventions to improve QOL or that seek QOL differences between modifiable transplant practices should be the new standard. Only by moving to the next level of research studies will we be able to actually improve QOL and return the investment of so many patients who faithfully fill out our surveys.

REFERENCES

1. Grant M. Assessment of quality of life following hematopoietic cell transplantation. In: Thomas ED, Blume KG, Forman SJ, eds. *Hematopoetic Cell Transplantation*. Malden, UK: Blackwell Sciences, 1999:407–413.
2. Slevin ML, Plant H, Lynch D, et al. Who should measure quality of life, the doctor or the patient? *Br J Cancer* 1988;57:109–112.
3. King CR, Ferrell BR, Grant M, et al. Nurses' perceptions of the meaning of quality of life for bone marrow transplant survivors. *Cancer Nurs* 1995;18:118–129.
4. Ferrell B, Grant M, Schmidt GM, et al. The meaning of quality of life for bone marrow transplant survivors. Part 1. The impact of bone marrow transplant on quality of life. *Cancer Nurs* 1992;15:153–160.
5. Ferrell B, Grant M, Schmidt GM, et al. The meaning of quality of life for bone marrow transplant survivors. Part 2. Improving quality of life for bone marrow transplant survivors. *Cancer Nurs* 1992;15:247–253.
6. Haberman M, Bush N, Young K, et al. Quality of life of adult long-term survivors of bone marrow transplantation: a qualitative analysis of narrative data. *Oncol Nurs Forum* 1993;20:1545–1553.
7. Baker F, Zabora J, Polland A, et al. Reintegration after bone marrow transplantation. *Cancer Pract* 1999;7:190–197.
8. Altmaier EM, Gingrich RD, Fyfe MA. Two-year adjustment of bone marrow transplant survivors. *Bone Marrow Transplant* 1991;7:311–316.
9. Baker F, Wingard JR, Curbow B, et al. Quality of life of bone marrow transplant long-term survivors. *Bone Marrow Transplant* 1994;13:589–596.
10. Andrykowski MA. Psychosocial factors in bone marrow transplantation: a review and recommendations for research. *Bone Marrow Transplant* 1994;13:357–375.
11. Bush NE, Haberman M, Donaldson G, et al. Quality of life of 125 adults surviving 6-18 years after bone marrow transplantation. *Soc Sci Med* 1995;40:479–490.
12. Sutherland HJ, Fyles GM, Adams G, et al. Quality of life following bone marrow transplantation: a comparison of patient reports with population norms. *Bone Marrow Transplant* 1997;19:1129–1136.
13. Kiss TL, Abdolell M, Jamal N, et al. Long-term medical outcomes and quality-of-life assessment of patients with chronic myeloid leukemia followed at least 10 years after allogeneic bone marrow transplantation. *J Clin Oncol* 2002;20:2334–2343.

14. Syrjala KL, Chapko MK, Vitaliano PP, et al. Recovery after allogeneic marrow transplantation: prospective study of predictors of long-term physical and psychosocial functioning. *Bone Marrow Transplant* 1993;11:319–327.
15. Belec RH. Quality of life: perceptions of long-term survivors of bone marrow transplantation. *Oncol Nurs Forum* 1992;19:31–37.
16. Andrykowski MA, Brady MJ, Greiner CB, et al. "Returning to normal" following bone marrow transplantation: outcomes, expectations and informed consent. *Bone Marrow Transplant* 1995;15:573–581.
17. McQuellon RP, Russell GB, Rambo TD, et al. Quality of life and psychological distress of bone marrow transplant recipients: the "time trajectory" to recovery over the first year. *Bone Marrow Transplant* 1998;21:477–486.
18. Zittoun R, Suciu S, Watson M, et al. Quality of life in patients with acute myelogenous leukemia in prolonged first complete remission after bone marrow transplantation (allogeneic or autologous) or chemotherapy: a cross-sectional study of the EORTC-GIMEMA AML 8A trial. *Bone Marrow Transplant* 1997;20:307–315.
19. Hjermstad M, Holte H, Evensen S, et al. Do patients who are treated with stem cell transplantation have a health-related quality of life comparable to the general population after 1 year? *Bone Marrow Transplant* 1999;24:911–918.
20. Heinonen H, Volin L, Uutela A, et al. Quality of life and factors related to perceived satisfaction with quality of life after allogeneic bone marrow transplantation. *Ann Hematol* 2001;80:137–143.
21. Neitzert CS, Ritvo P, Dancey J, et al. The psychosocial impact of bone marrow transplantation: a review of the literature. *Bone Marrow Transplant* 1998;22:409–422.
22. McQuellon RP, Andrykowski MA. Psychosocial complications of hematopoietic stem cell transplantation. In: Atkinson K, ed. *Clinical Bone Marrow and Blood Stem Cell Transplantation*. Cambridge: Cambridge University Press, 2000:1045–1054.
23. Schimmer AD, Elliott MF, Abbey SE, et al. Illness intrusiveness among survivors of autologous blood and marrow transplantation. *Cancer* 2001;92:3147–3154.
24. Smith MY, Redd W, DuHamel K, Vickberg SJ, Ricketts P. Validation of the PTSD Checklist-Civilian Version in survivors of bone marrow transplantation. *J Trauma Stress* 1999;12:485–499.
25. Widows MR, Jacobsen PB, Fields KK. Relation of psychological vulnerability factors to posttraumatic stress disorder symptomatology in bone marrow transplant recipients. *Psychosom Med* 2000;62:873–882.
26. Fife BL, Huster GA, Cornetta KG, et al. Longitudinal study of adaptation to the stress of bone marrow transplantation. *J Clin Oncol* 2000;18:1539–1549.
27. Prieto JM, Blanch J, Atala J, et al. Psychiatric morbidity and impact on hospital length of stay among hematologic cancer patients receiving stem-cell transplantation. *J Clin Oncol* 2002;20:1907–1917.
28. Molassiotis A, Boughton BJ, Burgoyne T, et al. Comparison of the overall quality of life in 50 long-term survivors of autologous and allogeneic bone marrow transplantation. *J Adv Nurs* 1995;22:509–516.
29. Bush NE, Donaldson GW, Haberman MH, et al. Conditional and unconditional estimation of multidimensional quality of life after hematopoietic stem cell transplantation: a longitudinal follow-up of 415 patients. *Biol Blood Marrow Transplant* 2000;6:576–591.
30. Andrykowski MA, Cordova MJ, Hann DM, et al. Patients' psychosocial concerns following stem cell transplantation. *Bone Marrow Transplant* 1999;24:1121–1129.
31. Meyers CA, Weitzner M, Byrne K, et al. Evaluation of the neurobehavioral functioning of patients before, during, and after bone marrow transplantation. *J Clin Oncol* 1994;12:820–826.
32. Ahles TA, Tope DM, Furstenberg C, et al. Psychologic and neuropsychologic impact of autologous bone marrow transplantation. *J Clin Oncol* 1996;14:1457–1462.
33. Padovan CS, Yousry TA, Schleuning M, et al. Neurological and neuroradiological findings in long-term survivors of allogeneic bone marrow transplantation. *Ann Neurol* 1998;43:627–633.
34. Kramer JH, Crittenden MR, DeSantes K, et al. Cognitive and adaptive behavior 1 and 3 years following bone marrow transplantation. *Bone Marrow Transplant* 1997;19:607–613.
35. Wingard JR, Curbow B, Baker F, et al. Sexual satisfaction in survivors of bone marrow transplantation. *Bone Marrow Transplant* 1992;9:185–190.
36. Molassiotis A, van den Akker OB, Milligan DW, et al. Gonadal function and psychosexual adjustment in male long-term survivors of bone marrow transplantation. *Bone Marrow Transplant* 1995;16:253–259.
37. Syrjala KL, Roth-Roemer SL, Abrams JR, et al. Prevalence and predictors of sexual dysfunction in long-term survivors of marrow transplantation. *J Clin Oncol* 1998;16:3148–157.

38. Marks DI, Gale DJ, Vedhara K, et al. A quality of life study in 20 adult long-term survivors of unrelated donor bone marrow transplantation. *Bone Marrow Transplant* 1999;24:191–195.
39. Chiodi S, Spinelli S, Ravera G, et al. Quality of life in 244 recipients of allogeneic bone marrow transplantation. *Br J Haematol* 2000;110:614–619.
40. Lee SJ, Fairclough D, Parsons SK, et al. Recovery after stem-cell transplantation for hematologic diseases. *J Clin Oncol* 2001;19:242–252.
41. Wingard JR, Curbow B, Baker F, et al. Health, functional status, and employment of adult survivors of bone marrow transplantation. *Ann Intern Med* 1991;114:113–118.
42. Chao NJ, Tierney DK, Bloom JR, et al. Dynamic assessment of quality of life after autologous bone marrow transplantation. *Blood* 1992;80:825–830.
43. Schmidt GM, Niland JC, Forman SJ, et al. Extended follow-up in 212 long-term allogeneic bone marrow transplant survivors. Issues of quality of life. *Transplantation* 1993;55:551–557.
44. Hjermstad MJ, Kaasa S. Quality of life in adult cancer patients treated with bone marrow transplantation—a review of the literature. *Eur J Cancer* 1995;2:163–173.
45. Andrykowski MA, Greiner CB, Altmaier EM, et al. Quality of life following bone marrow transplantation: findings from a multicentre study. *Br J Cancer* 1995;71:1322–1329.
46. Duell T, van Lint MT, Ljungman P, et al. Health and functional status of long-term survivors of bone marrow transplantation. EBMT Working Party on Late Effects and EULEP Study Group on Late Effects. European Group for Blood and Marrow Transplantation. *Ann Intern Med* 1997;126:184–192.
47. Molassiotis A, Morris PJ. The meaning of quality of life and the effects of unrelated donor bone marrow transplants for chronic myeloid leukemia in adult long-term survivors. *Cancer Nurs* 1998;21:205–211.
48. Baker F, Curbow B, Wingard JR. Role retention and quality of life of bone marrow transplant survivors. *Soc Sci Med* 1991;32:697–704.
49. Molassiotis A, van den Akker OB, Milligan DW, et al. Quality of life in long-term survivors of marrow transplantation: comparison with a matched group receiving maintenance chemotherapy. *Bone Marrow Transplant* 1996;17:249–258.
50. de Lima M, Strom SS, Keating M, et al. Implications of potential cure in acute myelogenous leukemia: development of subsequent cancer and return to work. *Blood* 1997;90:4719–4724.
51. Andrykowski MA, Carpenter JS, Greiner CB, et al. Energy level and sleep quality following bone marrow transplantation. *Bone Marrow Transplant* 1997;20:669–679.
52. Curbow B, Somerfield MR, Baker F, et al. Personal changes, dispositional optimism, and psychological adjustment to bone marrow transplantation. *J Behav Med* 1993;16:423–443.
53. Fromm K, Andrykowski MA, Hunt J. Positive and negative psychosocial sequelae of bone marrow transplantation: implications for quality of life assessment. *J Behav Med* 1996;19:221–240.
54. Badell I, Igual L, Gomez P, et al. Quality of life in young adults having received a BMT during childhood: a GETMON study. Grupo Espanol de Trasplante de Medula Osea en el Nino. *Bone Marrow Transplant* 1998;21(suppl 2):S68–S71.
55. Johnson Vickberg SM, Duhamel KN, Smith MY, et al. Global meaning and psychological adjustment among survivors of bone marrow transplant. *Psychooncology* 2001;10:29–39.
56. Ferrell BR, Hassey Dow K. Quality of life among long-term cancer survivors. *Oncology (Huntingt)* 1997;11:565–568, 571; discussion 572, 575–576.
57. Van Eys J. Living beyond cure. Transcending survival. *Am J Ped Hematol/Oncol* 1987;9:114–118.
58. Brown HN, Kelly MJ. Stages of bone marrow transplantation: a psychiatric perspective. *Psychosom Med* 1976;38:439–446.
59. Andrykowski MA, Mcquellon RP. Psychological issues in hematpoietic cell transplantation. In: Thomas ED, Blume KG, Forman SJ, eds. *Hematopoetic Cell Transplantation*. Malden, UK: Blackwell Sciences, 1999.
60. Dermatis H, Lesko LM. Psychosocial correlates of physician–patient communication at time of informed consent for bone marrow transplantation. *Cancer Invest* 1991;9:621–628.
61. Baker F. Psychosocial sequelae of bone marrow transplantation. *Oncology (Huntingt)* 1994;8:87–92, 97; discussion, 97–101.
62. Leigh S, Wilson KC, Burns R, Clark RE. Psychosocial morbidity in bone marrow transplant recipients: a prospective study. *Bone Marrow Transplant* 1995;16:635–640.
63. Grassi L, Rosti G, Albertazzi L, et al. Psychological stress symptoms before and after autologous bone marrow transplantation in patients with solid tumors. *Bone Marrow Transplant* 1996;17:843–847.

64. Baker F, Marcellus D, Zabora J, et al. Psychological distress among adult patients being evaluated for bone marrow transplantation. *Psychosomatics* 1997;38:10–19.
65. Zittoun R, Achard S, Ruszniewski M. Assessment of quality of life during intensive chemotherapy or bone marrow transplantation. *Psychooncology* 1999;8:64–73.
66. Prieto JM, Saez R, Carreras E, et al. Physical and psychosocial functioning of 117 survivors of bone marrow transplantation. *Bone Marrow Transplant* 1996;17:1133–1142.
67. Kopp M, Schweigkofler H, Holzner B, et al. Time after bone marrow transplantation as an important variable for quality of life: results of a cross-sectional investigation using two different instruments for quality-of-life assessment. *Ann Hematol* 1998;77:27–32.
68. Horowitz MM. Uses and growth of hematopoietic cell transplantation. In: Thomas ED, Blume KG, Forman SJ, eds. *Hematopoetic Cell Transplantation*. Malden, UK: Blackwell Sciences, 1999.
69. Wolcott DL, Wellisch DK, Fawzy FI, et al. Adaptation of adult bone marrow transplant recipient long-term survivors. *Transplantation* 1986;41:478–484.
70. Broers S, Kaptein AA, Le Cessie S, et al. Psychological functioning and quality of life following bone marrow transplantation: a 3-year follow-up study. *J Psychosom Res* 2000;48:11–21.
71. Andrykowski MA, Altmaier EM, Barnett RL, et al. The quality of life in adult survivors of allogeneic bone marrow transplantation. Correlates and comparison with matched renal transplant recipients. *Transplantation* 1990;50:399–406.
72. Molassiotis A, van den Akker OB, Boughton BJ. Perceived social support, family environment and psychosocial recovery in bone marrow transplant long-term survivors. *Soc Sci Med* 1997;44:317–325.
73. Heinonen H, Volin L, Uutela A, et al. Gender-associated differences in the quality of life after allogeneic BMT. *Bone Marrow Transplant* 2001;28:503–509.
74. Hjermstad MJ, Evensen SA, Kvaloy SO, et al. Health-related quality of life 1 year after allogeneic or autologous stem-cell transplantation: a prospective study. *J Clin Oncol* 1999;17:706–718.
75. van Agthoven M, Vellenga E, Fibbe WE, et al. Cost analysis and quality of life assessment comparing patients undergoing autologous peripheral blood stem cell transplantation or autologous bone marrow transplantation for refractory or relapsed non- Hodgkin's lymphoma or Hodgkin's disease. a prospective randomised trial. *Eur J Cancer* 2001;37:1781–1789.
76. Lee SJ, Zahrieh D, Alyea EA, et al. Comparison of T-cell depled and non-T-cell depled unrelated donor transplantation for hematologic diseases: clinical outcomes, quality of life and costs. *Blood* 2002;100:2967–2702.
77. Colon EA, Callies AL, Popkin MK, et al. Depressed mood and other variables related to bone marrow transplantation survival in acute leukemia. *Psychosomatics* 1991;32:420–425.
78. Andrykowski MA, Brady MJ, Henslee-Downey PJ. Psychosocial factors predictive of survival after allogeneic bone marrow transplantation for leukemia. *Psychosom Med* 1994;56:432–439.
79. Murphy DJ, Burrows D, Santilli S, et al. The influence of the probability of survival on patients' preferences regarding cardiopulmonary resuscitation [see comments]. *N Engl J Med* 1994;330:545–549.
80. Jenkins PL, Lester H, Alexander J, Whittaker J. A prospective study of psychosocial morbidity in adult bone marrow transplant recipients. *Psychosomatics* 1994;35:361–367.
81. Loberiza FR Jr, Rizzo JD, Bredeson CN, et al. Association of depressive syndrome and early deaths among patients after stem-cell transplantation for malignant diseases. *J Clin Oncol* 2002;20:2118–2126.
82. Futterman AD, Wellisch DK, Bond G, et al. The Psychosocial Levels System. A new rating scale to identify and assess emotional difficulties during bone marrow transplantation. *Psychosomatics* 1991;32:177–186.
83. Twillman RK, Manetto C, Wellisch DK, et al. The Transplant Evaluation Rating Scale. A revision of the psychosocial levels system for evaluating organ transplant candidates. *Psychosomatics* 1993;34:144–153.
84. Presberg BA, Levenson JL, Olbrisch ME, Best AM. Rating scales for the psychosocial evaluation of organ transplant candidates. Comparison of the PACT and TERS with bone marrow transplant patients. *Psychosomatics* 1995;36:458–461.
85. Molassiotis A. Further evaluation of a scale to screen for risk of emotional difficulties in bone marrow transplant recipients. *J Adv Nurs* 1999;29:922–927.
86. Sullivan AK, Szkrumelak N, Hoffman LH. Psychological risk factors and early complications after bone marrow transplantation in adults. *Bone Marrow Transplant* 1999;24:1109–1120.

87. Litwins NM, Rodrigue JR, Weiner RS. Quality of life in adult recipients of bone marrow transplantation. *Psychol Rep* 1994;75:323–328.
88. Wellisch DK, Centeno J, Guzman J, et al. Bone marrow transplantation vs. high-dose cytorabine-based consolidation chemotherapy for acute myelogenous leukemia. A long-term follow-up study of quality-of-life measures of survivors. *Psychosomatics* 1996;37:144–154.
89. Hjermstad MJ, Loge JH, Evensen SA, et al. The course of anxiety and depression during the first year after allogeneic or autologous stem cell transplantation. *Bone Marrow Transplant* 1999;24:1219–1228.
90. Slevin ML, Stubbs L, Plant HJ, et al. Attitudes to chemotherapy: comparing views of patients with cancer with those of doctors, nurses, and general public [see comments]. *Br Med J* 1990;300:1458–1460.
91. Yellen SB, Cella DF, Leslie WT. Age and clinical decision making in oncology patients [see comments]. *J Natl Cancer Inst* 1994;86:1766–1770.
92. Yellen SB, Cella DF. Someone to live for: social well-being, parenthood status, and decision-making in oncology. *J Clin Oncol* 1995;13:1255–1264.
93. McQuellon RP, Muss HB, Hoffman SL, et al. Patient preferences for treatment of metastatic breast cancer: a study of women with early-stage breast cancer. *J Clin Oncol* 1995;13:858–868.
94. Singer DA, Donnelly MB, Messerschmidt GL. Informed consent for bone marrow transplantation: identification of relevant information by referring physicians. *Bone Marrow Transplant* 1990;6:431–437.
95. Jacoby LH, Maloy B, Cirenza E, et al. The basis of informed consent for BMT patients. *Bone Marrow Transplant* 1999;23:711–717.
96. Whedon M, Ferrell BR. Quality of life in adult bone marrow transplant patients: beyond the first year. *Semin Oncol Nurs* 1994;10:42–57.
97. Lesko LM, Dermatis H, Penman D, et al. Patients', parents', and oncologists' perceptions of informed consent for bone marrow transplantation. *Med Pediatr Oncol* 1989;17:181–187.
98. Perry D. Psychological and social preparation for bone marrow transplantation. *Soc Work Health Care* 2000;30:71–92.
99. Dimeo F, Bertz H, Finke J, et al. An aerobic exercise program for patients with haematological malignancies after bone marrow transplantation. *Bone Marrow Transplant* 1996;18:1157–1160.
100. Dimeo F, Fetscher S, Lange W, et al. Effects of aerobic exercise on the physical performance and incidence of treatment-related complications after high-dose chemotherapy. *Blood* 1997;90:3390–3394.
101. Dimeo FC, Stieglitz RD, Novelli-Fischer U, et al. Effects of physical activity on the fatigue and psychologic status of cancer patients during chemotherapy. *Cancer* 1999;85:2273–2277.
102. Gaston-Johansson F, Fall-Dickson JM, Nanda J, et al. The effectiveness of the comprehensive coping strategy program on clinical outcomes in breast cancer autologous bone marrow transplantation. *Cancer Nurs* 2000;23:277–285.
103. Syrjala KL, Donaldson GW, Davis MW, et al. Relaxation and imagery and cognitive-behavioral training reduce pain during cancer treatment: a controlled clinical trial. *Pain* 1995;63:189–198.
104. Matthes-Martin S, Lamche M, Ladenstein R, et al. Organ toxicity and quality of life after allogeneic bone marrow transplantation in pediatric patients: a single centre retrospective analysis. *Bone Marrow Transplant* 1999;23:1049–1053.
105. Dermatis H, Lesko LM. Psychological distress in parents consenting to child's bone marrow transplantation. *Bone Marrow Transplant* 1990;6:411–417.
106. Keogh F, O'Riordan J, McNamara C, et al. Psychosocial adaptation of patients and families following bone marrow transplantation: a prospective, longitudinal study. *Bone Marrow Transplant* 1998;22:905–911.
107. Buckner CD, Clift RA, Sanders JE, et al. Marrow harvesting from normal donors. *Blood* 1984;64:630–634.
108. Chang G, McGarigle C, Spitzer TR, et al. A comparison of related and unrelated marrow donors. *Psychosom Med* 1998;60:163–167.
109. Chern B, McCarthy N, Hutchins C, et al. Analgesic infiltration at the site of bone marrow harvest significantly reduces donor morbidity. *Bone Marrow Transplant* 1999;23:947–949.
110. Butterworth VA, Simmons RG, Bartsch G, et al. Psychosocial effects of unrelated bone marrow donation: experiences of the National Marrow Donor Program. *Blood* 1993;81:1947–1959.
111. Stroncek DF, Holland PV, Bartch G, et al. Experiences of the first 493 unrelated marrow donors in the National Marrow Donor Program. *Blood* 1993;81:1940–1946.
112. Simmons RG, Schimmel M, Butterworth VA. The self-image of unrelated bone marrow donors. *J Health Soc Behav* 1993;34:285–301.

113. Nishimori M, Yamada Y, Hoshi K, et al. Health-related quality of life of unrelated bone marrow donors in Japan. *Blood* 2002;99:1995–2001.
114. Sloan JA, Cella D, Frost M, et al. Assessing clinical significance in measuring oncology patient quality of life: introduction to the symposium, content overview, and definition of terms. *Mayo Clin Proc* 2002;77:367–370.
115. Litwin MS, McGuigan KA. Accuracy of recall in health-related quality-of-life assessment among men treated for prostate cancer. *J Clin Oncol* 1999;17:2882–2888.
116. Schluchter MD. Methods for the analysis of informatively censored longitudinal data. *Stat Med* 1992;11:1861–1870.
117. Fairclough DL, Hwang S, Chang V. Health related quality of life in terminal cancer patients: unbiased estimation in longitudinal studies with missing data due to morbidity and mortality. Boston: Dana-Farber Cancer Institute, 1996.
118. Andrykowski MA, Bruehl S, Brady MJ, et al. Physical and psychosocial status of adults one-year after bone marrow transplantation: a prospective study. *Bone Marrow Transplant* 1995;15:837–844.

Part III

Sources of Donor Stem Cells

15 Stem Cell Sources

Peripheral Blood Stem Cells and Bone Marrow for Allogeneic Transplantation

Corey Cutler, MD, MPH, FRCPC,
and Joseph H. Antin, MD

CONTENTS

1. INTRODUCTION

The discovery that human hematopoietic progenitors are found in the peripheral circulation and can be harvested for use in stem cell transplantation (SCT) has been both a scientifically enlightening and a clinically useful observation in SCT technology. Over the past decade, our understanding of peripheral blood stem cell (PBSC) properties has increased dramatically, and as a consequence, the use of PBSCs in autologous and allogeneic transplantation has increased exponentially. PBSCs have rapidly become the stem cell of choice for nearly all patients undergoing autologous transplantation because of their ease of collection and rapid engraftment. In the allogeneic setting, there have been dramatic increases in the use of PBSCs; however, many centers do not yet have adequate facilities to collect PBSCs from allogeneic donors and some centers have chosen not to adapt PBSCs as the main source for allogeneic stem cells for a variety of reasons. In the autologous setting, the broad adoption of peripheral blood stem cell transplantation (PBSCT) has been beneficial, with more rapid time to engraftment and less in-hospital morbidity noted after transplant. In the allogeneic setting, however, these data are less mature and there are observations that suggest that some of the putative advantages of PBSCT in the allogeneic setting may have substantial limitations.

Figure 1 demonstrates the overwhelming use of PBSCs for autologous transplantation and the dramatic increase in PBSC use for allogeneic transplantation in recent years. Greater than 90% of autologous transplants reported to the International Bone Marrow Transplant Registry

From: *Stem Cell Transplantation for Hematologic Malignancies*
Edited by: R. J. Soiffer

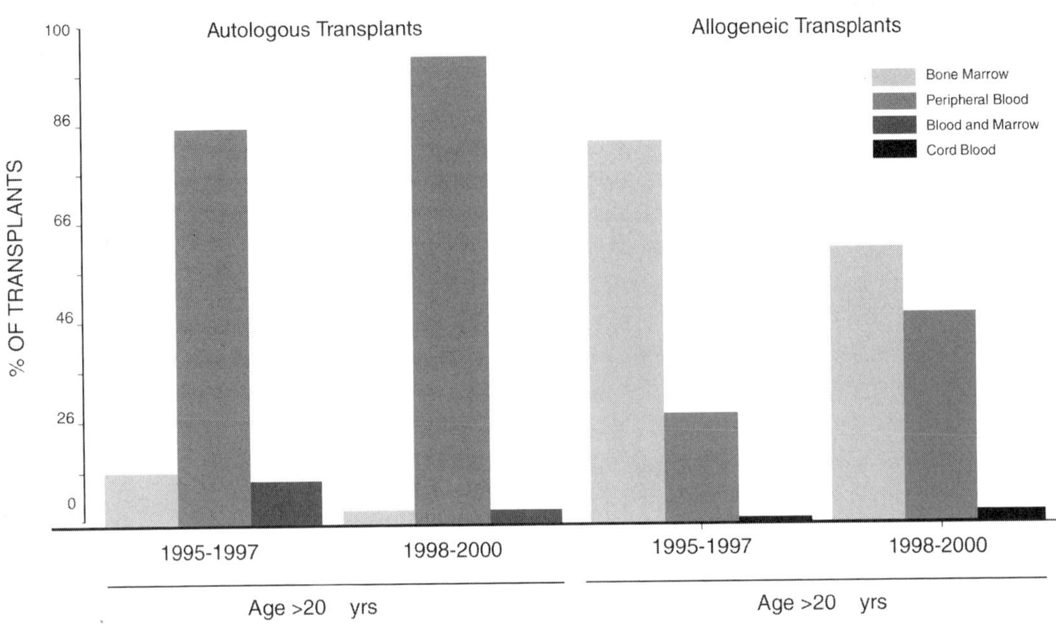

Fig. 1. Proportional uses of stem cells, 1995–2000, as reported to the IBMTR. (Modified from ref. *1*, with permission.)

(IBMTR) were performed with PBSCs, whereas over 40% of allogeneic transplants recently reported were performed with PBSC *(1)*. This proportion is expected to increase further in the coming years. The European Group for Blood and Marrow Transplant (EBMT) has noted similar increases in the use of PBSCs for allogeneic transplantation *(2)*. The use of cord blood as an alternative source of stem cell in adults has, to date, been limited and is discussed elsewhere in this text (Chapter 18).

Over the past number of years, the debate over the relative advantages and disadvantages of PBSCT when compared to traditional bone marrow transplantation (BMT) has prompted the completion of eight randomized clinical trials, with a number of additional studies nearing completion. In addition to the short- and intermediate-term end points reported in these clinical trials (such as engraftment, acute graft-vs-host disease [GVHD] and 100-d treatment-related mortality), long-term end points (such as chronic GVHD, immunologic reconstitution, and long-term survival) have become the major focus in the debate between these two stem cell sources. Other considerations, such as donor quality of life and economic factors, also affect upon the relative use of PBSCs.

2. STEM CELL MOBILIZATION AND ENGRAFTMENT KINETICS

Circulating PBSCs represent less than 0.001% of all nucleated cells in circulation *(3)*. These cells are in continuous recirculation from the marrow to the blood and back to random sites in the marrow cavity. Presumably, this process ensures an even distribution of hematopoiesis throughout the skeletal system. Levels of hematopoietic progenitors rise dramatically during the recovery phase after myelosuppressive chemotherapy and in response to exogenous recombinant human colony-stimulating factors (rhCSFs). Doses and schedules of different rhCSFs (i.e., G-CSF, GM-CSF) used for mobilization of PBSCs can vary and have ranged between 2 and 24 μg/kg/d for 1–5 d in reported studies *(4–6)*. Although different doses, schedules, and types of CSF have been examined in clinical trials prior to autologous transplantation (often in conjunction with myeloablative chemotherapy) *(7,8)*, trials in healthy PBSC donors have not been reported until recently *(9)*. Ten micrograms per kilogram per day of filgrastim administered for 5 consecutive days is the regimen recommended by the National Marrow Donor Program (NMDP) for healthy donors. Factors that may affect the cell yield from normal donors include the dose and duration of CSF administration and the timing of the apheresis procedure.

Progenitor cell mobilization is mediated through the downregulation and cleavage of adhesion molecules found on stem cell progenitors and marrow stromal endothelium. These adhesion molecules are expressed in high levels in the steady state and play an important role in the maintenance of localization of the stem cells in the endosteal regions of the marrow space. Once these critical adhesion interactions are disrupted, the progenitor cells migrate through the diaphragmed fenestra of the bone marrow (BM) endothelium into the peripheral circulation *(10)*. The VLA-4/VCAM-1 complex is thought to be the primary target of both downregulation *(11)* and neutrophil protease-mediated cleavage *(12)* in response to G-CSF, but other important interactions, such as those involving the selectin molecules, the kit–kit ligand interaction and hyaluronan with CD44 have been shown to be instrumental as well *(10)*.

Yields of PBSC harvests are generally superior to BM harvests when CD34+ progenitor numbers are compared. The differences in stem cell yields after dual collection of both BM and PBSCs from healthy donors was examined in one randomized trial. Forty healthy donors underwent BM harvesting followed by G-CSF-stimulated PBSC collection 1 wk later for their human leukocyte antigen (HLA)-identical siblings. The recipients were randomized in a blinded fashion to receive either the PBSCs or the BM collected from their siblings. Total nucleated cells, CD34+ cell yield, and colony-forming unit (CFU)–GM activity were 2.3, 3.7, and 3.7 times higher after PBSC harvesting when compared with BM harvesting. Furthermore, BM harvests were 6.8 times more likely to be insufficient for transplantation (defined as less than 2×10^6 CD34+ cells/kg of recipient weight, $p < 0.001$) *(13)*. This interpretation may not be valid, because traditionally, a range of $2–4 \times 10^8$ total nucleated cells/kg has been used as an arbitrary criterion for a sufficient marrow harvest. These results need to be interpreted with caution, because the BM harvest procedure may have artificially enhanced stem cell peripheralization and thus increased PBSC yields.

A relationship between the dose of CD34+ cells delivered with the transplant and the tempo of hematologic recovery has been demonstrated for both BMT *(14)* and PBSCT *(15–18)*. The use of higher doses of CD34+ cells leads to quicker engraftment, particularly when doses are greatly increased *(19,20)*. Platelet recovery appears to be more sensitive to CD34+ doses than neutrophil recovery *(20)*.

A convincing reduction in time to engraftment after both autologous and allogeneic PBSCT has been noted when compared to traditional BMT. This reduction is thought largely to be the result of the increased numbers of CD34+ progenitor cells delivered with PBSC grafts, although differences in the stem cells themselves may be implicated as well. In the allogeneic setting, neutrophil engraftment (to 0.5×10^9 cells/L on 3 consecutive days) occurred between 3 and 6 d earlier with PBSCT when compared with BMT in randomized trials (median time to engraftment: 12 vs 15 d and 15 vs 21 d, respectively [*21,22*]). Unsupported platelet counts of 20×10^9/L occurred between 5 and 8 d earlier (median time to platelet engraftment: 15 vs 19 d and 11 vs 18 d, respectively [*22,23*]). A comparison of the median times to neutrophil engraftment and stable platelet engraftment can be found in Fig. 2. Of note, all of the randomized trials dem-

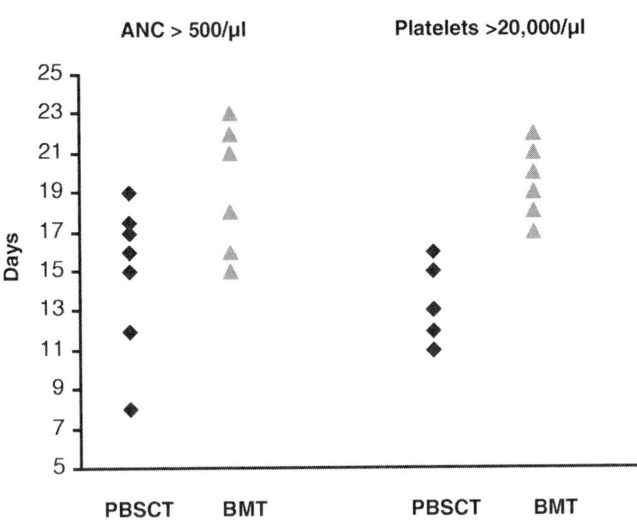

Fig. 2. Scatterplot of numbers of days to absolute neutrophil count greater than 500/µL (medians) and platelet count greater than 20,000/µL (medians) reported in randomized trials. (Platelets greater than 25,000/µL for the study was reported by Blaise [*21*]).

onstrated a decrease in the time to stable neutrophil and platelet engraftment. The results of a large database review are consistent with the results of the randomized trials (median time to neutrophil engraftment: 14 vs 19 d; median time to platelet engraftment: 18 vs 25 d; $p < 0.001$ for both comparisons) *(24)*.

The earlier engraftment seen after PBSCT has lead to earlier discharge from hospital *(23,25,26)*, fewer posttransplant transfusions *(22,25,27,28)* and total lower immediate costs associated with the transplant procedure *(21,29)*. The reduction in costs associated with the procedure is primarily the result of fewer dollars spent on hospital room charges, blood products, and other supportive measures. The costs of stem cell mobilization and collection procedures, however, are greater for PBSCT than for traditional BMT primarily the result of the use of recombinant human hematopoietic growth factors *(29)*. Long-term cost issues are more difficult to predict and will be influenced by GVHD outcomes after PBSCT (*see* Subheading 3).

3. TRANSPLANTATION OUTCOMES

3.1. Acute GVHD

Acute GVHD is caused by the complex interaction of donor T cells with the cytokine-mediated inflammatory milieu of the recipient. In comparison with BM grafts, there is an approx 10-fold increase in the number of CD3+ T cells delivered with PBSC grafts. The median T-cell dose delivered with PBSC grafts was 279×10^6/kg in comparison with only 23.8×10^6/kg delivered with BM grafts in one prospective trial *(27)*. Similar ratios were noted in many other clinical trials *(21–23,30)*. The increase in T cells delivered with PBSC products is one of the theoretical reasons for the increased rates of GVHD seen after PBSCT and explains, at least in part, the cautious adoption of PBSCT in the allogeneic setting. Preliminary phase II studies examining PBSCT did not support the notion that the incidence of acute GVHD would be increased *(31–34)*. Despite this, in addition to a large IBMTR/EBMT registry analysis *(24)* and a subgroup analysis by the EBMT *(2)*, there have been eight randomized trials that specifically address differences in acute GVHD incidence after PBSCT or BMT *(21,23,25,27,28,30, 35,36)*. The rates of acute GVHD from these trials can be found in Table 1. In the largest randomized trial involving 350 patients, both acute GVHD (grade II–IV) and severe acute GVHD (grade III–IV) were found to be significantly increased in the PBSCT group (52% vs 39%, $p = 0.013$; 28% vs 16%, $p = 0.0088$, respectively). In this trial however, an abbreviated course of methotrexate (three doses only) was used in both treatment arms for GVHD prophylaxis *(36)*. The Seattle group demonstrated a nonsignificant increase in the hazard ratio for both grade II–IV GVHD (hazard ratio-1.21, 95% confidence interval [CI]-0.81–1.81) and grade III–IV GVHD (hazard ratio-1.27, 95% CI-0.55–2.89) *(27)*. Similarly, the trials reported by Vigorito et al. *(37)* and Heldal et al. *(28)* demonstrated nonsignificant increases in the risk of acute GVHD. Of the remaining randomized trials examining acute GVHD, the relative risk of GVHD was similar in the PBSCT and BMT groups *(21,23,25)*. The notable exception is the randomized trial of only 30 individuals reported by Mahmoud et al., in which a statistically significant increase in acute GVHD in the BMT arm was noted *(35)*. The IBMTR/EBMT collaborative review of 288 PBSCT and 536 BMT procedures demonstrated a nonsignificant increase in the rate of grades II–IV acute GVHD (relative risk [RR] 1.19, 95% CI 0.9–1.56) *(24)*. Finally, a meta-analysis involving 15 studies (9 cohorts, 5 randomized trials, and 1 database review) demonstrated a significant increase in the risk of acute GVHD (RR 1.16, 95% CI 1.04–1.28). These results remained statistically significant when the randomized evidence was examined alone (RR 1.23, 95% CI 1.05–1.45) *(38)*.

There are many possible explanations for the discrepancies noted in the rates of acute GVHD noted in the clinical trials. Factors such as the age of patients and their donors *(39)*, the proportion of sex mismatches among donor–recipient pairs, the inclusion of higher-risk patients in some trials, the use of different conditioning or GVHD prophylaxis regimens, and discrepancies in GVHD scoring between transplant centers may influence GVHD occurrence. These differences may become less apparent in the unrelated setting, where rates of GVHD are expected to be higher than in the matched related setting. At the present time, there are no randomized trials available to support this assumption, and because not all donor centers can provide PBSCs for unrelated donors, there may be issues in designing studies to address these questions.

3.2. Chronic GVHD

Chronic GVHD is a significant contributor to the morbidity and mortality noted after allogeneic transplantation. There remains very little doubt that the incidence of chronic GVHD is increased after PBSCT in the matched, related-donor setting. Although none of the randomized trials were powered specifically to detect differences in chronic GVHD incidence, every trial has demonstrated at least a trend toward more chronic GVHD and some have demonstrated statistically significant results. Relative risks for chronic GVHD have ranged between a 1.29-fold and a 4.26-fold increase for PBSCT over BMT (*see* Table 2).The large EBMT randomized trial demonstrated a statistically significant increased risk of chronic GVHD in the PBSCT group (67% vs 54%, $p = 0.0066$) *(36,40)*. In contrast, the large American trial failed to demonstrate a statistical relationship between stem cell source and the occurrence of chronic GVHD, but a trend toward more chronic GVHD after PBSCT was observed (46% vs 35%) *(27)*. The Canadian trial demonstrated a trend toward increased chronic GVHD in the PBSCT group as well (85% vs 69%, p = NS) *(25)*. An updated meta-analysis *(38)* of the randomized trials (with available data) demonstrates an overall relative risk of 1.57 (95% CI-1.28–1.94) for chronic GVHD after

Table 1
Rates of Acute GVHD From Randomized Trials

First author, publication year	*Grade II–IV GVHD*					*Grade III–IV GVHD*				
	PBSCs		*BM*		*Relative risk*	*PBSCs*		*BM*		*Relativerisk*
Schmitz, 2002,	NA	52%	NA	39%	1.33*	NA	28%	NA	16%	1.75*
Couban, 2002	51/117	44%	47/107	44%	0.99	28/107	26%	21/117	18%	1.46
Bensinger, 2001	52/81	64%	52/91	57%	1.12[a]	12/81	15%	11/91	12%	1.23[b]
Vigorito, 2001, 1998	6/23	26%	5/23	22%	1.20	4/23	17%	3/23	13%	1.33
Blaise, 2000	21/47	45%	22/52	42%	1.06	8/47	17%	12/52	23%	0.74
Powles, 2000	10/20	50%	9/19	47%	1.06	NA	NA	NA	NA	NA
Heldal, 1999	6/28	21%	3/30	10%	2.14	NA	NA	NA	NA	NA
Mahmoud, 1999	1/15	7%	7/15	47%	0.14*	1/15	7%	6/15	40%	0.17*

[a]Hazard ratio = 1.21 by actuarial methods.
[b]Hazard ratio = 1.27 by actuarial methods.
*$p < 0.05$.

Table 2
Rates of Chronic GVHD From Randomized Trials

First author, publication year	*All chronic GVHD*					*Extensive chronic GVHD*				
	PBSCs		*BM*		*Relative risk*	*PBSCs*		*BM*		*Relative risk*
Schmitz, 2002	NA	67%	NA	54%	1.24	41/163	25%	19/166	11%	2.20*
Couban, 2002	NA	85%	NA	69%	1.09[a]	NA	40%	NA	30%	1.23[a]
Bensinger, 2001	NA	NA	NA	NA	NA	37/81	46%	32/91	35%	1.30
Vigorito, 2001, 1998	14/21	67%	11/20	55%	1.21*	14/21	67%	6/20	30%	2.22*
Blaise, 2000	24/44	55%	15/50	30%	1.82*	15/44	34%	4/50	8%	4.26*
Powles, 2000	8/20	40%	5/19	26%	1.52	NA	NA	NA	NA	NA
Heldal, 1999	15/27[b]	56%	8/30	27%	2.08	4/27	15%	2/30	7%	2.22

[a]Hazard ratios.
[b]Five had one antigen mismatch with donors.
*p 0.05.

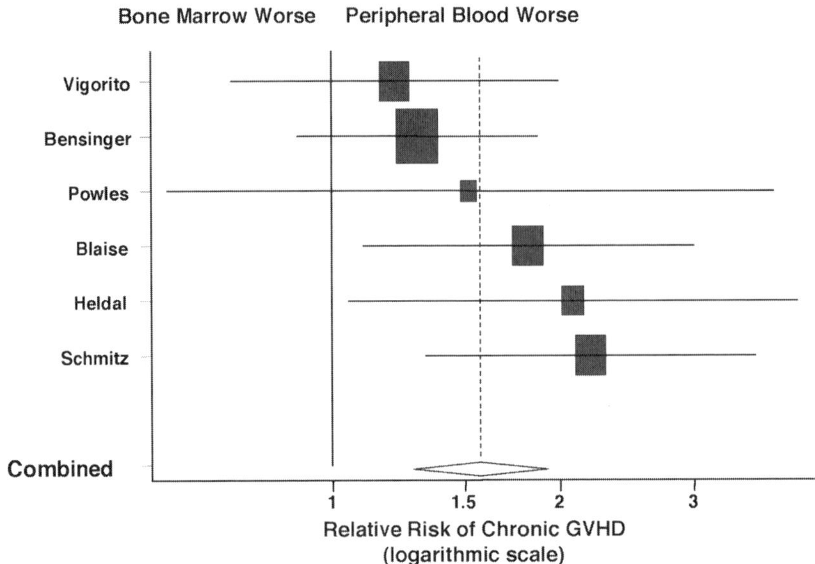

Fig. 3. Meta-analysis of chronic GVHD from published studies. Solid squares reflect study sample size and variance with 95% confidence intervals for relative risk. Solid line denotes relative risk of 1. Dotted line denotes combined relative risk across trials. Diamond reflects 95% confidence interval for the combined relative risk.

PBSCT when compared with BMT (*see* Fig. 3). Also, extensive chronic GVHD was more common after PBSCT. Similar to acute GVHD, the differences in the rates of chronic GVHD may be explained by a number of institution- and patient-specific factors.

The IBMTR/EBMT database review of 288 PBSCT procedures and 536 BMT procedures performed between 1995 and 1996 for acute myelogenous leukemia (AML), acute lymphoblastic leukemia (ALL), and chronic myelogenous leukemia (CML) demonstrated a significant increase in chronic extensive GVHD after PBSCT (65% vs 53% at 1 yr, $p = 0.02$) *(24)*. In another retrospective database review, univariate risk factors for chronic GVHD after PBSCT include the use of immunosuppressive regimens other than tacrolimus/methotrexate, prior acute GVHD, corticosteroids use 100 d after transplantation, and a high total nucleated cell dose in the PBSC graft *(41)*.

In the matched, unrelated-donor setting, no differences in the incidence of chronic GVHD was noted in a single published cohort study *(42)*. The lack of a difference in this group may be attributed to the relatively high rates of GVHD noted in this trial (61% and 76% for the PBSCT and BMT groups, respectively).

As previously discussed, CD34+ cell doses are increased in PBSC grafts. Recently, some groups have reported that the total CD34+ cell dose may influence the incidence of chronic GVHD. A retrospective analysis of 181 PBSC transplants performed between 1996 and 1999 demonstrated an increased hazard for chronic GVHD among patients who received more than 8.0×10^6 CD34+ cells/kg (hazard ratio 2.3, $p = 0.001$). This relationship was independent of the number of T cells delivered with the graft *(17)*. A trend for increased chronic GVHD was noted in the risk factor analysis reported by Przepiorka et al. *(41)*, but these findings were not confirmed in another similar study *(18)*. In an analysis of CD34+-selected PBSCT, increased mortality was associated with higher CD34+ cell doses, although the relationship with increased

GVHD in this group was not statistically significant *(43)*. Higher CD34+ cell doses have also been associated with an increased incidence of acute GVHD *(44)*. Until prospective studies document significant changes in mortality related to higher doses of CD34+ cells, it would be unwise to suggest minimum or maximum doses of stem cells required for transplantation, with the exception that a minimum number of cells (in the range of 2×10^6 CD34+ cells/kg) is required for prompt engraftment.

3.3. Relapse

There is sufficient evidence from nonmyeloablative transplantation, donor lymphocyte infusions (DLIs), and immunosuppression withdrawal studies to suggest that a potent graft-vs-leukemia (GVL) reaction can occur after SCT. With the exception of some experimental rodent studies *(45–49)*, separation of clinical GVL from GVHD has remained the elusive "holy grail" of transplantation. Despite the detrimental effects on survivorship that acute and chronic GVHD can cause, there is evidence to suggest that the presence of acute GVHD, chronic GVHD, or both correlates with disease-relapse prevention after BMT *(48,49)*. These findings have been confirmed after PBSCT as well, where the presence of chronic GVHD *(21,50)* or both acute and chronic GVHD *(51)* have been demonstrated to protect against relapse. Brunet et al., reporting on 136 patients who had undergone allogeneic PBSCT for advanced hematological malignancies, demonstrated a cumulative incidence of relapse of 47% in patients without any GVHD but only 14% for patients who experienced both acute and chronic GVHD ($p = 0.002$). This decrease in relapse translated into a long-term survival advantage *(51)*. Przepiorka et al. noted a nonsignificant trend for chronic GVHD to be protective from relapse in a retrospective review (hazard ratio 0.6, $p = 0.2$) *(41)*.

Körbling first noted the possible advantage of PBSCT over BMT for refractory leukemia and lymphoma *(52)*. Elmaagacli et al. demonstrated a lower incidence of molecular and cytogenetic relapse in a nonrandomized trial comparing matched related PBSCT and BMT for CML *(53)* and subsequently demonstrated improved survival after PBSCT when compared with BMT in the unrelated-donor setting *(54)*. Similar reductions in disease relapse after PBSC allografting for myeloma have been demonstrated *(55)*.

In the randomized setting, several studies have independently demonstrated a decrease in the rate of disease relapse after PBSCT when compared to BMT. Six of 20 patients relapsed in the BM arm, whereas none of 19 patients transplanted with PBSCs relapsed in the study reported by Powles et al. *(23,56)*. A trend toward decreased relapse in the PBSCT group was also noted in the studies reported by Blaise et al. *(20)* and Mahmoud et al. *(35)*. The hazard ratio for relapse in the study reported by Bensinger et al. was 0.49 (95% CI 0.38–1.28) among patients transplanted with PBSCs. In this trial, the decrease in relapse rates was associated with an increase in disease-free survival (DFS) for the PBSCT group (65% vs 45%, $p = 0.03$) *(27)*. A nonsignificant trend toward decreased relapse rates after PBSCT was noted in the published meta-analysis, where the relative risk of relapse was 0.81 (95% CI 0.62–1.05) *(38)*. Unfortunately, to date, the decrease in relapse rates noted with PBSCT have not translated into prolongation of overall survival (OS) after transplantation in the randomized trials (*see* below).

3.4. Immune Reconstitution

Immune reconstitution after allogeneic SCT is critical, because important morbidity and mortality can be ascribed to infectious complications in the posttransplant period. Complete immune reconstitution or, at a minimum, T-cell reconstitution may also be important for the development of an effective GVL response as well. Immune reconstitution can be assessed by enumeration of specific immune cell subclasses, by measurement of T-cell neogenesis *(57)*, by measurement of immune diversity through Vβ gene rearrangement spectrotyping *(58)*, and by functional assays of immune activity. These studies can be misleading when performed in the context of active infection, GVHD, and immunosuppression.

Despite seemingly normal numbers of mature lymphocytes and granulocytes within weeks to months of allogeneic transplantation, immunosuppressive medications, the occurrence of GVHD, and other clinical events may alter immune function. Impaired immune function has been noted in a number of studies after allogeneic BMT *(59)* as well as after PBSCT *(60)*. In a retrospective study of 115 healthy transplant recipients evaluated at least 1 yr after BMT, risk factors for impaired immune reconstitution (measured by T- and B-cell numbers, immunoglobulin levels, and T-cell proliferative responses) included the presence of chronic GVHD, cytomegalovirus (CMV) infection, mismatched transplantation, total-body irradiation (TBI) conditioning, and advanced recipient age *(61)*. Earlier studies had noted the correlation between lower T-cell counts *(62)* and lower B-cell and monocyte counts *(63)* with infectious complications after transplantation.

Two of the published randomized studies have addressed issues related to immune reconstitution comparing PBSCT with BMT. The French study documented higher levels of lymphocytes (total), B cells, T cells, and T-cell subpopulations after PBSCT when compared to BMT, whereas natural killer (NK) cells and monocyte numbers were not significantly different 30 d after transplantation *(64)*. Both CD56+ NK cells *(22)* and CD19+ B cells *(13)* have been shown to be found in greater quantities in PBSC collections than in BM harvests previously. In the Seattle study, transplantation with PBSC was associated with higher CD4+ T-cell counts ($CD45RA^{high}$ naïve and $CD45^{low/-}$ mature cells), higher CD8+ T-cell counts, and higher CD4– CD8– T-cell counts early after transplantation. The increase in T-cell number (without an increase in single T-cell function as measured by lymphoproliferation assays) was associated with a lower incidence of confirmed infections (RR=0.59, $p < 0.001$) and confirmed severe infections (RR=0.42, p=0.002) after transplantation *(65)*. In contrast to an earlier report by the same authors *(66)*, serum immunoglobulin levels were similar to those found in BMT patients. This study confirmed the results offered in smaller studies reported by Ottinger et al. *(67)* and Trenschel et al. *(68)*.

3.5. Survival

Although GVHD outcomes following transplantation are important in the short term, long-term survival differences will ultimately drive stem cell choice decision-making in allogeneic transplantation. With shorter time to engraftment following PBSCT and a reduction in length of first hospital stay, a reduction in treatment-related mortality (TRM), measured at 100 d posttransplant, was expected to be found in the randomized clinical trials, but generally has not been noted overall. The Canadian randomized trial demonstrated a reduction in TRM after PBSCT when compared to BMT (2.8% vs 7.6% TRM at 30 d, $p = 0.18$, and 7.4% vs 16.1% TRM at 100 d, $p = 0.07$) *(25)* (*see* Table 3). Similarly, a reduction in TRM after PBSCT was noted for individuals with high-risk disease in the IBMTR/EBMT review, where TRM was lower for individuals with advanced-stage AML and accelerated-phase CML, but not different for individuals with AML in first remission or CML in the chronic stable phase *(24)*.

Long-term survival after transplantation is affected by early TRM, relapse incidence, and mortality resulting from acute and chronic GVHD and infection. Because TRM and relapse

Table 3
Treatment-Related Mortality and Long-Term Survival From the Randomized Trials

First author, publication year	*Treatment-related mortality (at 100 d) PBSCs vs BM*	*Long-term survival PBSCs vs BM*
Schmitz, 2002	No differences noted	No differences noted
Couban, 2002	7.4% for PBSCs, 16.1% for BM at 100 d ($p = 0.07$)	68% vs 60% 30-mo survival ($p = 0.04$). Significant improvement for high-risk disease and CML. Trend for MDS. 66% vs 54% 2-yr survival ($p = 0.06$).
Bensinger, 2001	NA	Significant improvement for high-risk disease.
Vigorito, 2001, 1998	NA	56% vs 48% survival at 2000 d
Schmitz, 2002	No differences noted	No differences noted
Blaise, 2000	NA	67% vs 65% 2-yr survival (p = NS)
Powles, 2000	35% vs 32% (p = NS)	65% vs 47% at 4 yr (p = NS)
Heldal, 1999	13% vs 0% (p = NS)	80% vs 73% at a median of 34 and 36 mo (p = NS)
Mahmoud, 1999	27% vs 53% (p = NS)	NA

MDS, myelodysplastic syndrome.

may be reduced after PBSCT, GVHD may be more common after PBSCT and immune reconstitution may be more complete after PBSCT, it is unclear how these competing risks would translate into long-term survival differences. In the Canadian trial, an overall survival advantage was noted for the PBSCT group (68% vs 60% survival at 30 mo, $p = 0.04$). This advantage was largely attributed to the reduction in early TRM *(25)*. Despite an improvement in DFS for individuals transplanted with PBSC (65% vs 45%, $p = 0.03$), long-term survival differences did not reach statistical significance in the trial reported by Bensinger et al. *(27)*. In this trial, there was a very strong trend toward improved survival after PBSCT overall (66% vs 54% 2-yr survival, $p = 0.06$), whereas for individuals with more advanced malignancies, there was a significant improvement in overall survival (57% vs 33%, $p = 0.04$). One might be concerned that the relative survival advantage reported at 2 yr may diminish with time, because much of the mortality from chronic GVHD may occur after 2 yr. Small differences in survival favoring PBSCT were noted in several other randomized studies *(28,37,57)* but the EBMT trial has not yet demonstrated a survival advantage for PBSCT *(36)*. The IBMTR/EBMT review demonstrated a leukemia-free advantage for individuals with high-risk features at the time of transplantation (77% vs 57% for advanced AML, $p = 0.003$; 68% vs 23% for advanced CML, $p < 0.001$) but not for standard-risk malignancies (70% vs 61% for AML in first complete remission [CR], $p = 0.25$; 63% vs 74% for CML in first chronic phase, $p = 0.27$) *(24)*.

Once again, the impact of CD34+ cell dose has been explored with respect to overall survival. In a multivariate Cox analysis of predictive factors for TRM and long-term survival after PBSCT, a CD34+ cell dose greater than 3×10^6 cells/kg was associated with a reduction in 180-d TRM (hazard ratio 0.54, $p = 0.03$) and a reduction in overall mortality at a median of 3.4 yr after transplantation (hazard ratio-0.55, $p = 0.006$) *(17)*. Conversely, in a study of T-cell depleted-PBSCT, a higher CD34+ cell dose was associated with diminished survival, largely as a result of increased GVHD and infectious complications *(43)*.

4. LINKING BIOLOGY TO CLINICAL OUTCOMES: UNDERSTANDING THE DIFFERENCES BETWEEN PBSCT AND BMT

Mobilization and peripheralization of PBSCs, either with filgrastim, cytotoxic chemotherapy, or a combination of the two, is mediated through modulation of adhesion molecules found on steady-state BM progenitor cells. In response to intracellular signaling (through pathways such as JAK2) *(69)* from a variety of cytokines (i.e., G-CSF, GM-CSF, *flt*-3 ligand, and, interleukin [IL]-12) or chemokines (i.e., SDF-α *[69]* and IL-8 *[70]*), changes in the BM microenvironment, and changes in the repertoire of cellular adhesion molecules occur. As a result of the cytokine and chemokine-induced signaling that occurs upon mobilization, peripheralized hematopoietic progenitors are phenotypically different in comparison to their marrow stromal-bound counterparts. In fact, gene expression profiling studies have demonstrated that cell-cycle-promoting genes and genes regulating DNA synthesis and replication are expressed at significantly lower levels in PBSCs, whereas apoptosis-related genes are expressed at significantly higher levels in PBSCs *(71)*. These results corroborate earlier findings demonstrating PBSCs to be less metabolically active and less involved in active cell cycling by rhodamine-retention studies and S-phase analysis *(72)*. PBSCs have been shown to express higher levels of differentiation markers, such as CD13 and CD33. These committed progenitors may be responsible for the more rapid engraftment noted after PBSCT. In addition, mobilized PBSCs have been shown to composed of higher proportions of CD34+CD38– cells and CD34+Thy-1+ coexpressing cells, which are known to be enriched for long-term culture-initiating colonies (LTC-IC) subpopulations. Whether this in turn promotes enhanced graft stability and the earlier appearance of more diverse immune reconstitution is not known.

The inoculum of T cells delivered with a PBSC graft is roughly 10-fold greater than with a traditional marrow graft. In theory, this increase in cell load should be sufficient to explain the increase in GVHD noted with PBSCs; however, there is very little objective evidence to suggest that there is a relationship between T-cell dose and GVHD. In addition to quantitative changes in T cells in PBSC grafts, there may be qualitative changes in the T cells delivered as well. In animal studies, G-CSF administration has been shown to polarize mobilized T cells to a type 2 response *(73,74)*, largely as a result of type 2 dendritic cell stimulation *(75,76)*. This has led to diminished rates of GVHD noted in many mouse models, but it has not been confirmed in all studies. The etiology of the increase in GVHD in one mouse model was explored by examining regulatory T-cell subsets in a murine PBSC and marrow transplant model. In this study, regulatory T cells present in marrow but not in PBSC grafts were capable of mediating engraftment and GVL reactions, but were incapable of inciting GVHD *(77)*.

It is possible that in humans, despite a polarization of T cells to the type 2 phenotype, the increased number of T cells is still the driving force behind the increased rates of GVHD noted after PBSCT. Older studies demonstrated a relationship between CD3+ cell dose and GVHD after BMT *(78,79)*, but, interestingly, none of the recent analyses were able to demonstrate this correlation after PBSCT *(41,44)*. Despite the lack of correlation, it is clear that there are more potent GVL reactions with PBSCT, which correlates with the increased incidence of GVHD.

Owing to reduced thymic function in older individuals, the majority of mature T lymphocytes found in the circulation within the first year after transplantation are felt to have been transferred with the stem cell graft, because evidence of T cell neogenesis does not occur until 6 mo posttransplantation *(57)*. Tayebi et al. demonstrated a significant correlation between the infused T-cell dose, but not the infused CD34+ stem cell dose, and lymphocyte counts 30 d after transplantation *(64)*. Because PBSCT is associated with a log-fold increase in delivered T cells, the finding of increased T cell numbers after transplant is not surprising and may explain the differences noted in immune reconstitution studies.

5. IMPLICATIONS FOR STEM CELL DONORS AND THE ECONOMICS OF SCT

The procurement of stem cells from both related and unrelated marrow and PBSC donors must be performed with only minimal morbidity to the volunteer donors. Recombinant growth factors, which are used to peripheralize stem cells, at daily subcutaneous doses varying between 2 and 24 μg/kg have been administered to PBSC donors *(4–6)*, including donors over the age of 60 yr *(80)*. The induced leukocytosis, when maintained at levels below 70,000 cells/μL, has generally not been shown to be detrimental to the donor's health; however, importantly morbidity, including splenic rupture and death, has rarely been reported *(81,82)*. Common minor side effects caused by the administration of growth factors include bone pain, myalgia, headache, and fever, all of which respond to mild analgesics in over 80% of cases. Longer follow-up (up to 6 yr) has confirmed the safety of administration of rhG-CSF to healthy donors *(82,83)*. Almost all BM harvest procedures are performed without the administration of colony-stimulating factors.

Of 1337 PBSC apheresis procedures reported to the IBMTR/EBMT between 1994 and 1998, complications were reported to occur in 15 donors. One-third of these complications were related to central-line venous access (which was required in 20% of donors). Complications unrelated to line placement included pericarditis, back pain, hypercalcemia, alterations in blood pressure, nausea, diarrhea, and thrombocytopenia *(84)*. Complications related to BM harvesting include prolonged pain at the site of the harvest, infection, anemia requiring red cell transfusion, and complications related to either general or spinal anesthesia. There have been two fatalities reported to the IBMTR/EBMT after BM harvesting *(84)*.

Donor preference for either PBSC or BM donation has been examined, as the two procedures differ in the time required for donor preparation (several days for rhG-CSF administration), in the time needed for the procedure itself (between 1 and 3 d for PBSC donation, 1 d for marrow donation), and in the time to complete recovery (days to weeks for BM donors, nearly immediate for PBSC donors). No differences in self-reported quality-of-life measures were noted among healthy donors randomized to undergo PBSC or marrow donation *(85)*; however, patients randomized to donate autologous PBSCs or BM reported higher acceptance of the PBSC donation *(87)*. Health-related quality-of-life changes related to BM harvesting, as measured by the Short Form 36 (SF36), have demonstrated that the detrimental effects on quality of life after harvesting are predominantly related to pain at the site of marrow harvest *(87)*. There are some donors who, for personal reasons, prefer either not to receive G-CSF or not to undergo general anaesthesia.

Two economics analyses have demonstrated lower costs associated with PBSCT because of a reduction in first hospital stay and blood product support; however, both of these analyses did not include long-term costs that could be associated with increased rates of chronic GVHD *(29,88)*.

6. CONCLUSIONS AND FUTURE DIRECTIONS

Peripheral blood stem cell transplantation has widely become the standard of care in autologous transplantation and rapidly become more popular in the allogeneic setting. The major differences in outcomes between PBSCT and BMT include a reduction in the time required for stable neutrophil and platelet engraftment, a higher incidence of acute and chronic GVHD with decreased relapse rates, and at least a trend toward improved survival after PBSCT. A summary of the major findings from all of the published the randomized trials can be found in Table 4.

The major limitations to the broadened use of PBSCT is the fear of higher rates of GVHD and the potential negative impact on survival. In the related setting, the introduction of novel immunosuppressant medications (such as sirolimus and mycophenolate mofetil) may significantly lower the risk of GVHD to allow PBSCs to be used more widely. Furthermore, if GVHD is adequately controlled, the benefits of reduced disease relapse and improved DFS may outweigh the risks of GVHD. Novel immunosuppressive regimens may be particularly helpful in the unrelated setting where GVHD rates are slightly higher than in the related setting, although the rates of GVHD after PBSCT do not appear to be elevated in comparison to BMT in cohort studies *(42)*.

There are several investigational strategies designed to mimic the engraftment kinetics of PBSCs that are being tested. These strategies include the use of combined PBSC and BM transplants *(89,90)* and the use of rhG-CSF mobilized bone marrow for transplantation *(88,91–94)*. The latter approach may have the advantage of GVHD rates similar to traditional BMT *(92,93)*, but with neutrophil engraftment kinetics similar to those of PBSC transplants *(94)*.

Table 4
Clinical of Summary of Randomized Trials Comparing PBSCs to BM

First author, publication year	*Sample size*	*Time to neutrophil engraftment*	*Time to platelet engraftment*	*Acute GVHD*	*Chronic GVHD*	*Relapse*	*DFS*	*OS*
Schmitz, 2002	350	↓ PBSC	↓ PBSC	**↑ PBSC**	**↑ PBSC**	ND	ND	ND
Couban, 2002	228	↓ PBSC	↓ PBSC	ND[a]	↑ PBSC	ND	NA	↑ PBSC
Bensinger, 2001	172	↓ PBSC	↓ PBSC	↑ PBSC	↑ PBSC	↑ BM	↑ PBSC	↑ PBSC[b]
Vigorito, 2001, 1998	56	↓ PBSC	↓ PBSC	↑ PBSC	↑ PBSC	NA	↑ PBSC	↑ PBSC
Schmitz, 2002	350	↓ PBSC	↓ PBSC	↑ PBSC	↑ PBSC	ND	ND	ND
Blaise, 2000	101	↓ PBSC	↓ PBSC	ND	↑ PBSC	↑ BM	ND	ND
Powles, 2000	39	↓ PBSC	↓ PBSC	ND	↑ PBSC	↑ BM	NA	↑ PBSC
Heldal, 1999	61	↓ PBSC	↓ PBSC	↑ PBSC	↑ PBSC	↑ BM	↑ PBSC	↑ PBSC
Mahmoud, 1999	30	↓ PBSC	↓ PBSC	↑ BM	NA[c]	NA	NA	NA

[a]ND = no difference.
[b]Patients with advanced malignancy.
[c]NA = not applicable.
Note: Bold arrows and bold text represent statistically significant differences (p 0.05). Light arrows represent trends (p = NS).

In terms of deciding which stem cell source is the most appropriate for individual patients, a risk stratification approach may be useful. Taking into account factors such as patient age, disease stage (early vs advanced) and the evidence for an efficient GVL response, the age of the donor and recipient, recipient comorbidity, and future quality of life considerations may influence the stem cell choice. For example, for young individuals with stable-phase CML, the slightly prolonged period of neutropenia associated with BMT may be a preferable trade-off for a decreased rate of chronic GVHD, particularly in a disease where relapses are relatively rare and a potent GVL effect with marrow or DLI is observed. In contrast, patients with relapsed acute leukemia may benefit from the enhanced GVL effects of PBSCT, despite the increased risk of GVHD.

As more randomized trials near completion and data mature from previously reported trials, it may become evident that a survival advantage for PBSCT truly does exist, particularly when effective GVHD prophylaxis regimens are employed. When this occurs, the use of PBSCT will likely further increase, and traditional, unstimulated BM will no longer serve as an important source of stem cells in allogeneic transplantation.

REFERENCES

1. Eapen M. IBMTR/ABMTR Newslett 2002;9(1).
2. Ringdén O, Labopin M, Bacigalupo A, et al. Transplantation of peripheral blood stem cells as compared with bone marrow from HLA-identical siblings in adult patients with acute myeloid leukemia and acute lymphoblastic leukemia. *J Clin Oncol* 2002;20:4655–4664.
3. Abkowitz JL. Can human hematopoietic stem cells become skin, gut, or liver cells? *N Engl J Med* 2002;346(10):770–772.
4. Bensinger WI, Price TH, Dale DC, et al. The effects of daily recombinant human granulocyte colony-stimulating factor administration on normal granulocyte donors undergoing leukapheresis. *Blood* 1993;81(7):1883–1889.
5. McCullough J, Clay M, Herr G, et al. Effects of granulocyte-colony-stimulating factor on potential normal granulocyte donors. *Transfusion* 1999;39(10):1136–1140.
6. Murata M, Harada M, Kato S, et al. Peripheral blood stem cell mobilization and apheresis: analysis of adverse events in 94 normal donors. *Bone Marrow Transplant* 1999;24(10):1065–1071.
7. Demirer T, Ayli M, Ozcan M, et al. Mobilization of peripheral blood stem cells with chemotherapy and recombinant human granulocyte colony-stimulating factor (rhG-CSF): a randomized evaluation of different doses of rhG-CSF. *Br J Haematol* 2002;116(2):468–474.
8. Gazitt Y. Comparison between granulocyte colony-stimulating factor and granulocyte–macrophage colony-stimulating factor in the mobilization of peripheral blood stem cells. *Curr Opin Hematol* 2002;9(3):190–198.
9. Kröger N, Renges H, Sonnenberg S, et al. Stem cell mobilisation with 16 μg/kg vs 10 μg/kg of G-CSF for allogeneic transplantation in healthy donors. *Bone Marrow Transplant* 2002;29:727–730.
10. Thomas J, Liu F , Link DC. Mechanisms of mobilization of hematopoietic progenitors with granulocyte colony-stimulating factor. *Curr Opin Hematol* 2002;9(3):183–189.
11. Papayannopoulou T. Mechanisms of stem-/progenitor-cell mobilization: the anti-VLA-4 paradigm. *Semin Hematol* 2000;37(1, suppl 2):11–18.
12. Levesque JP, Takamatsu Y, Nilsson SK, et al. Vascular cell adhesion molecule-1 (CD106) is cleaved by neutrophil proteases in the bone marrow following hematopoietic progenitor cell mobilization by granulocyte colony-stimulating factor. *Blood* 2001;98(5):1289–1297.
13. Singhal S, Powles R, Kulkarni S, et al. Comparison of marrow and blood cell yields from the same donors in a double-blind, randomized study of allogeneic marrow vs. blood stem cell transplantation. *Bone Marrow Transplant* 2000;25:501–505.
14. Siena S, Schiavo R, Pedrazzoli P, et al. Therapeutic relevance of CD34 cell dose in blood cell transplantation for cancer therapy. *J Clin Oncol* 2000;18(6):1360–1377.

15. Mavroudis D, Read E, Cottler-Fox M, et al. CD34+ cell dose predicts survival, posttransplant morbidity, and rate of hematologic recovery after allogeneic marrow transplants for hematologic malignancies. *Blood* 1996;88(8):3223–3229.
16. Ilhan O, Arslan Ö, Arat M, et al. The impact of the CD34+ cell dose on engraftment in allogeneic peripheral blood stem cell transplantation. *Transfusion Sci* 1999;20:69–71.
17. Zaucha JM, Gooley T, Bensinger WI, et al. CD34 cell dose in granulocyte colony-stimulating factor-mobilized peripheral blood mononuclear cell grafts affects engraftment kinetics and development of extensive chronic graft-versus-host disease after human leukocyte antigen-identical sibling transplantation. *Blood* 2001;98(12):3221–3227.
18. Bittencourt H, Rocha V, Chevret S, et al. Association of CD34 cell dose with hematopoietic recovery, infections, and other outcomes after HLA-identical sibling bone marrow transplantation. *Blood* 2002;99(8):2726–2733.
19. Miflin G, Russell NH, Hutchinson RM, et al. Allogeneic peripheral blood stem cell transplantation for haematological malignancies—an analysis of kinetics of engraftment and GVHD risk. *Bone Marrow Transplant* 1997;19:9–13.
20. Shpall EJ, Champlin R, Glaspy JA. Effect of CD34+ peripheral blood progenitor cell dose on hematopoietic recovery. *Biol Blood Marrow Transplant* 1998;4:84–92.
21. Blaise D, Kuentz M, Fortanier C, et al. Randomized trial of bone marrow versus Lenograstim-primed blood cell allogeneic transplantation in patients with early-stage leukemia: a report from the Société Française de Greffe de Moelle. *J Clin Oncol* 2000;18(3):537–546.
22. Schmitz N, Bacigalupo A, Hasenclever D, et al. Allogeneic bone marrow transplantation vs. filgrastim-mobilised peripheral blood progenitor cell transplantation in patients with early leukaemia: first results of a randomised multicentre trial of the European Group for Blood and Marrow Transplantation. *Bone Marrow Transplant* 1998,21:995–1003.
23. Powles R, Mehta J, Kulkarni S, et al. Allogeneic blood and bone-marrow stem-cell transplantation in haematological malignant diseases: a randomised trial. *Lancet* 2000;335:1231–1237.
24. Champlin RE, Schmitz N, Horowitz MM, et al. Blood stem cells compared with bone marrow as a source of hematopoietic cells for allogeneic transplantation. *Blood* 2000;95(12):3702–3709.
25. Couban S, Simpson DR, Barnett MJ, et al. A randomized multicentre comparison of bone marrow and peripheral blood in recipients of matched sibling allogeneic transplants for myeloid malignancies. *Blood* (first edition paper), www.hematologyjournal.org, accessed on June 20, 2002.
26. Anderlini P, Körbling M, Dale D, et al. Allogeneic blood stem cell transplantation: considerations for donors. *Blood* 1997;90(3):903–908.
27. Bensinger WI, Martin PJ, Storer B, et al. Transplantation of bone marrow as compared with peripheral-blood cells from HLA-identical relatives in patients with hematologic cancers. *N Engl J Med* 2001;344(3):175–181.
28. Heldal D, Tjonnfjord G, Brinch L, et al. A randomised study of allogeneic transplantation with stem cells from blood or bone marrow. *Bone Marrow Transplant* 2000;25(11):1129–1136.
29. Bennett CL, Waters TM, Stinson TJ, et al. Valuing clinical strategies early in development: a cost analysis of allogeneic peripheral blood stem cell transplantation. *Bone Marrow Transplant* 1999;24:555–560.
30. Vigorito AC, Azevedo WM, Marques JFC, et al. A randomised, prospective comparison of allogeneic bone marrow and peripheral blood progenitor cell transplantation in the treatment of haematological malignancies. *Bone Marrow Transplant* 1998;22:1145–1151.
31. Bacigalupo A, Zikos P, Van Lint M-T, et al. Allogeneic bone marrow or peripheral blood cell transplants in adults with hematologic malignancies: a single-center experience. *Exper Hematol* 1998;26:409–414.
32. Russell JA, Larratt L, Brown C, et al. Allogeneic blood stem cells and bone marrow transplantation for acute myelogenous leukemia and myelodysplasia: influence of stem cell source on outcome. *Bone Marrow Transplant* 1999;24:1177–1183.
33. Storek J, Gooley T, Siadak M, et al. Allogeneic peripheral blood stem cell transplantation may be associated with a high risk of chronic graft-versus-host disease. *Blood* 1997;90(12):4705–4709.
34. Üstün C, Arslan Ö, Beksaç M, et al. A retrospective comparison of allogeneic peripheral blood stem cell and bone marrow transplantation results from a single center: a focus on the incidence of graft-vs.-host disease and relapse. *Biol Blood Marrow Transplant* 1999;5:28–35.
35. Mahmoud H, Fahmy O, Kamel A, et al. Peripheral blood vs bone marrow as a source for allogeneic hematopoietic stem cell transplantation. *Bone Marrow Transplant* 1999;24(4):355–358.
36. Schmitz N, Beksaç M, Hasenclever D, et al. Transplantation of mobilized peripheral blood cells to HLA-identical siblings with standard-risk leukemia. *Blood* 2002;100:761–767.

37. Vigorito AC, Marques Junior JF, et al. A randomized, prospective comparison of allogeneic bone marrow and peripheral blood progenitor cell transplantation in the treatment of hematologic malignancies: an update. *Haematologica* 2001;86(6):665–666.
38. Cutler C, Giri S, Jeyapalan S, et al. Acute and chronic graft-versus-host disease after allogeneic peripheral-blood stem-cell and bone marrow transplantation: a meta-analysis. *J Clin Oncol* 2001;19(16):3685–3691.
39. Kollman C, Howe CW, Anasetti C, et al. Donor characteristics as risk factors in recipients after transplantation of bone marrow from unrelated donors: the effect of donor age. *Blood* 2001;98(7):2043–2051.
40. Schmitz N, Barrett J. Optimizing engraftment-Source and dose of stem cells. *Semin Hematol* 2002;39(1):3–14.
41. Przepiorka D, Anderlini P, Saliba R, et al. Chronic graft-versus-host disease after allogeneic blood stem cell transplantation. *Blood* 2001;98(6):1695–1700.
42. Remberger M, Ringden O, Blau IW, et al. No difference in graft-versus-host disease, relapse, and survival comparing peripheral stem cells to bone marrow using unrelated donors. *Blood* 2001;98(6):1739–1745.
43. Urbano-Ispizua A, Carreras E, Marin P, et al. Allogeneic transplantation of CD34(+) selected cells from peripheral blood from human leukocyte antigen-identical siblings: detrimental effect of a high number of donor CD34(+) cells? *Blood* 2001;98(8):2352–2357.
44. Przepiorka D, Smith TL, Folloder J, et al. Risk factors for acute graft-versus-host disease after allogeneic blood stem cell transplantation. *Blood* 1999;94(4):1465–1470.
45. Chen BJ, Cui X , Liu C, et al. Prevention of graft-versus-host disease while preserving graft-versus-leukemia effect after selective depletion of host-reactive T cells by photodynamic cell purging process. *Blood* 2002;99(9):3083–3088.
46. Uckun FM, Roers BA, Waurzyniak B, et al. Janus kinase 3 inhibitor WHI-P131/JANEX-1 prevents graft-versus-host disease but spares the graft-versus-leukemia function of the bone marrow allografts in a murine bone marrow transplantation model. *Blood* 2002;99:4192–4199.
47. Baker J, Verneris MR, Ito M, et al. Expansion of cytolytic CD8(+) natural killer T cells with limited capacity for graft-versus-host disease induction due to interferon gamma production. *Blood* 2001;97(10):2923–2931.
48. Horowitz MM, Gale RP, Sondel PM, et al. Graft-versus-leukemia reactions after bone marrow transplantation. *Blood* 1990;75(3):555–562.
49. Sullivan KM, Weiden PL, Storb R, et al. Influence of acute and chronic graft-versus-host disease on relapse and survival after bone marrow transplantation from HLA-identical siblings as treatment of acute and chronic leukemia. *Blood* 1989;73(6):1720–1728.
50. Le Blanc R, Montminy-Metivier S, Belanger R, et al. Allogeneic transplantation for multiple myeloma: further evidence for a GVHD-associated graft-versus-myeloma effect. *Bone Marrow Transplant* 2001;28(9):841–848.
51. Brunet S, Urbano-Ispizua A, Ojeda E, et al. Favourable effect of the combination of acute and chronic graft-versus-host disease on the outcome of allogeneic peripheral blood stem cell transplantation for advanced haematological malignancies. *Br J Haematol* 2001;114(3):544–550.
52. Körbling M, Przepiorka D, Huh YO, et al. Allogeneic blood stem cell transplantation for refractory leukemia and lymphoma: potential advantage of blood over marrow allografts. *Blood* 1995;85(6):1659–1665.
53. Elmaagacli A, Beelen DW, Opalka B, et al. The risk of residual molecular and cytogenetic disease in patients with Philadelphia-chromosome positive first chronic phase chronic myelogenous leukemia is reduced after transplantation of allogeneic peripheral blood stem cells compared with bone marrow. *Blood* 1999;94(2):384–389.
54. Elmaagacli AH, Basoglu S, Peceny R, et al. Improved disease-free-survival after transplantation of peripheral blood stem cells as compared with bone marrow from HLA-identical unrelated donors in patients with first chronic phase chronic myeloid leukemia. *Blood* 2002;99(4):1130–1135.
55. Corradini P, Voena C, Tarella C, et al. Molecular and clinical remissions in multiple myeloma: role of autologous and allogeneic transplantation of hematopoietic cells. *J Clin Oncol* 1999;17(1):208–215.
56. Powles R, Mehta J, Treleaven J, et al. Blood or BM for allogeneic transplantation from HLA-identical siblings? Extended follow-up of a randomized study confirms significantly higher relapse with BM. *Blood* 2000;96(11):196a [Abstract].
57. Hochberg EP, Chillemi AC, Wu CJ, et al. Quantitation of T-cell neogenesis in vivo after allogeneic bone marrow transplantation in adults. *Blood* 2001;98(4):1116–1121.
58. Wu CJ, Chillemi A, Alyea EP, et al. Reconstitution of T-cell receptor repertoire diversity following T-cell depleted allogeneic bone marrow transplantation is related to hematopoietic chimerism. *Blood* 2000;95(1):352–359.
59. Fujimaki K, Maruta A, Yoshida M, et al. Immune reconstitution assessed during five years after allogeneic bone marrow transplantation. *Bone Marrow Transplant* 2001;27(12):1275–1281.

60. Shenoy S, Mohanakumar T, Todd G, et al. Immune reconstitution following allogeneic peripheral blood stem cell transplants. *Bone Marrow Transplant* 1999;23(4):335–346.
61. Maury S, Mary JY, Rabian C, et al. Prolonged immune deficiency following allogeneic stem cell transplantation: risk factors and complications in adult patients. *Br J Haematol* 2001;115(3):630–641.
62. Storek J, Gooley T, Witherspoon RP, et al. Infectious morbidity in long-term survivors of allogeneic marrow transplantation is associated with low CD4 T cell counts. *Am J Hematol* 1997;54(2):131–138.
63. Storek J, Espino G, Dawson MA, et al. Low B-cell and monocyte counts on day 80 are associated with high infection rates between days 100 and 365 after allogeneic marrow transplantation. *Blood* 2000;96(9):3290–3293.
64. Tayebi H, Tiberghien P, Ferrand C, et al. Allogeneic peripheral blood stem cell transplantation results in less alteration of early T cell compartment homeostasis than bone marrow transplantation. *Bone Marrow Transplant* 2001;27(2):167–175.
65. Storek J, Dawson MA, Storer B, et al. Immune reconstitution after allogeneic marrow transplantation compared with blood stem cell transplantation. *Blood* 2001;97(11):3380–3389.
66. Storek J, Witherspoon RP, Maloney DG, et al. Improved reconstitution of CD4 T cells and B cells but worsened reconstitution of serum IgG levels after allogeneic transplantation of blood stem cells instead of marrow. *Blood* 1997;89(10):3891–3893.
67. Ottinger HD, Beelen DW, Scheulen B, et al. Improved immune reconstitution after allotransplantation of peripheral blood stem cells instead of bone marrow. *Blood* 1996;88(7):2775–2779.
68. Trenschel R, Bernier M, Delforge A, et al. Myeloid and lymphoid recovery following allogeneic bone marrow transplantation: a comparative study between related, unrelated bone marrow and allogeneic peripheral stem cell transplantation. *Leuk Lymphoma* 1998;30(3–4):325–352.
69. Zhang XF, Wang JF, Matczak E, et al. Janus kinase 2 is involved in stromal cell-derived factor-1alpha-induced tyrosine phosphorylation of focal adhesion proteins and migration of hematopoietic progenitor cells. *Blood* 2001;97(11):3342–3348.
70. Link DC. Mechanisms of granulocyte colony-stimulating factor-induced hematopoietic progenitor-cell mobilization. *Semin Hematol* 2000;37(1, suppl 2):25–32.
71. Steidl U, Kronenwett R, Rohr UP, et al. Gene expression profiling identifies significant differences between the molecular phenotypes of bone marrow-derived and circulating human CD34(+) hematopoietic stem cells. *Blood* 2002;99(6):2037–2044.
72. Gyger M, Stuart RK, Perreault C. Immunobiology of allogeneic peripheral blood mononuclear cells mobilized with granulocyte-colony stimulating factor. *Bone Marrow Transplant* 2000;26:1–16.
73. Zeng D, Dejbakhash-Jones S, Strober S. Granulocyte colony-stimulating factor reduces the capacity of blood mononuclear cells to induce graft-versus-host disease: impact on blood progenitor cell transplantation. *Blood* 1997;90(1):453–463.
74. Pan L, Delmonte J Jr, Jalonen CK, et al. Pretreatment of donor mice with granulocyte colony-stimulating factor polarizes donor T lymphocytes toward type-2 cytokine production and reduces severity of experimental graft-versus-host disease. *Blood* 1995;86(12):4422–4429.
75. Arpinati M, Green CL, Heimfeld S, et al. Granulocyte-colony stimulating factor mobilizes T helper 2-inducing dendritic cells. *Blood* 2000;95:2484–2490.
76. Reddy V, Hill GR, Pan L, et al. G-CSF modulates cytokine profile of dendritic cells and decreases acute graft-versus-host disease through effects on the donor rather than the recipient. *Transplantion* 2000;69(4):691–693.
77. Zeng D, Hoffmann P, Lan F, et al. Unique patterns of surface receptors, cytokine secretion, and immune functions distinguish T cells in the bone marrow from those in the periphery: impact on allogeneic bone marrow transplantation. *Blood* 2002;99(4):1449–1457.
78. Atkinson K, Farrelly H, Cooley M, et al. Human marrow T cell dose correlates with severity of subsequent acute graft-versus-host disease. *Bone Marrow Transplant* 1987;2(1):51–57.
79. Kernan NA, Collins NH, Juliano L, et al. Clonable T lymphocytes in T cell-depleted bone marrow transplants correlate with development of graft-v-host disease. *Blood* 1986;68(3):770–773.
80. Anderlini P, Przepiorka D, Lauppe J, et al. Collection of peripheral blood stem cells from normal donors 60 years of age or older. *Br J Haematol* 1997;97(2):485–487.
81. Becker PS, Wagle M, Matous S, et al. Spontaneous splenic rupture following administration of granulocyte colony-stimulating factor (G-CSF): occurrence in an allogeneic donor of peripheral blood stem cells. *Biol Blood Marrow Transplant* 1997;3(1):45–49.
82. de la Rubia J, Martinez C, Solano C, et al. Administration of recombinant human granulocyte colony-stimulating factor to normal donors: results of the Spanish National Donor Registry. *Bone Marrow Transplant* 1999;24(7):723–728.

83. Cavallaro AM, Lilleby K, Majolino I, et al. Three to six year follow-up of normal donors who received recombinant human granulocyte colony-stimulating factor. *Bone Marrow Transplant* 2000;25:85–89.
84. Anderlini P, Rizzo JD, Nugent ML, et al. Peripheral blood stem cell donation: an analysis from the International Bone Marrow Transplant Registry (IBMTR) and European Group for Blood and Marrow Transplant (EBMT) databases. *Bone Marrow Transplant* 2001;27(7):689–692.
85. Rowley SD, Donaldson G, Lilleby K, et al. Experiences of donors enrolled in a randomized study of allogeneic bone marrow or peripheral blood stem cell transplantation. *Blood* 2001;97(9):2541–2548.
86. Auquier P, Macquart-Moulin G, Moatti JP, et al. Comparison of anxiety, pain and discomfort in two procedures of hematopoietic stem cell collection: leukacytapheresis and bone marrow harvest. *Bone Marrow Transplant* 1995;16:541–547.
87. Nishimori M, Yamada Y, Hoshi K, et al. Health-related quality of life of unrelated bone marrow donors in Japan. *Blood* 2002;99(6):1995–2001.
88. Couban S, Messner HA, Andreou P, et al. Bone marrow mobilized with granulocyte colony-stimulating factor in related allogeneic transplant recipients: a study of 29 patients. *Biol Blood Marrow Transplant* 2000;6(4A):422–427.
89. Link H, Arseniev L, Bahre O, et al. Combined transplantation of allogeneic bone marrow and CD34+ blood cells. *Blood* 1995;86(7):2500–2508.
90. Szer J, Curtis DJ, Bardy PG, et al. The addition of allogeneic peripheral blood-derived progenitor cells to bone marrow for transplantation: results of a randomised clinical trial. *Aust NZ J Med* 1999;29(4):487–493.
91. Morton J, Hutchins C, Durrant S. Granulocyte-colony-stimulating factor (G-CSF)-primed allogeneic bone marrow: significantly less graft-versus-host disease and comparable engraftment to G-CSF-mobilized peripheral blood stem cells. *Blood* 2001;98(12):3186–3191.
92. Ji SQ, Chen HR , Xun CQ, et al. The effect of G-CSF-stimulated donor marrow on engraftment and incidence of graft-versus-host disease in allogeneic bone marrow transplantation. *Clin Transplant* 2001;15(5):317–323.
93. Isola L, Scigliano E, Fruchtman S. Long-term follow-up after allogeneic granulocyte colony-stimulating factor-primed bone marrow transplantation. *Biol Blood Marrow Transplant* 2000;6:428–433.
94. Serody JS, Sparks SD, Lin Y, et al. Comparison of granulocyte colony-stimulating factor (G-CSF)-mobilized peripheral blood progenitor cells and G-CSF-stimulated bone marrow as a source of stem cells in HLA-matched sibling transplantation. *Biol Blood Marrow Transplant* 2000;6:434–440.

16 Allogeneic Unrelated Donor Blood and Marrow Transplantation

Daniel Weisdorf, MD

CONTENTS

1. INTRODUCTION

Allogeneic stem cell transplantation (alloSCT) can provide curative therapy for patients with hematologic malignancies, marrow failures states, severe immunodeficiencies, hemoglobinopathies, and inherited metabolic diseases *(1–8)*. Unfortunately, only approx 25–30% of patients will have a suitable human leukocyte antigen (HLA) genotypically identical sibling donor available to facilitate transplant therapy. An extensive family search may find a closely matched related donors for only 3–5% of patients; thus, in the 1970s, consideration was first given toward searching for coincidently HLA-matched unrelated donors (URD) *(1–3)*. In the early 1980s, registries of volunteer marrow donors were established in Europe and North America, but the extreme polymorphism of the HLA system and the immunodominant gene products of the major histocompatibility complex (MHC) as well as differential frequencies of HLA phenotypes in different populations indicated a requirement for volunteer donor registries of substantial size and great genetic diversity. Over 50 national registries exist in all continents, including the National Marrow Donor Program (NMDP) in the United States and the Anthony Nolan Research Centre Registry in the United Kingdom, which allow expedited searching for donors among well over 5 million registered volunteer donors.

After 15 yr experience, the US NMDP currently lists over 4.7 million donors with extensive HLA typing (HLA-A, -B, and DRB1) for nearly 3 million. Donor searching is facilitated by electronic communication, Internet access, and the multinational linkage of cooperating donor registries, including Bone Marrow Donors Worldwide. The extreme diversity of HLA could theoretically yield many millions of possible HLA phenotypes; yet, under 500,000 distinct

From: *Stem Cell Transplantation for Hematologic Malignancies*
Edited by: R. J. Soiffer © Humana Press Inc., Totowa, NJ

HLA-A, -B, and DRB1 phenotypes are represented in the several million donors available for searching.

Great efforts have been made to broaden the ethnic diversity of donor registry files. However, the nonrandom linkage disequilibrium associations of certain HLA phenotypes in specific ethnic groups and the somewhat greater diversity of HLA polymorphism in black and Hispanic individuals compared to northern and western European-derived Caucasians or other genetically more restricted populations such as Japanese donors yield differential chances of finding a donor for patients of different and racial ethnic background.

2. DONOR SELECTION

2.1. Chances of Finding a Donor

Currently, searching through the NMDP can identify at least one HLA-A, -B, and DRB1 matched donor for 78% of Caucasians, 38% of African-Americans, 55% of Hispanic, and 54% of Asian–Pacific Islander populations. Because donor availability and medical suitability for donation further limit these options, the likelihood of a medically suitable available HLA-A, -B, and DRB1 matched donor are somewhat lower. At present, through the NMDP, suitably matched and available donors are identifiable for approx 73% of Caucasians, 25% of African-Americans, 69% of Hispanics, and 65% Asian–Pacific Islanders *(9)*. Encouragingly, if initial searching identifies more than five donors potentially compatible, the chances of a well-matched, available donor are much greater, even for the racial and ethnic minorities.

2.2. Donor Searching

Although facilitated electronically and expedited through the experienced and committed network of the NMDP and similar cooperating donor registries worldwide, searching still requires an average of 6–8 wk to identify a donor and a total median time of 10–12 wk to proceed to transplant. Donor contact, counseling, medical evaluation, informed consent, precollection donation of autologous red cell units prior to marrow harvest as well as scheduling, logistics between transplant and donor center, medical complications, and preparation of the recipient all contribute to these delays. Ongoing efforts within all cooperating registries are continuing to expedite these logistical and administrative steps. Enhancing the rapid availability of donors for patients in urgent need have gradually shortened, but not eliminated these practical delays. Aggressive pilot studies at the NMDP have been able to shorten the search time to only 3–4 wk. Recognition of the time required for donor searching is an added element in the choices of alternative therapies and additional treatment options. This time must be considered in order to improve clinical decision-making, particularly for patients with acute leukemia or other pressing clinical conditions where remissions and thus the suitable period for transplantation may be brief.

2.3. Histocompatibility Matching

The highly polymorphic genes of the MHC defined two major classes relevant for donor selection. Class I antigens include HLA-A, -B, and -C, whereas class II includes HLA-DR, -DQ, and -DP antigens. Original typing techniques using allo-antisera have been, in large part, replaced with DNA-based typing as the gene products and protein structure of HLA alleles have been defined. Certain allelic polymorphisms are recognized by T cells with exquisite specificity and can elicit alloantigenic responses in response to alleles differing by only a single amino acid at appropriate components of an HLA epitope. HLA antigens inherited from a parent (one-half of the chromosome 6 pair) are referred as to as an HLA haplotype. Haplotype structure is preserved across extended haplotypes, which show positive linkage disequilibrium. Particularly within families or in racial and minority ethnic populations, linkage frequencies between specific antigens occur considerably more often than chance, thus increasing the likelihood of identifying common haplotypes even in unrelated individuals. Although initial definition of a satisfactory donor suggested that serologically defined matching at HLA-A and -B and later allele level matching at HLA-DRB1 was satisfactory, newer information has suggested the importance of matching at additional loci (HLA-C, HLA-DQ, and HLA-DP) and at higher resolution (matching at the allele level) *(2,10–25)*. Although earlier reports suggested that partial-matched, unrelated-donor transplantation, differing at only a single class I antigen or a single DRB1 allele, could yield satisfactory clinical results, following these partial-matched transplants increasing risks of graft failure and graft-vs-host disease (GVHD) have been recognized *(11,27,28)*. Recent analyses confirm the importance of closer matching. A recent analysis from the NMDP confirms the importance of matching at HLA-A, -B, -C, and -DRB1 to identify optimal outcome *(26)*. Mismatching at a single class I or DRB1 locus led to more frequent graft failure, more frequent GVHD, and poorer survival. Multiple mismatches led to even poorer results. Of greatest importance was the recognition that allele level matching at class I, similar to allele matching at HLA-DRB1, conferred added protection against the major posttransplant complications.

Importantly however, close, although still only partial-matched URD transplants (mismatched at a single class I allele or at a single DRB1 allele) led to results nearly as good as fully matched transplants and should not be regarded as imperfect or unsatisfactory matches *(19,20,26)*. Particularly for racial and ethnic minorities, where fully matched donors may be hard to identify and available, closely matched (but only single-allele-level mismatched) donors may yield satisfactory clinical outcomes. Transplants using serologically defined single-antigen mismatches, particularly for adults, may yield poorer results because unrecognized multiple-allele-level mismatches may exist unless high-resolution class I and DRB1 typing is performed.

3. APPLICATIONS OF ALLOGENEIC UNRELATED DONOR TRANSPLANTATION

Broad categories of hematologic malignancies, nonmalignant hematologic disorders, metabolic disorders, immunodeficiencies, and other malignant diseases have been treated with URD transplantation (*see* Table 1). Although experience is greatest in chronic myelogenous leukemia and acute leukemia, other illnesses have been studied. The quality of available data is based on the disease rarity and the international experience evaluating this technique.

3.1. Clinical Results

In general, URD transplantation has been performed using similar clinical approaches to HLA-identical sibling transplants, including combinations of high-dose chemotherapy and/or total-body irradiation for pretransplant conditioning and pharmacologic immunosuppression for graft-vs-host disease (GVHD) prophylaxis after transplantation (*see* Table 2). Numerous reports suggest that URD marrow transplantation yields high (90–95%) rates of engraftment but slightly higher risks of graft failure compared to HLA-identical sibling donor transplan-

Table 1
Diseases Treatable With Unrelated Donor Allogeneic Hematopoietic Stem Cell Transplantation

Nonmalignant diseases
Severe aplastic anemia
Hemoglobinopathy and thalassemia
Immune deficiencies
Metabolic storage diseases
Malignant diseases
Acute myeloid leukemia
Acute lymphoblastic leukemia
Chronic myelogenous leukemia
Juvenile myelomonocytic leukemia
Non-Hodgkin's lymphoma
Chronic lymphocytic leukemia
Multiple myeloma

tation *(1,11,39–41)*. Similarly, GVHD, peritransplant and posttransplant infectious complications, and treatment-related mortality may be substantively higher with URD transplantation compared to sibling donor transplants *(11,39–41)*. Initial series reporting results of URD transplantation described disease-free survival (DFS) for patients with well-matched donors of 40–60% for patients with favorable prognosis disease and 20–35% for those with more advanced, high-risk diseases *(1,3,4,7,10)*. Results were better for younger recipients, those with more closely matched URD, and those with favorable, pretransplant performance status.

3.2. Complications of Unrelated Donor Transplant

Using even well-matched URDs, primary graft failure of 1–7% and secondary graft failure of 3–5% have been reported *(11,27,28)*. Closer HLA matching, a higher nucleated cell dose, and, perhaps importantly, a graft containing a higher dose of CD34 positive cells may all be associated with rapid and sustained engraftment following URD transplantation *(7,42)*. Acute and chronic GVHD have been more frequent and possibly more therapy resistant in recipients of URD transplantation compared to those receiving sibling donor transplants *(1,11,39–43)*. Acute GVHD rates of 40–90% and chronic GVHD rates of 50–80% have been described. Lower risks of GVHD have been observed with closer HLA matching, T-lymphocyte depletion of the donor graft, non-allo-immune (by via pregnancy or transfusion) donors, younger recipients, and, intriguingly, younger donors as well *(44)*.

3.3. Infectious Morbidity

Severe early and late infections have been recognized more commonly after URD transplantation. Only limited formal studies of their immune reconstitution have been reported *(45–47)*. The greater incidence of acute and chronic GVHD as well as functionally delayed immune reconstitution following URD transplantation may necessitate more intensive and extended antibacterial, antiviral, and antifungal prophylaxis.

3.4. Immune Reconstitution

Immune recognition and protective immune response against foreign microbial peptides is most efficiently initiated when presented by self HLA, but not by allogeneic HLA molecules. This HLA-restricted interaction between antigen-presenting cells (APCs), naïve T cells, and effector immune cells (B lineage and T lineage) may be confounded in recipients of URD transplantation. Donor marrow-derived T cells, emanating from the transplanted hematopoietic stem cells, must be educated and directed to interact with host APCs, initially by host dendritic cells, and possibly by residual host thymic elements. Disruption of host antigen-presenting function and thymic epithelium by chemotherapy and radiation conditioning regimen may further deplete the capacity for this host and donor T-cell interaction, thereby compromising or delaying development of an effective multiparameter immune defense against infection. Further, the development of GVHD and its necessary immunosuppressive therapy prolongs the immuno-incompetence of the transplant recipient. Delay in development of antibody diversity, total antibody production, CD4 T-cell numbers and effective T-cell recognition, proliferation, and memory to mount an appropriate immune response may be delayed *(45–47)*. It takes up to 3–6 mo after transplantation for antibody development and 6–12 mo for an effective T-cell response. Donor/recipient HLA disparity, clinical GVHD, and extended immunosuppressive therapy may extend this recovery interval even further. Recent clinical recognition of late infections, both viral and fungal, even in the non-neutropenic host underscores the importance of this delayed immune reconstitution, which is more profound and longer in the URD recipient. Extended infectious disease prophylaxis and ongoing surveillance for opportunistic infection (particularly cytomegalovirus, fungi, and *Pneumocystis carinii*) is required.

Recognition of later posttransplant infections may be particularly important in URD recipients. One report from the University of Minnesota identified more frequent late infections, even in unrelated donor recipients without GVHD, compared to recipients of HLA-matched sibling donor transplantation *(48)*.

3.5. Protection Against Relapse

The greater donor/host disparity that might augment hazards of GVHD may, in turn, promote a more powerful graft-vs-leukemia (GVL) response and better protection against relapse. Clinically demonstrable GVL appears most frequent in those with clinically recognized GVHD, particularly chronic GVHD. Some series have corroborated the comparison of posttransplant relapse rates in sibling vs URD recipients *(11,28,39–41)*. After adjustment for GVHD incidence and severity, modestly better protection against relapse was observed after URD transplantation. This may differ in different disease settings that express inherently different sensitivity to the immunologically based GVL effect *(29–31,33,49–51)*. Chronic myelogenous leukemia (CML) is most sensitive to GVL and experience to date suggests a particularly low rate of relapse following URD transplantation, at least for transplants performed in the early chronic phase *(6,28,39,43)*. More advanced CML, acute lymphoblastic leukemia (ALL), and other aggressive malignancies may be less well contained by the URD GVL effect. Notably, however, unrelated donor lymphocyte infusions (DLIs) have demonstrable efficacy in inducing durable remissions when infused following relapse after URD bone marrow transplant (BMT) *(52)*.

Table 2
Clinical Results of Unrelated Donor Transplantation

Disease Author (ref.)	*n*	*Age (yr) median (range)*	*Acute GVHD*[a] *Grade III-IV*	*Nonrelapse mortality*	*Relapse*[a]	*Survival*[b]
CML						
Weisdorf *(28)*	2464	36 (1–62)	Matched 35%	N.R.	Chronic phase 5%	Matched 45% 5 yr
			Partial matched 49%		AP/BP 18%	Partial matched 31% 5 yr
AML						
Sierra *(7)*	74	20 (1–54)	47%	39%		
	CR1/2+ 21				CR1/2 20–22%	38–58% 5-yr DFS
	Rel 53				Rel 40–70%	15–18% DFS
ALL						
Corneissen *(29)*	127		31%	CR 54%	6%	32% 4 yr
	CR1 64	31 (16–54)		CR 2/3 75	8	17% 2 yr
	CR2/3 16	27 (17–51)		Rel 64	31	5% 2 yr
	Rel 47	36 (19–51)				
						5% 2 yr
Bunin *(30)*	363	9 (0–19)	29%	42%	22%	36% 5 yr DFS
Weisdorf *(31)*	517	14	—	42%	CR1 14%	CR1 51% 3 yr
					CR2 25%	CR2 40% 3 yr

(continued on on next page)

Woolfrey	88	9 (0–18)	Matched 43%	CR1 20%	10%	CR1 70%
			Partial matched 59%	CR2 22%	33%	CR2 46%
				CR3 60%	20%	CR3 20%
				Rel 41%	50%	Rel 9%
MDS						
Castro-Malaspina *(32)*	510	38 (1–62)	47% (II–IV)	54% (2 yr)	14% (2 yr)	29% 2-yr DFS
Arnold *(33)*	118	24 (0–53)	47% (II–IV)	58%	35%	28% 2-yr DFS
Aplastic anemia						
Deeg *(34)*	50	14 (0–46)	61% (II–IV)	—	—	58% 2 yr
Deeg *(35)*	141		52% (II–IV)	—	—	36% 3 yr
Kojima *(36)*	154	17 (1–46)	20%	—	—	56% 5 yr
Unrelated donor cord blood vs BM for acute leukemia						
Rocha *(37)*	UCB 99	6 (2.5–10)	22%	39% 100 d	38%	31% 2-yr DFS
	BM 442	8 (5–12)	30%	17% 100 d	44%	43% 2-yr DFS
Barker *(38)*[c]	UCB 31	6 (1–18)	19%	NR	—	53% 2-yr survival
	BM 31	7 (0–17)	8%	NR	—	41% 2-yr survival

[a]Cumulative incidence or Kaplan–Meier incidence.
[b]Survival or DFS, disease-free survival.
[c]Not all acute leukemia.
Abbreviations: CP, chronic phase; AP/BP, accelerated phase/blast phase; CR, complete remission; UCB, umbilical cord blood; BM, bone marrow; CML, chronic myelogenous leukemia; AML, acute myelogenous leukemia; ALL, acute lymphoblastic leukemia; MDS, myelodysplastic syndrome.

4. SURVIVAL AFTER TRANSPLANTATION

4.1. Aplastic Anemia and Nonmalignant Disease

Although most patients with aplastic anemia receive immunosuppressive therapy as initial treatment, URD transplantation can yield encouraging results and eradication of their aplasia for a sizable fraction of patients (*see* Table 2). In recent reports, 40–50% of patients survive after URD transplantation, offering encouraging options for those who fail initial immunosuppressive therapy *(35,36)*. Modification of conditioning regimens may reduce the peritransplant toxicity even further and increase the success of such treatment *(34)*. Severe childhood immunodeficiencies can be well contained after transplantation, particularly classical severe combined immunodeficiency (SCID); variant immunodeficiency states have been successfully treated as well *(5,47,53)*. Inherited metabolic disorders *(54,55)*, hemoglobinopathies, and thalassemia *(56)* have sometimes been treated with URD transplantation, although difficulties with sustained engraftment, hazards of GVHD, and peritransplant morbidity and mortality have limited more broad application of URD transplantation for these disorders.

4.2. Acute Myeloid Leukemia

Paralleling the successes of sibling donor transplants for acute leukemia, patients with acute myeloid leukemia (AML) and ALL have been successfully treated with URD transplantation *(7,42,49)*. AML patients in second complete remission (CR2) have been regularly treated with well-matched URD and 30–40% of adults enjoy long-term leukemia-free survival (LFS) (*see* Fig. 1). Outcomes in children are more favorable, with 40–60% of patients alive many years posttransplantation. For patients with AML in CR1 with high-risk characteristics, autologous transplantation or ongoing consolidation and maintenance chemotherapy have proven to be useful. A recent analysis comparing autologous transplantation from the Autologous Bone Marrow Transplant Registry to multicenter experience from the NMDP suggests a modest survival advantage for autotransplants both in first and second remissions compared to URD BMT *(57)*. The excessive morbidity and mortality accompanying GVHD and posttransplant infection overcame the profoundly better protection against relapse accompanying the URD transplants. Newer advances encompassing better donor selection, modifications of GVHD prevention, and granulocyte colony-stimulating factor (G-CSF)-mobilized peripheral blood stem cells may enhance the outcomes of URD transplantation and require revisiting comparisons with autografts.

Myelodysplastic syndromes (MDSs) have also been treated with URD transplantation *(32,33)*. Posttransplant relapse rates are low (14%), but, disappointingly, related mortality is high (54%). Overall 29% 5-yr DFS was reported in one large series from the NMDP *(32)*.

4.3. Acute Lymphoblastic Leukemia

In ALL, similar URD transplant experience has been extensively analyzed *(8,29–31,39,41,51,58)*. Whereas high-risk ALL [e.g., t(4;11), t(9;22)], extreme leukocytosis, or mature-B-cell ALL have inadequate results following conventional, even aggressive chemotherapy, allotransplantation from URD can protect against relapse and yield extended LFS for a sizable fraction of children and a modest number of adults. Several series of Philadelphia chromosome-positive (Ph+) ALL report 40-50% extended DFS after URD transplantation. For patients lacking a sibling donor, this is now recognized as the treatment of choice *(29,58)*.

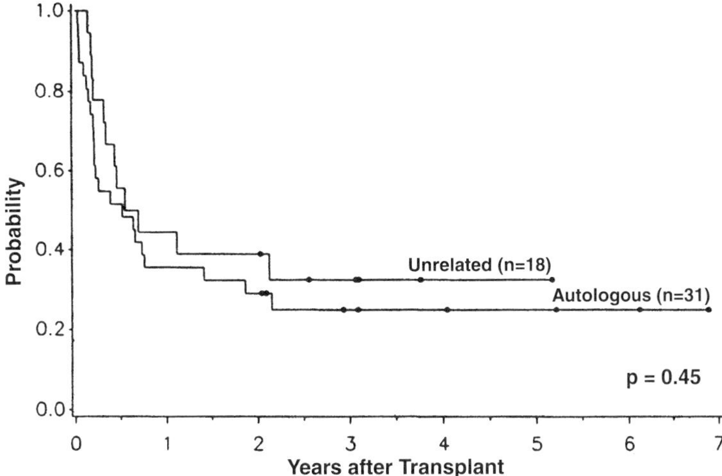

Fig. 1. Survival after URD BMT for AML Comparison with autologous transplantation is shown. (Adapted from ref. *49*.)

Autotransplantation, less widely used for ALL than for AML, has been contrasted with URD transplantation as well for patients lacking sibling donors. An earlier report from the University of Minnesota and Dana–Farber Cancer Institute compared autografts to URD experience through the NMDP *(8)*. In that analysis, similar outcomes were observed for most patients. Adjusted multivariate analysis could not define a particular cohort definitively benefiting from the allogeneic approach. A more recent report comparing ABMTR autograft experience vs NMDP URD transplants demonstrated superior DFS for standard-risk ALL in second or later remission compared to autotransplantation (*see* Fig. 2) *(31)*. Disappointingly, high-risk ALL (short initial remission, white blood cell [WBC] > 50,000/μL at diagnosis) was not better protected against relapse by the URD allograft. For this group, survival was unsatisfactory after both URD BMT and autotransplantation. Children and adults with high-risk ALL have been reported from the NMDP to have satisfactory outcomes after URD transplantation *(29,30,51)*. Thirty-six to 46% of children and 20–40% of adults with high-risk features are alive without relapse more than 3 yr following transplantation. As mentioned earlier, improvements in URD selection and peritransplant management may yield greater advances in their outcome.

4.4. Chronic Myelogenous Leukemia

Before imatinib (Gleevec) changed the initial management strategies for nearly all patients with CML, URD transplantation was the only curative option for those lacking a matched sibling donor *(6,28,43)*. Decision analyses suggested a survival advantage for the application of URD transplantation compared to extended interferon therapy *(59)* and some reports recognized the adverse impact of pretransplant interferon on the outcome of URD BMT *(60–62)*. Numerous series have documented the efficacy of URD BMT for treatment of CML, particularly in the chronic phase *(6,28,43)*, and cost analyses have supported its cost-effectiveness *(63)*. One report from the NMDP identified 63% of young, early chronic-phase patients surviving leukemia-free more than 3 yr posttransplantation *(6)*. Recent comparisons of URD to sibling transplantation suggested slightly, although statistically significantly superior survival

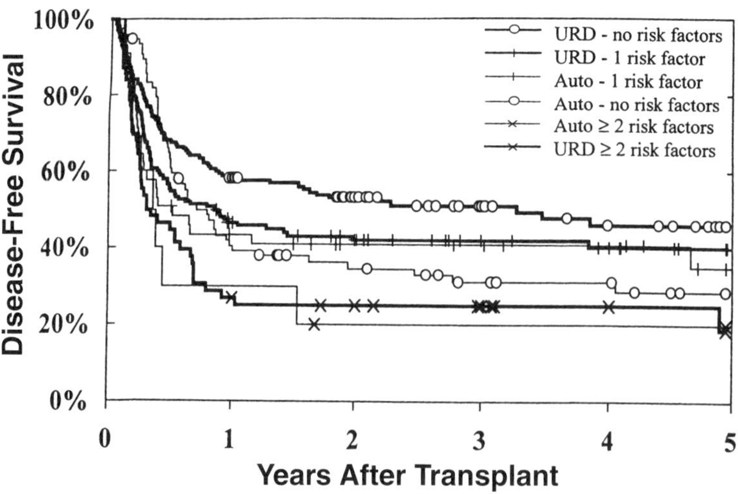

Fig. 2. Disease-free survival after autologous vs URD BMT for ALL. Superior outcome for URD BMT with standard-risk disease (WBC < 50,000/μL; CR1 > 1-yr duration; performance status 90%). (Adapted from ref. *31*.)

for recipients of sibling donor BMT compared to URD BMT *(28,40)*. Importantly, the well-recognized hazard of delay in time to transplantation exacted a greater reduction in survival after URD transplantation than sibling donor BMT for patients in several age cohorts *(28)*. As shown in Fig. 3, delay for between 1 and 2 yr postdiagnosis had little impact on survival after sibling donor transplantation, whereas 8% and 10% fewer patients survived with 1 and 2+ yr delay for recipients of unrelated donor transplantation. The pathophysiology of this added hazard resulting from delay from diagnosis to transplantation is uncertain. This complicates its application for clinical decision-making and further confounds the clinical dilemma facing patients with newly diagnosed CML. Young patients, expected to have a high clinical response rate to imatinib therapy, might similarly expect 60% 5-yr LFS after URD BMT if a well-matched URD donor is identified and the transplant is performed in the early chronic phase. Patients aged 30–40 or older than 40 can expect slightly poorer outcomes (40–50% 5-yr LFS after URD BMT) and may better accept the uncertainties of delay in contrast to the immediate hazards of an early transplant. Longer follow-up to assess the durability of response to imatinib is still awaited. In addition, longer experience will address any clinical impact of pretransplant imatinib on allotransplants for patients with CML. Cautious and careful analyses of these comparative treatments will still be required to guide the complex and sometimes anguished decision-making for asymptomatic patients with CML who have no sibling donor.

5. FUTURE MODIFICATIONS

Overall, peritransplant and nonrelapse mortality is substantially higher following URD transplant compared to sibling donor approaches. For good-risk patients with early disease, nonrelapse mortality of 20–40% has been described, but for patients with diagnoses other than CML, many series report nonrelapse mortality attributable to the complications of URD transplant up to 40–50%. Substantive advances in GVHD prophylaxis and management, interventions to facilitate and accelerate immune reconstitution, and more effective and longer duration

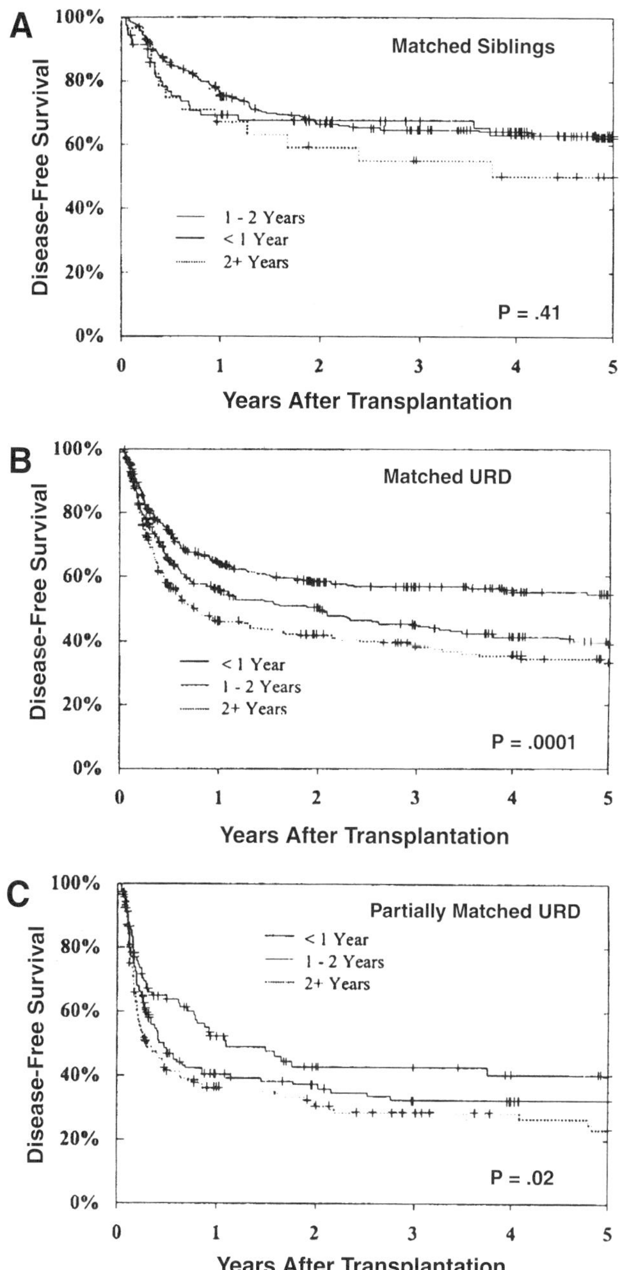

Fig. 3. Five-year disease-free survival after sibling vs URD BMT for CML in the chronic phase: poorer outcome with delayed URD transplantation. (Adapted from ref. *28*.)

infectious disease prophylaxis will be required to reduce these hazards and improve the safety of URD transplantation overall.

Changes in donor-selection criteria to identify better matched and potentially more suitable URD requires more study and more clinical experience. Defining the optimal histocompatibility criteria for matching may only identify a smaller cohort of patients able to enjoy the benefits of a well-matched donor while underscoring or actually increasing the minority populations inadequately aided by the donor search and identification process of the worldwide donor registries. New advances in umbilical cord blood transplants, which potentially permit safe transplantation across greater histocompatibility barriers and tolerating even two HLA antigen differences, require ongoing experience, particularly for larger children and adult recipients *(37,38,64–67)*. Application of URD transplantation using G-CSF-mobilized peripheral blood might realize the same advantages accompanying sibling donor PBSC allotransplantation *(68,69)*, yet the uncertainty of chronic GVHD risks and the accompanying extended morbidity are inadequately understood and represent a major obstacle to a broader application of URD blood SCT.

Unrelated donor transplantation is a fabulous clinical experiment. It taps the wealth of generosity manifest in the donation of hematopoietic stem cells from unrelated and anonymous distant volunteers and has been life-saving for many and hope-sustaining for an even greater number still searching for a donor. Advances in the clinical science will broaden these opportunities and enrich the outcomes of patients in years to come.

REFERENCES

1. Kernan NA, Bartsch G, Ash RC, et al. Analysis of 462 transplantations from unrelated donors facilitated by the National Marrow Donor Program. *N Engl J Med* 1993;328:593–602.
2. Hansen JA, Clift RA, Thomas ED, et al. Transplantation of marrow from an unrelated donor to a patient with acute leukemia. *N Engl J Med* 1980;303:565–567.
3. Ash RC, Casper JT, Chitambar CR, et al. Successful allogeneic transplantation of T-cell-depleted bone marrow from closely HLA-matched unrelated donors. *N Engl J Med* 1990;322:485–494.
4. Barker JN, Davies SM, DeFor TE, et al. Determinants of survival after human leucocyte antigen-matched unrelated donor bone marrow transplantation in adults. *Br J Haematol* 2002;118:101–107.
5. O'Reilly RJ, Dupont B, Pahwa S, et al. Reconstitution in severe combined immunodeficiency by transplantation of marrow from an unrelated donor. *N Engl J Med* 1977;297:1311–1318.
6. McGlave PB, Shu XO, Wen W, et al. Unrelated donor marrow transplantation for chronic myelogenous leukemia: 9 years experience of the National Marrow Donor Program. *Blood* 2000;95:2219–2225.
7. Sierra J, Storer B, Hansen JA, et al. Transplantation of marrow cells from unrelated donors for treatment of high-risk acute leukemia: the effect of leukemic burden, donor HLA matching and marrow cell dose. *Blood* 1997;89:4226–4235.
8. Weisdorf DJ, Billett AL, Hannan P, et al. Autologous versus unrelated donor allogeneic marrow transplantation for acute lymphoblastic leukemia. *Blood* 1997;90:2962–2968.
9. NMDP data; available at www@marrow.org.
10. Beatty PG, Anasetti C, Hansen JA, et al. Marrow transplantation from unrelated donors for treatment of hematologic malignancies: effect of mismatching for one HLA locus. *Blood* 1993;81:249–253.
11. Davies SM, Shu XO, Blazar BR, et al. Unrelated donor bone marrow transplantation: influence of HLA A and B incompatibility on outcome. *Blood* 1995;86:1636–1642.
12. Ferrara GB, Bacigalupo A, Lamparelli T, et al. Bone marrow transplantation from unrelated donors: the impact of mismatches with substitutions at position 116 of the human leukocyte antigen class I heavy chain. *Blood* 2001;98:3150–3155.
13. Morishima Y, Sasazuki T, Inoko H, et al. The clinical significance of human leukocyte antigen (HLA) allele compatibility in patients receiving a marrow transplant from serologically HLA-A, HLA-B, and HLA-DR matched unrelated donors. *Blood* 2002;99:4200–4206.
14. Petersdorf EW, Gooley T, Malkki M, et al. The biological significance of HLA-DP gene variation in haematopoietic cell transplantation. *Br J Haematol* 2001;112:988–994.
15. Petersdorf EW, Gooley TA, Anasetti C, et al. Optimizing outcome after unrelated marrow transplantation by comprehensive matching of HLA class I and II alleles in the donor and recipient. *Blood* 1998;92:3515–3520.

16. Petersdorf EW, Kollman C, Hurley CK, et al. Effect of HLA class II gene disparity on clinical outcome in unrelated donor hematopoietic cell transplantation for chronic myeloid leukemia: the US National Marrow Donor Program experience. *Blood* 2001;98:2922–2929.
17. Petersdorf EW, Longton GM, Anasetti C, et al. Association of HLA-C disparity with graft failure after marrow transplantation from unrelated donors. *Blood* 1997;89:1818–1823.
18. Petersdorf EW, Longton GM, Anasetti C, et al. Definition of HLA-DQ as a transplantation antigen. *Proc Natl Acad Sci USA* 1996;93:15,358–15,363.
19. Petersdorf EW, Longton GM, Anasetti C, et al. The significance of HLA-DRB1 matching on clinical outcome after HLA-A, B, DR identical unrelated donor marrow transplantation. *Blood* 1995;86:1606–1613.
20. Petersdorf EW. Major histocompatibility complex class I alleles and antigens in hematopoietic cell transplantation. *N Engl J Med* 2001;345:1794–1800.
21. Prasad VK, Heller G, Kernan NA, et al. The probability of HLA-C matching between patient and unrelated donor at the molecular level: estimations based on the linkage disequilibrium between DNA typed HLA-B and HLA-C alleles. *Transplantation* 1999;68:1044–1050.
22. Santamaria P, Reinsmoen NL, Lindstrom AL, et al. Frequent HLA class I and DP sequence mismatches in serologically (HLA-A, HLA-B, HLA-DR) and molecularly (HLA-DRB1, HLA-DQA1, HLA-DQB1) HLA-identical unrelated bone marrow transplant pairs. *Blood* 1994;83:280–287.
23. Sasazuki T, Juji T, Morishima Y, et al. Effect of matching of class I HLA alleles on clinical outcome after transplantation of hematopoietic stem cells from an unrelated donor. From the Japan Marrow Donor Program. *N Engl J Med* 1998;339:1177–1185.
24. Schreuder GM, Hurley CK, Marsh SG, et al. The HLA dictionary 2001: a summary of HLA-A, -B, -C, -DRB1/3/4/5, -DQB1 alleles and their association with serologically defined HLA-A, -B, -C, -CR, and -DQ antigens. *Hum Immunol* 2001:62:826–849.
25. Scott I, O'Shea J, Bunce M, et al. Molecular typing shows a high level of HLA class I incompatibility in serologically well matched donor/patient pairs: implications for unrelated bone marrow donor selection. *Blood* 1998;92:4864–4871.
26. Flomenberg N, Baxter-Lowe LA, Confer D, et al. Impact of HLA class I and class II high resolution matching on outcomes of unrelated donor bone marrow transplantation: HLA-C mismatching is associated with a strong adverse effect on transplant outcome. Submitted.
27. Davies SM, Kollman C, Anasetti C, et al. Engraftment and survival after unrelated donor bone marrow transplantation: a report from the National Marrow Donor Program (NMDP). *Blood* 2000;96:4096–4102.
28. Weisdorf DJ, Anasetti C, Antin JH, et al. Allogeneic bone marrow transplantation for chronic myelogenous leukemia: comparative analysis of unrelated versus matched sibling donor transplantation. *Blood* 2002;99:1971–1977.
29. Cornelissen JJ, Carston M, Kollman C, et al. Unrelated marrow transplantation for adult patients with poor-risk acute lymphoblastic leukemia: strong graft-versus-leukemia effect and risk factors determining outcome. *Blood* 2001;97:1572–1577.
30. Bunin N, Carston M, Wall D, et al. Unrelated marrow transplantation for children with acute lymphoblastic leukemia in second remission. *Blood* 2002;99:3151–3157.
31. Weisdorf D, Bishop M, Dharan B, et al. Autologous versus allogeneic unrelated donor transplantation for acute lymphoblastic leukemia: comparative toxicity and outcomes. *Biol Blood Marrow Transplant* 2002;8:213–220.
32. Castro-Malaspina H, Harris RE, Gajewski J, et al. Unrelated donor marrow transplantation for myelodysplastic syndromes: outcome analysis in 510 transplants facilitated by the national Marrow Donor Program. *Blood* 2002;99:1943–1951.
33. Arnold R, de Witte T, van Biezen A, et al. Unrelated bone marrow transplantation in patients with myelodysplastic syndromes and secondary acute myeloid leukemia: an EBMT survey. European Blood and Marrow Transplantation Group. *Bone Marrow Transplant* 1998;21:1213–1216.
34. Deeg HJ, Amylon ID, Harris RE, et al. Marrow transplants from unrelated donors for patients with aplastic anemia: minimum effective dose of total body irradiation. *Biol Blood Marrow Transplant* 2001;7:208–215.
35. Deeg HJ, Seidel K, Casper J, et al. Marrow transplantation from unrelated donors for patients with severe aplastic anemia who have failed immunosuppressive therapy. *Biol Blood Marrow Transplant* 1999;5:243–252.
36. Kojima S, Matsuyama T, Kato S, et al. Outcome of 154 patients with severe aplastic anemia who received transplants from unrelated donors: the Japan Marrow Donor Program. *Blood* 2002;100:799–803.

37. Rocha V, Cornish J, Sievers EL, et al. Comparison of outcomes of unrelated bone marrow and umbilical cord blood transplants in children with acute leukemia. *Blood* 2001;97:2962–2971.
38. Barker JN, Davies SM, DeFor T, et al. Survival after transplantation of unrelated donor umbilical cord blood is comparable to that of human leukocyte antigen-matched unrelated donor bone marrow: results of a matched-pair analysis. *Blood* 2001;97:2957–2961.
39. Saarinen-Pihkala UM, Gustafsson G, Ringden O, et al. No disadvantage in outcome of using matched unrelated donors as compared with matched sibling donors for bone marrow transplantation in children with acute lymphoblastic leukemia in second remission. *J Clin Oncol* 2001;19:3406–3414.
40. Davies SM, DeFor TE, McGlave PB, et al. Equivalent outcomes in patients with chronic myelogenous leukemia after early transplantation of phenotypically matched bone marrow form unrelated or unrelated donors. *Am J Med* 2001;110:339–346.
41. Al-Kasim FA, Thornley I, Rolland M, et al. Single-centre experience with allogeneic bone marrow transplantation for acute lymphoblastic leukaemia in childhood: similar survival after matched-related and matched-unrelated donor transplants. *Br J Haematol* 2002;116:483–490.
42. Sierra J, Storer B, Hansen JA, et al. Unrelated donor marrow transplantation for acute myeloid leukemia: an update of the Seattle experience. *Bone Marrow Transplant* 2000;26:397–404.
43. Hansen JA, Gooley TA, Martin PJ, et al. Bone marrow transplants from unrelated donors for patients with chronic myeloid leukemia. *N Engl J Med* 1998;338:962–968.
44. Kollman C, Howe CW, Anasetti C, et al. Donor characteristics as risk factors in recipients after transplantation of bone marrow from unrelated donors: the effect of donor age. *Blood* 2001;98:2043–2051.
45. Storek J, Dawson MA, Storer B, et al. Immune reconstitution after allogeneic marrow transplantation compared with blood stem cell transplantation. *Blood* 2001;97:3380–3389.
46. Moretta A, Maccario R, Fagioli F, et al. Analysis of immune reconstitution in children undergoing cord blood transplantation. *Exp Hematol* 2001;29:371–379.
47. Small TN, Papadopoulos EB, Boulad F, et al. Comparison of immune reconstitution after unrelated and related T-cell-depleted bone marrow transplantation: effect of patient age and donor leukocyte infusions. *Blood* 1999;93:467–480.
48. Ochs L, Shu XO, Miller J, et al. Late infections after allogeneic bone marrow transplantations: comparison of incidence in related and unrelated donor transplant recipients. *Blood* 1995;86:3979–3986.
49. Busca A, Anasetti C, Anderson G, et al. Unrelated donor or autologous marrow transplantation for treatment of acute leukemia. *Blood* 1994;83:3077–3084.
50. Smith FO, King R, Nelson G, et al. Unrelated donor bone marrow transplantation for children with juvenile myelomonocytic leukaemia. *Br J Haematol* 2002;116:716–724.
51. Woolfrey AE, Anasetti C, Storer B, et al. Factors associated with outcome after unrelated marrow transplantation for treatment of acute lymphoblastic leukemia in children. *Blood* 2002;99:2002–2008.
52. Porter DL, Collins RH Jr, Hardy C, et al. Treatment of relapsed leukemia after unrelated donor marrow transplantation with unrelated donor leukocyte infusions. *Blood* 2000;95:1214–1221.
53. van Burik JA, Weisdorf DJ. Infections in recipients of blood and marrow transplantation. *Hematol Oncol Clin North Am* 1999;13:1065–1089.
54. Hoogerbrugge PM, Brouwer OF, Bordigoni P, et al. Allogeneic bone marrow transplantation for lysosomal storage diseases. The European Group for Bone Marrow Transplantation. *Lancet* 1995;345:1398–1402.
55. Krivit W. Stem cell bone marrow transplantation in patients with metabolic storage diseases. *Adv Pediatr* 2002;49:359–378.
56. Sullivan KM, Anasetti C, Horowitz M, et al. Unrelated and HLA-nonidentical related donor marrow transplantation for thalassemia and leukemia. A combined report from the Seattle Marrow Transplant Team and the International Bone Marrow Transplant Registry. *Ann NY Acad Sci* 1998;850:312–324.
57. Lazarus HM, Pérez WS, Klein JP, et al. Autotransplantation versus HLA-matched unrelated donor transplantation for acute myeloid leukemia (AML): a retrospective comparison from the National Marrow Donor Program, the International Bone Marrow Transplant Registry and the Autologous Blood and Marrow Transplant Registry. *Blood*, in press.
58. Sierra J, Radich J, Hansen JA, et al. Marrow transplants from unrelated donors for treatment of Philadelphia chromosome-positive acute lymphoblastic leukemia. *Blood* 1997;90:1410–1414.
59. Lee SJ, Kuntz KM, Horowitz MM, et al. Unrelated door bone marrow transplantation for chronic myeloid leukemia: A decision analysis. *Ann Intern Med* 1997;127:1080–1088.

60. Morton AJ, Gooley T, Hansen JA, et al. Association between pretransplant interferon-alpha and outcome after unrelated donor marrow transplantation for chronic myelogenous leukemia in chronic phase. *Blood* 1998;92:394–401.
61. Hehlmann R, Hochhaus A, Kolb JH, et al. Interferon-alpha before allogeneic bone marrow transplantation in chronic myelogenous leukemia does not affect outcome adversely, provided it is discontinued at least 90 days before the procedure. *Blood* 1999;94:3668–3677.
62. Giralt S, Szydlo R, Goldman JM, et al. Effect of short-term interferon therapy on the outcome of subsequent HLA-identical sibling bone marrow transplantation for chronic myelogenous leukemia: an analysis from the International Bone Marrow Transplant Registry. *Blood* 2000;95:410–415.
63. Lee SJ, Anasetti C, Kuntz KM, et al. The costs and cost-effectiveness of unrelated donor bone marrow transplantation for chronic phase chronic myelogenous leukemia. *Blood* 1998;92:4047–4052.
64. Laughlin MJ, Barker J, Bambach B, et al. Hematopoietic engraftment and survival in adult recipients of umbilical-cord blood from unrelated donors. *N Engl J Med* 2001;344:1815–1822.
65. Ooi J, Iseki T, Takahashi S, et al. A clinical comparison of unrelated cord blood transplantation and unrelated bone marrow transplantation for adult patients with acute leukaemia in complete remission. *Br J Haematol* 2002:118:140–143.
66. Rubinstein P, Carrier C, Scaradavou A, et al. Outcomes among 562 recipients of placental blood transplants from unrelated donor. *N Engl J Med* 1998;339:1565–1577.
67. Locatelli F, Rocha V, Chastang C, et al. Factors associated with outcome after cord blood transplantation in children with acute leukemia. *Blood* 1999;93:3662–3671.
68. Remberger M, Ringden O, Blau IW, et al. No difference in graft-versus-host disease, relapse, and survival comparing peripheral stem cells to bone marrow using unrelated donors. *Blood* 2001;98:1739–1745.
69. Elmaagacli AH, Basoglu S, Peceny R, et al. Improved disease-free-survival after transplantation of peripheral blood stem cells as compared with bone marrow from HLA identical unrelated doors in patients with first chronic phase chronic myeloid leukemia. *Blood* 2002;99:1130–1135.

17 Haploidentical Stem Cell Transplantation

P. Jean Henslee-Downey, MD

Contents

1. INTRODUCTION

1.1. Historical Review

Once allogeneic bone marrow transplant (alloBMT) was shown to have efficacy, investigators began to seek ways to increase access to donors in order to make potential curative therapy available to patients who lacked human leukocyte antigen (HLA)-matched sibling donors. During the eighth decade of the 20th century, medical publications began to describe methods by which HLA histocompatibility barriers to transplantation could be overcome *(1–6)*, with the first clinical reviews dating back to experience in the late seventh decade *(7–10)*. The most successful early efforts at performing an HLA-haplotype-disparate, haploidentical stem cell transplant (SCT) was reported in the treatment of children with severe combined immunodeficiencies *(11–19)*.

1.2. Focus on Hematologic Malignancy

The greatest need for transplant is patients with hematologic malignancy; thus, this chapter will focus on the growing experience in treating such diseases. Often there is an immediate requirement for transplant. The process for identifying preferred donors from within the family will include consideration of the logistical advantages of this donor option. Transplant methods and developing technology, aimed at improving the outcome of haploidentical SCT, through prevention and/or management of clinical events that cause failure, will be examined. The most significant clinical challenges are the topic of many review articles and include (1)

From: *Stem Cell Transplantation for Hematologic Malignancies*
Edited by: R. J. Soiffer © Humana Press Inc., Totowa, NJ

rejection and/or graft failure, (2) acute and chronic graft-vs-host disease (GVHD), (3) immune incompetence and fatal infections, and (4) relapse of the underlying malignancy *(20–30)*. Briefly, haploidentical donors will be compared to the use of other alternative donors who are not HLA genotypically fully matched. Finally, future uses of allogeneic cells for cellular immunotherapy and regeneration will be explored in the context of lessons learned that may facilitate broad access through haploidentical donors.

2. DONOR SELECTION

2.1. HLA Disparity and Donor Factors

Serologic typing of family members has been the primary method to identify donor–recipient pairs who inherit in common a sixth chromosome containing the major histocompatibility complex (MHC) of genes that largely regulate immune response *(31,32)*. Because of homozygosity for MHC genes and/or phenotypic similarity or molecular identity on the opposite, genetically nonshared chromosome, haploidentical donors and recipients are found to be variably mismatched for the major "transplant" antigens: HLA-A, -B, and -DR. Mismatching for these major HLA antigens defines the degree of incompatibility in the recipient, which increases the risk of GVHD, and in the donor, which increases the risk of graft failure (GF). Thus, a donor–recipient pair could be 0 to 3 antigen mismatched in both immunological vectors or any combination of disparity including 0 in one vector and 3 in the opposing vector, with variation being quite common. This complicates examining the correlation between major HLA mismatch and clinical outcomes. Because these differences that create two sets of data are not always clearly defined in the medical literature, it is also difficult to compare results between studies.

Whereas choosing a donor was traditionally based on the degree of HLA compatibility *(33)*, advances in transplant technique that overcame GF and GvHD and the ability to analyze larger patient datasets led to the recognition that younger donor age is better correlated with improved outcome *(34,35)*. Given the choice, greater major HLA mismatch in the patient is more tolerable than in the donor, as graft failure is associated with a high mortality risk. Even though immunologic modulation of the recipient has permitted transplantation across a known antidonor humoral response *(36,37)*, it remains advisable to avoid donors when there is a positive crossmatch and donor-specific HLA antibodies are found in the recipient *(38)*. A large retrospective analysis of haploidentical transplants examined the effect of mismatched noninherited maternal antigens compared to paternal antigens *(39)*. Sibling transplants to a recipient mismatched for noninherited maternal antigens were shown to be associated with less acute GVHD. In addition, maternal grafts were associated with less GF and chronic GVHD. Thus, siblings mismatched for noninherited maternal antigens and mothers may be preferable donors *(39–41)*. Finally, for a patient with myeloid leukemia, a donor might be chosen based on the ability to demonstrate donor-vs-recipient NK alloreactivity shown to be associated with an effective graft-vs-leukemia (GVL) effect *(42)*. Many patients will have numerous related haploidentical donors so that the choice of donor can be guided by these considerations, the donor's health status (e.g., positive infectious disease screening or medical reasons pertinent to minimize donor risk), and ease of graft collection among acceptable family members.

Table 1
Rank Order of Alternative Donors for Allogeneic Stem Cell Transplant

Donor relationship	*Major HLA-A, -B, -DR low-resolution typing*	*Major HLA-DR high-resolution typing*
Related	3/3 genetic and 3/3 phenotypic	2/2
Unrelated	6/6 phenotypic	2/2
Related	3/3 genetic and 2/3 phenotypic	2/2
Unrelated	5/6 phenotypic	2/2
Related	3/3 genetic and 2/3 phenotypic	1/2
Unrelated	5/6 phenotypic	1/2
Related	3/3 genetic and 1/3 phenotypic	2/2
Related	3/3 genetic and 1/3 phenotypic	1/2
Unrelated	4/6 phenotypic	2/2
Related	3/6 genetic	1/2

2.2. Alternative Donor Considerations

Donor selection also involves consideration of other alternative donors *(22,24)*. Unrelated donor sources include adult volunteers or cord blood units found in national and international registries or storage banks. In practice, decisions are often influenced by (1) the expected outcomes based on correlates with HLA compatibility, (2) the urgency of the transplant, and (3) the experience of the transplant center. Based on current transplant outcome data and across-the-board donor availability, Table 1 displays a rank order of potential alternative donors centered on molecular HLA typing that favors high-resolution HLA class II identity *(25)*. Advantages unique to the haploidentical donor include (1) immediate and constant donor availability, shortening the time to transplant and creating the opportunity to use donor-derived immunotherapy, (2) ability to harvest and engineer superior graft composition, and (3) reduce graft acquisition cost.

3. TRANSPLANT TECHNIQUES

A review of the published literature on haploidentical SCT suggests that past and current approaches can be divided into five categories describing treatment techniques: (1) myeloablative conditioning, unmodified marrow, and posttransplant immunosuppression, (2) myeloablative conditioning, T-cell-depleted marrow, with or without posttransplant immunosuppression, (3) myeloablative conditioning, CD34+ megadose peripheral blood with or without marrow and with or without posttransplant immunosuppression, (4) myeloablative conditioning, immunologically modulated marrow, and posttransplant immunosuppression, and (5) reduced-intensity conditioning, CD34+ peripheral blood, mixed chimerism, with or without posttransplant immunosuppression and with or without posttransplant cell infusions. Each will be evaluated as a learning exercise to recognize both problems and clinical advances with the purpose of understanding where future research might be directed. All approaches will have in common the fact that many patients are at high risk for failure by virtue of poor medical status from both disease and treatment effects and a far advanced stage of the underlying hematologic malignancy. Even now, many patients undergo haploidentical SCT only as a "last resort." This compromises the ability to evaluate the true toxicity and efficacy of the transplant procedure and makes survival an often untenable primary endpoint.

3.1. Myeloablative Conditioning, Unmodified Marrow, and Posttransplant Immunosuppression

Following studies in animal models exploring more intense conditioning regimens and alternative or combined methods of immunosuppression *(1,4,6,43,44)*, haploidentical SCT was undertaken in Europe and the United States *(7–10,45–48)*. A small number of patients were shown to achieve cure and survive long term. In an analysis of the then largest patient cohort, at the Seattle Transplant Center, 105 haploidentical marrow recipients were compared to those receiving a matched sibling donor (MSD) transplant *(8)*. Delay in engraftment and the early onset and increased frequency of acute GVHD was observed and correlated with increasing HLA disparity. However, of interest, there was no statistically significant difference in survival between study and control patients who were in remission preceding transplant. In a subsequent, extended study of 269 patients, the higher risk of GF in haploidentical recipients (12.3% vs 2%, $p < 0.0001$) was well defined and, again, shown to correlate with increasing donor HLA disparity and a positive crossmatch *(48)*.

To improve the outcome with unmodified mismatched marrow grafts, methods to increase immunoablation, rather than cytotoxicity, in otherwise myeloablative conditioning regimens have been explored. The use of serotherapy, with an extended serum half-life, directed against lymphocytes can inhibit both host- and donor-derived immune responses when given pretransplant and, thus, improve engraftment and control GVHD *(49,50)*. However, when this strategy is employed, the dose and persistence of serum antibody levels can have a detrimental effect on immune reconstitution, resulting in a significant increase in serious opportunistic infections with an adverse effect on survival *(51)*.

New immunosuppressive or "blocking" therapies have been explored in animal models in a search for safer and more effective methods to prevent allorecognition and response to major HLA-antigenic stimulation. Townsend and colleagues showed promising results in reducing GVHD with a peptide, rD-mPGPtide, which inhibits CD4 T-cell-mediated immune responses in a MHC-haploidentical murine model *(52)*. In the same model, an additive inhibitory effect was seen when the peptide was combined with cyclosporine, which resulted in prolonged survival *(53)*. Continued work by these and other investigators may lead to the discovery of drugs that can be given to the recipient to modulate or block early host- or donor-mediated responses and allow the successful transplantation of unmodified haploidentical stem cells *(54)*.

3.2. Myeloablative Conditioning, T-Cell-Depleted Marrow, and Posttransplant Immunosuppression

Whether in murine, dog, or human experiments, the value in depleting T cells from marrow innoculum for the prevention of GVHD following allogeneic transplant caused considerable enthusiasm to develop the technique for use with MHC-mismatched donors where the risk of GVHD could exceed 80% using unmodified grafts *(8,55–57)*. Promptly, barriers to engraftment were recognized and were shown to be related to inadequate suppression of both host humoral and cytotoxic immune responses *(58–62)*. Investigators began to explore more intensive host conditioning and demonstrated a value in adding additional immunosuppressive and cytotoxic systemic therapy as well as improved methods for delivery of higher-dose total-body irradiation (TBI), with or without additional total-lymphoid irradiation (TLI) *(63–68)*.

A recent review of T-cell-depleted, alternative-donor recipients demonstrated an increased risk of GF when the graft processing technique involved broad specificities for hematopoietic cells, particularly all-embracing T-cell subsets *(69)*. Adopting a narrow specificity technique, Soiffer and coworkers combined a TLI-enhanced conditioning regimen with an anti-CD6 monoclonal antibody for T-cell depletion of haploidentical donor grafts without the use of posttransplant immune suppression *(70)*. Stable engraftment occurred early in 24 of 27 patients, of whom 40% developed grade II–IV acute GVHD. For mismatched patients, the probability of survival was 56% at 2 yr and was not correlated with the degree of HLA disparity. For patients with early disease status, the event-free survival was 69% at 2 yr.

Studies by Martin and colleagues showed that the presence of CD8 T cells help to prevent marrow graft rejection, whereas CD4 T cells are not required *(71)*. Further, their work highlighted the tight correlation between competing donor and host immunologic responses by demonstrating that any dose of donor CD8+ cells associated with less than a 5% risk of GF would produce a greater than 15% risk of severe acute GVHD. Recognizing the potential for this tightrope between successful engraftment and control of GVHD, Henslee-Downey and coworkers at the Univeristy of Kentucky initiated clinical trials beginning in the mid-1980s to examine sequential immunosuppression targeted at the recipient, donor graft, and posttransplant chimera *(72)*. The conditioning regimen was equally aimed at recipient immunoablation and leukemia eradication and combined fractionated TBI with multiagent high-dose chemotherapy. T-Cell depletion was aimed at delivering a CD3 cell dose less than 1 × 10^5/kg recipient weight, a dose shown to be associated with an increasing risk of acute GVHD in matched sibling T-cell-depleted transplants *(73)*. On average, such a dose was given by using an IgM, anti-αβTCR monoclonal antibody, T10B9, activated by complement. For additional GVHD prophylaxis, posttransplant immunosuppression using an anti-CD5 ricin-conjugated immunotoxin was targeted at lysis of T lymphocytes to prevent expansion of allo-reactive clones. Low-dose steroid therapy was given in preparation for immunotoxin infusion and gradually tapered thereafter. All leukemic patients developed stable engraftment, and when compared to historical control patients not given posttransplant lympholysis, the risk of grade II–IV acute GVHD was significantly reduced (100% vs 36%, $p = 0.0001$), reducing the risk to as low as 17% in a subgroup of patients given the immunotoxin within 5 d of transplant. The probability of 5-yr survival in the later group was 46% *(72)*.

In a separate analysis of patients with high-risk acute lymphoblastic leukemia (ALL), recipients of T-cell-depleted haploidentical donor grafts were compared with T-cell-replete MSD transplants *(74)*. No difference in rates of engraftment, acute GVHD, survival, and disease-free survival (DFS) were seen. Finally, long-term follow-up of 82 consecutive patients demonstrated a 47% 4-yr survival in patients transplanted at or less than 30 yr of age, who had early or intermediate disease status and less than a 3-antigen mismatch *(75)*.

This approach was further developed at the University of South Carolina in a series of clinical trials that tested alterations in each step of sequential immune modulation and ablation. An analysis of 72 patients examined a reduction followed by increase in TBI dose and a switch from posttransplant anti-CD5 immunotoxin to broader serotherapy using equine antithymocyte globulin (ATG) combined with low-dose cyclosporine and steroid taper *(76)*. The engraftment probability was 88% and was adversely affected by reduction in TBI dose, a 3-antigen HLA mismatch in the donor, and the diagnosis of chronic myelogenous leukemia (CML) *(77)*. In engrafted patients, the probability of grade II–IV acute GVHD was 16%. Chronic GVHD occurred in 35% of patients and most had only limited disease. There was a 7% risk of early death (<60 d) that could be ascribed to regimen-related toxicity, which occurred exclusively in high-risk patients. The risk of relapse at 2 yr was related to disease status at transplant: 21% in the low-risk, early disease group vs 58% in the high-risk, late advanced disease group. Similarly, survival was best in low-risk patients (55% vs 27%, respectively). Prognostic factors that affected outcome included (1) a lower TBI dose and 3-antigen donor mismatch decreased engraftment, (2) a higher T-cell dose increased acute GVHD, (3) a higher TBI dose increased chronic GVHD, and (4) a high-risk disease category increased treatment failure from relapse or death.

In an attempt to improve engraftment and reduce toxicity, the conditioning regimen was changed by lowering the TBI dose and adding noncytotoxic serotherapy using equine ATG. The use of an Food and Drug Administration (FDA)-approved reagent for T-cell depletion was considered desirable and OKT3 was adopted for marrow preparation. In a comparison of 110 consecutive recipients in the later trial with 100 recipients previously given a T10B9-depleted graft, graft composition was shown to include a lower mononuclear cell and higher T-cell dose in the OKT3 grafts. However, there was a significant improvement in engraftment (97% vs 91%, $p = 0.001$), without a change in the control of acute GVHD. These improvements were thought to be related to the addition of equine ATG to the conditioning regimen *(22,78–80)*. Subsequently, in an analysis of 219 patients treated in the later protocol, the probability of engraftment was shown to be 98%, occurring at a median of 15 d. There was a trend toward earlier engraftment associated with higher doses of mononuclear cells and a higher CD34 dose, the later also associated with less transplant-related toxicity and improved survival. In this study, the degree or type of HLA disparity was not associated with any major clinical outcome. Factors that affected survival included age of donor and recipient and disease status but not disease diagnosis at time of transplant. Five-year DFS was 44% in low-risk vs 11% in high-risk patients. The major cause of death was relapse, appropriate to the disease status, followed by infection *(35)*.

In tackling these problems, the investigators turned their attention to the development of highly specific cellular immunotherapy. Of interest, a small subset of patients were shown to have an increase in the proportion of gamma delta positive T lymphocytes during their first year of recovery after T10B9-depleted haploidentical transplantation *(81)*. All 10 patients were surviving beyond 2.5 yr posttransplant and only one relapsed. Additional studies in seven donor–recipient pairs demonstrated that Vδ1+CD4– CD8+ γδ+ T cells are activated and proliferate in response to recipient primary ALL cells but do not respond to HLA-mismatched unrelated cells. These unique observations suggested that haploidentical γδ+ T cells could be an effective form of immunotherapy without the risk of GVHD *(82)*. Clinical trials have now been launched to exploit this potential therapeutic option. A similar approach to infection was also underway through the development of an expansion technique that made it possible to generate sufficient quantities of cytomegalovirus (CMV)-specific cytotoxic T cells for adoptive immunotherapy using small quantities of donor blood *(83)*. Further, donor-derived Epstein–Barr virus (EBV)-specific cytotoxic T lymphocytes (CTLs) were demonstrated not to recognize haploidentical recipient cells, and the ability to scale production to a clinical grade made it feasible to pursue posttransplant prophylactic and/or treatment protocols *(84)*.

These advances, coupled with efforts to decrease toxicity of the conditioning regimen and alterations in graft preparation taking advantage of preclinical and preliminary clinical experience utilizing granulocyte colony-stimulating factor (G-CSF)-stimulated marrow, were considered promising methods to improve outcome *(85)*. However, major gains in survival would probably not be realistic without further restrictions regarding patient eligibility. This being said, the need to discover effective treatment for advanced and/or refractory leukemia remains.

3.3. Myeloablative Conditioning, CD34+ Megadose Peripheral Blood, and ± Posttransplant Immunosuppression

Observations made in murine models showed the ability to induce full donor-type engraftment using megadoses of T-cell-depleted incompatible bone marrow (BM) innoculum *(86–88)*. This, coupled with growing interest in the use of peripheral blood stem cells (PBSCs) for transplantation *(89)*, led to collaboration between the laboratories of The Weizmann Institute of Science in Israel and the clinical research programs of the University of Perugia resulting in the initiation of clinical trials using "megadose" stem cell marrow and/or peripheral blood (PB) grafts from haploidentical donors. Aversa and co-workers reported results in 17 patients who were conditioned with single-fraction TBI, ATG, cyclophosphamide (Cy), and thiotepa followed by T-cell-depleted marrow augmented with G-CSF-stimulated PB progenitor cells *(90)*. Most patients experienced early engraftment and few were observed to have grade II or higher acute GVHD. At the time of publication, 6 of 17 patients were surviving at a median follow-up of 230 d. However, further follow-up and expanded patient accrual indicated an approx 20% risk of both GF and grade II–IV acute GVHD *(29)*. Ultimately, regimen toxicity and transplant-related mortality led to disappointing survival outcome.

Based on preclinical murine studies showing that fludarabine could replace Cy in a TBI-based conditioning regimen *(91)*, this change was applied to the clinical protocol in an effort to reduce regimen-related toxicity. Further, the dose of T lymphocytes was reduced by processing PB with one-round of e-rosetting, followed by positive immunoselection of CD34 cells given with or without T-cell-depleted BM *(92)*. Forty-one of 43 patients established stable engraftment and no patient was observed to have acute GVHD. The prevention of GVHD is at least partially ascribed to persistence of highly potent rabbit ATG in serum, a form of posttransplant immunosuppression. Nonrelapse mortality was less associated with regimen-related toxicity and more often caused by fatal infections. The risk of relapse was higher in patients transplanted for ALL compared to acute myelogenous leukemia (AML) (63% vs 13%, $p = 0.004$). Continued follow-up of this patient cohort demonstrates a 4-yr DFS of 25% in AML and 17% in ALL *(29)*. Investigators were concerned that slow immune reconstitution was the result of the administration of G-CSF given to speed up granulocyte reconstitution *(93)*, and this drug was removed from subsequent protocols.

As primary clinical outcomes did not appear to be linked to the use of bone marrow, the investigators concluded that CD34-selected PB grafts would be sufficient for future haploidentical transplant trials. In a current ongoing trial, CD34 selection alone is used to prepare the graft. Patients are given a median of 12×10^6 CD34 and 1×10^4 CD3 cells/kg recipient weight. Preliminary review of this protocol indicates a 98% engraftment rate and only 4 of 53 patients developed acute GVHD. Sixteen (30%) experienced nonrelapse mortality. Patients transplanted in relapse did so more often than those in remission (12/25 vs 3/28). The current probability of DFS remains best in patients with AML compared to ALL (60% vs 38%). Further, AML patients who received grafts from donors who demonstrate natural killer (NK) cell alloreactivity have a decidedly superior survival compared to those who do not (70% vs 7%) *(42)*.

These investigators studied the immunophenotype of circulating lymphocytes posttransplant in haploidentical recipients. They demonstrated the presence of a large population of lymphocytes that exhibit NK-like function and lyse leukemic cells. The early expansion of these cells following transplant was associated with freedom from relapse, primarily in myeloid leukemias *(94)*. They showed that donor NK-cell killer inhibitory receptors (KIR) do not recognize certain recipient allotypes, do not exhibit tolerance to host, and appear to be highly reactive to

Table 2
Available Outcomes From Published Clinical Trials Seeking to Duplicate Haploidentical Transplant Using "Megadose" CD34-Selected Peripheral Blood Grafts[a]

First author	*No. of patients*	*Graft failure*	*Acute GvHD*[b]	*Survival*	*1E COD*
Kawano *(98)*	13	8	2	5	Graft failure
Peters *(99)*	14	4	0	8	Graft failure
Bunjes *(100)*	10	1	0	6	Infection
Passweg *(101)*	10	3	3	3	TRM
Handgretinger *(102)*	39	3	1	15	Relapse
Redei *(103)*	19	2	4	6	Infection
Totals	105	21	10	43	

Abbreviations: 1E, primary; COD, cause of death; TRM, transplant-related mortality.
[a]Ten or more patients, primarily for hematologic malignancy.
[b]Higher than grade I.

myeloid leukemic cells. The investigators postulate that ALL cells may lack appropriate stimulatory mechanisms to elicit this otherwise almost solely GVL response *(95–97)*.

Across the world, numerous investigators have sought to reproduce the results published from the University of Perugia. Table 2 shows identifiable outcomes from published clinical trials of 10 or more patients *(98–103)*. Unfortunately, many of the trials initiated in the United States closed without publication of outcomes. Taken together, although results appear to be improving in experienced centers when transplanting low-risk patients, problems are seen in centers initiating new trials. It is hard not to question whether one or more ingredient in the clinical protocol, which has produced good rates of engraftment and control of GVHD, is also blocking essential immune reconstitution and broad GVL effects. Clearly, there is enthusiasm to continue exploration of this approach to haploidentical transplant. Meetings held in Perugia, Italy and Chicago, IL (USA) resulted in a consensus recommendation regarding parameters for developing future trials *(104)*. These include details for patient eligibility, graft manipulation and cell composition of the graft, conditioning of the patient, and posttransplant treatments. These studies should help to clarify outcomes and possibly provide solutions to current problems.

3.4. Myeloablative Conditioning, Immunologically Modulated Marrow, and Posttransplant Immunosuppression

Although minimizing the T-cell content of an allogeneic marrow graft does reduce the risk of GVHD, problems with engraftment, delay in immune reconstitution, and lack of a GVL effect can result in failure of the transplant as a result of relapse and/or fatal infections. To avoid these untoward effects, investigators at the Dana-Farber Cancer Institute sought methods to alter donor T cells by blocking recipient allo-recognition so that the remaining T-cell repertoire would be preserved. Interference with signal pathways between the B7 family of proteins on antigen-presenting cells and the CD28 receptor on T cells produces anergy *(105,106)*. Soluble CTLA-4 has a higher affinity for B7 than CD28 and, thus, blocks T-cell activation, resulting in anergy shown to be sufficient to permit successful histoincompatible transplantation *(107,108)*. After completion of preclinical marrow studies, a phase I clinical trial was initiated using haploidentical donors for allogeneic transplant at the Dana-Farber Cancer Institute

(109,110). Prior to conventional myeloablative condition therapy, recipient blood was obtained and subsequently irradiated and cocultured with donor marrow and CTLA-4-Ig, producing a graft shown to have a significant reduction in the frequency of T cells capable of recognizing the recipient. Additional GVHD prophylaxis included a standard methotrexate and cyclosporine combination. All evaluable patients engrafted and 3 of 11 developed acute GVHD. At the time of publication, 5 of 12 patients were alive in remission. Of interest, surviving patients established normalization of lymphocyte recovery in less than 1 yr posttransplant. The lack of further investigation of this approach to haploidentical transplant is thought to be at least partiallycaused by drug inaccessibility.

Another approach to modulating the T cell rather that removing it has been explored at The General Hospital of Air Force in Beijing, China, where investigators have embarked on a series of clinical trials using haploidentical donors to meet the great need of patients who usually have no siblings. Based on favorable results using G-CSF to stimulate and enrich marrows from matched sibling donors *(111,112)*, the approach was applied to the preparation of haploidentical grafts, unmodified other than the influence from systemically administered G-CSF. Marrow was considered preferable to blood because of the significantly lower T-cell content. Pretransplant and posttransplant sequential immunosuppression was given to prevent rejection and GVHD. The conditioning regimen was broad, including cytarabine, Cy, moderate-dose TBI, and rabbit ATG. Donors received 7 consecutive days of G-CSF prior to marrow harvest. Posttransplant GVHD prophylaxis included cyclosporine, methotrexate, and mycophenolate mofetil (MMF) *(113)*. Quantification of graft characteristics before and after G-CSF stimulation revealed a significant increase in total nucleated cells, CD34, and colony-forming units granulocyte-macrophage cells, a decrease in lymphocytes, and a decrease in the CD4 : CD8 ratio. All patients obtained successful early engraftment, with full donor chimerism and sustained engraftment at median follow-up of 22 mo. Five patients developed grade II–IV acute GVHD, three of whom died of severe GVHD. Only one patient relapsed and few patients suffered serious infections. At the time of publication, 9 of 15 patients were surviving between 13 and 35 mo with 100% Karnofsky performance. The estimated disease-free survival at 2 yr was 60%.

In the subsequent study, additional posttransplant immunosuppression using CD25 monoclonal antibody was tested for better control of acute GVHD *(114)*. Study patients were given CD25 2 h prior to transplant and repeated on d 4 after transplant. The study group received, on average, larger doses of CD34 and CD3 cells. All patients engrafted and established full donor chimerism. Compared with the prior historical control group, no study patient developed grade II–IV acute GVHD. This improvement was ascribed to be a direct effect of CD25 administration. At a median 8 mo follow-up, 12 of 13 patients survived disease-free. Projected survival for both groups of patients combined at 2 yr is 72%. These rather remarkable results seem most compelling to continue and expand this research effort. In addition, the methods utilized are not complicated and could easily be transportable *(115)*.

3.5. Reduced-Intensity Conditioning, CD34+ Peripheral Blood, Mixed Chimerism, ± Posttransplant Immunosuppression, and ± Cell Add-Back

Initially, reduced-intensity conditioning therapy prior to allogeneic transplant was primarily offered to older or infirm patients, who did not otherwise qualify for a transplant procedure, in the hope that a GVL effect might be therapeutic *(116–118)*. As techniques evolved, investigators are now actively looking at new methods and applications to exploit this form of immunotherapy. Almost surprising, this mechanism has been embraced for conducting allogeneic transplants from alternative donors, which would have seemed almost impossible in the prior decade, and, yet, publications are now available from both animal models and small clinical trials using haploidentical donors *(119)*.

Some of the first efforts at establishing hematopoietic engraftment across HLA barriers were focused on the induction of mixed chimerism for tolerance to solid organ transplantation *(120,121)*. Next, building on the theme of mixed chimerism, Spitzer, Sykes, and co-workers sought a platform for producing GVL without significant GVHD in patients with advanced lymphoma *(122,123)*. Extending the work to patients with hematologic malignancy, O'Donnell and co-workers performed a phase I clinical trial to examine minimal conditioning using intensely lympholytic immunosuppression that combined fludarabine and single-fraction TBI before transplant and Cy, MMF, and tacrolimus after transplant *(124)*. Engraftment was poor until the Cy dose was escalated. In the later group, 6 of 10 patients were surviving at 191 d posttransplant. This trial demonstrates feasibility and encouragement promise for continued research efforts.

Currently, in the development of "mini" haploidentical transplant, acute and chronic GVHD remains the most significant cause of morbidity and mortality. In an effort to diminish this risk, genetically modified donor T cells with an inducible "suicide" gene have been studied *(125)*. Of interest, transduced, ex vivo expanded CTLs maintained function, enhanced engraftment of dog leukocyte antigen-haploidentical marrow, and caused severe acute GvHD. Whether a part of the primary graft or donor leukocyte infusion (DLI) therapy, this approach would only be clinically relevant if the suicide gene mechanism could be precisely controlled. Another approach to achieve engraftment, control GVHD, and achieve immune reconstitution, is under development at the National Institutes of Health. Burrett and coworkers are exploring techniques for graft preparation using host-reactive T-cell-depleted, expanded cells combined with G-CSF-mobilized, CD34-selected T-cell-depleted PB *(126)*. Finally, in the clinical setting, investigators have demonstrated effective yet sometimes transient antileukemic effects using haploidentical DLI therapy posttransplant, not infrequently associated with notable toxicity, including marrow suppression and GVHD in a dose-dependent fashion *(127,128)*. However, highly specific cellular therapy targeted at both leukemia and infection has been developed and noted in previous sections *(82–84,129)*.

4. FUTURE PERSPECTIVES

In this last decade, progress moved forward in developing the capability to perform haploidentical transplantation. However, the pace is unacceptable. There are daunting accomplishments yet needed. This will require a highly organized research effort—one that will cast a wide net to encourage innovation and collaboration. In return, a "universal" donor could be made available. No patient in need would be without opportunity.

The challenges to the research scientists and physicians are immense but attainable. Attention needs to be focused on every aspect of patient and transplant management. We need new ways to harness the immune system and, at the same time, less complex ways to deliver care to the patient. New drugs and cellular therapies are critical to making the cure of the underlying malignancy a reality. Methods for prevention and treatment of each threatening complication, whether it be disordered immune function or life-threatening infection, must be perfected. Attention must also be directed to facilitating healthy recovery and obtaining quality survivorship.

5. CONCLUSION

For patients with hematologic malignancies who are in need of transplant and/or cellular immunotherapy and do not have a matched sibling donor, haploidentical SCT is an acceptable therapeutic option. The risks and benefits for most disease and patient conditions are not notably different than transplant using an unrelated alternative donor. Striking advantages of haploidentical SCT include universal and rapid access to donors who can repeatedly donate cells for a wide range of purposes for and following transplantation.

How to best perform haploidentical SCT is not yet clear. Rather, the state of the science and art are a work in progress. Unmistakably, continuation of effort needs to be encouraged and supported in order to achieve total access to stem cells, tissue, and organs for restorative and/or replacement therapy. Thus, all patients could realize the potential promise of curative intervention for many life-threatening and fatal conditions using hematopoietic stem cell transplant and cellular therapies that would provide highly specific targeted immunotherapy, immune reconstitution, tissue repair and regeneration, and cell or organ transplantation.

ACKNOWLEDGMENT

The content of this publication does not necessarily reflect the views or policies of the Department of Health and Human Services, nor does mention of trade names, commercial products, or organizations imply endorsement by the US Government.

The author would like to express gratitude to Kathy Fain for her invaluable assistance in preparing the manuscript.

REFERENCES

1. Kolb HJ, Bodenberger U, Rodt HV, et al. Bone marrow transplantation in DLA-haploidentical canine littermates: fractionated total body irradiation (FTBI) and in vitro treatment of the marrow graft with anti-T-cell globulin (ATGCG). *Hematol Bluttransfus* 1980;25:61–71.
2. Vallera DA, Soderling CC, Carlson GJ, et al. Bone marrow transplantation across major histocompatibility barriers in mice. Effect of elimination of T cells from donor grafts by treatment with monoclonal Thy-1.2 plus complement or antibody alone. *Transplantation* 1981;31:218–222.
3. Reisner Y, Kapoor N, Kitkpatrick D, et al. Transplantation for acute leukaemia with HLA-A and B nonidentical parental marrow cells fractionated with soybean agglutinin and sheep red blood cells. *Lancet* 1981;2:327–331.
4. Deeg HJ, StorbR, Raff RF, et al. Marrow grafts between phenotypically DLA-identical and haploidentical unrelated dogs: additional antigens controlling engraftment are not detected by cell-mediated lympholysis. *Transplantation* 1982;33:17–21.
5. Good RA, Kapoor N, Reisner Y. Bone marrow transplantation—an expanding approach to treatment of many diseases. *Cell Immunol* 1983;82:36–54.
6. Deeg HJ, Storb R, Appelbaum FR, et al. Combined immunosuppression with cyclosporine and methotrexate in dogs given bone marrow grafts from DLA-haploidentical littermates. *Transplantation* 1984;37:62–65.
7. Filipovich AH, Ramsay NK, Arthur DC, et al. Allogeneic bone marrow transplantation with related donors other than HLA MLC-matched siblings, and the use of antithymocyte globulin, prednisone, and methotrexate for prophylaxis of graft-versus-host disease. *Transplantation* 1985;39:282–285.
8. Beatty PG, Clift RA, Mickelson EM, et al. Marrow transplantation from related donors other than HLA-identical siblings. *N Engl J Med* 1985;313:765–771.
9. Filipovich AH. Progress in broadening the uses of marrow transplantation: donor availability. *Vox Sang* 1986;51(suppl 2):95–103.
10. Kolb HJ, Bender-Gotze C, Holler E, et al. Improved survival following HLA-incompatible bone marrow transplantation. Munich Cooperative Group of Bone Marrow Transplantation. *Folia Haematol Int Mag Klin Morphol Blutforsch* 1989;116(3–4):421–425.

11. O'Reilly RJ, Kapoor N, Kirkpatrick D, et al. Transplantation of hematopoietic cells for lethal congenital immunodeficiencies. *Birth Defects Orig Artic Ser* 1983;19:129–137.
12. Reisner Y, Kapoor N, Kirkpatrick D, et al. Transplantation for severe combined immunodeficiency with HLA-A, B, D, DR incompatible parental marrow cells fractionated bysoybean agglutinin and sheep red blood cells. *Blood* 1983;61:341–348.
13. Friedrich W, Goldmann SF, Vetter U, et al. Immunoreconstitution in severe combined immunodeficiency after transplantation of HLA-haploidentical, T-cell-depleted bone marrow. *Lancet* 1984;1:761–764.
14. Cowan MJ, Wara DW, Weintrub PS, et al. Haploidentical bone marrow transplantation for severe combined immunodeficiency disease using soybean agglutinin-negative, T-depleted marrow cells. *J Clin Immunol* 1985;5:371–376.
15. Morgan G, Linch DC, Knott LT, et al. Successful haploidentical mismatched bone marrow transplantation in severe combined immunodeficiency: T cell removal using CAMPATH-I monoclonal antibody and E-rosetting. *Br J Haematol* 1986;62:421–430.
16. Buckley RH, Schiff SE, Sampson HA, et al. Development of immunity in human severe primary T cell deficiency following haploidentical bone marrow stem cell transplantation. *J Immunol* 1986;136:2398–2407.
17. Fischer A, Durandy A, de Villartay JP, et al. HLA-haploidentical bone marrow transplantation for severe combined immunodeficiency using E rosette fractionation and cyclosporine. *Blood* 1986;67:444–449.
18. Parkman R. Antibody-treated bone marrow transplantation for patients with severe combined immune deficiency. *Clin Immunol Immunopathol* 1986;40:142–146.
19. Moen RC, Horowitz SD, Sondel PM, et al. Immunologic reconstitution after haploidentical bone marrow transplantation for immune deficiency disorders: treatment of bone marrow cells with monoclonal antibody CT-2 and complement. *Blood* 1987;70:664–669.
20. Henslee-Downey PJ. Mismatched bone marrow transplantation. *Curr Opin Oncol* 1995;7:115–121.
21. Aversa F, Martelli MM, Reisner Y. Use of stem cells from mismatched related donors. *Curr Opin Hematol* 1997;4:419–422.
22. Henslee-Downey PJ. Allogeneic related partially mismatched transplantation. In: Barrett J, Treleaven J, eds. *The Clinical Practice of Stem Cell Transplantation*, 2nd ed. Oxford: Isis Medical Media, 1998:391–417.
23. Henslee-Downey PJ. Haploidentical transplantation. *Cancer Treat Res* 1999;101:53–77.
24. Henslee-Downey PJ, Gluckman E. Allogeneic transplantation from donors other than HLA-identical siblings. *Hematol Oncol Clin North Am* 1999;13:1017–1039.
25. Henslee-Downey PJ. Allogeneic transplantation across major HLA barriers. *Best Pract Res Clin Haematol* 2001;14:741–754.
26. Rowe JM, Lazarus HM. Genetically haploidentical stem cell transplantation for acute leukemia. *Bone Marrow Transplant* 2001;27:669–676.
27. Walker IR. Workshop on haploidentical stem cell transplantation: Chicago, Illinois, USA, 18–19 November 1999. *Leukemia* 2002;16:424–426.
28. Berneman ZN. Second European Workshop on haploidentical stem cell transplantation (12–14 October 2000—Perugia, Italy). *Leukemia* 2002;16:418–423.
29. Aversa F, Tabilio A, Velardi A, et al. Allogeneic transplantation across the HLA barriers. *Rev Clin Exp Hematol* 2001;5.2:147–161.
30. Martelli MF, Aversa F, Bachar-Lustig E, et al. Transplants across human leukocyte antigen barriers. *Semin Hematol* 2002;39:48–56.
31. Dupont B. O'Reilly RJ, Pollack MS, et al. Histocompatibility testing for clinical bone marrow transplantation and prospects for identification of donors other than HLA genotypically identical siblings. *Hematol Bluttransfus* 1980;25:121–134.
32. Agrawal S, Bhardwaj U. HLA and bone marrow transplant donor search strategies. *J Assoc Physicians India* 2002;50:937–945.
33. Henslee-Downey PJ. Choosing an alternative bone marrow donor among available family members. *Am J Pediatr Hematol Oncol* 1993;15:150–161.
34. Godder KT, Hazlett LJ, Abhyankar SH, et al. Partially mismatched related-donor marrow transplantation for pediatric patients with acute leukemia: younger donors and absence of peripheral blasts improve outcome. *J Clin Oncol* 2000;18:1856–1866.
35. van Rhee F, Adams S, Godder K, et al. Allogeneic transplantation from partially mismatched related donors: use of younger donors improves outcome. *Blood* 2000;96(suppl 1):208.

36. Braun N, Faul C, Wernet D, et al. Successful transplantation of highly selected CD34+ peripheral blood cells in a HLA-sensitized patient treated with immunoadsorption onto protein A. *Transplantation* 2000;69:1742–1744.
37. Abhyankar SH, Geier SS, Parrish R, et al. Effect of crossmatch reactions and HLA typed cell panel antibody response on engraftment using plasmapheresis and Prosorba column absorption during partially mismatched related donor BMT. *Blood* 1995;86(suppl 1):564.
38. Richter KV. Histocompatibility and bone marrow transplantation. *Folia Haematol Int Mag Klin Morphol Blutforsch* 1989;116:445–450.
39. van Rood JJ, Lobeiza FR Jr, Zhang M-J, et al. Effect of tolerance to noninherited maternal antigens on the occurrence of graft-versus-host disease after bone marrow transplantation from a parent or an HLA-haploidentical sibling. *Blood* 2002;99:1572–1577.
40. Tamaki S, Ichinohe T, Matsuo K, et al. Superior survival of blood and marrow stem cell transplants given maternal grafts over recipients given paternal grafts. *Bone Marrow Transplant* 2001;28:375–380.
41. Ochiai N, Shimazaki C, Fuchida S, et al. Successful non-T cell-depleted HLA haploidentical three-loci mismatched hematopoietic stem cell transplantation from mother to son based on the feto-maternal microchimerism in chronic myleogenous leukemia. *Bone Marrow Transplant* 2002;30:793–796.
42. Aversa F, Terenzi A, Felicini R, et al. Haploidentical stem cell transplantation for acute leukemia. *Int J Hematol* 2002;76(suppl 1):165–168.
43. Raff RF, Storb R, Graham T, et al. Succinyl acetone plus methotrexate as graft-versus-host disease prophylaxis in DLA-haploidentical canine littermate marrow grafts. *Transplantation* 1992;54:813–820.
44. Deeg HJ, Severns E, Raff RF, et al. Specific tolerance and immunocompetence in haploidentical but not in completely allogeneic, canine chimeras treated with methotrexate and cyclosporine. *Transplantation* 1987;44:621–632.
45. Chan KW, Fryer CJ, Denegri JF, et al. Allogeneic bone marrow transplantation using partially-matched related donors. *Bone Marrow Transplant* 1987;2:27–32.
46. Anasetti C, Martin PJ, Storb R, et al. Prophylaxis of graft-versus-host disease by administration of the murine anti-IL-2 receptor antibody 2A3. *Bone Marrow Transplant* 1991;7:375–381.
47. Polchi P, Lucarelli G, Galimberti M, et al. Haploidentical bone marrow transplantation from mother to child with advanced leukemia. *Bone Marrow Transplant* 1995;16:529–535.
48. Anasetti C, Amos D, Beatty PG, et al. Effect of HLA compatibility on engraftment of bone marrow transplants in patients with leukemia or lymphoma. *N Engl J Med* 1989;320:197–204.
49. Remberger M, Svahn B-M, Hentschke P, et al. Effect on cytokine release and graft-versus-host disease of different anti-T cell antibodies during conditioning for unrelated haematopoietic stem cell transplantation. *Bone Marrow Transplant* 1999;24:823–830.
50. Byrne JL, Stainer C, Cull G, et al. The effect of the serotherapy regimen used and the marrow cell dose received on rejection, graft-versus-host disease and outcome following unrelated donor bone marrow transplantation for leukemia. *Bone Marrow Transplant* 2000;25:411–417.
51. Duval M, Pedron B, Rohrlich P, et al. Immune reconstitution after haematopoietic transplantation with two different doses of pre-graft antithymocyte globulin. *Bone Marrow Transplant* 2002;30:421–426.
52. Townsend RM, Briggs C, Marini JC, et al. Inhibitory effect of a CD4-CDR3 peptide analog on graft-versus-host disease across a major histocompatibility complex-haploidentical barrier. *Blood* 1996;88:3038–3047.
53. Townsend RM, Gilbert MJ, Korngold R. Combination thrapy with a CD4-CDR3 peptide analog and cyclosporin A to prevent graft-vs-host disease in a MHC-haploidentical bone marrow transplantation model. *Clin Immunol Immunopathol* 1998;86:115–119.
54. Hsieh MH, Varadi G, Flomenberg N, et al. Leucyl-leucine methyl ester-treated haploidentical donor lymphocyte infusions can mediate graft-versus-leukemia activity with minimal graft-versus-host disease risk. *Biol Blood Marrow Transplant* 2002;8:303–315.
55. Schumm M, Gunther W, Kolb HJ, et al. Prevention of graft-versus-host disease in DLA-haplotype mismatched dogs and hemopoietic engraftment of CD6-depleted marrow with and without cG-CSF treatment after transplantation. *Tissue Antigens* 1994;43:170–178.
56. O'Reilly RJ, Collins N, Dinsmore R, et al. Transplantation of HLA-mismatched marrow T-depleted of T-cells by lectin agglutination and E-rosette depletion. *Tokai J Exp Clin Med* 1985;10:99–107.

57. Trigg ME, Sondel PM, Billing R, et al. Mismatched bone marrow transplantation in children with hematologic malignancy using T lymphocyte depleted bone marrow. *J Biol Response Mod* 1985;4:602–612.
58. Sondel PM, Hank JA, Trigg ME, et al. Transplantation of HLA-haploidentical T-cell-depleted marrow for leukemia: autologous marrow recovery with specific immune sensitization to donor antigens. *Exp Hematol* 1986;14:278–286.
59. Kernan NA, Flomenberg N, Dupont B, et al. Graft rejection in recipients of T-cell-depleted HLA-nonidentical marrow transplants for leukemia. Identification of host-derived antidonor allocytotoxic T lymphocytes. *Transplantation* 1987;43:842–847.
60. Bierer BE, Emerson SG, Antin J, et al. Regulation of cytotoxic T lymphocyte-mediated graft rejection following bone marrow transplantation. *Transplantation* 1988;46:835–839.
61. Soderling CC, Song CW, Blazar BR, et al. A correlation between conditioning and engraftment in recipients of MHC-mismatched T cell-depleted murine bone marrow transplants. *J Immunol* 1985;135:941–946.
62. Ishii E, Gengozian N, Good RA. Influence of dimethyl myleran on tolerance induction and immune function in major histocompatibility complex-haploidentical murine bone-marrow transplantation. *Proc Natl Acad Sci USA* 1991;88:8435–8439.
63. Bozdech MJ, Sondel PM, Trigg ME, et al. Transplantation of HLA-haploidentical T-cell-depleted marrow for leukemia: addition of cytosine arabinoside to the pretransplant conditioning prevents rejection. *Exp Hematol* 1985;13:1201–1210.
64. Kernan NA, Emanuel D, Castro-Malaspina H, et al. Posttransplant immunosuppression with antithymocyte globulin and methylpredisolone prevents immunologically mediated graft failure following a T-cell depleted marrow transplant. *Blood* 1989;74(suppl 1):123.
65. Soiffer RJ, Mauch P, Tarbell NJ, et al. Total lymphoid irradiation to prevent graft rejection in recipients of HLA non-identical T cell-depleted allogeneic marrow. *Bone Marrow Transplant* 1991;7:23–33.
66. Terenzi A, Aristei C, Aversa F, et al. Efficacy of fludarabine as an immunosuppressor for bone marrow transplantation conditiong: preliminary results. *Transplant Proc* 1996;28:3101.
67. Henslee-Downey PJ, Lee CG, Hazlett LJ, et al. Rare failure to engraft following haploidentical T-cell depleted marrow transplantation using enhanced host immunoablation and OKT3 graft purging. *Exp Hematol* 1997;25:183.
68. D'Costa S, Hurwitz JL. Antibody and pre- plus post-transplant prednisone treatments support T-cell depleted stem cell engraftment without drug-induced morbidity. *Bone Marrow Transplant* 2002;29:553–556.
69. Champlin RE, Passweg JR, Zhang M-J, et al. T-Cell depletion of bone marrow transplants for leukemia from donors other than HLA-identical siblings: advantage of T-cell antibodies with narrow specificities. *Transplantation* 2000;95:3996–4003.
70. Soiffer RJ, Mauch P, Fairclough D, et al. CD6+ T cell depleted allogeneic bone marrow transplantation from genotypically HLA nonidentical related donors. *Biol Blood Marrow Transplant* 1997;1:11–17.
71. Martin PJ, Rowley SD, Anasetti C, et al. A phase I–II clinical trial to evaluate removal of CD4 cells and partial depletion of CD8 cells from donor marrow for HLA-mismatched unrelated recipients. *Blood* 1999;94:2192–2199.
72. Henslee-Downey PJ, Parrish RS, Macdonald JS, et al. Combined in vitro and in vivo T lymphocyte depletion for the control of graft-versus-host disease following haploidentical marrow transplant. *Transplantation* 1996;61:738–745.
73. Kernan NA, Collins NH, Juliano L, et al. Clonable T lymphocytes in T cell-depleted bone marrow transplants correlate with development of graft-v-host disease. *Blood* 1986;68:770–773.
74. Fleming DR, Henslee-Downey PJ, Romond EH, et al. Allogeneic bone marrow transplantation with T cell-depleted partially matched related donors for advanced acute lymphoblastic leukemia in children and adults: a comparative matched cohort study. *Bone Marrow Transplant* 1996;17:917–922.
75. Munn RK, Henslee-Downey PJ, Romond EH, et al. Treatment of leukemia with partially matched related bone marrow transplantation. *Bone Marrow Transplant* 1997;19:421–427.
76. Henslee-Downey PJ, Abhyankar SH, Parrish RS, et al. Use of partially mismatched related donors extends access to allogeneic marrow transplant. *Blood* 1997;89:3864–3872.
77. Lee C, Brouillette M, Lamb L, et al. Use of a closed system for V alpha beta-positive T cell depletion of marrow for use in partially mismatched related donor (PMRD) transplantation. *Prog Clin Biol Res* 1994;389:523–532.
78. Lamb LS, Gee AP, Parrish RS et al. Acute rejection of marrow grafts in patients transplanted from a partially mismatched related donor: clinical and immunologic characteristics. *Bone Marrow Transplant* 1996;17:1021–1027.
79. Lee C, Henslee-Downey PJ, Brouillette M, et al. Comparison of OKT3 and T10B9 for ex vivo T-cell depletion of partially mismatched related donor bone marrow transplants. *Blood* 1995;86(suppl 1):625a.

80. Henslee-Downey PJ, Godder K, Abhyankar S, et al. Sequential immunomodulation to achieve engraftment an control graft-versus-host disease across mismatched MHC barriers. In: Schechter G, Hoffman R, Schrier S eds. *Hematology*. Washington, DC: American Society of Hematology, 1999:389–395.
81. Lamb L, Henslee-Downey PJ, Parrish RS, et al. Increased frequency of TCR-γδ+ T-cells in disease-free survivors following T-cell depleted partially mismatched bone marrow transplantation for leukemia. *J Hematother* 1996;5:503–509.
82. Lamb LS, Musk P, Ye Z, et al. Human γδ+ T lymphocytes have in vitro graft vs leukemia activity in the absence of an allogeneic response. *Bone Marrow Transplant* 2001;27:601–606.
83. Szmania S, Galloway A, Bruorton M, et al. Isolation and expansion of cytomegalovirus-specific cytotoxic T lymphocytes to clinical scale from a single blood draw using dendritic cells and HLA-tetramers. *Blood* 2001;98:505–512.
84. Musk P, Szmania S, Galloway A, et al. In Vitro generation of Epstein–Barr virus-specific cytotoxic T cells in patients receiving haplo-identical allogeneic stem cell transplantation. *J Immunother* 2001;24:312–322.
85. Chiang K-Y, Lamb L, Worthington-White D, et al. Assessment of G-CSF stimulated BM hematopoietic stem cells in normal donors. *Cytotherapy* 2002;4:55–63.
86. Lapidot T, Terenzi A, Singer TS, et al. Size of bone marrow inoculum versus number of donor-type cells used for presensitization: a murine model for bone marrow allograft rejection in leukemia patients. *Blood* 1987;70:309.
87. Uharek L, Gassmann W, Glass B, et al. Influence of cell dose and graft-versus-host reactivity on rejection rates after allogeneic bone marrow transplantation. *Blood* 1992;79:1612–1621.
88. Bachar-Lustig E, Rachamim N, Li HW, et al. Megadose of T cell-depleted bone marrow overcomes MHC barriers in sublethally irradiated mice. *Nature Med* 1995;1:1268–1273.
89. Bensinger WI, Berenson RJ. Peripheral blood and positive selection of marrow as a source of stem cells for transplantation. *Prog Clin Biol Res* 1990;337:93–98.
90. Aversa F, Tabilio A, Terenzi A, et al. Successful engraftment of T-cell-depleted haploidentical "three-loci" incompatible transplants in leukemia patients by addition of recombinant human granulocyte colong-stimulating factor-mobilized peripheral blood progenitor cells to bone marrow inoculum. *Blood* 1994;84:3948–3955.
91. Terenzi A, Aristei C, Aversa F, et al. Efficacy of fludarabine as an immunosuppressor for bone marrow transplantation conditioning: preliminary results. *Transplant Proc* 1996;28:3101.
92. Aversa F, Tabilio A, Terenzi A, et al. Treatment of high risk acute leukemia with T-cell-depleted stem cells from related donors with one fully mismatched HLA haplotype. *N Engl J Med* 1998;339:1186–1193.
93. Volpi I, Perruccio K, Tosti A, et al. Post-grafting granulocyte colony-stimulating factor administration impairs functional immune recovery in recipients of HLA haplotype-mismatched hematopoietic transplants. *Blood* 2001;97:1483–1490.
94. Albi N, Ruggeri L, Aversa F, et al. Natural killer (NK)-cell function and antileukemic activity of a large population of CD3/CD8 T cells expressing NK receptors for major histocompatibility complex class I after "three-loci" HLA-incompatible bone marrow transplantation. *Blood* 1996;87:3993–4000.
95. Ruggeri L, Capanni M, Casucci M, et al. Role of natural killer cell alloreactivity in HLA-mismatched hematopoietic stem cell transplantation. *Blood* 1999;94:333–339.
96. Velardi A, Ruggeri L Alessandro, et al. NK cells: a lesson from mismatched hematopoietic transplantation. *Trends Immunol* 2002;23:438–444.
97. Ruggeri L, Capanni M, Urbani E, et al. Effectiveness of donor natural killer cell alloreactivity in mismatched hematopoietic transplants. *Science* 2002;295:2097–2100.
98. Kawano Y, Takaue Y, Watanabe A et al. Partially mismatched Pediatric transplants with allogeneic CD34+ blood cells from a related donor. *Blood* 1998;92:3123–3130.
99. Peters C, Matthes-Martin S, Fritsch G, et al. Transplantation of highly purified peripheral blood CD34+ cells from HLA-mismatched parental donors in 14 children: evaluation of early monitoring of engraftment. *Leukemia* 1999;13:2070–2078.
100. Bunjes D, Duncker C, Wiesneth M, et al. CD34+ selected cells in mismatched stem cell transplantation: a single centre experience of haploidentical peripheral blood stem cell transplantation. *Bone Marrow Transplant* 2000;25:(suppl 2):9–11.
101. Passweg JR, Kuhne T, Gregor M, et al. Increased stem cell dose, as obtained using currently available technology, may not be sufficient for engraftment of haploidentical stem cell transplants.
102. Handgretinger R, Lkingebiel T, Lang P, et al. Megadose transplantation of purified peripheral blood CD34 (+) progenitor cells from HLA-mismatched parental donors in children. *Bone Marrow Transplant* 2001;27:777–783.

103. Redei I, Langston AA, Lonial S, et al. Rapid hematopoietic engraftment following fractionated TBI conditioning and transplantation with CD34+ enriched hematopoietic progenitor cells from partially mismatched related donors. *Bone Marrow Transplant* 2002;30:335–340.
104. Champlin R, Hesdorffer C, Lowenberg B, et al. Haploidentical "megadose" stem cell transplantion in acute leukemia: recommendations for a protocol agreed upon at the Perugia and Chicago meetings. *Leukemia* 2001;16:427–428.
105. Bretscher P, Cohn M. A theory of self-nonself discrimination. *Science* 1970;169:1042–1049.
106. Boussiotis VA, Gribben JG, Freeman GJ, et al. Blockade of the CD28 costimulatory pathway: a means to induce tolerance. *Curr Opin Immunol* 1994;6:797–807.
107. Lin H, Bolling SF, Linsley PS, et al. Long-term acceptance of major histocompatibility complex mismatched cardiac allografts induced by CTLA-4Ig plus donor-specific transfusion. *J Exp Med* 1993;178:1801–1806.
108. Lenschow DJ, Zeng Y, Thistlethwaite JR, et al. Long-term survival of xenogreneic pancreatic islet grafts induced by CTLA-4Ig. *Science* 1992;257:789–792.
109. Gribben JG, Guinan ED, Boussiotis VA, et al. Complete blockade of B7 family-mediated costimulation is necessary to induce human alloantigen-specific anergy: a method to ameliorate graft-versus-host disease and extend the donor pool. *Blood* 1996;87:4887–4893.
110. Guinan EC, Boussiotis VA, Neuberg D, et al. Transplantation of anergic histoincompatible bone marrow allografts. *N Engl J Med* 1999;340:1704–1714.
111. Ji SQ, Chen HR, Xu CQ, et al. The effect of G-CSF-stimulated donor marrow on engraftment and incidence of graft-versus-host disease in allogeneic bone marrow transplantation. *Clin Transplant* 2001;15:317–323.
112. Ji SG, Chen HR, Wang HX, et al. Comparison outcome of allogeneic bone marrow transplantation with and without granulocyte colony stimulating factor (G-CSF) (lenograstim) donor marrow priming in patients with chronic myelogenous leukemia (CML). *Biol Blood Marrow Transpl* 2002;8:261–267.
113. Ji S-Q, Chen H-R, Wang H-X, et al. G-CSF-primed haploidentical marrow transplantation without ex vivo T-cell depletion: an excellent alternative for high-risk leukemia. *Bone Marrow Transplant* 2002;30:861–866.
114. Ji SQ, Chen HR, Wang HX, et al. A clinical study of haploidentical and G-CSF primed bone marrow transplantation by using CD25 for aGvHD prophylaxis. *Zhongguo Shi Yan Xue Ye Xue Za Zhi* 2002;5:447–451.
115. Xun C, Ji S, Chen H, et al. A successful approach of G-CSF primed haploidentical bone marrow transplantation without ex-vivo T cell depletion for high-risk leukemia.*Biol Blood Marrow Transpl* 2003;9:63.
116. Khouri IF, Keating M, Korbling M, et al. Transplant-lite: induction of graft-versus-malignancy using fludarabine-based nonablative chemotherapy and allogeneic blood progenitor-cell transplantation as treatment for lymphoid malignancies. *J Clin Oncol* 1998;16:2817–2824.
117. Slavin S, Nagler A, Naparstek E, et al. Nonmyeloablative stem cell transplantation and cell therapy as an alternative to conventional bone marrow transplantation with lethal cytoreduction for the treatment of malignant and non-malignant hematologic diseases. *Blood* 1998;91:756–763.
118. McSweeney PA, Niederwieser D, Shizuru JA, et al. Hematopoietic cell transplantation in older partients with hematologic malignancies: replacing high-dose cytotoxic therapy with graft-versus-tumor effects. *Blood* 2001;97:3390–3400.
119. Luznik L, O'Donnell P, Fuchs EJ. Nonmyeloablative alternative donor transplants. *Curr Opin Oncol* 2003;15:121–126.
120. Sharabi Y, Sachs DH. Mixed chimerism and permanent specific transplantation tolerance induced by a nonlethal preparative regimen. *J Exp Med* 1989;169:493–502.
121. Wekerle T, Sykes M. Mixed chimerism as an approach for the induction of transplantation tolerance. *Transplantation* 1999;68:459–467.
122. Sykes M, Preffer F, McAfee S, et al. Mixed lymphohaemopoietic chimerism and graft-versus-lymphoma effects after non-myeloablative therapy and HLA-mismatched bone marrow transplantation. *Lancet* 1999;353:1755–1759.
123. Spitzer TR. Nonmyeloablative allogeneic stem cell transplant strategies and the role of mixed chimerism. *Oncologist* 2000;5:215–223.
124. O'Donnell PV, Luznik L, Jones RJ, et al. Nonmyeloablative bone marrow transplantation from partially HLA-mismatched related donors using posttransplantation cyclophosphamide. *Biol Blood Marrow Transplant* 2002;8:377–386.
125. Georges GE, Storb R, Bruno B, et al. Engraftment of DLA-haploidentical marrow with ex vivo expanded, retrovirally transduced cytotoxic T lymphocytes. *Blood* 2001;98:3447–3455.

126. Solomon SR, Tran T, Carter CS, et al. Optimized clinical-scale culture conditions for ex vivo selective depletion of host-reative donor lymphocytes: a trategy for GvHD prophylaxis in allogeneic PBSC transplantation. *Cytotherapy* 2002;4:395–406.
127. Ferster A, Bujan W, Mouraux T, et al. Complete remission following donor leukocyte infusion in ALL relapsing after haploidentical bone marrow transplantation. *Bone Marrow Transplant* 1994;14:331–332.
128. Pati AR, Godder K, Lamb L, et al. Immunotherapy with donor leukocyte infusions for patients with relapsed acute myeloid leukemia following partially mismatched related donor bone marrow transplantation. *Bone Marrow Transplant* 1995;15:979–981.
129. Nagler A, Ackerstein A, Or R, et al. Adoptive immunotherapy with haplidentical allogeneic peripheral blood lymphocytes following autologous bone marrow transplantation. *Exp Hematol* 2000;28:1225–1231.

18 Umbilical Cord Hematopoietic Stem Cell Transplantation

Timothy F. Goggins, MD *and Nelson J. Chao,* MD

CONTENTS

1. INTRODUCTION

Umbilical cord blood (UCB) transplantation has been successful for a variety of malignant and nonmalignant hematopoietic diseases *(1–5)*. Since the first related donor UCB transplant for Fanconi's anemia in 1988 and the first unrelated donor UCB transplant (UCBT) in 1993, more than 2000 patients have undergone UCBT. Prior to and since the first successful UCBT, numerous studies have been performed looking at the suitability of this stem cell source for patients of all ages. Additionally, numerous UCBTs have been performed for a variety of diseases, ranging from nonmalignant hematologic disorders, enzyme deficiencies, congenital metabolic disorders to hematologic malignancies, and, recently, nonmyeloablative stem cell transplantation (SCT) *(6)*.

The investigation of cord blood as a potential source began because of the lack of suitable matched related donors for patients who could benefit from allogeneic transplantation. Unfortunately, only 25–30% of potential recipients have a human leukocyte antigen (HLA)-identical sibling who can participate as a donor. To address this particular problem, the National Marrow Donor Program (NMDP) was established in 1986 to facilitate the finding and procurement of suitable marrow from unrelated donors for patients lacking a matched sibling *(7)*. In the first 4 yr of the program, 462 patients benefited from transplants from unrelated donors. However, despite this program's success, many patients remain without suitable donors. Since the introduction of UCBT in 1988 and the first unrelated-donor (URD) placental blood transplants in 1993, the Placental Blood Project was developed to determine the feasibility of a larger-scale use of this source of stem cells in unrelated settings. The program focused on factors relevant to successful recovery, testing, and storage of cord blood *(8)*. Cord blood has now become a

From: *Stem Cell Transplantation for Hematologic Malignancies*
Edited by: R. J. Soiffer © Humana Press Inc., Totowa, NJ

feasible source of hematopoietic progenitor cells in children, and research is currently ongoing for its role in adult transplantation.

2. CORD BLOOD BANKING

The use of cord blood as an alternative source of hematopoietic stem cells for bone marrow (BM) reconstitution has been shown to be as successful as allogeneic stem cell transplants (alloSCTs) *(4,9–14)*. Cord blood is a potential source to overcome some of the limitations of the current system for finding an unrelated matched donor. Cord blood banks would not depend on recruitment and continued collaboration with the large numbers of volunteer donors and on the necessary continued updating of the "bank" because of the unavoidable attrition by retired donors. The ease and speed of obtaining typed, tested, and frozen cord blood makes cord blood banks necessary *(15)*. Numerous banks now exist with the goal of providing stem cells for transplantation. Also, there has been a proliferation of for profit cord blood banks storing cord blood cells for possible future use of the child.

2.1. Consent Process

Written consent should be obtained from the mother, authorizing the use of cord blood for transplantation. The preferred time to obtain consent would be prior to delivery of the infant. Informational material should be made available to mothers through their obstetrician and hospital obstetric units and during birthing classes. The option of collecting and storing cord blood prior to obtaining consent would put undo pressures on the mother, as well as resulting in excessive cost to the health care system. The unfortunate barrier to obtaining consent would be the lack of prenatal care obtained by the mother.

Some articles have proposed not obtaining consent to store and transplant cord blood stem cells (CBSCs). This proposal is primarily a result of routine hospital policy to dispose of the cord blood and placenta as waste. Thus, the argument exists that material being discarded can be salvaged for the beneficence of society, and consent would not be necessary. Additionally, some donor groups may be reluctant to donate cord blood, thus providing benefit by alleviating the consent process *(16)*. However, in the current health care environment focusing on altruism, it would be important to obtain consent from the donor.

The purpose of obtaining consent would also allow further testing of the mother and donor cord cells. The necessary testing to provide maximal safety can have social, psychological, and medical implications to the donor. These testing strategies are necessary in today's health care environment.

2.2. Regulatory Issues

The regulation of cord blood banks has come under regulations by the Food and Drug Administration (FDA) noted in a 1995 draft document concerning UCB stem cell products intended for transplantation. The FDA identifies cord blood as a biologic product, applicable to the prevention and treatment/cure of disease. The regulation of biologic products currently includes product applications and establishment of license applications *(17–22)*.

In 1995, the National Heart Lung and Blood Institute (NHLBI) funded three cord blood banks, six transplant centers, and one medical coordinating center to establish standard operating procedure for cord blood collection, processing, and investigation into its use. The NHLBI developed the standard operating procedure and preliminarily published recommendations in July 1998 *(17,18)*.

2.3. Ethical Issues

Cord blood presents numerous potential ethical issues to the transplant community related to harvesting of cord blood, banking, confidentiality, recruitment, informed consent, allocation, and clinical research. Many of these issues have yet to be explored, and only recently have some of these dilemmas been addressed. In a recent JAMA article, Sugarman et al. *(23)* summarized a Working Group on Ethical Issues in Umbilical Cord Blood Banking conclusions. The conclusions included the following:

1. Cord blood technology has multiple investigational aspects.
2. Confidentiality of the donor should be maintained during the investigational phase of UCBT.
3. Umbilical cord blood banking for autologous use is more uncertain than allogeneic use.
4. The private-sector marketing practices need to be closely monitored.
5. Recruitment for banking of cord blood must be investigated further to ensure equitable donor groups.
6. Informed consent should occur in the perinatal period.

Further committee reviews of these ethical issues are now becoming necessary as we come closer to improving the success of transplantation.

2.4. Histocompatibility Testing

Cord blood placed in the bank needs to have HLA-A, -B, and -DR testing prior to the freezing process to define the antigens necessary to perform successful searches for potential recipients. Appropriate storage of cells should also be available for more extensive histocompatibility testing of the donor to optimize obtaining more successful matches. Additionally, future testing of cord stem cells may be necessary by the transplant center to assess engraftment, graft-vs-host disease (GVHD), or graft failure. The importance of conserving the maximal number of cells for transplant must be weighed against the need for future testing. The data obtained from these samples could be beneficial in the clinical setting as well as for future studies.

2.5. Maternal and Donor Data

Both the infant and mother should be considered the donor; thus, information regarding both is important to obtain, including medical history of the mother and donor. Also, important would be obtaining the medical history of family members for rare genetic disorders, as well as documenting newborn medical screening for disorders such as sickle cell anemia, galactosemia, phenylketonuria (PKU), and other metabolic disorders.

2.5.1. Infectious Agent Testing

Infectious organisms can be transferred to recipients of cord blood (Table 1) *(15,16)*. The risk of congenital infections depends on the prevalence and incidence in the pregnant women and the variability of the placental barrier to allow the fetus, and thus the cord blood, to pass the infectious agent. The congenital infections that can be passed from mother to infant are vast and include such agents as human immunodeficiency virus (HIV), cytomegalovirus (CMV), syphilis, and rubella. The data regarding these infectious agents vary with subpopulations, but general risks are known. For example, mothers with primary CMV infection during pregnancy can transmit the virus to the fetus in up to 40% of patients. HIV has a prevalence of transmission to the fetus in up to 30% of maternal patients not treated with antiretroviral drugs. Primary toxoplasmosis and rubella infections have also been widely known to cross the placental

Table 1
Common Tests Performed on UCB

ABO and Rh blood groups and types
Antibody screen
Alanine aminotransferase
Alanine aminotransferase in international units
Cholesterol level
Cytomegalovirus (CMV) antibody
Hepatitis B core antibody
Hemoglobin S (hemoglobin electropheresis)
Hepatitis B surface antigen
Hepatitis C virus antibody
Human immunodeficiency virus 1/2 combo test
Human immunodeficiency virus-1 antigen p24
Human T-lymphotropic virus type I and type II
Nucleic acid test for HIV-1 and HCV
Serological test for syphilis
Bacterial culture/contamination

barrier and infect the fetus, causing numerous congenital anomalies. Infections such as hepatitis B, herpes simplex, and varicella zoster rarely cross the placenta during gestation, but, rather, are acquired perinatally *(15)*. This certainly could be an important route by which infectious agents are transmitted to cord blood. Additionally, during vaginal delivery, the umbilical cord and placenta come into contact with vaginal, cervical, and perineal skin, which could be sources of contamination with infectious agents such as *Candida albicans*, an important known infectious agent in transplant patients.

Cytomegalovirus, the most common life-threatening infection in BM transplant (BMT) patients *(24)*, affects up to 2% of newborns in the United States, with a majority arising from women with primary CMV infection during pregnancy. The virus can reliably be detected from urine and saliva samples of the newborn, and rarely is it detected in the serum of congenitally infected infants. IgM antibody in the newborn or placental blood is diagnostic, yet it fails to detect up to 40% of cases. Therefore, testing of the infant may need to be necessary *(15)*.

Human immunodeficiency virus infection, as indicated earlier, can be transmitted to the fetus in up to one-third of infected mothers not treated with antiretroviral medications. Polymerase chain reaction (PCR)-detectable HIV-1 sequences have been found in peripheral blood of about two-thirds of newborns documented to have the virus. HIV infection can be acquired by the fetus in numerous ways, including perinatally, during fetal life by vertical transmission, or by breast-feeding. Serologic testing could identify most infants at risk, except in mothers with early HIV infection who have not yet developed antibodies. This necessitates testing of maternal blood using PCR for HIV, which can determine infection earlier in the process.

Hepatitis B infections are usually transmitted perinatally to the infant. The risk of infection depends on maternal viremia, particularly at delivery. Hepatitis B surface antigen is known not to cross the placental barrier. Additionally, accurate testing of the fetus for hepatitis B is currently not readily available. This makes the testing of the mother necessary.

Hepatitis C is a known complication of BMT. The route of transmission of the hepatitis C virus (HCV) to the infant has not been elucidated clearly. Seroconversion during the first year of life suggests that most infections are acquired perinatally or postnatally. This, again, makes the testing of the mother necessary.

Table 2
Relevant Genetic Diseases

Hemoglobinopathies
Sickle cell anemia
Thalassemias
Erythrocyte enzyme deficiencies
G6PD deficiency
Adenosine deaminase (ADA) deficiency
Dihydrofolate reductase deficiency
Pyruvate kinase deficiency
Formamino transferase deficiency
Congenital Anemias
Fanconi's anemia
Dyserythropoietic syndromes
Rh-null disease
Congenital immunologic defects
Severe combined immunodeficiency
ADA deficiency
Wiskott–Aldrich syndrome
X-Linked lymphoproliferative disorder
Leukocyte adhesion defects
Glycogen storage disorders
Hurler syndrome
Hunter syndrome
Aplastic anemia
Adrenoleukodystrophies
Metachromatic leukodystrophy
Infantile leukodystrophy
Juvenile leukodystrophy

Other maternal infections must also be taken into account when testing cord blood. These include mothers chronically infected with streptococcus B in the cervix and who have undergone vaginal delivery. The implications of this infection are currently unclear. However, of note is the benefit of cord blood having a lower frequency of latent and chronic infections acquired throughout adult life, including CMV. This clearly gives cord blood a benefit when considered for use as a stem cell source.

2.5.2. Genetic and Metabolic Disorders

Prenatal testing of chorionic villus sampling and amniocentesis are available for prenatal diagnosis of genetic disorders. Some of these include metabolic storage diseases, combined immunodeficiencies, thallasemia, sickle cell, cystic fibrosis, and fragile X (*see* Table 2). However, many women and the institution of medicine would likely be reluctant to perform such procedures for the sole purpose of cord blood harvest. Other possibilities for obtaining this information include state newborn screening tests, which are routinely done on newborns in all 50 states. However, these screening tests would require consent from the parents to obtain cord blood for future use. Additionally, not all states screen for the same disorders, making information obtained through these sources incomplete. Testing on the newborn several months after birth may be necessary, yet several parents may be reluctant to have blood testing performed on their infant. This reluctance mostly stems from trauma inflicted from blood draws as well as information generated that some parents do not desire. Another strategy to obtain this information is to retain DNA from the original cord blood for testing when a match has been found. This manner of screening could minimize costs to the cord bank. The costs of such testing could add substantially to the transplantation, which the blood bank may be unwilling to absorb. Also, if any genetic or metabolic testing is to be done, it would be necessary again to obtain the mother's consent, maintain records of identity of both the mother and infant, and notify the parents of any abnormal test results. Obviously, this could add a great deal of labor to the processing of cord blood.

2.5.3. Maternal Blood Contamination of UCB

Contamination of cord blood with maternal cells was initially thought to possibly result in increased GVHD. However, this theory has not been supported in subsequent studies. Socie et al. *(25)*, using PCR amplification of two minisatellite sequences, first point out the low incidence of contamination of UCB by maternal cells. His study detected maternal cells in only 1 of 47 cases. Most important, however, was that even though they were detected, only a small level was present in the lymphocyte fraction (0.1–1%). The cells from this same group were then later studied using a highly sensitive PCR method *(26)*. Repeating the study revealed maternal cells present in 10 cases, a maternal allele could be discriminated from a neonatal allele. The cells amounted to 10^{-4}–10^{-5} of cord blood nucleated cells. Maternal cells at such low levels in cord blood samples is less likely to have any effect on GVHD in a clinical setting of transplantation. Additional studies utilizing fluorescence *in situ* hybridization has been performed on UCB. Hall et al. *(27)* noted contamination of maternal cells in only 7 of 49 cord blood samples, analyzing a minimum of 1000 nucleated cells. The level of contamination ranged from 0.4% to 1%. CD8 and CD38 cells were also analyzed from cord blood; again, only minimal contamination was present in 5 of 39 CD8 cells and in 1 of 27 CD34 cells.

Studies of maternal cell contamination have also revealed that expansion of UCB ex vivo using interleukin (IL)-3, IL-6, erythropoietin (EPO), and granulocyte colony-stimulating factor (G-CSF) failed to result in an increase in the maternal cell population *(28)*. This indicates that cells possibly with the capability of inducing GVHD would fail to proliferate to large enough levels to have any effect on inducing GVHD. Based on the above reviewed data, cord testing for maternal blood contamination cannot be routinely recommended.

2.5.4. Harvesting of UCB

The number of nucleated cells available from a cord blood sample has emerged, particularly in the adult population, as the most important factor determining the chance of engraftment. Numerous techniques have been utilized to harvest cord blood, including harvesting after placental delivery and harvesting prior to placental delivery. These harvesting methods have been studied to determine the optimal manner to collect cord blood cells. Wong et al. *(29)* noted a decrease in the number of nucleated cells harvested after placental delivery compared to before placental delivery. The median number of nucleated cells and colony-forming units (CFU) was significantly lower in cord blood collected after delivery by 9.5% and 11.6%, respectively, when compared to before placental delivery. The reduction of nucleated cells in samples collected after placental delivery included granulocytes, monocytes, and CD19+ B cells. The importance of harvesting the maximal number of nucleated cells was further reinforced by Broxmeyer et al. *(30)*, who indicated the lowest number of cord cells transplanted successfully to engraftment was 1×10^7/kg body weight of the recipient. Gluckman et al. *(31)* further refined this number in adult patients to include 2×10^7 nucleated cells per kg, noting an engraftment rate of only 69% in patients who received less than this number.

The size of UCB cell harvest is also affected by the infant's size, longer gestational age, and women with fewer previous live births *(32)*. Larger infants have a higher cell count, and more colony-forming units granulocyte macrophage (CFU-GM) as well as CD34+ cells. Additionally, every 500 g increase in birth weight increased the number of CD34+ cells by 28%. Women with fewer previous live births also had higher cells counts and more CFU-GM and CD34+ cells. Ballen et al. *(32)* also noted a decrease in CD34+ cell counts with each additional week of gestation and each previous birth. Conclusions regarding the optimal time and patient to harvest remains controversial and, at times, difficult because of numerous other factors relating to the donor and consent of the procedure. It is optimal to provide the safest environment for both mother and fetus as well as the harvesting the UCB at the best time to maximize the number of cells.

Additionally, the delivery of an infant can affect the numbers of leukocytes, leukocyte subpopulations, and hematopoietic progenitor cells. UCB leukocytes was highest with a prolonged second stage of labor, a likely result of granulocytosis. Stress during delivery decreased the number of T cells in the UCB than in peripheral blood, mostly the result of a relative decrease of CD3+/CD4+ cells. UCB, regardless of delivery, tends to have a higher number of T cells per milliliter of UCB than adult peripheral blood. A prolonged secondary stage of labor resulted in an increase in the absolute number of CD34+ cells and hematopoietic progenitor cells. The relative and absolute concentration of CD56+ was higher in UCB as well. Hasan et al. *(33)* first reported that vaginal deliveries had higher white blood cell counts than newborns born by cesarean section, which was confirmed in a study by Lim et al. *(34)* on the influence of delivery on cord blood.

Shipping of the harvested cord blood to the bank also must be considered. Broxmeyer et al. *(35)* noted that cord blood could be left at 4°C and room temperature for up to 3 d without much loss in numbers of progenitor cells responsive to IL-3, GM-CSF, G-CSF, and M-CSF. These results imply that cord blood could be shipped from a distant obstetrical unit and sent by express mail and arrive in a viable form for transplantation.

The volume of the unit of cord blood matters significantly. UCB volumes in excess of 60 mL are associated with a cell count of 700,000 or more stem and progenitor cells, the number thought to be required for transplantation. The New York Blood Center *(8)* now routinely does not do cell counts on volumes over 60 mL. Units under 40 mL are discarded, and units between 40 and 60 mL undergo cell counts.

2.6. Cryopreservation and Thawing

An initial 10- to 15-cm^3 aliquot is removed from the UCB sample for testing purposes. The unit of UCB is then ready for processing and cryopreservation. The New York Blood Center *(8)* processes the UCB sample initially with the addition of 20% dimethyl sulfoxide (DSMO); the amount of DSMO is equal to the UCB volume minus the aliquot removal plus the addition of anticoagulant. Both acid–citrate–dextrose and citrate–phosphate–dextrose have been used successfully as anticoagulants *(16)*.

Progenitor cell recovery is critically important to the transplantation process. Recovery has been improved by adding DNAse (20 U/mL) to the unit as soon as possible in the thawing process *(36)*. Clinical dextran (40,000–80,000 molecular weight [MW]) has also been shown to improve progenitor cell recovery *(8)*. The proportion of viable progenitor mononuclear cell recovery may exceed 85% with rapid thawing. Previous studies have shown increased progenitor cell loss with a slow thawing process *(37)*. Many transplant centers receive cryopreserved donor cord blood units. Most centers rapidly thaw the units, which are then diluted and washed in equal volumes of dextran 40/5% albumin solution (added over 2 min); samples are removed again, and then further diluted in 100 cm^3 of dextran/albumin solution. The entire process is widely accepted at many cord blood banks; however, only recently have studies begun to evaluate cord blood thawing and dilution for progenitor cell loss. Lane et al. *(38)*, in a recent abstract, concluded that thawing and washing cryopreserved cord blood was associated with approx 25% loss of the total nucleated cells and reduction in overall cell viability. Preliminary data indicate CD34 cells are well maintained. Recently, with the advent of attempts at ex vivo expansion, one study *(39)* analyzed repeated freezing and thawing, again using rapid thawing followed by dilution/washing with a dextran/albumin solution; no significant change in long-term culure-initiating cell (LTC-IC), CFU-GM, burst-forming unit-erythroid (BFU-E), or ccolony-forming unit-mixed (CFU-MIX) cell populations was noted. The study did note an increase in CD34+38– cell percentage of volume.

Red cell depletion has been proposed as desirable to avoid hemolysis in cases of ABO incompatibility and to reduce the volume of cord blood necessary to store. Reducing the volume would likely decrease storage costs and decrease the amount of DMSO transfused, reducing risk of severe reactions *(16)*. Broxmeyer et al. *(35)* noted an unfavorable loss of stem cell progenitor cells with red cell depletion. More recently, some studies have favored alternative approaches to red cell depletion. Denning-Kendall et al. *(40)* compared the efficiencies of these methods: Ficoll, Percoll, methylcellulose, gelatin, starch, and lysis to remove red cells and recover nucleated cells, colony-forming cells (CFCs), and CD34+ cells from UCB. The Ficoll and Percoll density gradient separation uses dilution of UCB in 1:1 Hank's solution and layered onto equal volumes of the density gradient, centrifuged, and then low-density cells are collected by pipet. The resultant cell pellet represents the progenitor cells. Percoll and Ficoll processing contained an average of 76% lymphocytes and more than 93% lymphocytes plus monocytes estimated morphologically. The Ficoll method yielded approx 1% CD34+ cells *(41–43)*. The gelatin method requires more steps to red cell depletion than either the Ficoll or Percoll method. Gelatin sedimentation prepares cord blood with 1 : 1 Hank's balanced salt solution (HBSS) and mixing it prewarmed to 30°C in 3% gelatin. The sample then is allowed to settle, with the supernatant collected by pipet. The remaining cells are resedimented using gelatin in the same manner except the volume lost from the first sedimentation is replaced with albumin. This method consistently, in Denning-Kendall's study, gave the best results, recovering CFC of $19.7 \pm 11.8 \times 10^5/70\ cm^3$ cord blood and CD34+ of $32.4 \pm 18.3 \times 10^5/70\ cm^3$ cord blood *(40)*. Starch sedimentation again requires 1 : 1 dilution in HBSS with cord blood and a volume of 6% Hetastarch *(40,44)*. The red cells sediment for up to 45 min at 30°C. This is repeated a second time before the cells undergo centrifuging, washing, and counting. The methylcellulose method adds HBSS to give a cord blood hematocrit of 25%; methycellulose is then added to give a final concentration of 0.1%. The sample is then mixed and allowed to sediment at room temperature for 40 min. The leukocyte-rich plasma layer is then harvested. The red cell lysis method mixes UCB with cold lysis fluid (8.29 g ammonium chloride, 1.00 g potassium hydrogen carbonate, and 37 mg disodium EDTA per liter of water); after 15 min at room temperature, the sample is then centrifuged for 10 min. Supernatant fluid containing lysed cells is removed, leaving the white cell pellet. Methylcellulose cell recovery was disappointing, whereas starch, gelatin, and lysis processes consistently removed greater than 95% red blood cells. Percoll and Ficoll were the most efficient in removing red cells. The Percoll and Ficoll methods recovered 23.2–21.4% of nucleated cells in UCB samples, which was not as good in terms of progenitor cell recovery as gelatin and the most expensive technique.

Gelatin appears to give the best recovery of nucleated cells in the original UCB sample (76.9 ± 13.5%) *(40)*. At least one transplant has been done successfully using gelatin red blood cell-depleted UCB *(45)*. Additional studies have supported cryopreservation using the Percoll method of red blood cell depletion and advocate the use of DNase I in the thawing process *(36)*.

2.7. Computerized HLA-Matching Algorithm

Rubinstein et al. *(8)* described the New York Blood Center's Placental Blood project data storage and processing. This center currently uses a computer network ORACLE database. The program, according to Rubinstein et al. *(8)*, performs the following functions: stores questionnaires and test results, stores volume of cryoprotectant to be added to each unit, compares HLA type of mother to UCB to determine the genetic relationship, generates labels for samples and testing trays, provides periodic reports regarding units and mothers and monitors missing data, maintains information of inventories (volume of UCB, lymphocytes, DNA), stores data on all requests for searches, performs the search for unit patient matches, and provides information on compatible matches. This computer system increases the ease of recalling data regarding each sample and prospective transplants and is a valuable tool to monitor each UCB transplantation.

3. BIOLOGICAL CHARACTERISTICS OF CORD BLOOD

3.1. Cellular Content of Cord Blood

The types of cell present in cord blood samples correlates with those present in BM and peripheral blood, although they differ widely in percentage of cellular composition of their lymphocyte compartments. The yields and distribution of lymphocyte progenitors, lymphocyte subsets, and hematopoeitic stem cells vary among allografts. The yields of CD34+CD38– hematopoietic stem cells (HSCs) appears to be lowest in cord blood allografts when compared to leukapheresis products and BM grafts *(46)*. Lymphocyte subsets tended to be lowest in cord blood grafts. However, the relative frequencies of the naïve CD45RA+CD45RO– phenotypes among CD4+ and CD8^{high} T cells were highest in cord blood grafts. CD3+ T cells, which have demonstrated to facilitate engraftment in murine models, demonstrated a tendency toward lower frequencies in cord blood grafts. Additionally, the cord blood grafts contained a significantly higher percentage of CD34+CD7+CD3–T-cell progenitors than other allografts. The CD34-positive population is quite heterogeneous, with a higher percentage of CD34+CD38– pluripotent stem cells present in cord blood. Cord blood contained the highest fraction of natural killer (NK) cells (CD3–CD16/56+) and almost no NK T cells (CD3+CD16/56+) compared to adult cell sources *(46)*.

3.2. Primitive Cells

Numerous studies have been performed on the cellular characteristics of primitive cells. Assays of colony-forming unit blast (CFU-blast), high proliferative potential colony-forming cell (HPP-CFC), and long-term culture initiating cells (LTC-IC) demonstrate the ability of cell fractions to form erythroid, granulocyte/monocyte, and macrophage precursors over an extended period of time in an in vitro environment *(47)*. Cord blood, as described previously, has several characteristics of BM and peripheral blood stem cells (PBSCs). The characteristics of these primitive cells, present in both BM and cord blood, has undergone extensive investigation over the last several years.

The CD34+CD38– cells present in BM and UCB generate early progenitor cells in long-term culture. The fraction of these cells present in UCB accounts for 4% of the CD34+ fraction, whereas in the BM, it represents only 1%. Cardoso et al. *(48)* estimated this population from a typical UCB sample could produce equivalent numbers of colony-forming units (CFU)–granulocyte/erythrocyte/macrophage/megakaryocyte, twice as many CFU–granulocyte/macrophage (GM), and three times as many burst-forming units–erythroid as the same population from an average BM sample used in adult transplantation. They also noted a fourfold lower production of CFU-GM among later progenitor cells (CD34+CD38+). The CD34+CD38– hematopoietic progenitor cells have a higher cloning efficiency, are more proliferative to cytokine stimulation, and generate approximately sevenfold more progeny than BM cells *(49)*. Mouse models have further attempted to clarify this subpopulation. The nonobese diabetic/severe combined immunodeficient (NOD/SCID) recipients noted that SCID-repopulating cells (SRCs) were exclusively found in the CD34+CD38– cell population *(50)*. Mice transplanted with 1 SRC could produce approximately 400,000 progeny 6 wk after transplantation. The human CD34+ cells infused into mice partitioned into a manner consistent with normal hematopoiesis and did not randomly distribute throughout the mice hematopoietic organs *(47)*.

New data have focused on the different ploidy levels of megakaryocytes (MKs) generated in cord blood CD34+ cells *(51)*. Cord blood MKs showed reduced number and polyploidization when compared to peripheral blood MKs, although, phenotypically, the platelets had similar membranes. The amount of DNA present in peripheral blood MKs during the late stage of culture showed a high content of polyploidy (up to 64 times), whereas cord blood rarely showed greater than two times the normal DNA content. The lesser degree of polyploidy present in cord blood MKs indicated the presence of a more primitive cell compared with peripheral blood MKs; this was further supported because cord blood MKs survived in culture longer than peripheral blood MKs. However, this is at the expense of decreased numbers of platelets developing early in the transplantation process *(51)*.

The CD34+CD38– population of cells has been further delineated using several antigenic markers. CD34+ cells in cord blood, which are HLA-DR+, are more primitive. They are enriched for primitive blast-cell-containing colonies, HPP-CFCs, and LTC–ICs. The opposite holds true in BM cells, where the HLA-DR^{-} cell population is the more primitive cell *(41)*. Traycoff et al. *(41)* further delineated this subpopulation to include cells containing the Rh123^{dull} cells (CD34+HLA–DR+RH123^{dull} cells), which are presumably cord blood cells capable of producing long-term cord blood culture-initiating cells (LTCBC-ICs). CD34+ Rh123^{high} cells form significantly more granulocytic/macrophages, erythroids, and mixed colonies than their counterparts. These findings were analogous to human BM *(52)*. Rh-123 is supravital fluorochrome dye reported to bind specifically to the mitochondria of a variety of living cells without accumulating in other organelles *(53)*. The more primitive cell populations also have low or undetectable levels of CD45RA and CD71 *(43,54)*. Further characteristics of hematopoietic progenitor cells (HPC) include Thy-1 expression, which is noted to be particularly enriched for HPP-CFCs *(55)*. Thy-1 is a cell surface molecule expressed on hematopoietic cells capable of reconstituting SCID mice and initiating long-term hematopoiesis in vitro *(55)*. C-kit expression can characterize primitive hematopoietic progenitors, the population of cells with a low expression of c-kit are cycle-dormant progenitors, and high expression indicates more rapidly cycling cells *(57)*. The majority of blast cell CFCs are in the c-kit^{low} population, whereas the opposite exists for CFCs. A similar pattern of c-kit expression is seen in adult marrow cells *(57)*.

The study of T-cell repopulation after UCBT has been more difficult. One of the major problems with the mouse model was the absence of T-cell development. Only recently has Kerre et al. *(58)* proposed a method to support T-cell development in the NOD/SCID mouse. Treatment with a monoclonal antibody against the murine interleukin-2RB resulted in human thymopoiesis in up to 60% of the mice. T-Cell development in these mice was phenotypically normal and resulted in functional T cells. Mice that continued to have ongoing thymopoiesis developed naïve CD45RA+ cells. The study of T-cell repopulation is also halted by recovery following myeloablative regimens, which usually occurs between 18 mo and 3 yr after transplantation. UCBT usually requires up to 2–3 yr to reconstitute T cells, both in children and adults *(59)*. Interestingly, nonmyeloablative regimens tend to reconstitute T-cell populations over a faster time period (12 mo). Chao et al. *(60)*. noted a remarkably different pattern of recovery of the T-cell pool following nonmyeloablative regimens compared to myeloablative ones. A naïve rapidly expanding population of T cells outnumbered the memory cells in recipients of nonmyeloablative regimens. This cell population resulted in normal range T-cell counts 1 yr after transplantation.

3.3. Implications of the Cell Cycle

The cell cycle phase in which cells reside has important implications in proliferative capacity and gene transduction. In both the BM and cord blood, the percentage of CD34-positive cells in the proliferative phase (S-G_2/M phase) of the cell cycle increased with CD38 expression. A lower percentage of more primitive cells were cycling than later progenitor cells *(49)*. The earliest cord blood cells tended to be in G_0/G_1 phase of the cell cycle, compared to more rapid cycling cells in the bone marrow. Additionally, BM hematopoietic progenitor cells tended to be more responsive than cord blood cells to negative regulation by cytokines, although cells stimulated into the cell cycle regardless of the site of origin can be inhibited equally *(61–66)*. Cord blood cells also respond more favorably to growth factors, increasing the number of progeny several-fold compared to BM cells, implying that cord blood progenitors are a superior source of stem cells for transplantation. Cord blood cells have been noted to rapidly exit G0/G1 phases of the cell cycle in response to the steel factor, which has further implications on enhancing ex vivo expansion of progenitor cells.

Loss of telomeric DNA has also been shown to trigger cellular senescence with exponential increases in somatic cell division *(67)*. Cells produced in cultures of purified adult BM precursors tended to have shorter telomere lengths than cord blood cells or purified fetal liver. Vaziri et al. *(67)* suggest that this indicated reduced proliferative potential as cells age. These findings clearly have implications on future directions of treatment, including the source of progenitor cells as well as gene therapy.

3.4. Ex Vivo Expansion of CBSCs

Numerous laboratory studies have reinforced that cord blood cells can be expanded ex vivo using culture conditions similar to those used for BM or peripheral blood cells. As previously indicated, several studies support expansion of the most primitive cells, which are believed to be in higher concentration in cord blood samples. Extensive research looking for the optimal cytokine "cocktail" has been performed and, currently, there are active ongoing trials of ex vivo-expanded progenitor cells. The goal of these studies is to prevent graft failure in adult recipients following cord blood transplantation.

Initial studies described mouse hemopoietic progenitors capable of differentiation in three cell lineages when stimulated in spleen-conditioned medium without detectable erythropoietin *(68)*. Eventually, mononuclear cells isolated from UCB were noted to form blast cells after incubation in methylcellulose, erythropoietin, and medium conditioned by phytohemagglutinin-stimulated leukocytes *(69)*. Replating of the blast cells revealed secondary regeneration in 100% of primary colonies. However, replating of GEMM (granulocyte–erythrocyte–macrophage–megakaryocyte) colonies had less capacity for secondary colony formation.

Later, high replating efficiency of cord blood and BM CFU-GEMM was noted in response to erythropoietin and c-kit ligand with increased number of secondary colonies formed with replated primary colonies *(70)*. The c-kit ligand is an early-acting cytokine variously referred to as stem cell factor (SCF), mast cell growth factor (MGF), kit ligand (KL), and now mostly termed steel factor (SLF) *(63)*. The SLF alone has minimal proliferative capacity on hemopoietic progenitor cells in terms of colony numbers and size, although when used in combination with other cytokines, it has a synergistic effect *(71)*. SLF appears to enhance integrin–fibronectin-dependent tyrosine phosphorylation, which has implications in both growth of cells as well as localization to the BM environment *(72)*. SLF synergizes with GM-CSF, G-CSF, numerous interleukins, and erythropoietin (Epo) to enhance granulocyte macrophage colony formation and erythroid as well as multipotential colony units, respectively *(63,71)*. Additionally, it synergizes with interleukin-7 to stimulate pre-B-lymphocyte colony formation of mouse bone marrow cells. The SLF has also been shown to synergize with other interleukins. The limiting factor of SLF appears to be the ability to stimulate growth of leukemic blasts. The variability of responsiveness of malignant cells has cautioned its use in human subjects.

Cord blood plasma, when compared with fetal bovine serum (FBS), appears to enhance the human multipotential progenitor cells' (CFU-GEMM) ability to form secondary CFU-GEMM when replated *(73)*. When cord blood plasma was used in combination with FBS, the replating efficiency of cord blood CFU-GEMM was further enhanced. However, the average number of secondary colonies per replated primary CFU-GEMM colony was significantly greater with cord blood plasma alone *(65,73)*. Additionally, FBS in combination with other cytokines has noted impressive expansion of HPP-CFCs, CFU-GM, and erythroid (CFU-E and BFU-E) progenitor cells *(65)*. Ruggieri et al. *(74)* noted combinations of cord blood plasma, SLF, and cytokines induced maximal cumulative nucleated cell expansion (1044-fold), with the least expansion (142-fold) occurring with the FBS and cytokine combination. This was particularly true among mature cell subsets; however, expansion of immature subsets appeared to be equivalent when comparing cord blood plasma with peripheral blood plasma. The effects of cord blood plasma on ex vivo expansion remains poorly understood; it is unclear whether this is secondary to known or unknown factors or to the synergy of these cytokines. The use of FBS and cord blood plasma appears promising with ex vivo expansion and may impact the use of cord blood transplantation in the adult population.

Recent studies have noted platelet-derived growth factor enhances ex vivo expansion of megakaryocytic progenitors from UCB, without promoting in vitro maturation of megakaryocytes *(75)*. Thrombopoietin (TPO) has also shown evidence of ex vivo expansion of cord blood CD34+ cells as well as apoptosis *(10,76)*. The implications of TPO and its use in ex vivo expansion continues to be delineated.

Flt-3 ligand (FL), an early-acting growth factor, promotes ex vivo expansion of hematopoietic stem and progenitor cells. The effect and mechanism of FL is unclear. FL, when used in combination with SLF and other growth factors, promotes ex vivo expansion and differentiation of cord blood hematopoietic cells *(77)*. Recent data on the promotion of the megakaryocytic lineage has shown beneficial results in the presence of FL, further reinforcing its use as an ex vivo expansion of cord blood cells *(78)*.

Studies further focused on the proliferative capacity of CD34+ cells. Xiao et al. *(79)* reinforced the expansion capacity of these cells, noting that a single CD34+ cell could expand several-fold when combined with various cytokines, including SLF. Fourteen days of expansion of UCB CD34+ cells can result in a progenitor yield exceeding conventional BM harvest or three cytokine-elicited peripheral blood aphereses used in autologous transplantation by as much as 1000-fold *(80)*. This implies the greater potential for ex vivo expansion of UCB CD34+ cells.

The use of bioreactors, continuous perfusion culture, to enhance ex vivo expansion of populations of cord blood cells has noted significant expansion of UCB cells. Yields of progenitor cells from perfusion cultures with SLF-containing medium (with or without stroma) averaged 40- to 60-fold expansion of CFU-GM colonies *(81)*. Continuous perfusion culture medium attempts to mimic the biologic compartment (BM) optimizing physiologic growth of cells. The continuous perfusion culture bioreactors have noted large-scale expansion of human progenitor mononuclear cells from BM *(82)*. Application of perfusion culture technology offers potentially attractive means to increase efficacy and safety of transplantation while reducing complexity and cost.

3.5. Gene Therapy of CBSCs

Since the first successful transduction of genetic material into a hematopoietic stem cell, several studies have been published evaluating various vehicles of transduction, transduction into murine stem cells, and several case reports of transduced genetic material for cure of various genetic disorders. Cord blood hematopoietic progenitor cells are obvious vehicles for genetic material to be disseminated, because these are the earliest progenitor cells and are likely capable of lifetime expression of genetic material *(83)*.

The initial studies on murine models utilizing retroviral gene transduction have been favorable. The transduction of murine pluripotential cell have been shown to provide progeny in secondary and even tertiary recipients *(84)*. However, the genetic transduction has been less successful in larger animals. The process remains inefficient based on the low frequency of progeny cells found to have the transduced material *(84)*. Recently, several case studies of transduced ADA deficiency recombinant vectors have been successfully performed, with continued production of the deficient enzyme *(85,86)*. Moritz et al. initially compared the efficiency of transduction of LTC-ICs from cord blood and adult BM and noted a higher frequency of cord blood cells with transduced material *(87)*. This was further confirmed by Lu et al., demonstrated high efficiency of retroviral vector transduction of the Fanconi anemia complementation C (FACC) gene into normal cryopreserved blood, with greater than 50% of cells showing PCR evidence of the FACC gene *(88)*.

The future of clinical trials will inevitably focus of the vehicles/vectors used to transduce genetic material into pluripotential cells. It is likely to focus of continued efficacy and production of the transduced material.

3.6. Localization of CBSCs

Chemoattractants and/or extracellular matrix proteins have a role in directing migration of hematopoietic stem cells and progenitor cells to the BM. Extracellular matrix proteins have been implicated on the involvement of localization of stem and progenitor cells to the BM. Major extracellular matrix proteins, found in BM include collagens, glycoporteins (fibronectin and laminin), and proteoglycans *(89)*. G-CSF and GM-CSF appear to have no chemotactic or chemokinetic effects on hematopoietic progenitor cells, whereas SLF, interleukin (IL)-3, and IL-11 have been reported to be chemoattractants in murine HPCs.

Lectins, carbohydrate recognition molecules, appear to play a significant role in localization of stem cells to BM *(89,90)*. Both long-term marrow culture studies in vitro and transplantation studies implicate galactosyl and mannosyl moieties to be involved in BM localization. These same moieties have not been implicated in other studies involving localization to the spleen *(91)*. CD34+ hematopoietic cells are heavily glycosylated surface sialomucin receptors and contain up to nine sites for glycosylation *(92)*. Therefore, it has been hypothesized that CD34 plays a role in leukocyte adhesion and localization during the inflammatory processes, and it has been implicated to play a role in stem/progenitor cell localization to BM *(92)*. CD34-positive progenitors express a set of receptors for extracellular matrix (ECM) proteins. CD29 (*B1*-integrin) is expressed in over 90% of CD34-positive cells. CD29 forms a heterodimer, which acts as a receptor for fibronectin *(93)*. CD34 receptors display weak similarities to cell adhesion molecules, including LAM-1, ELAM-1, and membrane cofactor proteins. These studies and more raise the possibility that CD34+ cells may localize to the marrow compartment as a result of binding to an L-selectin-like molecule. A recent study comparing the presence of two cell adhesion molecules (CAMs) on both cord blood and BM CD34+ cells found that there is a significant difference between the two cell populations. Although the results were not statistically significant, BM cells had a greater number of VLA-5 receptors than cord blood cells *(94)*.

Additionally, growth factors have been recently implicated to be involved in the localization of stem/progenitor cells to the BM microenvironment. Kim et al. *(95)* reported on an in vitro study of steel factor (SLF), stromal cell-derived factor-1 (SDF-1), and the BM environment. They found that SDF-1 and SLF act synergistically to mobilize cells and are believed to cooperatively result in migration of HPCs to the BM. Thrombopoietin supports survival and proliferation of megakaryocytic cells and primitive cells *(91,96)*. Both thrombopoietin and erythopoietin have been shown to stimulate adhesion and binding of progenitor cells to the extracellular matrix (ECM), indicating that cooperation between hematopoietic growth factors and ECM in the microenvironment might influence migration, localization, mobilization, and proliferation of stem/progenitor cells.

The process of HPC/stem cell localization to the BM has not been clearly defined and remains an exciting area of research.

3.7. Immune Responses and Tolerance: GVHD and Graft-vs-Tumor

Cord blood transplant recipients, particularly in complete HLA matches, have a low incidence of GVHD *(1,3,97)*. The low incidence may in part reflect cord blood T lymphocytes, which appear to have less lytic activity than adult T cells. Cord blood T cells after primary allogeneic antigen presentation demonstrate an increase in proliferation, although a decrease in cytotoxic activity on subsequent challenges are observed *(98–102)*. The proliferative capacity of T cells in cord blood appears to be as much as 100-fold less than peripheral blood lymphocytes. Cord blood mononuclear cells have been shown to respond poorly to IL-2, mitogen, or alloantigen in a mixed lymphocyte culture *(101)*. Interestingly, the phenotypic analysis of cord blood T cells appears similar to adult T cells. However, cord blood T cells are CD3+CD45RA+ -indicating naïve cells, in contrast to peripheral blood, which has mostly CD3+CD45RO+ T cells *(100)*. CD45RO+ memory T cells synthesize higher cytokine (IL-4, IL-5, interferon-γ) levels compared to its more naïve cell *(103,104)*. Interleukin-10 is increased in production after primary antigen presentation in cord blood; yet, repeated stimulation is required prior to increased production in adult T cells. This may represent a mechanism for increased induction of tolerance *(104)*. Of note, the production of cytokines relevant to T-cell development, particularly tumor necrosis factor-α (TNF-α) and interferon (IFN)-γ, are rarely detected in cord blood samples. This may contribute to the decreased response to allogeneic antigens, as well as less ability of cord blood to present these as foreign to CTLs in cord blood *(98,99)*. Additionally, cord blood T cells appear to develop a tolerance for maternal HLA antigens *in utero*; cord blood cells were unresponsive to noninherited maternal HLA antigens *(98,99)*. Clearly, these results would imply increased tolerance to familial cord blood samples. Cord blood does express NK-cell activity, which appears equivalent to peripheral blood lympocytes *(98,99)*. Although, it appears that NK cytolytic activity is not detectable in newly isolated cord blood samples *(99)*. In general, the mechanism of secondary unresponsiveness of cord blood T lymphocytes remains poorly understood. Recent evidence by Porcu et al. *(102)* implies a defective activation of Ras as a major reason for alloantigen-induced unresponsiveness in cord blood T cells.

The graft-vs-tumor (GVT) effect appears to be intact in cord blood transplants as well. Cord blood appears as capable as peripheral blood lymphocytes to lyse a wide variety of tumor cells in vitro *(98)*. Cord blood was able to purge cell cultures of up to 50% tumor cells in less than 5 d.

4. CLINICAL RESULTS

4.1. Related Donor Transplantation

The amount of published data for related UCB transplantation remains limited. Wagner et al. *(105)* published the first report on UCB from sibling donors for transplantation (*see* Table 3). The study analyzed data from 44 sibling donor UCBTs prior to September 1994. The probability of engraftment in HLA-identical (total 34 patients) or 1 HLA locus-disparate matches (total 4 patients) was 85% 50 d posttransplantation; the overall probability of engraftment of all UCBTs was 82% (two HLA disparate [1], three HLA disparate [5]) at 50 d posttransplantation. The median to neutrophil recovery was 22 d (range: 12–46 d) and to platelet recovery was 49 d (range: 15–117 d). Growth factors in this group had no impact on time to recovery of hematologic cell lines. Additionally, the time to neutrophil recovery did not correlate with the number of nucleated cells infused on the basis of body weight. Graft failure occurred predominately in patients transplanted for nonmalignant disease. An increased risk of graft failure has been reported in patients with aplastic anemia, β-thallasemia, and HLA-disparate grafts. The probability of GVHD grade II–IV was 3% at d 100; no patient had grade III–IV. The probability of chronic GVHD was 6% at 1 yr, and only 2 of the 39 patients with identical HLA matches or one HLA locus disparate developed chronic GVHD. The probability of survival in this group was 72%.

The Eurocord experience was published initially by Gluckman et al. *(1)* and followed by Rocha et al. *(106)*. The Eurocord group analyzed 78 patients who received cord blood between 1988 and 1996. The donor was HLA identical in 60 cases. Thirty-two patients had nonmalignant disease and 46 had malignant disease. One-year survival was 63%. GVHD grade II–IV occurred in 9% of HLA–matched transplants. Neutrophil engraftment occurred in 85% of patients receiving greater than 3.7×10^7 nucleated cells. Patients receiving less than 3.7×10^7 nucleated cells had a 73% engraftment rate. The 1-yr survival comparing these two groups was 57% and 68% respectively. Although engraftment was increased with higher cell dose, the 1-yr survival among both groups was not statistically significant, with a *p*-value of 0.29. Age, weight, HLA identity, and negative CMV status were favorable prognostic factors.

Table 3
Related Donor Umbilical Cord Blood Transplantation

	Wagner et al. (105)	*Eurocord Experience (1,106)*
Number of patients (*n*)	44	78
Median age (yr)	4	5
Nucleated cells (median number/kg)	5.2×10^7	3.9×10^7
CD34+ cells	NA	3.8×10^6
CFU-GM (medikan number/kg	2.4×10^4	4.4×10^4
Engraftment		
ANC>500/μL	22	30
Platelet count>50,000/μL	56	NA
No. engrafted	36	62
HLA disparity		
0	34	60
1	4	3
2	1	5
3	5	9
GVHD		
Grade III–IV	3	5
Chronic	6	14
Survival (Percentage)	62	63

NA, not reported
CFU-GM, colon-forming units-granulocyte macrophage

4.2. Unrelated Donor Transplantation

The published data on URD cord blood transplantation continues to be limited and its role in adult patients continues to be studied (*see* Table 4). The information from these studies is difficult to interpret primarily because of the heterogeneous nature of the study groups as well as the conditioning regimens. Many of studies are limited to registries, a small series of adult patients, single institutional reports, and anecdotal case reports. The majority of knowledge comes from pediatric populations. Only recently has a single, large multicenter trial been published, and the database continues to lack a randomized controlled trial *(107)*. Barker et al. *(13)* first attempted to compare BM to UCB via a matched-pair analysis. The study noted that neutrophil recovery was slower in UCBT, although the probability of survival at 2 yr was comparable. The comparison among BMT–T-cell depleted, BM–methotrexate immune suppression for GVHD, and UCB noted comparable incidences of acute GVHD, with less chronic GVHD in UCBT. Rocha et al. *(12)* attempted to further clarify the comparison of UCB (99 patients), T-cell-depleted BM (180 patients), and unmanipulated BM (262 patients) in a retrospective review of 541 patients. Nonadjusted estimates of 2-yr survival and event-free survival rates were comparable among the groups. The main differences in adjusted outcomes among the three groups appeared in the first 100 d after transplantation. Delayed and failure of engraftment of UCBT resulted in greater treatment-related mortality. Although the three

Table 4
Unrelated Donor Umbilical Cord Blood Transplants

	Kurtzbeg et al. (108)	*Wagner et al. (109)*	*Long et al. (110)*	*Sanz et al. (9)*	*Laughlin et al. (107)*
Patients (*n*)	25+	18++	42	22	68
Nucleated celss (median number/kg)	3.0×10^7	8.1×10^7	1.37×10^7	1.7×10^7	1.6×10^7
$CD34^+$ cells (median number/kg)	1.43×10^6	NA	1.61×10^5	$.79 \times 10^5$	1.2×10^5
Engraftment (median, days)					
ANC>500/μL	22	24	23	22	27
Platelets>50,000/μL	82	67	67**	105	99
No. neutrophil graft	23	13	36	20	60
HLA Disparity					
0	1	7	2	1	2
1	20	7	5	13	18
2	3	3	32	8	37
3	1	1	3	0	11
GVHD (No.)					
Acute Grade III–IV	2	2	13*	7	11
Chronic	2	NA	NA	9	12
Disease Free Survival (No.)	16	12	11	12	18

*Includes grade II GVHD
+Age range .8 to 23.5 yr
**Time to platelet independence
++Age range .1 to 21.3 yr
NA, not available

groups achieved similar results in terms of relapse, chronic GVHD occurred less frequently with UCBT.

One of the first studies focusing on URD-UCBT published by Kurtzberg et al. *(108)* noted the ability of cord blood to reconstitute HLA-mismatched recipients. The preliminary data shows engraftment in 23 of 25 transplant recipients with HLA mismatches of one to three HLA antigens. The absolute neutrophil count reached 500 mm^3 in a median of 22 d (range: 14–37 d). Platelet transfusions became unnecessary at a median of 56 d (range: 35–89 d) in 16 patients who could be evaluated. Red cell transfusions could be stopped after a median of 55 d (range: 32–90 d). Acute grade III GVHD occurred in only 2 of 21 patients evaluated, and chronic GVHD occurred in 2 patients. The overall 100-d survival rate among these patients was 64%, with an overall event-free survival of 48%. However, the median age transplant recipient was 7 yr (range: 0.8–23.5 yr), and median weight was 19.4 kg (range: 7.5–79 kg). Primary graft failure occurred only in those who underwent transplantation during leukemic relapse.

Following this study was a single-institution review of 18 patients with a median age of 0.1–21.3 yr, weighing 3.3–78.8 kg with acquired or congenital lympho-hematopoietic disorders or metabolic disease. Patients received HLA-matched (7 patients) or 1 to 3 HLA antigen-disparate (11 patients) grafts *(109)*. The probability of engraftment was 100%. For the 13 patients surviving more than 30 d, the probability of neutrophil-donor-derived recovery at 60 d after transplantation was 100%, with a median time to absolute neutrophil count (ANC) greater than 500/μL was 24 d. Platelet recovery was delayed for the 13 evaluable patients, with 10 patients becoming transfusion dependent. The median time to platelet count greater than 2×10^{10} was 54 d. Grade II–IV acute GVHD by 100 d after transplantation was 50%. The probability of grade III–IV acute GVHD by 100 d after transplant was 11%. Notably, the two recipients of HLA-2 antigen-disparate unrelated UCB grafts had only grade II disease. The probability of survival at 3 and 6 mo was 65%.

The Duke University UCB transplant experience *(110)* has currently enrolled 42 adult patients with high-risk disease; only 2 patients experienced autologous recovery and 6 died from infection 18–89 d after transplantation with no evidence of engraftment. Forty of 42 patients were mismatched in 1–3 HLA antigens, and only 13 patients (34%) developed grade II–IV acute GVHD. The median survival of the entire group was 104 d. The actuarial projected 3-yr survival was 22% (unpublished data).

Another single-institution study by Sanz et al. *(9)* involved URD UCBT in 22 patients with hematologic malignancies. The median age was 29 yr (range: 18–46) and the median weight was 69.5 kg (range: 41–85 kg). HLA match ranged from 4/6 (8 cases) to 6/6 (1 case); the median number of nucleated cells infused was 1.71×10^7/kg (range: [1.01–4.96] $\times 10^7$ kg). All 20 patients surviving more than 30 d had myeloid engraftment, and only 1 developed secondary graft failure. The median time to reach an absolute neutrophil count of 0.5×10^9/L was 22 d (range: 13–52 d). The median time to platelet recovery of 20×10^9/L was 69 d (range: 49–153 d). Disease-free survival (DFS) at 1 yr was 53%; DFS among patients younger than age 30 was 73%. Only one patient did not develop acute GVHD. Grade I GVHD occurred in five cases, grade II in nine cases, grade III in three cases, and grade IV in four cases. Nine of 10 patients at risk developed chronic GVHD. The median time to development was 121 d (range: 100–325); four cases were extensive and five cases were limited. Twelve of 22 patients remained alive and disease free, with full donor chimerism, 3–45 mo after transplantation (median follow-up was 8 mo). The cumulative probability of transplantation-related mortality at 100 d was 43%, indicating, again, that long-term follow-up is lacking for unrelated UCBT.

Laughlin et al. *(107)* published one of the first multicenter studies of 68 adult patients with life-threatening hematologic disorders receiving HLA-mismatched unrelated UCBT. Sixty patients survived more than 28 d after transplantation, with a median neutrophil engraftment of 27 d (range: 13–59 d). The estimated probability of neutrophil recovery in 68 patients was 90%. DFS at 40 mo after transplantation was 26%. The presence of a high number of CD34+ cells in the graft was associated with improved event-free survival; additionally, the presence of a large number of nucleated cells in UCB before cryopreservation was associated with faster neutrophil recovery. The median number of nucleated cells in the grafts, prior to cryopreservation, was 2.1×10^7/kg recipient body weight (range: 1.0–6.3×10^7/kg), and the median number measured after thawing was 1.6×10^7 (range: [0.6–4.0] $\times 10^7$/kg). In 30 patients who could be evaluated, platelet recovery took a median of 58 d (range: 35–152 d); the median time to platelet recovery of 50,000 was 99 d and of 100,000 was 124 d. HLA mismatch occurred in 66 of 68 grafts; 2 patients had 6 of 6 matches, 5 of 6 in 18 patients, 4 of 6 in 37 patients, and 3 of 6 in 11 patients. Among the 55 patients in whom engraftment occurred and who survived 28 d or more, only 11 patients developed grade III–IV GVHD by 100 d after transplantation. There was no statistically significant association between the grade of acute GVHD and the degree of HLA mismatching, mismatching in HLA class II alleles, seropositivity for CMV in the recipient before transplantation, or use of total-body irradiation or busulfan as conditioning regimens, although the overall number of patients are small.

4.3. Immune Reconstitution

Limited data are available on the kinetics of hematological and immunological reconstitution of UCBT recipients. Immune reconstitution following cord blood transplant is of concern both on a short-term and long-term basis. The short-term recovery of neutrophils after transplantation generally averages longer than the more traditional sources of peripheral stem cells or BM for transplantation. Neutrophil recovery in an assortment of studies averaged 13–29 d. Additionally, platelet count recovery is often delayed for up to 100+ d to reach a level greater than 50,000. A majority of studies have focused on the number of nucleated cells infused, influencing the speed of recovery of immune function.

Long-term recovery of lymphocytes after related or UCBT has only recently drawn some attention. Absolute numbers of T cells (CD3+, CD4+, CD8+) increased slowly after UCBT. The median time to both CD3+ and CD4+ cell reconstitution was 11.7 mo, whereas the median time of CD8+ cell reconstitution was 7.9 mo *(112)*. Much faster recovery of CD8+ cells than CD4+ cells with a characteristic inversion of the CD4 : CD8 ratio often is observed after BMT *(93,111)*. CD3+ T cells tend to be sizable in number early in the transplant process, with a gradual decrease in the percentage of cells as CD4/CD8 T-cells recovery *(94)*.

Natural killer cells generally recover faster than B cells, taking less than the 5.9 mo average of B cells. NK cells do not appear to change significantly in the posttransplant period *(112)*. CD2+ and CD7+ receptors are expressed on the on the cell surface of NK cells and immature T lymphocytes. The NK cells tend to remain relatively stable throughout the posttransplant period. The majority of cord blood samples have less NK lytic activity than adult peripheral blood samples; IL-2 or IL-12 can increase the NK activity and induce lymphokine-activated killer activity in mononuclear cells, increasing the number of NK cells. Lytic activity of NK cells appears to be related to subsets defined by integrelins, CD16+56– has less lytic activity than cord blood CD16+56+ NK cells, and the greatest lytic activity is present in peripheral blood CD16+56+ *(113)*. CD16+56– NK cells appear to be a novel subset located in cord blood.

Cord blood NK cells also appear to have similar capabilities of lytic activity compared to peripheral blood NK cells—both contain similar lytic molecules perforin and granzyme B and both can be artificially stimulated to secrete these granules *(114)*. The differences in lytic activity between cord blood and peripheral blood NK cells continues to be investigated.

B Cells recover quickly, generally at a median of 5.9 mo *(112)*. Additionally, CD19+ B cells, starting around 2 mo posttransplant, appear to increase significantly. These lymphocytes, in one study, were noted to express CD20 antigen, with most of them bearing sIgM and the others sIgG and/or sIgA. This increase in B cells does not appear to be related to infectious agents *(93)*.

Interestingly, HbF levels after UCBT have been observed to be elevated; a subsequent decline in HbF levels is less pronounced than in the first year of life. HbF levels increased steadily during the first 3 mo posttransplanation *(93)*.

5. FUTURE DIRECTIONS

The knowledge of CBSCs and their role in transplantation is rapidly expanding. The future likely will include improved ex vivo expansion of cord cells prior to transplantation as well as the possible use of tandem units of cord blood, both of which are currently undergoing clinical trials. The role of cord blood in nonmyeloablative regimens also is expanding, and randomized trials are necessary to further validate the use of cord blood as a stem cell source.

Cord blood certainly has its benefits, including decreased infectious risk and severity of GVHD. Additionally, the primitive nature of its stem cells appears to conjure significant advantages to the recipient. Regardless of its benefit, further investigation will be necessary to perfect the use of cord blood in transplantation.

REFERENCES

1. Gluckman E, Rocha V, Boyer-Chammard A, et al. Outcome of cord-blood transplantation from related and unrelated donors. *N Engl J Med* 1997;337:373–381.
2. Barker J, Wagner JE. Umbilical cord blood transplantation: current state of the art. *Curr Opin Oncol* 2002;14(2):160–164.
3. Fleitz J, Rumelhart S, Goldman F, et al. Successful allogeneic hematopoietic stem cell transplantation (HSCT) for Shwachman–Diamond syndrome. *Bone Marrow Transplant* 2002;29(1):75–79.
4. Li CK, Shing MMK, Chik KW, et al. Haematopoietic stem cell transplantation for thalassaemia major in Hong Kong: prognostic factors and outcome. *Bone Marrow Transplant* 2002;29:101–108.
5. Gluckman E, Broxmeyer HA, Auerbach AD, et al. Hematopoietic reconstitution in a patient with Fanconi's anemia by means of umbilical cord blood from an HLA-identical sibling. *Ne Engl J Med* 1989;321:1174–1178.
6. Rizzieri DA, Long GD, Vredenburgh JJ, et al. Successful allogeneic engraftment of mismatched unrelated cord blood following a nonmyeloablative preparative regimen. *Blood* 2001;98(12):3486–3488.
7. Kernan NA, Barsch G, Ash RC,et al. Analysis of 462 transplantations from unrelated donors facilitated by the National Marrow Donor Program. *N Engl J Med* 1993;328:593–602.
8. Rubinstein P, Taylor P, Scaradavou A, et al. Unrelated placental blood for bone marrow reconstitution: organization of the Placental Blood Program. *Blood Cells* 1994;20l:587–600.
9. Sanz GF, Saavedra S, Planelles D, et al. Standardized, unrelated donor cord blood transplantation in adults with hematologic malignancies. *Blood* 2001;98:2332–2338.
10. Fukuda S, Pelus L. Regulation of the inhibitor-of-apoptosis family member survivin in normal cord blood and bone marrow CD34+ cells by hematopoietic growth factors: implication of surviving expression in normal hematopoiesis. *Blood* 2001;98:2091–2100.
11. Korbling M, Anderlini P. Peripheral blood stem cell versus bone marrow allotransplantation: does the source of hematopoietic stem cells matter? *Blood* 2001;98:2900–2908.
12. Rocha V, Cornish J, Sievers E, et al. Comparison of outcomes of unrelated bone marrow and umbilical cord blood transplants in children with acute leukemia. *Blood* 2001;97:2962–2970.

13. Barker JN, Davies S, DeFor T, et al. Survival after transplantation of unrelated donor umbilical cord blood is comparable to that of human leukocyte antigen-matched unrelated donor bone marrow: results of a matched-pair analysis. *Blood* 2001;97:2957–2961.
14. Sanz GF, Saavedra S, Jimenez C, et al. Unrelated donor cord blood transplantation in adults with chronic myelogenous leukemia: results in nine patients from a single institution. *Bone Marrow Transplant* 2001;27:693–701.
15. Rubinstein P, Rosenfeld R, Adamson J, et al. Stored placental blood for unrelated bone marrow reconstitution. *Blood* 1993;81:1679–1690.
16. McCullough J, Clay M, Fautsch S, et al. Proposed policies and procedures for the establishment of a cord blood bank. *Blood Cells* 1994;20:609–626.
17. Fraser JK, Cairo MS, Wagner EL, et al. Cord Blood Transplantation Study (COBLT): cord blood bank standard operating procedures. *J Hematother* 1998;7:521–561.
18. Wagner JE, Kurtzberg J. Banking and transplantation of unrelated donor umbilical cord blood: status of the National Heart, Lung, and Blood Institute-sponsored trial. *Transfusion* 1998;38:807–809; Comment: *Transfusion* 1998;38:867–873.
19. Weber-Nordt RM, Schott E, Finke J, et al. Umbilical cord blood: an alternative to the transplantation of bone marrow stem cells. *Cancer Treat Rev* 1996;22:381–391.
20. Menitove JE. Current problems in obstetrics. *Gynecol Fertil* 1996;19:70–73.
21. Fredrickson JK. Umbilical cord blood stem cells: my body makes them, but do I get to keep them? Analysis of the FDA proposed regulations and the impact on individual constitutional property rights. *J Contemp Health Law Policy* 1998;14:477–502.
22. O'Neil B. Implementing a validation program in a cord blood bank. *J Hematother* 1996;5:139–143.
23. Sugarman J, Kaalund V, Kodish E, et al. Ethical issues in umbilical cord blood banking. *JAMA* 1997;278:938–943.
24. Hao Q, Shah A, Thiemann F, et al. A functional comparison of CD34+CD38– cells in cord blood and bone marrow. *Blood* 1995;86:3745–3753.
25. Socie G, Gluckman E, Carosella E, et al. Search for maternal cells in human umbilical cord blood by polymerase chain reaction amplification of two minisatellite sequences. *Blood* 1994;83:340–344.
26. Clapp DW, Williams DA. The use of umbilical cord blood as a cellular source for correction of genetic diseases affecting the hematopoietic system. *Stem Cells* 1995;13:613–621.
27. Hall J, Lingenfeiter P, Adams S, et al. Detection of maternal cells in human umbilical cord blood using fluorescence in situ hybridization. *Blood* 1995;86:2829–2832.
28. Fietz T, Hilgenfeld E, Berdel WE, et al. Ex vivo expansion of human umbilical cord blood does not lead to co-expansion of contaminating maternal mononuclear cells. *Bone Marrow Transplant* 1997;20:1019–1026.
29. Wong A, Yuen PMP, Li K, et al. Cord blood collection before and after placental delivery: levels of nucleated cells, haematopoietic progenitor cells, leukocyte subpopulations and macroscopic clots. *Bone Marrow Transplant* 2001;27:133–138
30. Broxmeyer HE. Questions to be answered regarding umbilical cord blood hematopoietic stem and progenitor cells and their use in transplantation. *Transfusion* 1995;35:694–672.
31. Gluckman E, Rocha V, Chastang C. Cord blood banking and transplant in Europe. Eurocord. *Vox Sang* 1998;74(suppl 2):95–101.
32. Ballen KK, Wilson M, Wuu J, et al. Bigger is better: maternal and neonatal predictors of hematopoietic potential of umbilical cord blood units. *Bone Marrow Transplant* 2001;27:7–14.
33. Hasan R, Inoue S, Banarjee A. Vaginally delivered newborns have higher white cells and band counts than cesarean section delivered newborns. *Blood* 1991;78(suppl):433.
34. Lim F, Winsen L, Willlemze R, et al. Influence of delivery on numbers of leukocytes, leukocyte subpopulations, and hematopoietic progenitor cells in human umbilical cord blood. *Blood Cells* 1994;20:547–559.
35. Broxmeyer HE, Douglas GW, Hangoc G, et al. Human umbilical cord blood as a potential source of transplantable hematopoietic stem/progenitor cells. *Proc Natl Acad Sci USA* 1989;86:3828–3832.
36. Newton I, Charbord P, Schaal JP, et al. Toward cord blood banking: density-separation and cryopreservation of cord blood progenitors. *Exp Hematol* 1993;21:671–674.
37. Takahashi T, Hirsch A, Erbe E, et al. Mechanism of cryoprotection by extracellular polymeric solutes. *Biophys J* 1988;54:509–518.

38. Lane TA, Plunkett M, Buenviaje J, et al. Recovery of leukocytes in cord blood units after cryopreservation by controlled rate freeze in DMSO and storage in vapor phase liquid nitrogen. *Blood* 2001;98:761a.
39. Timeus F, Crescenzio N, Saracco P, et al. Recovery of cord blood hematopoietic progenitors after successful freezing and thawing procedures. *Blood* 2001;98:757a.
40. Denning-Kendall P, Donaldson C, Nicol A, et al. Optimal processing of human umbilical cord blood for clinical banking. *Exp Hematol* 1996;24:1394–1401.
41. Traycoff CM, Abboud MR, Laver J, et al. Evaluation of the in vitro behavior of phenotypically defined populations of umbilical cord blood hematopoietic progenitor cells. *Exp Hematol* 1994;22:215–222.
42. Traycoff C, Abboud MR, Laver J, et al. Rapid exit from G0/G1 phases of cell cycle in response to stem cell factor confers on umbilical cord blood CD34+ cells an enhanced ex vivo expansion potential. *Exp Hematol* 1994;22:1264–1272.
43. Mayani H, Dragowska W, Lansdorp PM. Cytokine-induced selective expansion and maturation of erythroid versus myeloid progenitors from purified cord blood precursors. *Blood* 1993;81:3252–3277.
44. Rubinstein P, Dobrila L, Rosenfield RE, et al. Processing and cryopreservation of placental/umbilical cord blood for unrelated bone marrow reconstitution. *Proc Natl Acad Sci USA* 1995;92:10,119–10,122.
45. Pahwa R, Fleischer A, Shih S, et al. Erythrocyte-depleted allogeneic umbilical cord blood transplantation. *Blood Cells* 1994;20:267–274.
46. Theilgaard-Monch K, Raaschou-Jensen K, Palm H, et al. Flow cytometric assessment of lymphocyte subsets, lymphoid progenitors, and hematopoietic stem cells in allogeneic stem cell grafts. *Bone Marrow Transplant* 2001;28:1073–1082.
47. Hogan C, Shpall E, NcNulty O, et al. Engraftment and development of human CD34+-enriched cells from umbilical cord blood in NOD/LtSz-scid/scid mice. *Blood* 1997;90:85–96.
48. Cardosa AA, Li M, Batard P, et al. Release from quiescence of CD34+ CD38– human umbilical cord blood cells reveals their potentiality to engraft adults. *Proc Natl Acad Sci USA* 1993;90:8707–8711.
49. Hao Q, Shah A, Thiemann F, et al. A functional comparison of CD34+CD38– cells in cord blood and bone marrow. *Blood* 1995;86:3745–3753.
50. Bhatia M, Wang JC, Kapp U, et al. Purification of primitive human hematopoietic cells capable of repopulating immune-deficient mice. *Proc Natl Acad Sci USA* 1997;94:5320–5325.
51. Mattia G, Vulcano F, Milazzo L, et al. Different ploidy levels of megakaryocytes generated from peripheral or cord blood CD34+ cells are correlated with different levels of platelet release. *Blood* 2002;99:888–897.
52. Udomsakdi C, Eaves CJ, Sutherland HK, et al. Separation of functionally distinct subpopulations of primitive human hematopoietic cells using rhodamine-123. *Exp Hematol* 1991;19:338.
53. Cicuttini FM, Welch KL, Boyd AW. The effect of cytokines on CD34+Rh-123high and low progenitor cells from human umbilical cord blood. *Exp Hematol* 1994;22:1244–1251.
54. Lansdorp PM, Dragowska W. Long-term erythropoiesis from constant numbers of CD34+ cells in serum-free cultures initiated with highly purified progenitor cells from human bone marrow. *J Exp Med* 1992;175:1501.
55. Mayani H, Lansdorp PM. Thy-1 expression is linked to functional properties of primitive hematopoietic progenitor cells from human umbilical cord blood. *Blood* 1994;83:2410–2417.
56. Laver JH, Abboud MR, Kawashima I, et al. Characterization of c-kit expression by primitive hematopoietic progenitors in umbilical cord blood. *Exp Hematol* 1995;23:1515–1519.
57. Gunji Y, Nakamura M, Osawa H, et al. Human primitive hematopoietic progenitor cells are more enriched in kit^{low} cells than in kit^{high} cells. *Blood* 1993;82:2353.
58. Kerre TCC, De Smet M, Zippelius A, et al. Adapted NOD/SCID model supports development of phenotypically and functionally mature T cells from human umbilical cord blood CD34+ cells. *Blood* 2002;99:1620–1626.
59. Klein A, Patel DD, Gooding ME, et al. Central versus peripheral mechanisms of T-cell recovery in adults and children following umbilical cord blood transplant. *Biol Blood Marrow Transplant* 2001;7:454–466.
60. Chao NJ, Liu CX, Rooney B, et al. Non-myeloablative regimens preserves "niches" allowing for peripheral expansion of donor T-cells. In progress. *Biol Blood Marrow Transplant* 2002;8(5):249–256.
61. Broxmeyer HE, Kurtzberg J, Gluckman E, et al. Umbilical cord blood hematopoietic stem and repopulating cells in human clinical transplantation. *Blood Cells* 1991;17:313–329.
62. Broxmeyer HE, Benninger L, Yip-Schneider M, et al. Expansion in bioreactors of human progenitor populations from cord blood and mobilized peripheral blood. *Blood Cells* 1994;20:492–497.
63. Broxmeyer HE, Maze R, Miyazawa K, et al. The kit receptor and its ligand, steel factor, as regulators of hemopoiesis. *Cancer Cells* 1991;3:480–487.

64. Broxmeyer HE, Cooper S, Hague N, et al. Human chemokines: enhancement of specific activity and effects in vitro on normal and leukemic progenitors and a factor-dependent cell line and in vivo in mice. *Ann Hematol* 1995;71:235–246.
65. Lu L, Xiao M, Shan R, et al. Enrichment, characterization, and responsiveness of single primitive CD34+++ human umbilical cord blood hematopoietic progenitors with high proliferative and replating potential. *Blood* 1993;81:41–48.
66. Lu L, Xiao M, Grigsby S, et al. Comparative effects of suppressive cytokines on isolated single CD34++ stem/ progenitor cells from human bone marrow and umbilical cord blood plated with and without serum. *Exp Hematol* 1993;21:1442–1446.
67. Vaziri H, Dragauska W, Allsopp RC, et al. Evidence for a mitotic clock in human hematopoietic stem cells: loss of telomeric DNA with age. *Pro Natl Acad Sci USA* 1994;91:9857–9860.
68. Johnson GR, Metcalf D. Pure and mixed erythroid colony formation in vitro stimulated by spleen conditioned medium with no detectable erythropoietin. *Proc Natl Acad Sci USA* 1977;74:3879–3882.
69. Nakahata T, Ogawa M. Hematopoietic colony-forming cells in umbilical cord blood with extensive capability to generate mono- and multipotential hemopoietic progenitors. *J Clin Invest* 1982;70:1324–1328.
70. Carow C, Hangoc G, Cooper S, et al. Mast cell growth factor (c-kit ligand) supports the growth of human multipotential progenitor cells with a high replating potential. *Blood* 1991;78(9):2216–2221.
71. Broxmeyer HE, Hangoc G, Cooper S, et al. Growth characteristics and expansion of human umbilical cord blood and estimation of its potential for transplantation in adults. *Proc Natl Acad Sci USA* 1992;89:4109–4113.
72. Takahira H, Gotch A, Ritchie A, et al. Steel factor enhances integrin-mediated tyrosine phosphorylation of focal adhesion kinase (pp125fak) and paxillin. *Blood* 1997;89:1574–1584.
73. Carow C, Hangoc G, Broxmeyer HE. Human multipotential progenitor cells (CFU-GEMM) have extensive replating capacity for secondary CFU-GEMM: an effect enhanced by cord blood plasma. *Blood* 1993;81:942–949.
74. Ruggieri L, Heimfeld S, Broxmeyer H. Cytokine-dependent ex vivo expansion of early subsets of CD34+ cord blood myeloid progenitors is enhanced by cord blood plasma, but expansion of the more mature subsets of progenitors is favored. *Blood Cells* 1994;20:436–454.
75. Su RJ, Li K, Yang M, et al. Platelet-derived growth factor enhances ex vivo expansion of megakaryocytic progenitors from human cord blood. *Bone Marrow Transplant* 2001;27:1075–1080.
76. Woo SY, Kie JH, Ruy KH et al. Megakaryothrombopoiesis during ex vivo expansion of human cord blood CD34+ cells using thrombopoietin. *Scand J Immunol* 2002;55:88–95.
77. Zhang X, Cai H, Zhao J, et al. Influence of FL on ex vivo expansion of hematopoietic cells from cord blood in long term liquid cultures. *Chin J Biotechnol* 1999;15:189–194.
78. Li K, Yang M, Lam AC, et al. Effects of flt-3 ligand in combination with TPO on the expansion of megakaryocytic progenitors. *Cell Transplant* 2000;9:125–131.
79. Xiao M, Broxmeyer H, Horie M, et al. Extensive proliferative capacity of single isolated CD34+++ human cord blood cells in suspension culture. *Blood Cells* 1994;20:455–467.
80. Moore M, Hoskins I. Ex vivo expansion of cord blood-derived stem cells and progenitors. *Blood Cells* 1994;20:468–481.
81. Van Zant G, Rummel S, Koller M, et al. Expansion in bioreactors of human progenitor populations from cord blood and mobilized peripheral blood. *Blood Cells* 1994;20:482–491.
82. Koller MR, Emerson SG, Palsson B. Large scale expansion of human stem and progenitor cells from bone marrow mononuclear cells in continuous perfusion culture. *Blood* 1993;82:378–384.
83. Williams DA, Moritz T. Umbilical cord blood stem cells as targets for genetic modification: new therapeutic approaches to somatic gene therapy. *Blood Cells* 1994;20:504–516.
84. Petit T, Gluckman E, Carosella E, et al. A highly sensitive polymerase chain reaction method reveals the ubiquitous presence of maternal cells in human umbilical cord blood. *Exp Hematol* 1995;23:1601–1605.
85. Bodine DM, Moritz T, Donahue RE, et al. Long term expression of a murine adenosine deaminase (ADA) gene in rhesus multilineage hematopoietic cells following retroviral mediated gene transfer into CD34+ bone marrow cells. *Blood* 1993;82:1975–1980.
86. Hanley ME, Nolta JA, Parkman R, et al. Umbilical cord blood cell transduction by retroviral vectors. Preclinical studies to optimize gene transfer. *Blood Cells* 1994;20:539–546.
87. Moritz T, Keller D, Williams D. Human cord blood cells as targets for gene transfer: potential use in genetic therapies of severe combined immunodeficiency disease. *J Exp Med* 1993;178:529–536.

88. Lu L, Yue G, Zhi-Hua L, et al. CD34+++ stem/progenitor cells purified from cryopreserved normal cord blood can be transduced with high efficiency by a retroviral vector and expanded ex vivo with stable integration and expression of Fanconi anemia complementation C gene. *Cell Transplant* 1995;4:493–503.
89. Gordon MY. Extracellular matrix of the bone marrow microenvironment. *Br J Haematol* 1988;70:1–4.
90. Hardy Cl. The homing of hematopoietic stem cells to the bone marrow. *Am J Med Sci* 1995;309:260–266.
91. Gotoh A, Ritchie A, Takahira H, et al. Thrombopoietin and erythropoietin activate inside-out signaling of integrin and enhance adhesion to immobilized fibronectin in human growth-factor-dependent hematopoietic cells. *Ann Hematol* 1997;75:207–213.
92. Krause D, Fackler MJ, Civin C, et al. CD34: structure, biology, and clinical utility. *Blood* 1996;87:1–13.
93. Locatelli F, Maccario R, Comoli P, et al. Hematopoietic and immune recovery after transplantation of cord blood progenitor cells in children. *Bone Marrow Transplant* 1996;18:1095–1101.
94. Pafumi C, Mancari R, Parisi G, et al. VLA-2 and VLA-5 cell adhesion molecules expression in CD34+ cells from umbilical cord blood and from bone marrow. *Blood Purif* 2002;20:174–176.
95. Kim CH, Broxmeyer HE. In vitro behavior of hematopoietic progenitor cells under the influence of chemoattractants: stromal cell-derived factor-1, steel factor, and the bone marrow environment. *Blood* 1998;91:100–110.
96. Johnson GR, Metcalf D. Pure and mixed erythroid colony formation in vitro stimulated by spleen conditioned medium with no detectable erythropoietin. *Proc Natl Acad Sci USA* 1977;74:3879–3882.
97. Gotch A, Takahira H, Geahlen R, et al. Cross-linking of integrins induces tyrosine phosphorylation of the proto-oncogene product Vav and the protein tyrosine kinase Syk in human factor-dependent myeloid cells. *Cell Growth Differ* 1997;8:721–729.
98. Harris D. Cord blood transplantation: implications for graft vs. host disease and graft vs. leukemia. *Blood Cells* 1994;20:560–565.
99. Risdon G, Gaddy J, Broxmeyer H. Allogeneic responses of human umbilical cord blood. *Blood Cells* 1994;20:566–572.
100. Roncarolo M, Bigler M, Ciuti E, et al. Immune responses by cord blood cells. *Blood Cells* 1994;20:573–586.
101. Risdon G, Gaddy J, Stehman FB, et al. Proliferative and cytotoxic responses of human cord blood T lymphocytes following allogeneic stimulation. *Cell Immunol* 1994;154:14–24.
102. Porcu P, Gaddy J, Broxmeyer HE. Alloantigen-induced unresponsiveness in cord blood T lymphocytes is associated with defective activation of Ras. *Proc Natl Acad Sci USA* 1998;95:4538–4543.
103. Rainsford E, Reen DJ. Interleukin 10, produced in abundance by human newborn T cells, may be the regulator of increased tolerance associated with cord blood stem cell transplantation. *Br J Haematol* 2002;116:702–709.
104. Broxmeyer HE. Questions to be answered regarding umbilical cord blood hematopoietic stem and progenitor cells and their use in transplantation. *Transfusion* 1995;35:694–672.
105. Wagner JE, Kernan NA, Steinbuch M, et al. Allogeneic sibling umbilical-cord-blood transplantation in children with malignant and non-malignant disease. *Lancet* 1995;346:214–219.
106. Rocha V, Chastang C, Souillet G, et al. Related cord blood transplants: the Eurocord experience from 78 transplants. Eurocord Transplant Group. *Bone Marrow Transplant* 1998;3(suppl):S59–S62.
107. Laughlin MJ, Barker J, Bambach B, et al. Hematopoietic engraftment and suvival in adult recipients of umbilical cord blood from unrelated donors. *N Engl J Med* 2001;344:1815–1822.
108. Kurtzberg J, Lauglin M, Graham M, et al. Placental blood as a source of hematopoietic stem cells for transplantation into unrelated recipients. *N Engl J Med* 1996;335:157–166.
109. Wagner JE, Rosenthal J, Sweetman R, et al. Successful transplantation of HLA-matched and HLA-mismatched umbilical cord blood from unrelated donors: analysis of engraftment and acute graft-versus-host disease. 1996;88:795–802.
110. Long G, Madan B, Kurtzberg J, et al. Unrelated umbilical cord blood transplantation in adult patients with hematological malignancies or genetic disorders. *Blood* 1999;94:570a [Abstract].
111. Lum LG. The kinetics of immune reconstitution after human marrow transplantation. *Blood* 1987;69:369–380.
112. Niehues T, Rocha V, Filipovich A, et al. Factors affecting lymphocyte subset reconstitution after either related or unrelated cord blood transplantation in children-a Eurocord analysis. *Br J Haematol* 2001;114:42.
113. Gaddy J, Broxmeyer HE. Cord blood CD16+56– cells with low lytic activity are possible precursors of mature natural killer cells. *Cell Immunol* 1997;180:132–142.

Part IV Graft Engineering

19 Tumor Contamination of Stem Cell Products

The Role of Purging

John G. Gribben, MD, DSc

Contents

1. INTRODUCTION

Despite the success of the use of combination chemotherapy for the treatment of advanced-stage malignancies, the majority of these patients die of their disease. In an attempt to overcome drug resistance, there has been increasing use of high-dose therapy (HDT) with a curative attempt both in patients with previously relapsed disease and increasingly as consolidation therapy in first complete remission. The myeloablation induced by HDT can be reversed by autologous or allogeneic hematopoietic cell transplantation (autoHCT and alloHCT, respectively). Autologous cells have several potential advantages over allogeneic cells for HCT. Autologous HCT overcomes the need for an human leukocyte antigen (HLA)-identical donor, eliminates the risk of graft-vs-host-disease (GVHD) and has, therefore, enabled the use of chemotherapy dose escalation for a large number of patients with hematologic and solid tumors *(1–4)*.

The major obstacle to the use of autologous HCT after high-dose chemotherapy (HDC) is that contaminating tumor cells will be infused back to the patient and would then contribute to subsequent relapse. To enable the use of autoHCT, a variety of methods have been developed

From: *Stem Cell Transplantation for Hematologic Malignancies*
Edited by: R. J. Soiffer © Humana Press Inc., Totowa, NJ

to "purge" malignant cells. The aim of purging is to eliminate any contaminating malignant cells and leave intact the hematopoietic stem cells that are necessary for engraftment. The development of purging techniques has led subsequently to a number of studies of autoHCT in patients with either a previous history of bone marrow (BM) infiltration or even overt marrow infiltration at the time of BM harvest *(2,5–7)*. These clinical studies have demonstrated that purging can deplete malignant cells in vitro without significantly impairing hematologic reconstitution. The rationale for removing tumor cells from hematopoietic cells might therefore appear compelling, yet the issue of purging remains highly controversial. To date, there have been no clinical trials testing the efficacy of purging by comparison of the infusion of purged versus unpurged autologous BM. In addition, the finding that the majority of patients who relapse after autologous BM transplantation (autoBMT) do so at sites of prior disease has led to the widespread view that purging of autologous marrow could contribute little to subsequent outcome.

In assessing the value of purging, three basic questions must be addressed. First, what is the evidence that residual malignant cells are contained within autologous BM or peripheral blood stem cell (PBSC) collections? Second, can we purge these tumor cells using available techniques? Third, do reinfused tumor cells contribute to relapse and does removal of these cells lead to improved outcome after treatment?

2. EVIDENCE FOR TUMOR CELL CONTAMINATION IN AUTOLOGOUS STEM CELL COLLECTIONS

The likelihood that autologous hematopoietic cells are contaminated with neoplastic cells is determined by a number of clinical variables. BM involvement is extremely rare in some tumors, such as testicular or ovarian cancers, more common in non-Hodgkin lymphoma and in solid tumors such as small-cell lung cancer, neuroblastoma, and breast cancer, and invariable in the leukemias. Generally, the higher the stage of the tumor, the more likely the BM is to be involved. In addition, the ability to detect malignant cells within the BM is dependent on the sensitivity of the assay used.

3. IMMUNOCYTOCHEMISTRY

Immunocytochemical techniques have been most widely used to detect minimal residual disease (MRD) in solid tumors. Detection rates and levels of sensitivity vary widely depending on the tumor type, the stage of disease in the patient population being studied, and the methodology used to detect the tumor cells. The use of monoclonal antibodies that recognize cytokeratins is one of the most widely used methods, particularly in breast cancer *(8)*. An advantage of immunocytochemical techniques is that it allows morphologic examination of the positively stained cells, although it is not always possible to determine whether a stained cell is malignant. Because there are no true tumor antigens that are recognized using these techniques, great care must be taken in the interpretation of data to ensure that normal cells that express these antigens are not also scored as tumor cells. Additional markers that stain cycling cells, such as Ki-67, may improve the ability to discern malignant cells from background normal cells.

4. MOLECULAR BIOLOGIC TECHNIQUES

The underlying principle for the application of molecular biological techniques to the diagnosis of human malignancies lies in the detection of the clonal proliferation of tumor-specific chromosomal translocations or gene rearrangements. These have been studied most widely in the lymphoproliferative malignancies because of the specific nature of gene rearrangements occurring at the antigen receptors. The use of the polymerase chain reaction (PCR) has greatly increased the sensitivity of detection of MRD. Nonrandom chromosomal translocations are ideal candidates for PCR amplification if the DNA sequences at the chromosomal breakpoints. For example, cloning of the t(14;18) breakpoints involving the bcl-2 proto-oncogene on chromosome 18 and the immunoglobulin heavy-chain locus on chromosome 14 has made it possible to use polymerase chain reaction (PCR) amplification to detect lymphoma cells containing this translocation *(9)*. Using this technique, residual lymphoma cells were detected in the BM at the time of initial assessment and following induction or salvage therapy of all patients with advanced-stage non-Hodgkin's lymphomas containing the bcl-2 translocation *(9–11)*. However, the majority of malignancies, especially the solid tumors, do not demonstrate nonrandom chromosomal translocations and are, therefore, less suitable for detection by PCR amplification.

5. CELL CULTURE TECHNIQUES

The greatest disadvantage of molecular and immunocytochemical techniques in the detection of MRD is that these techniques do not differentiate between clonogenic tumor cells and cells that that have lost the potential to proliferate. Clonogenic tumor assays have the capacity to detect the tumor cells that are likely to be most relevant for subsequent relapse. Unfortunately, the conditions for clonogenic tumor growth have not been well characterized in the majority of tumors. However, sensitive culture techniques have demonstrated clearly that clonogenic malignant cells can be grown from BM with no morphologic evidence of infiltration *(12–17)*. At least for breast cancer, there appears to be good association between immunocytochemical and clonogenic assays for detection of MRD *(16,17)*.

6. RESIDUAL TUMOR CELLS IN PERIPHERAL BLOOD STEM CELL COLLECTIONS

There is the presumption that peripheral blood stem cells (PBSCs) provide a source of stem cells that contains fewer tumor cells than harvested BM, although this has been poorly studied. However, a number of studies have now demonstrated that PBSCs are often contaminated with tumor cells so that this source of hematopoietic cells may also require further processing to separate the hematopoietic cells from tumor cells. In a multi-institutional study of PBSC transplantation (PBSCT) in patients with advanced multiple myeloma receiving myeloablative chemotherapy tumor cells were detected in leukopheresis products from 8–14 unselected patients and ranged from 1.13×10^4 to 2.14×10^6 malignant cells/kg *(18)*. After CD34 selection, a residual tumor was detected in only three patients' products. Overall, a greater than 2.7- to 4.5-log reduction in contaminating multiple myeloma cells was achieved. In a retrospective analysis, cryopreserved BM aspirates from 83 patients with high-risk stage II, III, and IV breast cancer were obtained after induction chemotherapy but before BM harvest. All samples had no evidence of BM infiltration by morphologic assessment. PCR for cytokeratin 19 was performed and results correlated with the probability of relapse following HDT and autoHCT. The incidence of detection of cytokeratin 19 positivity assessed by PCR analysis in BM increased significantly with advancing stage: 52% for 19 stage II, 57% for 14 stage III, and 82% for 50 stage IV patients ($p = 0.0075$) *(19)*. Paired PBSCs and BM samples from 48 patients were analyzed using immunocytochemical and clonogenic tumor colonies techniques *(16)*. Immunocytochemistry detected tumor cells at a significantly higher rate in BM than in PBSCs ($p < 0.005$). Tumor cells were detected in 13 of 133 PBSC specimens (9.8%) from 9 of 48 patients (18.7%) and in 38 of 61 BM specimens (62.3%) from 32 of these 48 patients (66.7%). Clonogenic tumor colonies grew in 21 of 26 immunocytochemically positive specimens. No tumor colony growth was detected in 30 of 32 immunocytochemically negative specimens. Immunocytochemical detection of tumor involvement in BM and PBSCs was correlated significantly with in vitro clonogenic growth ($p < 0.0001$). PBSCs appear to contain fewer tumor cells than paired BM specimens from patients with advanced breast cancer, but these tumor cells appear to be capable of clonogenic growth in vitro.

Although it seems clear that in the resting state, peripheral blood contains fewer tumor cells than BM in some malignancies, a number of factors must be taken into account. First, there is now considerable evidence that mobilization with chemotherapy and growth factors mobilizes tumor cells as well as stem cells *(20)*. Second, a greater number of PBSCs than BM cells must be collected so that the cell dose infused becomes an important determinant, in that the total number of tumor cells rather than the concentration of such cells is likely to be more relevant. In patients with non-Hodgkin's lymphoma, although the concentration of tumor cells was higher than in peripheral blood, there was less than 1-log difference, and when allowance was made for the greater number of PBSCs required, there was no difference in the total number of tumor cells within the collected products *(21)*. This issue was also addressed in a study of patients with multiple myeloma (MM) *(22)*. Quantitative PCR analysis of the Ig heavy-chain variable region sequence of the patient's myeloma cells was performed to assess tumor burden in samples from PBSC collections and BM harvests from 13 patients with MM. The percentage of tumor cells contaminating the BM harvest (median: 0.74%) was higher than in the PBSC specimens (median: 0.0024%). However, because of the increased total number of cells required for PBSCT the increase in total number of contaminating cells in the BM vs PBSC autografts was less pronounced.

Taken together, these data demonstrate that it is naive to assume that PBSC collections are free from contaminating tumor cells. Clinical trials examining the question of tumor contamination and its clinical significance for subsequent outcome after HCT using PBSCs are needed.

7. IMMUNOLOGIC PURGING OF MALIGNANT CELLS

At the same time that techniques were being developed to demonstrate the existence of MRD, attempts were being made to develop methodologies to deplete such contaminating malignant cells without impairing hematopoietic progenitor cells. Because of their specificity, monoclonal antibodies (MAbs) make ideal agents to identify and target such malignant cells. The principle for the selective depletion of contaminating residual tumor cells from hematopoietic stem cells is illustrated in Fig. 1. The most likely mechanism of failure of immunologic purging antigenic heterogeneity such that not all tumor cells express the targeted antigen.

7.1. Characteristics of Ideal MAbs for Purging

The most important factor to be determined is that the MAbs target the malignant cell as specifically as possible but have no effect on hematopoietic stem cells necessary for marrow engraftment. The ideal characteristics of MAbs for purging are shown in Table 1. The targeted antigen should be present at a high density on the cell surface to increase the efficiency of subsequent cell killing or removal. To limit the effect of antigenic heterogeneity of expression on the target cell, multiple MAb cocktails are employed, targeting multiple antigens.

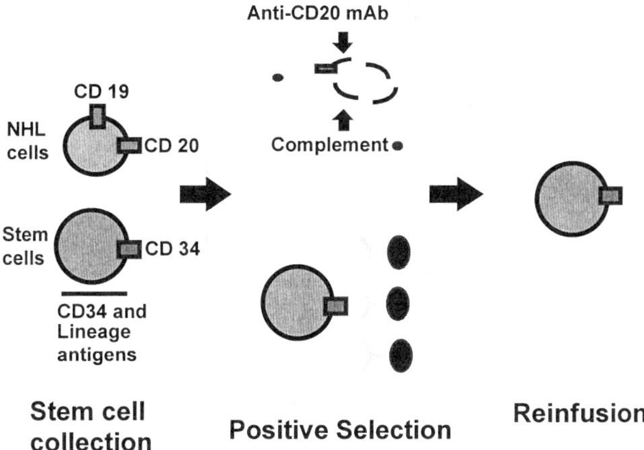

Fig. 1. Principles of immunologic purging. Targeted antigens are present on the surface of malignant cells but are not expressed on hematopoietic progenitors. Malignant cells escaping the purging procedure are likely not to express or express only weakly the targeted antigens. Purging may be by positive selection of CD34+ stem cells or by negative depletion of tumor cells.

7.2. Selection of Purging Methods

Because MAbs are not, by themselves, toxic, they must be used in combination with other agents to kill the targeted cell. The most widely studied methods of immunologic purging are complement-mediated lysis, immunomagnetic bead depletion, and immunotoxins.

7.2.1 Complement-Mediated Lysis

Early preclinical studies utilized the ability of MAbs to fix complement to the MAb-coated cells, which were then eliminated by complement-mediated cytotoxicity. Complement-mediated cytolysis was the most commonly employed method for immunologic purging, in part because of its efficiency, specificity, and relatively low cost, although this is used much less frequently because the use of animal products in the manipulation of human cells is not viewed favorably by the Food and Drug Administration (FDA). In most studies, rabbit complement was been used to circumvent the problem of homologous species restriction whereby cells are generally resistant to lysis by complement from the same species. The ideal complement source must be toxic to cells coated with MAb but not toxic to cells that have not been coated with antibody. However, there were major disadvantages to using complement. There is considerable variability among different lots of complement so that each new lot must be tested for nonspecific toxicity. There are nonspecific cell losses that occur because of the need for cell washing steps. In addition, complement-mediated lysis is inefficient when the neoplastic cells only weakly express the targeted antigen.

Among the factors that may influence the efficiency of complement-mediated lysis are the density of surface antigen expression, antigen modulation, and resistance to complement lysis. Failure of immunologic purging using complement-mediated lysis could be attributed to three possible mechanisms. First, the clonogenic tumor cells might not express, or only express weakly, the surface antigens expressed by the majority of tumor cells. Second, modulation of one or more of the surface antigens following attachment of the MAb to its ligand might limit complement-mediated lysis. Third, a subgroup of patients may have malignancies that are

Table 1
Ideal Characteristics of MAbs for Immunologic Purging

Not expressed on hematopoietic progenitors
Expressed on clonogenic tumor cells
High density of expression on tumor cells
Limited heterogeneity of expression on tumor cells
Lineage restriction
Depending on strategy for purging, ability to modulate

intrinsically more resistant to complement-mediated lysis. Anticomplementary factor has been described in normal BM cells that limits the activation of complement, not only on the cells that produce the factor but also on antibody-coated cells within the normal marrow *(23)*. Anticomplementary effects may be overcome by repeated treatments with complement, and previous studies have suggested that the use of repeated treatment cycles is more efficient in removing contaminating tumor cells than single treatment cycles. However, this approach is time-consuming, increases the expense of the procedure in both reagents and in laboratory staff effort, and may increase the nonspecific loss of hematopoietic stem cells. Recent work has focused on the identification and neutralization of membrane-bound regulators of complement activation, notably CD46, CD55, and CD59. Populations of cells that survive following MAb purging appear to be more resistant to subsequent treatments with the same MAb and complement, associated with the emergence of subpopulations of cells with a relative decrease in the surface expression of the targeted antigens.

7.2.2. Magnetic Bead Depletion

The use of immunomagnetic beads has the advantage that there is no biologic variability between lots as has been observed with complement. Most studies have utilized magnetic microspheres coated with affinity-purified sheep anti-mouse antibodies directed against the Fc portion of the MAb (Dynabeads; Dynal, Oslo, Norway). More recently, a number of particles have been developed that are directly attached to the primary MAbs used for purging. These reagents have the advantage of allowing more rapid and simpler purging procedures. Instruments to remove the immunomagnetic beads are now available commercially.

Immunomagnetic bead depletion is used increasingly as a method of eliminating malignant cells for HCT. The use of immunomagnetic beads was originally developed to facilitate depletion of neuroblastoma cells because the available MAb did not fix complement *(24)*. A number of studies have been performed for a variety of other malignancies, including small-cell lung cancer, breast cancer, acute lymphoblastic leukemia (ALL), myeloma, and lymphomas as described later in the chapter. Treatment of BM samples from lymphoma patients with either a three- or four-MAbs cocktail followed by immunomagnetic bead depletion resulted in the loss of all PCR-detectable cells after three cycles of treatment in all patients studied *(25)*. Immunomagnetic bead depletion had no significant effect on myeloid colony-forming assays, suggesting that repeated cycles of immunomagnetic bead depletion might be performed safely.

7.2.3. Immunotoxins

Purging of autologous marrow in vitro using immunotoxins is a particularly promising approach. Several exquisitely effective candidate toxins have been identified that mediate their cytotoxic function by inhibiting cellular protein synthesis. Because the mechanism of killing by toxins is different from that of chemotherapeutic agents, they are capable of killing cells that are resistant to chemotherapy *(26)*. However, these toxins are cytotoxic to both normal and malignant cells and must be targeted to the malignant cell to demonstrate specificity. The combination of these toxins with a MAb to target delivery specifically to the neoplastic cells is therefore a theoretically attractive proposition. If native toxins were to be conjugated to MAbs, the resultant immunotoxin would still be capable of binding to nonspecific targets by binding to the toxin-binding site on normal cells. This nonspecific binding is overcome by modification of the toxin moiety to delete the binding site but leave the toxin domains intact. The most widely studied toxins have been ricin, *pseudomonas* exotoxin, and *Diphtheria* toxin. Most experience of in vitro marrow purging has been with ricin. Multiple anti-T-cell intact ricin immunotoxins have been evaluated as potential purging agents *(27)*. The cocktail containing all four immunotoxins in equimolar concentrations eliminated more than 4 logs of clonogenic leukemic cells at a dose that spared more than 70% of the pluripotent hematopoietic stem cells.

7.3. Positive Selection of CD34+ Cells

Most studies performed have utilized immunologic maneuvers to remove malignant cells from the autologous marrow by a process of negative selection. An alternative and highly attractive strategy would be to select positively the hematopoietic stem cell. These studies have been hampered largely by the relative inefficiency of CD34 selection *(28)*. Preclinical and early clinical studies are underway in many centers examining the potential role of positive selection of CD34 cells followed by negative depletion steps to remove residual contaminating tumor cells.

7.4. Assessment of the Efficacy of Purging

The identical techniques that can be used to assess whether a hematopoietic cell collection contains residual tumor cells can be used to assess whether tumor cells remain present after immunologic purging. Culture systems have been used to examine the efficacy of different complement sources and to demonstrate synergy between chemotherapeutic agents and MAb-mediated purging *(29,30)*. PCR has been used to assess the efficacy of immunologic purging both in models using cell lines and patient samples *(11,31)*. Clonogenic lymphoma cell assays have demonstrated that different anti-B-cell MAbs differ in their efficiency of depleting lymphoma cells *(32)*. Treatment of harvested BM samples from lymphoma patients with either a three- or a four-MAb cocktail followed by immunomagnetic bead depletion resulted in the loss of all PCR-detectable cells after three cycles of treatment in all patients studied *(25)*. This study suggested that immunomagnetic bead depletion is significantly more efficient than complement-mediated lysis in depleting lymphoma cells but that multiple cycles of immunomagnetic bead depletion may still be required to remove PCR-detectable lymphoma cells.

Using a single cycle of treatment with multiple MAbs and beads, approx 2.5 logs of small-cell lung cancer lines could be depleted, although there was variability in the efficiency of purging different cell lines *(33)*. In parallel studies, there was no significant toxicity to myeloid progenitors noted. Using two small-cell lung cancer lines, immunomagnetic bead depletion was shown to result in a 4- to 5-log reduction of cancer cells and did not adversely affect BM colony growth *(34)*. Anti-CD15 MAb, expressed on a variety of human cancer cell lines, was capable of depleting up to 3 logs of breast cancer cells from normal contaminated marrow using immunomagnetic bead depletion, but it affected normal hematopoietic progenitors minimally *(35)*. The combination of 4-hydroperoxycyclophosphamide and immunomagnetic bead depletion removed 4–5 logs of clonogenic breast cancer cells.

8. CONTRIBUTION OF INFUSED TUMOR CELLS TO RELAPSE

The finding that the majority of patients who relapse after autoHCT do so at sites of prior disease has led to the widespread view that purging of autologous marrow could contribute little to subsequent outcome after autoHCT. Although no direct study has been made comparing the infusion of purged vs unpurged marrow, indirect approaches can be made to assess the clinical significance of immunologic purging.

8.1. Clinical Studies of Immunologic Purging

Immunologic purging was first performed in non-Hodgkin's lymphoma and has been most widely studied in this disease *(5,7,11,36,37)*. Additional studies have been performed in MM *(28,38,39)*, ALL *(40,41)*, acute myelogenous leukemia (AML) *(3,42)*, breast cancer *(43)*, small-cell lung cancer *(44)*, and neuroblastoma *(45,46)* among others. No randomized prospective study has demonstrated whether the removal of occult or overt neoplastic cells resulted in improved disease-free survival (DFS) *(28,39)*. Whether the failure to demonstrate an advantage of purging is the result of the relative inefficiency of the purging technique or the intrinsic resistance of the myeloma cells to the HDC approach used is not clear. However, these studies have confirmed that immunologic purging can be performed safely and that subsequent hematopoietic engraftment is not significantly delayed.

8.2. Complement-Mediated Lysis

In a clinical trial of 138 patients with AML, BM purging was performed using two MAbs and complement-mediated lysis *(3)*. One hundred ten patients were in complete remission (CR) at the time of transplantation (23 in first CR, 87 in second or third CR). Engraftment was faster in those patients infused with larger numbers of colony-forming units (CFUs). This study did not compare results obtained using purged vs unpurged marrow, but the relapse-free survival (RFS) of the patients in second and third CR was encouraging and appears to be comparable to that obtained following allogeneic transplantation in similar-risk patients. At the Dana–Farber Cancer Institute, anti-CD33 MAbs and complement-mediated lysis were used to purge the BM of 12 patients with AML *(42)*. Patients had durable but delayed engraftment, and platelet engraftment was particularly delayed in some patients. Of note, CFU-granulocyte-macrophage (GM) colony growth was markedly reduced following purging. In a multicenter study, autoHCT was used in 54 patients with ALL *(40)*. The BM was purged using as anti-CD10, anti-CD19 and anti-CD7 MAbs and rabbit complement. The transplant-related mortality was 5% and engraftment was rapid. Although the study was not designed to show efficacy, the clinical results appear promising.

Long-term follow-up was reported on 153 patients with B-cell non-Hodgkin's lymphoma who were treated at the Dana–Farber Cancer Institute with purged autoBMT when they were in CR or minimal disease state *(2)*. Notably, 47% of patients had overt marrow disease at the time of BM harvest. This study was associated with an encouragingly low treatment-related mortality. Engraftment was rapid in all cases.

8.3. Immunomagnetic Bead Depletion

The first clinical studies of purging using immunomagnetic beads were performed for children with neuroblastoma *(46)*. Immunomagnetic bead depletion was used to purge 123 marrows before autoHCT in 91 cases of neuroblastoma *(47)*. In this study, 59 patients received a single graft and 32 patients received 2 sequential procedures. Although the procedure resulted in a significant loss of mononuclear cells, there was little evidence of additional toxic effects on myeloid progenitors. Immunomagnetic beads were used to deplete leukemic cells from the marrows of patients with ALL *(46)*. In this study, the marrows of 18 patients were purged using a cocktail of three MAbs, although only 8 of these patients were subsequently treated with HDT and autoHCT. Engraftment was rapid in all cases, although reduced compared to that observed in patients with neuroblastoma.

8.4. Immunotoxins

Fewer clinical trials have been reported using immunotoxins for purging. Seven patients with high-risk T-cell ALL and six patients with T-cell lymphoma were treated by autoBMT following purging with anti-CD7 ricin A immunotoxin (WT1-ricin A) *(48)*. Incubation of the marrow with up to 10^{-8} mol/L had no significant effect on hematopoietic stem cell progenitors as assessed by colony assay growth or by subsequent delay of engraftment. Using a different approach, autologous marrow from 14 consecutive patients with T-cell ALL was purged with a combination of 2 immunotoxins, anti-CD5 and anti-CD7 linked to intact ricin, plus 4-hydroperoxycyclophosphamide *(49)*. The efficacy of purging was assessed using multiparameter flow analysis, cell sorting, and leukemic progenitor cell colony assay. Following purging, no blast colonies were observed in the marrows of 11 of 13 evaluable patients. Engraftment occurred in 13 of the 14 patients and the median time to reach an absolute neutrophil count greater than 500/µL was 27 d. Despite the apparent efficiency of purging, nine patients relapsed, the majority of them shortly after transplantation. In this study, relapse after transplantation was most likely the result of failure of the HDT to ablate endogenous disease in these high-risk patients.

8.5. Successful Immunologic Purging May Result in Improved Outcome

In studies at the Dana–Farber Cancer Institute, PCR amplification of the t(14;18) was used to detect residual lymphoma cells in the BM before and after purging to assess whether efficient purging had any impact on DFS *(11)*. In this study, 114 patients with B-cell non-Hodgkin's lymphoma and the bcl-2 translocation were studied. Residual lymphoma cells were detected in all patients in the harvested autologous BM. Following three cycles of immunologic purging using the anti-B-cell MAbs and complement-mediated lysis, PCR amplification detected residual lymphoma cells in 57 of these patients. The incidence of relapse was significantly increased in patients who had residual detectable lymphoma cells compared to those in whom no lymphoma cells were detectable. Patients who were infused with a source of hematopoietic cells that was free of detectable lymphoma cells had improved outcome compared to those who had residual detectable lymphoma. This finding was independent of the histology of the lymphoma, the degree of BM infiltration at the time of BM harvest, or remission status at the time of autoBMT. In non-Hodgkin's lymphoma, two additional studies have demonstrated that the presence of residual lymphoma cells within the stem cell product was associated with poorer outcome *(15,50)*. Even in metastatic breast cancer, under circumstances where it is likely that endogenous disease in the patient contributes highly to subsequent failure, the presence of contaminating breast cancer cells may be associated with poor outcome after HDT. In a retrospective analysis, cryopreserved BM aspirates from 83 patients with high-risk stage II, III, and IV breast cancer were obtained after induction chemotherapy but before BM harvest *(19)*. In this study, there was no evidence of BM infiltration by morphologic assessment. PCR for cytokeratin 19 was performed and results correlated with the probability of relapse following HDT and autoBMT. The incidence of detection of cytokeratin 19 positivity assessed by PCR analysis in BM increased significantly with advancing stage. Furthermore, in patients with advanced-stage breast cancer, detection of message for cytokeratin 19 in BM was associated with a significantly higher (p = 0.0002) incidence of subsequent relapse. The probability of relapse at 3 yr after autoBMT for PCR-positive patients was 32% for stage II/III and 94% and stage IV patients, respectively. Patients with no PCR-detectable disease had better outcome, having a probability of relapse of 10% for stage II/III patients and 14% for stage IV patients.

None of the studies listed here provide definitive proof that infusion of residual cells at the time of autoHCT contributes to relapse because it is possible that the detection of residual cancer cells at the time of HCT is associated with inherently worse prognosis in these patients. Irrespective of the mechanism, the finding of residual malignant cells in autologous hematopoietic cells does appear to provide a powerful prognostic marker, independent of other clinical parameters.

A retrospective analysis of the European Blood and Marrow Transplant Lymphoma Registry compared the outcome of 270 patients whose BM had been purged and compared the outcome with 270 case-matched control patients *(51)*. A variety of purging methodologies was used. In this study, there was no advantage in outcome if patients received purged BM. Patients with low-grade lymphoma did not have a significantly improved progression-free survival if the BM was purged (p = 0.1757), but they did have a significantly improved overall survival (p = 0.00184). In this study, time to hematologic engraftment, response to autoBMT, and number of procedure-related deaths were similar in purged and unpurged patients, further demonstrating that purging can be performed safely. In multiple myeloma, a phase III randomized trial using purged vs unpurged autologous PBSCs was performed using CD34 selection *(28)*. After CD34 selection, tumor burden was reduced by a median of 3.1 log, with 54% of CD34 selected, products having no detectable tumor. There was no improvement in DFS or overall survival.

8.6. Marker Gene Studies Demonstrate That Infused Cells Contribute to Relapse

Transfection of a marker gene into clonogenic malignant cells ex vivo provides a method to assess the fate of malignant cells within the autologous hematopoietic cells. If the majority of cells at the site of relapse expressed the marker gene, this would provide compelling evidence that infused malignant cells contribute to relapse. Because the efficiency of transfection is low using existing technology, a negative result would still not be definitive. However, results to date have demonstrated that when relapse occurs, there is evidence of malignant cells with the marker gene, suggesting strongly that the reinfused malignant cells contributed to relapse *(52–55)*.

8.7. In Vivo Purging

The availability of humanized antibodies allows the use of MAbs to perform purging in vivo at the time of collection of stem cells *(56,57)*. This clearly has the advantage that it is easier to perform, does not require a cell manipulation laboratory, and allows treatment not only of the collected stem cells but also of the whole patients. Moreover, this approach can be repeated following infusion of the autologous stem cells. A disadvantage at present is the limited availability of suitable antibodies such that only one antigen is being targeted. Ongoing clinical trials are assessing the efficacy of this approach to obtain tumor-free sources of stem cells.

9. SUMMARY

Immunologic methods exist that are capable of eradicating minimal and overt disease from autologous hematopoietic stem cells. The evidence that such eradication of tumor cells results in improved DFS or overall survival is circumspect at best. Techniques are also now available to assess whether such purging techniques have successfully eradicated tumor cells from the autologous hematopoietic stem cell from a variety of tumor types. It is important to continue to assess whether successful eradication of detectable tumor from the source of autologous hematopoietic stem cell results in improved outcome. Although purging procedures remain suboptimal, it may not be possible to perform adequate studies to resolve fully whether purging has any benefit. Therefore, such procedures should be continued only in the clinical trial setting because it is under these circumstances that it will eventually be possible to determine the clinical impact of immunologic purging.

REFERENCES

1. Craddock C. Haemopoietic stem-cell transplantation: recent progress and future promise. *Lancet Oncol* 2000;1:227–234.
2. Freedman AS, Neuberg D, Mauch P, et al. Long-term follow-up of autologous bone marrow transplantation in patients with relapsed follicular lymphoma. *Blood* 1999;94:3325–3333.
3. Ball ED, Wilson J, Phelps V, et al. Autologous bone marrow transplantation for acute myeloid leukemia in remission or first relapse using monoclonal antibody-purged marrow: results of phase II studies with long-term follow-up. *Bone Marrow Transplant* 2000;25:823–829.
4. Nieto Y, Champlin RE, Wingard JR, et al. Status of high-dose chemotherapy for breast cancer: a review. *Biol Blood Marrow Transplant* 2000;6:476–495.
5. Freedman AS, Gribben JG, Neuberg D, et al. High dose therapy and autologous bone marrow transplantation in patients with follicular lymphoma during first remission. *Blood* 1996;88:2780–2786.
6. Hurd DD, LeBien TW, Lasky LC, et al. Autologous bone marrow transplantation in non-Hodgkin's lymphoma: monoclonal antibodies plus complement for ex vivo marrow treatment. *Am J Med* 1988;85:829–834.
7. Freedman AS, Takvorian T, Anderson KC, et al. Autologous bone marrow transplantation in B-cell non-Hodgkin's lymphoma: very low treatment-related mortality in 100 patients in sensitive relapse. *J Clin Oncol* 1990;8:784–791.
8. Braun S, Pantel K, Muller P, et al. Cytokeratin-positive cells in the bone marrow and survival of patients with stage I, II, or III breast cancer. *N Engl J Med* 2000;342:525–533.
9. Gribben JG, Neuberg D, Freedman AS, et al. Detection by polymerase chain reaction of residual cells with the bcl-2 translocation is associated with increased risk of relapse after autologous bone marrow transplantation for B-cell lymphoma. *Blood* 1993;81:3449–3457.
10. Gribben JG, Freedman A, Woo SD, et al. All advanced stage non-Hodgkin's lymphomas with a polymerase chain reaction amplifiable breakpoint of bcl-2 have residual cells containing the bcl-2 rearrangement at evaluation and after treatment. *Blood* 1991;78:3275–3280.
11. Gribben JG, Freedman AS, Neuberg D, et al. Immunologic purging of marrow assessed by PCR before autologous bone marrow transplantation for B-cell lymphoma. *N Engl J Med* 1991;325:1525–1533.
12. Benjamin D, Magrath IT, Douglass EC, et al. Derivation of lymphoma cell lines from microscopically normal bone marrow in patients with undifferentiated lymphoma: evidence of occult bone marrow involvement. *Blood* 1983;61:1017–1019.

13. Estrov Z, Grunberger T, Dube ID. Detection of residual acute lymphoblastic leukemia cells in cultures of bone marrow obtained during remission *N Engl J Med* 1986;315:538–542.
14. Sharp JG, Joshi SS, Armitage JO, et al. Significance of detection of occult non-Hodgkin's lymphoma in histologically uninvolved bone marrow by culture technique. *Blood* 1992;79:1074–1080.
15. Sharp JG, Kessinger A, Mann S, et al. Outcome of high dose therapy and autologous transplantation in non-Hodgkin's lymphoma based on the presence of tumor in the marrow or infused hematopoietic harvest. *J Clin Oncol* 1996;14:214–219.
16. Ross AA, Cooper BW, Lazarus HM, et al. Detection and viability of tumor cells in peripheral blood stem cell collections from breast cancer patients using immunocytochemical and clonogenic assay techniques. *Blood* 1993;82:2605–2610.
17. Ross RE, Jeter EK, Gazitt Y, et al. Predictive factors for the rate of engraftment of neuroblastoma patients autotransplanted with purged marrow. *Prog Clin Biol Res* 1994;389:139–143.
18. Schiller G, Vescio R, Freytes C, et al. Transplantation of CD34+ peripheral blood progenitor cells after high-dose chemotherapy for patients with advanced multiple myeloma. *Blood* 1995;86:390–397.
19. Fields KK, Elfenbein GJ, Trudeau WL, et al. Clinical significance of bone marrow metastases as detected using the polymerase chain reaction in patients with breast cancer undergoing high-dose chemotherapy and autologous bone marrow transplantation. *J Clin Oncol* 1996;14:1868–1876.
20. Brugger W, Bross KJ, Glatt M, et al. Mobilization of tumor cells and hematopoietic progenitor cells into peripheral blood of patients with solid tumors. *Blood* 1994;83:636–640.
21. Leonard BM, Hetu F, Busque L, et al. Lymphoma cell burden in progenitor cell grafts measured by competitive polymerase chain reaction: less than one log difference between bone marrow and peripheral blood sources. *Blood* 1998;91:331–339.
22. Vescio RA, Han EJ, Schiller GJ, et al. Quantitative comparison of multiple myeloma tumor contamination in bone marrow harvest and leukapheresis autografts. *Bone Marrow Transplant* 1996;18:103–110.
23. Gee AP, Bruce KM, Morris TD, et al. Evidence for an anticomplementary factor associated with human bone marrow cells. *J Natl Cancer Inst* 1985;75:441–445.
24. Treleaven J, Gibson F, Udelstad J. Removal of neuroblastoma cells from bone marrow with monoclonal antibodies conjugated to magnetic microsphere. *Lancet* 1984;ii:70–76.
25. Gribben JG, Saporito L, Barber M, et al. Bone marrows of non-Hodgkin's lymphoma patients with a bcl-2 translocation can be purged of polymerase chain reaction-detectable lymphoma cells using monoclonal antibodies and immunomagnetic bead depletion. *Blood* 1992;80:1083–1089.
26. Fitzgerald DJ, Willingham MC, Cardarelli CO, et al. A monoclonal antibody–Pseudomonas toxin conjugate that specifically kills multidrug-resistant cells. *Proc Natl Acad Sci USA* 1987;84:4288–4292.
27. Strong RC, Uckun F, Youle RJ, et al. Use of multiple T cell-directed intact ricin immunotoxins for autologous bone marrow transplantation. *Blood* 1985;66:627–635.
28. Stewart AK, Vescio R, Schiller G, et al. Purging of autologous peripheral-blood stem cells using CD34 selection does not improve overall or progression-free survival after high-dose chemotherapy for multiple myeloma: results of a multicenter randomized controlled trial. *J Clin Oncol* 2001;19:3771–3779.
29. Roy DC, Felix M, Cannady WG, et al. Comparative activities of rabbit complements of different ages using an in-vitro marrow purging model. *Leukemia Res* 1990;14:407–416.
30. De Fabritiis P, Bregni M, Lipton J, et al. (1985). Elimination of clonogenic Burkitt's lymphoma cells from human bone marow using 4-hydroperoxycyclophosphamide in combination with monoclonal antibodies and complement. *Blood* 1985;65:1064–1070.
31. Negrin RS, Kiem HP, Schmidt WI, et al. Use of the polymerase chain reaction to monitor the effectiveness of ex vivo tumor cell purging. *Blood* 1991;77:654–660.
32. Kvalheim G, Sorensen O, Fodstad O, et al. Immunomagnetic removal of B-lymphoma cells from human bone marrow: a procedure for clinical use. *Bone Marrow Transplant* 1988;3:31–41.
33. Elias AD, Pap SA, Bernal SD. Purging of small cell lung cancer-contaminated bone marrow by monoclonal antibodies and magnetic beads. *Prog Clin Biol Res* 1990;333.263–275.
34. Vrendenburgh JJ, Ball ED. Elimination of small cell carcinoma of the lung from human bone marrow by monoclonal antibodies and immunomagnetic beads. *Cancer Res* 1990;50:7216–7120.
35. Vrendenburgh JJ, Simpson W, Memoli VA, et al. Reactivity of anti-CD15 monoclonal antibody PM-81 with breast cancer and elimination of breast cancer cell lines from human bone marrow by PM-81 and immunomagnetic beads. *Cancer Res* 1991;51:2451–2455.

36. Freedman AS, Takvorian T, Neuberg D, et al. Autologous bone marrow transplantation in poor-prognosis intermediate-grade and high-grade B-cell non-Hodgkin's lymphoma in first remission: a pilot study. *J Clin Oncol* 1993;11:931–936.
37. Freedman AS, Neuberg D, Gribben JG, et al. High-dose chemoradiotherapy and anti-B-cell monoclonal antibody-purged autologous bone marrow transplantation in mantle-cell lymphoma: no evidence for long-term remission [see comments]. *J Clin Oncol* 1998;16:13–18.
38. Anderson KC, Andersen J, Soiffer R, et al. Monoclonal antibody-purged bone marrow transplantation therapy for multiple myeloma. *Blood* 1993;82:2568–2576.
39. Vescio R, Schiller G, Stewart AK, et al. Multicenter phase III trial to evaluate CD34(+) selected versus unselected autologous peripheral blood progenitor cell transplantation in multiple myeloma [in process citation]. *Blood* 1999;93:1858–1868.
40. Simonsson B, Burnett AK, Prentice HG, et al. Autologous bone marrow transplantation with monoclonal antibody purged marrow for high risk acute lymphoblastic leukemia. *Leukemia* 1989;3:631–636.
41. Billett AL, Kornmehl E, Tarbell NJ, et al. Autologous bone marrow transplantation after a long first remission for children with recurrent acute lymphoblastic leukemia. *Blood* 1993;81:1651–1657.
42. Robertson MJ, Soiffer RJ, Freedman AS, et al. Human bone marrrow depleted of CD33-positive cells mediates delayed but durable reconstitution of hematopoiesis: clinical trial of My9 monoclonal antibody-purged autografts for the treatment of acute myeloid leukemia. *Blood* 1992;79:2229–2236.
43. Shpall EJ, Jones RB, Bearman S. High-dose therapy with autologous bone marrow transplantation for the treatment of solid tumors [review]. *Curr Opin Oncol* 1994;6:135–138.
44. Humblet Y, Feyens AM, Sekhavat M, et al. Immunological and pharmacological removal of small cell lung cancer cells from bone marrow autografts. *Cancer Res* 1989;49:5058–5061.
45. Kemshead JT, Heath L, Gibson FM, et al. Magnetic microspheres and monoclonal antibodies for the depletion of neuroblastoma cells from bone marrow: experiences, improvements and observations. *Br J Cancer* 1986;54:771–778.
46. Kemshead JT, Treleaven J, Heath L, et al. Monoclonal antibodies and magnetic microspheres for the depletion of leukemic cells from bone marrow harvested for autologous transplantation. *Bone Marrow Transplant* 1987;2:133–139.
47. Combaret V, Favrot MC, Chauvin F, et al. Immunomagnetic depletion of malignant cells from autologous bone marrow graft: from experimental models to clinical trials. *J Immunogenet* 1989;16:125–136.
48. Preijers FWMB, De Witte T, Wessels JMC, et al. Autologous transplantation of bone marrow purged in vitro with anti-CD7-(WT1-) ricin A immunotyoxin in T-cell lymphoblastic leukemia and lymphoma. *Blood* 1989;74:1152–1158.
49. Uckun F, Kersey JH, Vallera DA, et al. Autologous bone marrow transplantation in high risk remission T-lineage acute lymphoblastic leukemia using immunotoxins plus 4-hydroperoxycyclophosphamide for marrow purging. *Blood* 1990;76:1723–1733.
50. Corradini P, Astolfi M, Cherasco C, et al. Molecular monitoring of minimal residual disease in follicular and mantle cell non-Hodgkin's lymphomas treated with high dose chemotherapy and peripheral blood progenitor cell autografting. *Blood* 1997;89:724–731.
51. Williams CD, Goldstone AH, Pearce RM, et al. Purging of bone marrow in autologous bone marrow transplantation for non-Hodgkin's lymphoma: a case-matched comparison with unpurged cases by the European Blood and Marrow Transplant Lymphoma Registry. *J Clin Oncol* 1996;14:2454–2464.
52. Brenner MK, Rill DR, Holladay MS, et al. Gene marking to determine whether autologous marrow infusion restores long-term haemopoiesis in cancer patients. *Lancet* 1993;342:1134–1137.
53. Rill DR, Buschle M, Foreman NK, et al. Retrovirus-mediated gene transfer as an approach to analyze neuroblastoma relapse after autologous bone marrow transplantation. *Hum Gene Ther* 1992;3:129–136.
54. Rill DR, Moen RC, Buschle M, et al. An approach for the analysis of relapse and marrow reconstitution after autologous marrow transplantation using retrovirus-mediated gene transfer. *Blood* 1992;79:2694–2700.
55. Rill DR, Santana VM, Roberts WM, et al. Direct demonstration that autologous bone marrow transplantation for solid tumors can return a multiplicity of tumorigenic cells. *Blood* 1994;84:380–383.
56. Flinn IW, O'Donnell PV, Goodrich A, et al. Immunotherapy with rituximab during peripheral blood stem cell transplantation for non-Hodgkin's lymphoma. *Biol Blood Marrow Transplant* 2000;6:628–632.
57. Ladetto M, Zallio F, Vallet S, et al. Concurrent administration of high-dose chemotherapy and rituximab is a feasible and effective chemo/immunotherapy for patients with high-risk non-Hodgkin's lymphoma. *Leukemia* 2001;15:1941–1949.

20 T-Cell Depletion to Prevent Graft-vs-Host Disease

Vincent Ho, MD *and Robert J. Soiffer,* MD

CONTENTS

1. INTRODUCTION

The development of moderate to severe graft-vs-host disease (GVHD) has a negative impact upon the survival of patients after hematopoietic stem cell transplant (HSCT) *(1–4)*. Patients may die as a direct result of organ damage produced by GVHD or from opportunistic infections associated with the administration of immune suppressive medications. Acute and chronic GVHD can also produce substantial morbidity among survivors, severely compromising quality of life. Donor T cells have clearly been implicated in the pathogenesis of GVHD. Although traditional pharmacologic prophylaxis with calcineurin inhibitors and methotrexate limits T-cell function, GVHD can still occur in 25–50% of matched sibling transplants and at even higher frequencies in recipients of unrelated or mismatched transplants. Clearly, the most effective means of preventing GVHD has been the actual removal of T lymphocytes from the

From: *Stem Cell Transplantation for Hematologic Malignancies*
Edited by: R. J. Soiffer © Humana Press Inc., Totowa, NJ

Table 1
Pros and Cons of T-Cell Depletion

Advantages	*Disadvantages*
Decreased incidence of acute and chronic GVHD	Higher incidence of graft failure
Reduced or no requirement for posttransplant immune suppression as GVHD prophylaxis	Loss of graft-vs-leukemia activity (higher incidence of disease relapse, especially with chronic myelogenous leukemia)
Decreased organ toxicity	Delayed immune reconstitution
Lower early transplant-related mortality	Increased risk for posttransplant Epstein–Barr virus-associated lymphoproliferative disorder

donor graft *(5)*. However, in some studies, these reductions in GVHD have been counterbalanced by unexpectedly high rates of graft failure, immune deficiency, and disease recurrence (*see* Table 1). Preventing clinically significant GVHD without compromising engraftment, infectious surveillance, or antitumor activity is the most sought-after goal of allogeneic transplant research.

2. ANIMAL MODELS OF T-CELL DEPLETION

The first successful animal study of ex vivo T-cell depletion (TCD) was reported in the late 1960s. Using differential centrifugation on a discontinuous albumin gradient to separate lymphocytes from hematopoietic precursors, investigators demonstrated that irradiated mice given spleen cell fractions devoid of small lymphocytes resulted in 80–100% survival without evidence of GVHD. Mice innoculated with fractions that contained increased numbers of small lymphocytes all died from severe GVHD *(6)*. Similar beneficial results of TCD were observed when mouse bone marrow (BM) and spleen cell suspensions were depleted of T cells using soybean and/or peanut agglutination *(7)*. Incubation of marrow with both antilymphocyte sera (ALS) or antithymocyte globulin (ATG) ex vivo could deplete T-cell number and facilitated transplantation across major histocompatibility barriers in several animal systems by reducing the incidence of GVHD *(8–12)*. The development of monoclonal antibody technology permitted specific targeting of T cells and their subsets, expanding the potential of TCD as a strategy for GVHD prophylaxis in experimental transplantation *(13)*.

3. METHODS OF TCD

T-Cell depletion strategies include the ex vivo removal of T cells or T-cell subsets from the donor stem cell product or an in vivo reduction in T-cell number through anti-T-cell antibody administration. Ex vivo removal of T cells from the donor graft can be achieved either by negative anatomic selection of T cells or by positive selection of CD34+ stem cells. In ex vivo negative selection TCD, the T-cell population is removed from marrow or mobilized peripheral blood by physical separation or antibody-based techniques. Two of the more successful physical separation approaches are lectin agglutination followed by rosetting with sheep red blood cells *(14)* or counterflow centrifugal elutriation *(15,16)*. Monoclonal antibodies have been used alone *(17–19)*, with homologous or rabbit complements *(20–25)*, as immunotoxins *(26–28)* or as immunomagnetic beads *(29)*.

The development of anti-CD34 antibody-coated columns to select hematopoietic progenitors provides an alternative to traditional negative selection strategies of TCD. CD34 columns were initially developed to purge autologous grafts of tumor contaminants. These antibody-coated columns positively select hematopoietic progenitors, and by allowing nonadherent cells to be washed out, they effectively reduce the lymphocyte content by 4–5 logs in the peripheral blood stem cell (PBSC) graft *(30–34)*. Theoretically, positive stem cell selection techniques can be followed by antibody-based negative selection to further deplete specific T-cell populations. The increased utilization of mobilized peripheral blood rather than BM for allogeneic transplantation makes CD34-positive selection attractive as a means for TCD as the larger volume and T-lymphocyte content in mobilized peripheral blood poses some logistical difficulties for traditional negative selection antibody-based techniques.

The availability of humanized anti-T-cell antibodies permit effective in vivo TCD without cumbersome and time-consuming ex vivo manipulations. TCD with ATG preparations or humanized anti-T-cell antibodies such as Campath-1H (altemuzumab) administered in vivo before and after donor stem cell infusion can target both recipient T cells that could mediate graft rejection and donor T cells that might induce GVHD *(35–38)*. These antibodies have been particularly used for nonmyeloablative transplants as well as for haploidentical transplants in which both GVHD and graft rejection are of concern.

4. T-CELL DOSE AND GVHD

There does not appear to be a direct relationship between the number of T cells infused and the development of GVHD. Variability in the threshold T-cell GVHD dose likely depends on the degree of minor human leukocyte antigen (HLA) disparity and other potential polymorphisms between donor–recipient pairs *(39)*. Limiting dilution analyses have suggested a threshold of approx (1–3) × 10^5 T cells/kg for development of GVHD in recipients of HLA-identical related BM in the absence of exogenous immune suppression *(40,41)*. Studies of recipients of HLA-matched CD34-selected mobilized peripheral blood indicate significantly higher rates of GVHD when the CD3+ T-cell count exceeds 1 × 10^5 T cells/kg *(42)*. Because the extent of T cell removal by different TCD techniques may vary from 2 to 5 logs, it is not surprising that the capacity to prevent GVHD depends on the specific TCD strategy. In general, the more exhaustive the TCD, the lower the risk of GVHD.

More extensive TCD is required to prevent GVHD for recipients of unrelated or HLA-mismatched transplants than for recipients of HLA-matched siblings. In patients receiving TCD haplomismatched PBSCs, the incidence of acute GVHD is low if the number of infused T cells is below (1–2) × x10^4 T cells/kg *(43)*. The threshold number of T cells that leads to GVHD for unrelated or haploidentical graft recipients appears to be a log lower than the threshold for recipients HLA-matched sibling cells. In a single-institution analysis utilizing anti-CD6 antibodies as the sole form of TCD, the incidence of GVHD for recipients of unrelated marrow was more than twice as great as that observed in related marrow recipients despite an equal number of T cells infused (42% vs 20%) *(44)*.

5. SPECIFICITY OF TCD

Graft manipulation techniques also commonly differ in the specificity of depletion. Some strategies may also eliminate natural killer (NK) cells, immature thymocytes, B cells, and dendritic cells, as well as T cells. These cellular elements likely play an important role in immune surveillance, engraftment, and elimination of minimal residual disease. Within the T-cell compartment, it is also still unclear what contributions distinct T-cell subsets make to the pathogenesis of GVHD *(45)*.

T-cell depletion techniques may have narrow or broad spectra of reactivity. Examples of narrow-specificity depletion include depletion with antibodies targeting mature T cells only, such as anti-TCR, anti-CD6, or anti-CD5, or T cells with specific functional roles (e.g., anti-CD-8). Broad-specificity techniques that indiscriminately deplete T cells and other cellular elements include treatment with Campath antibodies, which target the widely expressed CD52 antigen, multiple antibody combinations, and soybean lectin agglutination. A retrospective registry study of alternative donor transplantation performed by the International Bone Marrow Transplant Registry (IBMTR) reported that depletion with narrow-specificity anti-T-cell antibodies resulted in superior leukemia-free survival than broad-specificity approaches *(46)*.

6. TCD AND ACUTE GVHD

6.1. Matched Related Transplantation

Most negative selection ex vivo TCD methods used for the past 20 yr have been associated with reductions in the incidence of grades II–IV acute GVHD to less than 20% after matched sibling bone marrow transplantation (BMT), often without additional immune suppression *(15,22–28,47–49)*. Studies have reported wide variations in rates of acute GVHD *(30–34)*. In these studies, the number of CD3+ cells infused, the number of CD34+ cells infused, and the use of additional immune suppressive agents appear to influence the incidence of GVHD *(42)*. There have been several devices developed for CD34 selection. A study comparing three products (CEPRATE, Isolex 300i, CliniMACs) found no apparent differences in allograft composition or outcome among the three, although ease of processing did differ among the units *(50)*. The availability of humanized anti-T-cell antibodies such as humanized Campath-1H (altemuzumab) or ATG preparations has allowed centers to offer TCD allogeneic transplantation without a cell processing facility. Prevention of GVHD on a scale similar to ex vivo TCD techniques has been reported, although little data on engraftment and disease relapse are available.

6.2. Transplantation From Unrelated Donors

Transplantation from donors other than HLA-identical siblings carries a higher risk of GVHD. Reports from the NMDP and other sources indicate that the incidence of acute GVHD after unrelated TCD BMT is 20–50% *(51–54)* compared to the 40–75% incidence of acute GVHD observed in series of unrelated donor (URD) BMT, where TCD is not employed. In the initial report from the National Marrow Donor Registry (NMDP), the use of TCD was the most significant factor predicting for freedom from severe (grade III–IV) acute GVHD *(51)*. A subsequent analysis from the IBMTR of 1868 leukemia patients who received marrow transplants from donors other than HLA-identical siblings revealed an incidence of grade II–IV GVHD between 34% and 38% in the TCD group compared to 57% in the non-TCD group ($p < 0.0001$) *(46)*. Only one large prospective randomized trial of TCD in unrelated marrow transplantation has been reported. Patients were randomized to receive either TCD (by the monoclonal antibody, $T_{10}B_9$, or by soybean lectin agglutination) or immune suppression with cyclosporine/methotrexate. The incidence of grades III–IV acute GVHD was lower in patients receiving TCD marrow plus cyclosporine compared with those receiving cyclosporine/methotrexate (15% vs 27%, $p < 0.01$) *(55)*.

6.3. Haploidentical Transplantation

T-cell depletion has permitted successful transplantation of fully haplotype mismatched related donors. Despite the fact that early studies of TCD in HLA-mismatched related marrow transplants were complicated by high rates of graft failure, recent series have yielded better results *(56)*. In single-institution studies, grade II–IV GVHD incidence has ranged from 20% to 40% in recipients of HLA-mismatched bone marrow after TCD using monoclonal antibody or in vivo TCD *(57,58)*. The most promising results have come from Italy, where patients receive large numbers of CD34+ selected mobilized peripheral blood cells with GVHD rates less than 20% when less than 1×10^4 T cells/kg are infused *(43)*.

6.4. Nonmyeloablative Transplantation

The use of nonmyeloablative transplantation has increased steadily over the past several years. Reduced-intensity conditioning regimens have extended the potential eligibility for transplantation to those previously considered too fragile for conventional transplantation, including both older patients and patients with compromised organ function. Conditioning is administered with chemotherapy or radiotherapy at doses adequate to permit engraftment of allogeneic hematopoietic stem cells, but likely not sufficient to kill significant numbers of tumor cells. Thus, the major therapeutic benefit comes from the allogeneic graft-vs-tumor (GVT) effect. Unfortunately, although reduced-intensity regimens have been less toxic in the peritransplant period, they have been associated with rates of acute GVHD equal to those noted after conventional ablative allo-transplantation. TCD could be problematic in this setting for two reasons. First, reduced-intensity conditioning might not be immune suppressive enough to prevent rejection of TCD stem cells or marrow. Second, because the therapeutic benefit of nonmyeloablative transplantation depends on GVT effects, TCD in the absence of additional immunotherapy might defeat the purpose of the transplant. Only a few attempts to reduce GHVD with ex vivo manipulation through CD34-positive selection or CD8-negative selection have been reported *(59)*. However, in vivo TCD with altemuzumab or ATG preparations have been more intensely studied, as these antibodies can serve the dual purpose of host immune suppression to prevent rejection and donor immune suppression to block GVHD. Comparative studies from Europe demonstrate less GVHD than in patients who do not receive antibody infusion, although with higher risks of infectious complications and disease relapse *(38)*.

6.5. Donor Lymphocyte Infusions

Donor lymphocyte infusions (DLIs) can produce remissions in some patients who relapse after transplantation *(60,61)*. Unfortunately, DLI is often associated with GVHD. The initial studies of DLI were performed with the intention of inducing GVHD in order to obtain graft-vs-leukemia (GVL) activity. It has been subsequently observed that remissions can be achieved in the absence of GVHD. Therefore, attempts to prevent GVHD without impacting GVL have been undertaken. One such approach has been by selective T-cell infusion. Phase II trials of CD8 TCD lymphocyte infusions in patients with relapsed hematologic malignancies have resulted in GVHD rates of 15–35%, lower than the 40–70% reported in series of patients receiving unmanipulated DLI *(62,63)*. In a prospective randomized study for patients at high risk of relapse given prophylactic DLI, six of nine (67%) patients given conventional DLI developed GVHD compared with none of nine (0%) patients receiving CD8 depleted DLI *(64)*. No differences in relapse rates or immune reconstitution were noted. An alternative approach to the problem of GVHD after DLI involves engineering donor cells ex vivo prior to infusion to be sensitive to elimination in vivo. This is accomplished by inserting the herpes simplex virus (HSV)–thymidine kinase into T cells *(65)*. If GVHD develops after DLI, the donor T cells responsible for GVHD can be destroyed in vivo by exposure to ganciclovir, to which they have now been rendered susceptible.

7. CHRONIC GVHD

It is more difficult to assess the effect of TCD upon chronic GVHD because many reported TCD studies have not included sufficient follow-up to determine whether chronic GVHD has developed. Several TCD approaches in use for many years (e.g., soybean lectin agglutination, Campath antibodies, and anti-CD6 antibody + complement) have reported very low rates of chronic GVHD (< 15%) in matched sibling transplantation. The results in unrelated transplantation are less clear. In a small randomized trial of rabbit ATG at 15 mg/kg in URD transplantation, patients receiving the ATG had a lower incidence of chronic GVHD than controls (39% vs 62%, $p = 0.04$) *(66)*. In contrast to these results, the recently reported randomized trial of TCD (using $T_{10}B_9$ or soybean lectin agglutination) plus cyclosporine vs cyclosporine/methotrexate demonstrated no significant difference in chronic GVHD (24% vs 29%) *(55)*.

8. ORGAN DYSFUNCTION AFTER TCD BMT

There are very few series that have focused on the effects of TCD on organ toxicity. However, in several single-institution studies, TCD has produced less hepatic, renal, and pulmonary complications than conventional transplantation *(67,68)*. In a recent analysis of 199 allogeneic transplants, the incidence of life-threatening pulmonary complications within the first 60 d of BMT was 8% among those who received TCD as the sole form of GVHD prophylaxis, but it was 33% among those who received cyclosporine and methotrexate ($p < 0.0001$) *(69)*. The protective effect of TCD against pulmonary complications was independent of the diagnosis of acute GVHD. Reductions in organ toxicity were also observed in a randomized trial of TCD plus cyclosporine vs cyclosporine/methotrexate. Pulmonary, hepatic, renal, central nervous system (CNS), and mucosal toxicity as assessed by the Bearman toxicity scale revealed a significantly lower incidence and severity of organ damage in the TCD cohort *(55)*. It is possible that the reduction in organ toxicity after TCD transplant relates to a partial or complete absence of pharmacologic agents like methotrexate or cyclosporine for GVHD prophylaxis. Alternatively, decreases in allogeneic reactions after TCD transplantation could result in reductions in the levels of elaborated cytokines that could be damaging to hepatic, renal, or pulmonary parenchyma.

9. TRANSPLANT-RELATED MORTALITY

For TCD to be useful in allogeneic transplantation, it must do more than just protect against GVHD. It has been suggested that if TCD can substantially prevent GVHD and reduce organ dysfunction after BMT, it should also result in lower rates of transplant-related mortality (TRM). Some matched sibling TCD transplant series have reported the incidence of TRM to be between 2% and 15% *(70–72)*. In a case-control study involving unrelated marrow recipients in Stockholm and Seattle, those receiving in vivo TCD with rabbit ATG experienced lower nonrelapse mortality than patients not given ATG (19% vs 35%, $p = 0.005$) *(73)*. However, other TCD studies have reported TRM rates from 25% to 40% even after matched sibling transplants, with many deaths being secondary to infection and Epstein–Barr virus (EBV)–lymphoproliferative disease (LPD) *(74–76)*. In a randomized trial evaluating TCD in unrelated marrow recipients, no difference in TRM between the groups could be detected, suggesting that elements other than GVHD, such as the intensity of conditioning, posttransplant immune suppression, graft failure, and immune reconstitution, play major roles in determining TRM *(55)*.

10. COSTS AND QUALITY OF LIFE

Few studies have been performed to assess the impact of TCD on quality of life (QOL) or costs after transplantation. One retrospective single-institution series did demonstrate a decrease in inpatient early hospitalization costs in patients receiving TCD BMT. However, no significant differences in overall QOL could be detected *(77)*. Future prospective trials should incorporate these parameters in their specific aims.

11. TCD AND GRAFT FAILURE

Early TCD BMT series reported higher incidences of graft failure than had been noted in prior experience with transplantation of unmanipulated marrow *(78–82)*. The IBMTR found TCD to be associated with a ninefold increased risk for graft failure compared to unmanipulated marrow transplantation ($p < 0.0001$) *(83)*. It is unlikely that failure of initial engraftment is caused by injury to hematopoietic progenitors or auxiliary cells during marrow manipulation because autologous marrow processed with T- or B-cell monoclonal antibodies engraft without significant difficulty *(84,85)*.

There is evidence that early graft failure (within the first few weeks after TCD transplantation) results from immunologic rejection of donor hematopoietic elements by host lymphoid elements that have survived the conditioning process. Host T lymphocytes with donor-specific cytotoxic activity have been recovered from the blood of patients at the time of graft rejection *(79,86–95)*. It is likely that TCD or marrow manipulation removes cells that promote engraftment, perhaps by suppressing host-derived T lymphocytes or dendritic cells that could participate in the rejection process. Some murine models have suggested that NK cells are critical to engraftment *(96)*, whereas others have implicated CD8+ T cells *(97)*. However, in a recent human trial using TCD donor grafts with the addition of a graded dose of CD4+ and CD8+ cells, it appeared that depletion of donor CD8+ cells, but not CD4+ cells, was associated with increased graft rejection *(98)*.

The mechanism behind late graft failure (several months posttransplant) remains uncertain. Host-derived cells with antidonor cell activity have not been isolated. Mixed lymphoid and myeloid chimerism is often observed after TCD BMT, suggesting a state of immune tolerance between the graft and host *(99–104)*. Graft failure conceivably may result when host lymphoid tolerance of the graft is broken by some event. It has been proposed that viral infections, such as cytomegalovirus (CMV) or human herpes virus 6 (HHV-6), may contribute to late graft failure after BMT *(105–108)*. Although TCD graft recipients have a higher risk of CMV reactivation *(109–111)*, there is no direct clinical evidence linking these viruses to graft failure.

Attempts to reduce the risk of graft failure have included increased myeloablation, increased host-directed immune suppression, modulation of T-cell removal, narrowing of the breadth of TCD, and infusion of increased numbers of hematopoietic precursors. Intensifying the myeloablative regimen with additional chemotherapy may empty out the host marrow more effectively and thus increase "hematopoietic space" for the incoming donor graft, but the benefit of decreased graft failure may be offset by increased regimen-related toxicity *(112–115)*. Increased immunosuppression with additional radiation (total lymphoid or body irradiation), corticosteroids, or in vivo anti-T-cell antibodies to target host alloreactive T cells has been reportedly successful in preventing graft rejection in phase II trials *(36,116–121)*. T-Cell add-back following marrow processing may promote engraftment but has the potential to precipitate GVHD *(122,123)*. Selective removal of T cells using narrow-spectrum antibodies, such as anti-CD5, anti-CD6, and anti-TCRαβ ($T_{10}B_9$) antibodies, have produced graft failure rates of 1–3% with a 15–20% risk of acute GVHD *(25–28,46)*. The unrelated BMT randomized trial of TCD vs cyclosporine/methotrexate found no difference between groups with respect to neutrophil or platelet engraftment *(55)*. Administering large numbers of CD34+ stem cells may be another effective way to overcome graft failure. Preclinical models have shown that mice given "megadoses" of TCD marrow engrafted despite only low doses of conditioning irradiation *(124)*. In human studies, the addition of CD34+ cells to TCD marrow to augment stem cell dose has permitted reliable engraftment in leukemia patients despite full HLA haplotype mismatches *(125)*. A subset of CD34 + progenitor cells with "veto" activity may help prevent rejection *(126)*. It may be that ex vivo TCD of mobilized peripheral blood progenitor cells may not carry the same risk of graft failure because of the increased number of CD34 cells infused with peripheral blood compared to BMT. In contrast to studies previously performed with CD8 depletion of bone marrow, recent experience with CD8 depletion of mobilized peripheral blood has not been associated with graft rejection *(48,127)*.

12. DELAYED IMMUNE RECONSTITUTION

Because TCD marrow contains less T cells than unmanipulated marrow grafts, delayed T-cell immune reconstitution is a concern after TCD BMT *(128–134)*. Total lymphocyte numbers are somewhat lower early after BMT in recipients of TCD marrow transplants compared to those who receive unmanipulated grafts. Most TCD BMT patients will have a deficit in CD4+ cells, with an inverted CD4+ to CD8+ ratio for up to 2 yr *(130)*. Functional recovery of T cells is also delayed after TCD BMT. The proliferative response of T cells to mitogenic stimulation can be impaired for over 18 mo post-BMT in recipients of TCD marrow *(130)*. The T-cell compartment after transplantation is largely expanded from lymphocytes cotransfused with the marrow; therefore, recipients of TCD transplants would have much fewer precursors with which to reconstitute their repertoire than recipients of conventional BMT. Impairment of T-cell neogenesis as assessed by generation of T-cell-receptor (TCR) excision circles (TREC) has been noted after TCD BMT and has correlated to increased risk of infection *(135,136)*. T Lymphocytes from recipients of TCD BMT also have restricted variability in their TCR repertoires *(132,137)*. Patients with persistent mixed chimerism after TCD BMT have marked abnormal TCR repertoires, whereas others who had converted to full donor hematopoiesis possess a normal spectrum of TCR variability *(137)*. The delayed reconstitution in numbers of CD4+ cells and impaired recovery of T-cell repertoire diversity has not been associated with a higher probability of reactivation for herpesviruses, such as CMV, but not with an increased risk of bacterial or fungal infections *(55,109–111,138,139)*.

13. POSTTRANSPLANT LYMPHOPROLIFERATIVE DISEASE

Posttransplant lymphoproliferative disease (PTLD), usually associated with Epstein–Barr virus, is a recognized complication in patients after solid-organ transplantation. However, it is uncommon after conventional BMT despite the use of immune suppressive agents similar to those prescribed to organ graft recipients. In contrast to recipients of unmanipulated marrow, PTLD is a concern after TCD BMT, with an incidence as high as 20–30% in some circumstances *(140,141)*. Recipients of TCD transplants using HLA-mismatched or unrelated donor marrow appear to be at particularly high risk, as are patients with severe GVHD and those treated with certain anti-T-cell monoclonal antibodies *(140,142)*. PTLD is thought to arise from virally infected donor B cells which have been cotransplanted with the allograft. If immune surveillance has been compromised by the removal of donor EBV-specific cytotoxic T cells, then those B cells may proliferate in the host and develop into a polyclonal or monoclonal process.

Strengthening anti-EBV immunity through the administration of unselected bulk DLIs *(143)* or EBV-specific cytotoxic T lymphocytes (CTLs) cultivated in vitro from donor lymphocytes has been effective in some cases of PTLD *(144,145)*. Recent data would suggest that treatment with anti-B-cell antibodies, such as the anti-CD20 monoclonal antibody rituximab, can induce durable remissions in some patients with PTLD *(146–148)*.

Prevention of PTLD after TCD transplantation may be achieved by using methods of purging that also remove B cells (e.g., Campath antibodies or CD34+ cell selection) or by purging with B-cell monoclonal antibodies in addition to specific T-cell antibodies *(149,150)*. Prophylactic administration of EBV-specific CTLs has also seemed effective *(145)*. Early detection of EBV reactivation with polymerase chain reaction (PCR)-based methods may help identify patients appropriate for pre-emptive therapy with either cellular or antibody-based therapies *(151,152)*.

14. TCD AND LEUKEMIA RELAPSE

Multiple studies have demonstrated that disease relapse is indeed more frequent after TCD BMT compared to conventional transplantation, particularly for chronic myelogenous leukemia (CML) *(153–158)*. The increased rate of leukemia relapse after TCD BMT has been linked, as least in part, to the reduction in GVHD and concomitant loss of graft-vs-leukemia (GVL) activity. It is well established from conventional transplantation experience that the development of GVHD is associated with a lower incidence of leukemia relapse *(159–161)*. The direct relationship between T cells and GVL has been established in DLI studies of patients with CML who have relapsed after BMT, where complete remission rates of 70–80% are achieved *(60,61)*.

In contrast to CML, TCD has only a modest effect on the relapse rates of patients transplanted for acute leukemia *(70,74,162–164)*. Retrospective data from the IBMTR have indicated that TCD was associated with a 1.5- to 2.0-fold increased risk for recurrence in patients with acute lymphoblastic leukemia (ALL) in any phase and in patients with AML who are transplanted in relapse or in first complete remission (CR) *(83)*. In this same analysis, AML patients transplanted in second CR actually had a lower risk of relapse with TCD. In two separate randomized trials comparing TCD with methotrexate and cyclosporine as GVHD prophylaxis for leukemia patients undergoing HLA-matched related or unrelated BMT, a higher relapse rate was observed after TCD BMT only in patients with CML, not in patients with acute leukemia *(55,165)*.

The effect of TCD on relapse is less marked after unrelated BMT compared to related BMT *(52,53,166–168)*. A single-institution experience of 146 patients found similar relapse rates after CD6-depleted or unmanipulated unrelated BMT *(77)*. A multivariable analysis of unrelated transplantation from the EBMT found no increase in relapse rates among TCD transplant recipients *(169)*. The 410-patient prospective randomized trial of TCD vs cyclosporine/methotrexate as GVHD prophylaxis could demonstrate only a modest increase in relapse incidence associated with TCD in CML patients (16% vs 6%) in the TCD arm, but no effect in acute leukemia *(55)*.

The extent and specificity of TCD may influence its effect on relapse rates. In a large retrospective IBMTR analysis, TCD with "narrow-specificity" antibodies (e.g., anti-CD5, CD6, anti-TCRαβ, etc.) was associated with a lower relapse rate than TCD with "broad-specificity" antibodies (e.g., anti-CD2, ATG, Campath antibodies, elutriation, or lectin/sheep red blood cells [SRBC] agglutination) *(46)*. The 5-yr relapse rate in recipients of "narrow-specificity" TCD BMT was similar to that observed in recipients of unmanipulated BMT, suggesting that, at least in the setting of unrelated or mismatched BMT, TCD using "narrow-specificity" antibodies can reduce GVHD without significant loss of GVL activity.

It would be ideal if cellular subsets that mediate GVL and GVH could be distinguished so that those cells that cause GVHD could be removed from the graft, leaving intact the population responsible for GVL activity. The T-cell subsets with the most clearly distinct functional capacities are CD4+ and CD8+ cells. In murine systems, both CD4 and CD8 cells have been implicated in GVHD and GVL, dependent on the genetic strain combinations under study. In humans, CD8+ T cells have been implicated in GVHD development, whereas the role of CD4+ cells has been less clear. Infiltrates of CD8+ T cells are often found in target organs of patients with GVHD. As well, the presence of high numbers of CD8+ T cells in peripheral blood early post-BMT has been associated with the subsequent development of GVHD *(170)*. A randomized trial of patients receiving either CD8-depleted or unmanipulated BM demonstrated that those receiving CD8+-depleted marrow experienced significantly less grade II–IV GVHD. The leukemia relapse rate was similar between the two groups, suggesting that CD8+ depletion reduced GVHD without abolishing GVL *(76)*. CD8+-depleted DLI has been shown to significantly reduce the incidence of GVHD but retain important GVL activity with preserved clinical responses in patients with relapsed CML *(62,63)*. A randomized study of CD8 depletion in patients receiving DLI demonstrated a reduction in acute GVHD from 66% to 0% without loss of GVL activity *(64)*. Although these studies have been encouraging, separating GVH from GVL is likely to be far more complicated.

The administration or manipulation of cytotoxic effectors cells after TCD transplantation to reduce relapse rates is under investigation. Compared to recipients of unmanipulated marrow, patients undergoing TCD-related donor transplantation for CML have similar disease-free survival (DFS) after salvage therapy with DLI despite a comparatively high initial relapse rate *(71,171)*. A retrospective analysis of CML patients receiving CD34+ peripheral blood cells with T-cell add-back demonstrated a lower rate of GVHD and superior 3-yr survival (90%) compared with recipients of unmanipulated mobilized peripheral blood (68%, $p < 0.03$) or bone marrow (63%, $p < 0.01$) *(172)*. These results suggest that TCD BMT followed by posttransplant DLI at or even before disease relapse could be a reasonable option for patients with CML. For this strategy to be optimally effective, DLI must reduce relapse rates without inducing GVHD. This may be accomplished by lowering the dose of lymphocytes infused, selectively depleting cell subsets from the lymphocyte pool, or suicide gene insertion *(62,63,65,173–175)*.

The success of DLI in salvaging CML patients after BMT has led to investigation of T-cell infusions after TCD BMT in other diseases. Patients with myeloma who underwent a TCD BMT were given DLI 6 mo post-BMT. Of the patients in that series who had persistent myeloma 6 mo after transplant, 10/11 responded (6 CR, 4 partial remission [PR]) to DLI. The 2-yr progression-free survival for all 14 patients who received DLI was significantly improved compared to a comparable historical cohort who received TCD BMT without DLI *(176)*. However, not all patients could receive DLI at 6 mo in this study, as some suffered early relapse, some developed significant GVHD, and some had morbidity from infection. The appropriate timing of DLI after TCD BMT has not yet been established.

The role of natural killer (NK) cells in preventing relapse after TCD transplantation is also under study. The ability to expand or activate NK cells in vivo or ex vivo with cytokines such as interleukin (IL)-2 has prompted several clinical trials after TCD BMT. Prolonged infusion of low-dose recombinant IL-2 (rIL-2) following TCD allogeneic BMT can safely expand the number of circulating cytotoxic NK cells without inducing GVHD, although the effect on the prevention of relapse was never firmly established *(177)*. The identification of killer immunoglobulinlike receptors (KIR) on NK cells has generated renewed interest in their role in controlling relapse. These receptors recognize groups of HLA class I (particularly HLA-Bx4 and HLA-C) alleles and, when engaged, result in inhibition of NK reactivity. The absence of recognition of these alleles on a cell can trigger NK-cell destruction of that target. In an analysis of patients who received allografts mismatched at the HLA-C or -Bw4 allele in the direction of GVHD, donor vs recipient alloreactive NK cell clones could be isolated posttransplant in patients without evidence of GVHD *(178)*. These alloreactive NK-cell clones could lyse pretransplant cryopreserved leukemia cells in vitro, suggesting that GVL activity mediated by NK cells exists in these patients without GVHD. In the setting of haploidentical transplantation under conditions of exhaustive T-cell depletion, donor NK activity appears to protect against relapse of AML without inducing GVHD, perhaps in part by eliminating host antigen-presenting cells *(179,180)*. Such a role for NK cells may be limited to conditions of haploidentical transplantation and extensive TCD, as one analysis of KIR incompatibility as assessed by HLA-Bw4 and -C discrepancies in unrelated transplants showed no advantage in terms of relapse or GVHD *(181)*.

15. ALTERNATIVE APPROACHES FOR GRAFT ENGINEERING

15.1. Functional TCD

Some investigators have turned their attention to TCD techniques in which only alloreactive T cells are removed from the graft either through photoinactivation *(182)* or immunologic purging. After priming by recipient mononuclear cells in vitro, alloreactive donor cells can be identified by expression of activation markers, such as CD25, CD69, CD71, or HLA-DR. These cells can then be separated from the remaining cells by immunomagnetic cell sorting *(183–185)*.

An alternative prophylactic approach has focused not upon removal of activated T cells, but upon induction of host-directed antigen-specific anergy through the blockade of costimulatory pathways (e.g., CD28/B7, LFA-1/ICAM, CD40/CD40L) (186–188). In a small pilot series, patients transplanted with HLA-mismatched BM that had been treated in vitro with CTLA4-Ig in the presence of donor antigen-presenting cells engrafted with a 27% incidence of acute GVHD *(189)*. If distinct targets for GVHD and GVL can be identified, it may ultimately be possible to induce GVHD-specific anergy while preserving the T-cell response to tumor antigens for a full GVL effect.

15.2. Suicide Gene Insertion

The insertion of herpes simplex thymidine kinase (HS-TK) gene into donor T lymphocytes renders them susceptible to destruction with ganciclovir. Recipients of engineered T cells who develop GVHD after infusion can theoretically be treated systemically with ganciclovir to eliminate the infused T cells *(65,175,190)*. The use of "suicide" gene therapy may also be applicable in conjunction with TCD BMT. HS-TK gene-modified T lymphocytes infused along with TCD marrow at the time of transplantation do not interfere with engraftment *(190)*. These gene-modified cells can be detected for months after infusion. In two of three patients who received engineered cells and who developed acute GVHD, a CR was observed upon treatment with ganciclovir. A case of chronic cutaneous GVHD responsive to ganciclovir has been reported in a patient who had received T cells bearing the HS-TK gene at the time of BMT *(191)*.

15.3. T-Cell Modification

CD4 and CD8 T cells can be broadly divided into Th1 and Th2 subsets and CD8 T cells into Tc1 and Tc2 populations. The type 1 and 2 cells secrete different sets of cytokines (IL-2 and interferon-γ [type 1] and IL-4, IL-5, IL-10 [type 2]) that contribute differently to promotion of cytotoxic and humoral immunity. Animal data suggest that skewing T-cell populations to the Th2 and Tc2 group may help suppress GVHD *(192,193)*. Clinical trials evaluating the additions of Th2 cells after nonablative transplantation are underway *(194)*.

15.4. Regulatory Cells and GVHD

The recent recognition of CD4+CD25+ cells with regulatory activity has prompted interest in isolating and expanding these cells for clinical use. Murine models have indicated that these cells may play a role in reducing lethality resulting from GVHD *(195–198)*. The isolation and characterization of these regulatory cells in humans is under investigation.

15.5. Vaccine Strategies

As new leukemia antigens are identified that are potential targets for the GVL response, allogeneic tumor vaccines may be developed to stimulate specific antitumor activity without GVHD after TCD. It is not clear whether TCD will render patients immune incompetent so that they unable to respond to vaccination. In a murine model, mice that had undergone TCD transplantation could mount a donor cell-mediated antitumor response without GVHD after vaccination with irradiated tumor cells genetically engineered to secrete granulocyte-macrophage colony-stimulating factor *(199)*. Rather than vaccinating recipients, it may be possible to vaccinate donors in vivo or perhaps donor cells in vitro prior to graft infusion, thereby transferring immune effectors to the host. Still to be determined are the precise antigen and adjuvants needed for optimal immunization and whether TCD will completely eliminate transfer of protective effector populations.

16. CONCLUSIONS

T-cell depletion to reduce the incidence of GVHD has been studied in clinical trials for over 20 yr. There is no debate that TCD can reduce the risk and severity of GVHD and, in most cases, reduce transplant related mortality. However, it has yet to be shown that TCD improves overall survival after transplantation. The optimal way to manipulate grafts to minimize GVHD while preserving immunologic integrity to fight infection and destroy residual tumor remains undetermined and awaits further delineation of the mechanisms underlying GVH and GVL.

REFERENCES

1. Ferrara JL, Levy R, Chao NJ. Pathophysiologic mechanisms of acute graft-versus-host disease. *Biol Blood Marrow Transplant* 1999;5:347–356.
2. Martin PJ, Schoch G, Fisher L, et al. A retrospective analysis of therapy for acute graft-versus-host disease: intitial treatment. *Blood* 1990;76:1464–1472.
3. Weisdorf D, Haake R, Blazar B, et al. Treatment of moderate/severe acute graft-versus-host disease after allogeneic bone marrow transplantation: an analysis of clinical risk features and outcome. *Blood* 1990;75:1024–1030.
4. Sullivan KM, Agura E, Anasetti C, et al. Chronic graft-versus-host disease and other late complications of bone marrow transplantation. *Semin Hematol* 1991;28:250–259.
5. Ho VY, Soiffer RJ. The history and future of T-cell depletion as graft-versus-host disease prophylaxis for allogeneic hematopoietic stem cell transplantation. *Blood* 2001;98:3192–3204.
6. Dicke KA, van Hoot JIM, van Bekkum DW. The selective elimination of immunologically competent cells from bone marrow and lymphatic cell mixtures. II. Mouse spleen cell fractionation on a discontinuous albumin gradient. *Transplantation* 1968;6:562–568.
7. Reisner Y, Itzicovitch L, Meshorer A, et al. Hematopoietic stem cell transplantation using mouse bone marrow and spleen cells fractionated by lectins. *Proc Natl Acad Sci USA* 1978;75:2933–2936.
8. Trentin JJ, Judd KP. Prevention of acute graft-versus-host (GVH) mortality with spleen-absorbed antithymocyte globulin (ATG). *Transplant Proc* 1973;5:865–868.
9. Rodt H, Kolb HJ, Netzel B, et al. GVHD suppression by incubation of bone marrow grafts with anti-T-cell globulin: effect in canine model and application to clinical bone marrow transplantation. *Transplant Proc* 1979;11:962–966.
10. Korngold R, Sprent J. Lethal graft-versus-host disease after bone marrow transplantation across minor histocompatibilty barriers in mice. Prevention by removing mature T cells from marrow. *J Exp Med* 1978;148:1687–1698.
11. Rodt H, Theirfelder S, Eulitz M. Antilymhpocyte antibodies and marrow transplantation. III. Effect of heterologous anti-brain antibodies on acute secondary disease in mice. *Eur J Immunol* 1974;4:15–19.
12. Kolb HJ, Rieder I, Rodt H, et al. Antilymphocyte antibodies and marrow transplantation. VI. Graft-versus-host tolerance in DLA-incompatible dogs after in vitro treatment of bone marrow absorbed with antithymocyte globulin. *Transplantation* 1979;27:242–245.
13. Vallera DA, Soderling CC, Carlson GJ, et al. Bone marrow transplantation across major histocompatibility barriers in mice. *Transplantation* 1981;31:218–222.
14. Reisner Y, Kapoor N, Kirkpatrick D, et al. Transplantation for acute leukemia with HLA-A and B nonidentical parental marrow cells fractionated with soybean agglutinin and sheep red blood cells. *Lancet* 1981;2(8242):327–331.
15. De Witte T, Hoogenhout J, de Pauw B, et al. Depletion of donor lymphocytes by counterflow centrifugation successfully prevents acute graft-versus-host disease in matched allogeneic marrow transplantation. *Blood* 1986;67:1302–1308.
16. Noga SJ, Donnenberg AD, Schwartz CL, et al. Development of a simplified counterflow centrifugation elutriation procedure for depletion of lymphocytes from human bone marrow. *Transplantation* 1986;41:220–225.
17. Prentice HG, Blacklock HA, Janossy G, et al. Use of anti-T-cell monoclonal antibody OKT3 to prevent acute graft versus host disease in allogeneic bone marrow transplantation for acute leukemia. *Lancet* 1982;1(8274):700–703.
18. Filipovich AH, McGlave PB, Ramsay NKC, et al. Pretreatment of donor bone marrow with monoclonal antibody OKT3 for prevention of acute graft versus host disease in allogeneic histocompatible bone marrow transplantation. *Lancet* 1982;1(8284):1266–1269.
19. Martin PJ, Hansen JA, Thomas ED. Preincubation of donor bone marrow cells with a combination of murine monclonal anti-T-cell antibodies without complement does not prevent graft-versus-host disease after allogeneic marrow trasnplantation. *J Clin Immunol* 1984;4:18–22.
20. Waldmann HG, Polliak A, Hale G, et al. Elimination of graft-versus-host disease by in vitro depletion of alloreactive lymphocytes with a monoclonal rat anti-human lymphocyte antibody (Campath-1). *Lancet* 1984;2(8401):483–486.

21. Martin PJ, Hansen JA, Buckner CD, et al. Effects of in vitro depletion of T cells in HLA-identical allogeneic marrow grafts. *Blood* 1985;66:664–672.
22. Herve P, Cahn JY, Flesch M, et al. Successful graft-versus-host disease prevention without graft failure in 32 HLA-identical allogeneic bone marrow transplantations with marrow depleted of T cells by monoclonal antibodies and complement. *Blood* 1987;69:388–393.
23. Trigg ME, Billing R, Sondel PM, et al. Clinical trial depleting T lymphocytes from donor marrow for matched and mismatched allogeneic bone marrow transplants. *Cancer Treat Rep* 1985;69:377–386.
24. Mitsuyasu RT, Champlin RE, Gale RP, et al. Treatment of donor bone marrow with monoclonal anti-T-cell antibody and complement for the prevention of graft versus host disease. *Ann Intern Med* 1986;105:20–26.
25. Soiffer RJ, Murray C, Mauch P, et al. Prevention of graft-versus-host disease by selective depletion of CD6-positive T lymphocytes from donor bone marrow. *J Clin Oncol* 1992;10:1191–2000.
26. Laurent G, Maraninchi D, Gluckman E, et al. Donor bone marrow treatment with T101 Fab fragment-ricin A-chain immunotoxin prevents graft-versus-host disease. *Bone Marrow Transplant* 1989;4:367–372.
27. Filipovich AH, Vallera D, McGlave P, et al. T cell depletion with anti-CD5 immunotoxin in histocompatible bone marrow transplantation. *Transplantation* 1990;50:410–414.
28. Antin JH, Bierer BE, Smith BR, et al. Selective depletion of bone marrow T lymphocytes with anti-CD5 monoclonal antibodies: effective prophylaxis for graft-versus-host disease in patients with hematologic malignancies. *Blood* 1991;78:2139–2144.
29. Vartdal F, Kvalheim G, Lea TE, et al. Depletion of T lymphocytes from human bone marrow. Use of magnetic monosized polymer microspheres coated with T-lymphocyte-specific monoclonal antibodies. *Transplantation* 1987;43:366–371.
30. Dreger P, Viehmann K, Steinmann J, et al. G-CSF-mobilized peripheral blood progenitor cells for allogeneic transplantation: comparison of T cell depletion strategies using different CD34+ selection systems or CAMPATH-1. *Exp Hematol* 1995;23:147–154.
31. Finke J, Brugger W, Bertz H, et al. Allogeneic transplantation of positively selected peripheral blood CD34+ progenitor cells from matched related donors. *Bone Marrow Transplant* 1996;18:1081–1085.
32. Socie G, Cayuela JM, Raynal B, et al. Influence of CD34 cell selection on the incidence of mixed chimaerism and minimal residual disease after allogeneic unrelated donor transplantation. *Leukemia* 1998;12:1440–1446.
33. Urbano-Ispizua A, Solano C, Brunet S, et al. Allogeneic transplantation of selected CD34+ cells from peripheral blood: experience of 62 cases using immunoadsorption or immunomagnetic technique. *Bone Marrow Transplant* 1998;22:519–524.
34. Vij R, Brown R, Shenoy S, et al. Allogeneic peripheral blood stem cell transplantation following CD34+ enrichment by density gradient separation. *Bone Marrow Transplant* 2000;25:1223–1228.
35. Hale G, Jacobs P, Wood L, et al. CD52 antibodies for prevention of graft-versus-host disease and graft rejection following transplantation of allogeneic peripheral blood stem cells. *Bone Marrow Transplant* 2000;26:69–75.
36. Henslee-Downey PJ, Parrish RS, MacDonald JS, et al. Combined in vitro and in vivo T lymphocyte depletion for the control of graft-versus-host disease following haploidentical marrow transplant. *Transplantation* 1996;61:738–743.
37. Spitzer TR, McAfee S, Sackstein R, et al. Intentional induction of mixed chimerism and achievement of antitumor responses after nonmyeloablative conditioning therapy and HLA-matched donor bone marrow transplantation for refractory hematologic malignancies. *Biol Blood Marrow Transplant* 2002;6:309–315.
38. Perez-Simon JA, Kottaridis PD, Martino R, et al. Nonmyeloablative transplantation with or without alemtuzumab: comparison between 2 prospective studies in patients with lymphoproliferative disorders. *Blood* 2002;100:3121–3127.
39. Goulmy E, Schipper R, Pool J, et al. Mismatches of minor histocompatibilitiy antigens between HLA-identical donors and recipients and development of graft-versus-host disease after bone marrow transplantation. *N Engl J Med* 1996;334:281–285.
40. Kernan NA, Collins NM, Juliano L, et al. Clonable T lymphocytes in T cell-depleted bone marrow transplants correlate with development of graft-v-host disease. *Blood* 1986;68:770–773.
41. Martin PJ, Hansen JA. Quantitative assays for detection of residual T cells in T-depleted human marrow. *Blood* 1985;65:1134–1139.
42. Urbano-Ispizua A, Rozman C, Pimentel P, et al. Risk factors for acute graft-versus-host disease in patients undergoing transplantation with CD34+ selected blood cells from HLA-identical siblings. *Blood* 2002;100:724–727.

43. Aversa F, Tabilio A, Velardi A, et al. Treatment of high-risk acute leukemia with T-cell-depleted stem cells from related donors with one fully mismatched HLA haplotype. *N Engl J Med* 1998;339:1186–1193.
44. Alyea EP, Weller E, Fisher DC, et al. Comparable outcome with T-cell-depleted unrelated-donor versus related-donor allogeneic bone marrow transplantation. *Biol Blood Marrow Transplant* 2002;8:601–607.
45. Kawanishi Y, Passweg J, Drobyski WR, et al. Effect of T cell subset dose on outcome of T cell-depleted bone marrow transplantation. *Bone Marrow Transplant* 1997;19:1069–1074.
46. Champlin RE, Passweg JR, Zhang MJ, et al. T-Cell depletion of bone marrow transplants for leukemia from donors other than HLA-identical siblings: advantage of T-cell antibodies with narrow specificities. *Blood* 2000;95:3996–4002.
47. Hale G, Cobbold S, Waldmann H. T-Cell depletion with Campath-1 in allogeneic bone marrow transplantation. *Transplantation* 1988;45:753–759.
48. Champlin R, Ho W, Gajewski J, et al. Selective depletion of CD8+ T lymphocytes for prevention of graft-versus-host disease after allogeneic bone marrow transplantation. *Blood* 1990;76:418–423.
49. Wagner JE, Santos GW, Noga SJ, et al. Bone marrow graft engineering by counterflow elutriation: results of a phase I–II clinical trial. *Blood* 1990;75:1370–1375.
50. O'Donnell PV, Myers B, Edwards J, et al. CD34 selection using three immunoselection devices: comparison of T-cell depleted allografts. *Cytotherapy* 2001;3:483–488.
51. Kernan NA, Bartsch G, Ash RC, et al. Analysis of 462 transplantations from unrelated donors facilitated by the National Marrow Donor Program. *N Engl J Med* 1993;328:593–602.
52. Soiffer RJ, Weller E, Alyea EP, et al. CD6+ donor marrow T-cell depletion as the sole form of graft-versus-host disease prophylaxis in patients undergoing allogeneic bone marrow transplant from unrelated donors. *J Clin Oncol* 2001;19:1152–1159.
53. Drobyski WR, Ash RC, Casper JT, et al. Effect of T-cell depletion as graft-versus-host disease prophylaxis on engraftment, relapse, and disease-free survival in unrelated marrow transplantation for chronic myelogenous leukemia. *Blood* 1994;83:1980–1986.
54. Marks DI, Bird JM, Vettenranta K, et al. T Cell-depleted unrelated donor bone marrow transplantation for acute myeloid leukemia. *Biol Blood Marrow Transplant* 2000;6:646–653.
55. Wagner JE, Thompson JS, Carter S, et al. Impact of graft-versus-host disease (GVHD) prophylaxis on 3-year disease-free survival (DFS): results of a multi-center, randomized phase II–III trial comparing T cell depletion/cyclosporine (TCD) and methotrexate/cyclosporine (M/C) in 410 recipients of unrelated donor bone marrow (BM). *Blood* 2002;100(11):75a.
56. Ash RC, Horowitz MM, Gale RP, et al. Bone marrow transplantation from related donors other than HLA-identical siblings: effect of T cell depletion. *Bone Marrow Transplant* 1991;7:443–452.
57. Soiffer RJ, Mauch P, Fairclough D, et al. CD6+ T cell depleted allogeneic bone marrow transplantation from genotypically HLA nonidentical related donors. *Biol Blood Marrow Transplant* 1997;3:11–17.
58. Henslee-Downey PJ, Abhyankar SH, Parrish RS, et al. Use of partially mismatched related donors extends access to allogeneic marrow transplant. *Blood* 1997;89:3864–3872.
59. Baron F, Baudoux E, Frere P, et al. Nonmyeloablative stem cell transplantation with CD8-depleted or CD34-selected peripheral blood stem cells. *J Hematother Stem Cell Res* 2002;11:301–314.
60. Kolb HJ, Schattenberg A, Goldman JM, et al., the European Group for Blood and Marrow Transplantation Working Party Chronic Leukemia : graft-versus-leukemia effect of donor lymphocyte transfusions in marrow grafted patients. *Blood* 1995;86:2041–2050.
61. Collins R, Shpilberg O, Drobyski W, et al. Donor leukocyte infusions in 140 patients with relapsed malignancy after allogeneic bone marrow transplantation. *J Clin Oncol* 1997;15:433–444.
62. Giralt S, Hester J, Huh Y, et al. CD8-depleted donor lymphocyte infusion as treatment for relapsed chronic myelogenous leukemia after allogeneic bone marrow transplantation. *Blood* 1995;86:4337–4343.
63. Alyea EP, Soiffer RJ, Canning C, et al. Toxicity and efficacy of defined doses of CD4(+) donor lymphocytes for for treatment of relapse after allogeneic bone marrow transplant. *Blood* 1998;91:3671–3680.
64. Soiffer RJ, Alyea EP, Hochberg E, et al. Randomized trial of CD8+ T-cell depletion in the prevention of graft-versus-host disease associated with donor lymphocyte infusion. *Biol Blood Marrow Transplant* 2002;8:625–632.
65. Link CJ, Burt RK, Traynor AE, et al. Adoptive immunotherapy for leukemia: donor lymphocytes transduced with the herpes simplex thymidine kinase gene for remission induction. HGTRI 0103. *Hum Gene Ther* 1998;9:115–134.
66. Bacigalupo A, Lamparelli T, Bruzzi P, et al. Antithymocyte globulin for graft-versus-host disease prophylaxis in transplants from unrelated donors: 2 randomized studies from Gruppo Italiano Trapianti Midollo Osseo (GITMO). *Blood* 2001;98:2942–2947.

67. Soiffer RJ, Dear K, Rabinowe SN, et al. Hepatic dysfunction following T-cell-depleted allogeneic bone marrow transplantation. *Transplantation* 1991;52:1014–1019.
68. Breuer R, Or R, Lijovetzky G, et al. Interstitial pneumonitis in T cell-depleted bone marrow transplantation. *Bone Marrow Transplant* 1988;3:625–630.
69. Ho VT, Weller E, Lee SJ, et al. Prognostic factors for early severe pulmonary complications after hematopoietic stem cell transplantation. *Biol Blood Marrow Transplant* 2001;7:223–229.
70. Soiffer RJ, Fairclough D, Robertson M, et al. CD6-depleted allogeneic bone marrow transplantation for acute leukemia in first complete remission. *Blood* 1997;89:3039–3047.
71. Drobyski WR, Hessner MJ, Klein JP, et al. T-Cell depletion plus salvage immunotherapy with donor leukocyte infusions as a strategy to treat chronic-phase chronic myelogenous leukemia patients undergoing HLA-identical sibling marrow transplantation. *Blood* 1999;94:434–441.
72. Hale G, Zhang MJ, Bunjes D, et al. Improving the outcome of bone marrow transplantation by using CD52 monoclonal antibodies to prevent graft-versus-host disease and graft rejection. *Blood* 1998;92:4581–4590.
73. Remberger M, Storer B, Ringden O, et al. Association between pretransplant thymoglobulin and reduced non-relapse mortality rate after marrow transplantation from unrelated donors. *Bone Marrow Transplant* 2002;29:391–397.
74. Papadopoulos EB, Carabasi MH, Castro-Malaspina H, et al. T-Cell-depleted allogeneic bone marrow transplantation as postremission therapy for acute myelogenous leukemia: freedom from relapse in the absence of graft-versus-host disease. *Blood* 1998;91:1083–1090.
75. Hale G, Waldmann H, et al. Control of graft-versus-host disease and graft rejection by T cell depletion of donor and recipient with Campath-1 antibodies. Results of matched sibling transplants for malignant diseases. *Bone Marrow Transplant* 1994;13:597–603.
76. Nimer SD, Giorgi J, Gajewski JL, et al. Selective depletion of CD8+ cells for prevention of graft-versus-host disease after bone marrow transplantation. A randomized controlled trial. *Transplantation* 1994;57:82–87.
77. Lee SJ, Zahrieh D, Alyea EP, et al. Comparison of T-cell-depleted and non-T-cell-depleted unrelated donor transplantation for hematologic diseases: clinical outcomes, quality of life, and costs. *Blood* 2002;100:2697–2702.
78. Patterson J, Prentice HG, Brenner MK, et al. Graft rejection following HLA matched T-lymhpocyte depleted bone marrow transplantation. *Br J Haematol* 1986;63:221–230.
79. Bordignon C, Kernan NA, Keever CA, et al. The role of residual host immunity in graft failures following T-cell-depleted marrow transplants for leukemia. *Ann NY Acad Sci* 1987;511:442–446.
80. Martin PJ, Hansen JA, Torok-Storb B, et al. Graft failure in patients receiving T cell-depleted HLA-identical allogeneic marrow transplants. *Bone Marrow Transplant* 1988;3:445–456.
81. Delain M, Cahn JY, Racadot E, et al. Graft failure after T cell depleted HLA identical allogeneic bone marrow transplantation: risk factors in leukemic patients. *Leuk Lymphoma* 1993;11:359–368.
82. Kernan NA, Bordignon C, Heller G, et al. Graft failure after T-cell-depleted leukocyte antigen identical marrow transplants for leukemia: I. Analysis of risk factors and results of secondary transplants. *Blood* 1989;74:2227–2234.
83. Marmont A, Horowitz MM, Gale RP, et al. T-Cell depletion of HLA-identical transplants in leukemia. *Blood* 1991;78:2120–2130.
84. Gerritsen WR, Wagemaker G, Jonker M, et al. The repopulation capacity of bone marrow grafts following pretreatment with monoclonal antibodies against T lymphocytes in rhesus monkeys. *Transplantation* 1988;45:301–307.
85. Freedman AS, Gribben JG, Neuberg D, et al. High dose therapy and autologous bone marrow transplantation in patients with follicular lymphoma during first remission. *Blood* 1996;88:2780–2786.
86. Sondel PM, Hank JA, Trigg ME, et al. Transplantation of HLA-haploidentical T cell-depleted marrow for leukemia: autologous marrow recovery with specific immune sensitization to donor antigens. *Exp Hematol* 1986;14:278–286.
87. Bunjes D, Heit W, Arnold R, et al. Evidence for the involvement of host derived OKT8-positive T cells in the rejection of T-depleted, HLA-identical bone marrow grafts. *Transplantation* 1987;43:501–505.
88. Bunjes D, Theobald M, Wiesneth M, et al. Graft rejection by a population of primed CDw52-host T cells after in vivo/ex vivo T-depleted bone marrow transplantation. *Bone Marrow Transplant* 1993;12:209–215.
89. Kernan NA, Flomenberg N, Dupont B, et al. Graft rejection in recipients of T cell depleted HLA-nonidentical marrow transplants for leukemia. *Transplantation* 1987;43:842–847.
90. Bierer BE, Emerson SG, Antin J, et al. Regulation of cytotoxic T lymphocyte-mediated graft rejection following bone marrow transplantation. *Transplantation* 1990;49:714–771.

91. Bordignon C, Keever CA, Small TN, et al. Graft failure after T-cell-depleted leukocyte antigen identical marrow transplants for leukemia: II. In vitro analysis of host effector mechanisms. *Blood* 1989;74:2237–2242.
92. Bosserman LD, Murray C, Takvorian T, et al. Mechanism of graft failure in HLA-matched and HLA-mismatched bone marrow transplant recipients. *Bone Marrow Transplant* 1989;4:239–245.
93. Voogt PJ, Fibbe WE, Marijt WA, et al. Rejection of bone marrow graft by recipient derived cytotoxic T lymphocytes against minor histocompatibility antigens. *Lancet* 1990;335(2):131–134.
94. Fleischauer K, Kernan NA, O'Reilly RJ, et al. Bone marrow-allograft rejection by T lymphocytes recognizing a single amino acid difference on HLA-B44. *N Engl J Med* 1990;323:1818–1825.
95. Donohue J, Homge M, Kernan NA. Characterization of cells emerging at the time of graft failure after bone marrow transplantation from an unrelated bone marrow donor. *Blood* 1993;82:1023–1029.
96. Manilay JO, Sykes M. Natural killer cells and their role in graft rejection. *Curr Opin Immunol* 1998;10:532–539.
97. Martin PJ. Donor CD8 cells prevent allogeneic marrow graft rejection in mice: potential implications for marrow transplantation in humans. *J Exp Med* 1993;178:703–709.
98. Martin PJ, Rowley SD, Anasetti C, et al. A phase I–II clinical trial to evaluate removal of CD4 cells and partial depletion of CD8 cells from donor marrow for HLA-mismatched unrelated recipients. *Blood* 1999;94:2192–2199.
99. Bertheas MF, Lafage M, Levy P, et al. Influence of mixed chimerism on the results of allogeneic bone marrow transplantation for leukemia. *Blood* 1991;78:3103–3111.
100. Offit K, Burns JP, Cunningham I, et al. Cytogenetic analysis of chimerism and leukemia relapse in chronic myelogenous leukemia patients after T cell-depleted bone marrow transplantation. *Blood* 1990;75:1346–1354.
101. Mackinnon S, Barnett L, O'Reilly RJ. Minimal residual disease is more common in patients who have mixed T-cell chimerism after bone marrow transplantation for chronic myelogenous leukemia. *Blood* 1994;83:3409–3415.
102. van Leeuwen JEM, van Tol MJD, Joosten AM, et al. Mixed T-lymphoid chimerism after allogeneic bone marrow transplantation for hematologic malignancies of children is not correlated with relapse. *Blood* 1993;82:1921–1928.
103. Butturini A, Seeger RC, Gale RP. Recipient immune-competent T lymphocytes can survive intensive conditioning for bone marrow transplantation. *Blood* 1986;68:954–959.
104. Kedar E, Or R, Naparstek E, et al. Preliminary characterization of functional residual host-type T lymphocytes following conditioning for allogeneic HLA-matched bone marrow transplantation (BMT). *Bone Marrow Transplant* 1988;3:129–134.
105. Mutter W, Reddehase MJ, Busch FW, et al. Failure in generating hemopoietic stem cells is the primary cause of death from cytomegalovirus disease in the immunocompromised host. *J Exp Med* 1988;167:1645–1650.
106. Steffens HP, Podlech J, Kurz S, et al. Cytomegalovirus inhibits the engraftment of donor bone marrow cells by downregulation of hemopoietin gene expression in recipient stroma. *J Virol* 1998;72:5006–5012.
107. Johnston RE, Geretti AM, Prentice HG, et al. HHV-6-related secondary graft failure following allogeneic bone marrow transplantation. *Br J Haematol* 1999;105:1041–1045.
108. Rosenfeld CS, Rybka WB, Weinbaum D, et al. Late graft failure due to dual bone marrow infection with variants A and B of human herpesvirus-6. *Exp Hematol* 1995;23:626–630.
109. Couriel D, Canosa J, Engler H, et al. Early reactivation of cytomegalovirus and high risk of interstitial pneumonitis following T-depleted BMT for adults with hematological malignancies. *Bone Marrow Transplant* 1996;18:347–352.
110. Hertenstein B, Hampl W, Bunjes D, et al. In vivo/ex vivo T cell depletion for GVHD prophylaxis influences onset and course of active cytomegalovirus infection and disease after BMT. *Bone Marrow Transplant* 1995;15:387–393.
111. Broers AEC, van der Holt R, van Esser JWJ, et al. Increased transplant-related morbidity and mortality in CMV-seropositive patients despite highly effective prevention of CMV disease after allogeneic T-cell-depleted stem cell transplantation. *Blood* 2000;95:224–231.
112. Ash RC, Casper JT, Chitambar CR, et al. Successful allogeneic transplantation of T-cell-depleted bone marrow from closely HLA-matched unrelated donors. *N Engl J Med* 1990;322:485–494.
113. Aversa F, Pelicci PG, Terenzi A, et al. Results of T-depleted BMT in chronic myelogenous leukaemia after a conditioning regimen that included thiotepa. *Bone Marrow Transplant* 1991;7(suppl 2):24–26.

114. Schaap N, Schattenberg A, Bar B, et al. Outcome of transplantation for standard-risk leukaemia with grafts depleted of lymphocytes after conditioning with an intensified regimen. *Br J Haematol* 1997;98:750–756.
115. Schattenberg A, Schaap N, Preijers F, et al. Outcome of T cell-depleted transplantation after conditioning with an intensified regimen in patients aged 50 years or more is comparable with that in younger patients. *Bone Marrow Transplant* 2000;26:17–22.
116. Guyotat D, Dutou L, Ehrsam A, et al. Graft rejection after T cell-depleted marrow transplantation: role of fractionated irradiation. *Br J Haematol* 1987;65:499–500.
117. Burnett AK, Hann IM, Robertson AG, et al. Prevention of graft-versus-host disease by ex vivo T cell depletion: reduction in raft failure with augmented total body irradiation. *Leukemia* 1988;2:300–303.
118. Soiffer RJ, Mauch P, Tarbell NJ, et al. Total lymphoid irradiation to prevent graft rejection in recipients of HLA non-identical T cell-depleted allogeneic marrow. *Bone Marrow Transplant* 1991;7:23–33.
119 Ganem G, Kuentz M, Beaujean F, et al. Additional total lymphoid irradiation in preventing graft failure of T-cell depleted bone marrow transplantation from HLA-identical siblings. *Transplantation* 1987;45:244–249.
120. Cobbold S, Martin G, Waldmann H. Monoclonal antibodies for the prevention of graft-versus-host disease and marrow graft rejection. The depletion of T cell subsets in vitro and in vivo. *Transplantation* 1986;42:239–244.
121. Castro-Malaspina H, Childs B, Laver J, et al. Hyperfractionated total lymphoid irradiation and cyclophosphamide for preparation of previously transfused patients undergoing HLA-identical marrow transplantation for severe aplastic anemia. *Int J Radiat Oncol Biol Phys* 1994;29:847–852.
122. Potter MN, Pamphilon DH, Cornish JM, et al. Graft-versus-host disease in children receiving HLA-identical allogeneic bone marrow transplants with a low adjusted T lymphocyte dose. *Bone Marrow Transplant* 1991;8:357–362.
123. Barrett AJ, Mavroudis D, Tisdale J, et al. T Cell-depleted bone marrow transplantation and delayed T cell add-back to control acute GVHD and conserve a graft-versus-leukemia effect. *Bone Marrow Transplant* 1998;21:543–551.
124. Bachar-Lustig E, Rachamim N, Li HW, et al. Megadose of T cell-depleted bone marrow overcomes MHC barriers in sublethally irradiated mice. *Nature Med* 1995;1:1268–1272.
125. Aversa F, Tabilio A, Terenzi A, et al. Successful engraftment of T-cell-depleted haploidentical transplants in leukemia patients by addition of recombinant human granulocyte colony-stimulating factor-mobilized peripheral blood progenitor cells to bone marrow inoculum. *Blood* 1994;84:3948–3953.
126. Reisner Y, Martelli MF. Tolerance induction by 'megadose' transplants of CD34+ stem cells: a new option for leukemia patients without an HLA-matched donor. *Curr Opin Immunol* 2000;12:536–541.
127. Soiffer RJ, Alyea EP, Kim H, et al. Engraftment, graft-vs-host disease (GVHD), and survival after CD8+ T cell depleted allogeneic peripheral blood stem cell transplantation (PBSCT). *Blood* 2002;100(11):418a.
128. Ault KA, Antin JH, Ginsburg D, et al. Phenotype of recovering lymphoid cell populations after marrow transplantation. *J Exp Med* 1985;161:1483–1488.
129. Keever CA, Small TN, Flomenberg N, et al. Immune reconstitution following bone marrow transplantation: comparison of recipients of T-cell depleted marrow with recipients of conventional marrow grafts. *Blood* 1989;73:1340–1346.
130. Soiffer RJ, Bosserman L, Murray C, et al. Reconstitution of T-cell function after CD6-depleted allogeneic bone marrow transplantation. *Blood* 1990;75:2076–2084.
131. Parreira A, Smith J, Hows JM, et al. Immunological reconstitution after bone marrow transplant with Campath-1 treated bone marrow. *Clin Exp Immunol* 1987;67:142–148.
132. Roux E, Helg C, Dumont-Girard F, et al. Analysis of T-cell repopulation after allogeneic bone marrow transplantation: significant differences between recipients of T-cell depleted and unmanipulated grafts. *Blood* 1996;87:3984–3990.
133. Roux E, Dumont-Girard F, Starobinski M, et al. Recovery of immune reactivity after T-cell-depleted bone marrow transplantation depends on thymic activity. *Blood* 2000;96:2299–2305.
134 Small TN, Papadopoulos EB, Boulad F, et al. Comparison of immune reconstitution after unrelated and related T-cell-depleted bone marrow transplantation: effect of patient age and donor leukocyte infusions. *Blood* 1999;93:467–480.
135. Lewin SR, Heller G, Zhang L, et al. Direct evidence for new T-cell generation by patients after either T-cell-depleted or unmodified allogeneic hematopoietic stem cell transplantations. *Blood* 2002;100:2235 2242.
136. Hochberg EP, Chillemi AC, Wu CJ, et al. Quantitation of T-cell neogenesis in vivo after allogeneic bone marrow transplantation in adults. *Blood* 2001;98:2116–2121.

137. Wu CJ, Chillemi A, Alyea EP, et al. Reconstitution of T-cell receptor repertoire diversity following T-cell depleted allogeneic bone marrow transplantation is related to hematopoietic chimerism. *Blood* 2000;95:352–359.
138. Engelhard D, Or R, Strauss N, et al. Cytomegalovirus infection and disease after T cell depleted allogeneic bone marrow transplantation for malignant hematologic diseases. *Transplant Proc* 1989;21:3101–3105.
139. Martino R, Rovira M, Carreras E, et al. Severe infections after allogeneic peripheral blood stem cell transplantation: a matched-pair comparison of unmanipulated and CD34+ cell-selected transplantation. *Haematologica* 2001;86:1075–1080.
140. Zutter MM, Martin PJ, Sale GE, et al. Epstein–Barr virus lymphoproliferation after bone marrow transplantation. *Blood* 1988;72:520–529.
141. Gerritsen EJ, Stam ED, Hermans J, et al. Risk factors for developing EBV-related B cell lymphoproliferative disorders (BLPD) after non-HLA-identical BMT in children. *Bone Marrow Transplant* 1996;18:377–383.
142. Martin PJ, Shulman HM, Schubach WH, et al. Fatal Epstein–Barr virus associated proliferation of donor B-cells after treatment of acute graft-versus-host disease with a murine anti-T-cell antibody. *Ann Intern Med* 1984;101:310–315.
143. Papadapoulos EB, Ladanyi M, Emmanuel D, et al. Infusions of donor leukocytes to treat Epstein–Barr-associated lymphoproliferative disorders after allogeneic bone marrow transplantation. *N Engl J Med* 1994;330:1185–1191.
144. Rooney CM, Smith CA, Ng CY, et al. Use of gene-modified virus-specific T lymphocytes to control Epstein–Barr-virus-related lymphoproliferation. *Lancet* 1995;345:9–13.
145. Rooney CM, Smith CA, Ng CY, et al. Infusion of cytotoxic T cells for the prevention and treatment of Epstein–Barr virus-induced lymphoma in allogeneic transplant recipients. *Blood* 1998;92:1549–1556.
146. Fischer A, Blanche S, Le Bidois J, et al. Anti-B-cell monoclonal antibodies in the treatment of severe B-cell lymphoproliferative syndrome following bone marrow and organ transplantation. *N Engl J Med* 1991;324:1451–1457.
147. McGuirk JP, Seropian S, Howe G, et al. Use of rituximab and irradiated donor-derived lymphocytes to control Epstein–Barr virus-associated lymphoproliferation in patients undergoing related haplo-identical stem cell transplantation. *Bone Marrow Transplant* 1999;24:1253–1257.
148. Kuehnle I, Huls MH, Liu Z, et al. CD20 monoclonal antibody (rituximab) for therapy of Epstein–Barr virus lymphoma after hemopoietic stem-cell transplantation. *Blood* 2000;95:1502–1509.
149. Hale G, Waldmann H. Risks of developing Epstein–Barr virus-related lymphoproliferative disorders after T-cell-depleted marrow transplants. *Blood* 1998;91:3079–3084.
150. Cavazzana-Calvo M, Bensoussan D, Jabado N, et al. Prevention of EBV-induced B-lymphoproliferative disorder by ex vivo marrow B-cell depletion in HLA-phenoidentical or non-identical T-depleted bone marrow transplantation. *Br J Haematol* 1998;103:543–547.
151. Gustafsson A, Levitsky V, Zou JZ, et al. Epstein–Barr virus (EBV) load in bone marrow transplant recipients at risk to develop posttransplant lymphoproliferative disease: prophylactic infusion of EBV-specific cytotoxic T cells. *Blood* 2000;95:807–813.
152. Rooney CM, Loftin SK, Holladay MS, et al. Early identification of Epstein–Barr virus-associated post-transplantation lymphoproliferative disease. *Br J Haematol* 1995;89:98–102.
153. Goldman JM, Gale RP, Horowitz MM, et al. Bone marrow transplantation for chronic myelogenous leukemia in chronic phase. Increased risk for relapse associated with T-cell depletion. *Ann Intern Med* 1988;108:806–812.
154. Martin P, Clift RA, Fisher LD, et al. HLA-identical marrow transplantation during accelerated-phase chronic myelogenous leukemia: analysis of survival and remission duration. *Blood* 1988;72:1978–1984.
155. Marks DI, Hughes TP, Szydlo R, et al. HLA-identical sibling donor bone marrow transplantation for chronic myeloid leukaemia in first chronic phase: influence of GVHD prophylaxis on outcome. *Br J Haematol* 1992;81:383–387.
156. Wagner JE, Zahurak M, Piantadosi S, et al. Bone marrow transplantation of chronic myelogenous leukemia in chronic phase: evaluation of risks and benefits. *J Clin Oncol* 1992;10:779–785.
157. Gratwohl A, Hermans J, Niderwieser D, et al. Bone marrow transplantation for chronic myeloid leukemia: long-term results. *Bone Marrow Transplant* 1993;12:509–514.
158. Apperley JF, Mauro FR, Goldman JM, et al. Bone marrow transplantation for chronic myeloid leukaemia in first chronic phase. Importance of a graft-versus-leukaemia effect. *Br J Haematol* 1988;69:239–244.

159. Weiden PL, Flournoy N, Thomas ED, et al. Antileukemic effect of graft-versus-host disease in recipients of allogeneic-marrow grafts. *N Engl J Med* 1979;300:1068–1074.
160. Sullivan KM, Weiden PL, Storb R, et al. Influence of acute and chronic graft-versus-host disease on relapse and survival after bone marrow transplantation from HLA-identical siblings as treatment of acute and chronic leukemia. *Blood* 1989;73:1720–1727.
161. Horowitz MM, Gale RP, Sondel PM, et al. Graft-versus-leukemia reactions after bone marrow transplantation. *Blood* 1990;75:555–565.
162. Bunjes D, Hertenstein B, Wiesneth M, et al. In vivo/ex vivo T cell depletion reduces the morbidity of allogeneic bone marrow transplantation in patients with acute leukaemias in first remission without increasing the risk of treatment failure: comparison with cyclosporin/methotrexate. *Bone Marrow Transplant* 1995;15:563–568.
163. Aversa F, Terenzi A, Carotti A, et al. Improved outcome with T-cell-depleted bone marrow transplantation for acute leukemia. *J Clin Oncol* 1999;17:1545–1552.
164. Novitzky N, Thomas V, Hale G, et al. Ex vivo depletion of T cells from bone marrow grafts with CAMPATH-1 in acute leukemia: graft-versus-host disease and graft-versus-leukemia effect. *Transplantation* 1999;67:620–626.
165. Remberger M, Ringden O, Aschan J, et al. Long-term follow-up of a randomized trial comparing T-cell depletion with a combination of methotrexate and cyclosporine in adult leukemic marrow transplant recipients. *Transplant Proc* 1994;26:1829–1833.
166. Enright H, Davies SM, DeFor T, et al. Relapse after non-T-cell-depleted allogeneic bone marrow transplantation for chronic myelogenous leukemia: early transplantation, use of an unrelated donor, and chronic graft-versus-host disease are protective. *Blood* 1996;88:714–721.
167. McGlave P, Bartsch G, Anasetti C, et al. Unrelated donor marrow transplantation therapy for chronic myelogenous leukemia: initial experience of the National Marrow Donor Program. *Blood* 1993;81:543–549.
168. Hessner MJ, Endean DJ, Casper JT, et al. Use of unrelated marrow grafts compensates for reduced graft-versus-leukemia reactivity after T-cell-depleted allogeneic marrow transplantation for chronic myelogenous leukemia. *Blood* 1995;86:3987–3993.
169. Devergie A, Apperley JF, Labopin M, et al. European results of matched unrelated donor bone marrow transplantation for chronic myeloid leukemia. Impact of HLA class II matching. Chronic Leukemia Working Party of the European Group for Blood and Marrow Transplantation. *Bone Marrow Transplant* 1997;20:11–19.
170. Soiffer RJ, Gonin R, Murray C, et al. Prediction of graft-versus-host disease by phenotypic analysis of early immune reconstitution after CD6-depleted allogeneic bone marrow transplantation. *Blood* 1993;82:2216–2223.
171. Sehn LH, Alyea EP, Weller E, et al. Comparative outcomes of T-cell-depleted and non-T-cell-depleted allogeneic bone marrow transplantation for chronic myelogenous leukemia: impact of donor lymphocyte infusion. *J Clin Oncol* 1999;17:561–570.
172. Elmaagacli AH, Peceny R, Steckel N, et al. Outcome of transplantation of highly purified peripheral blod CD34+ cells with T-cell add-back compared with unmanipulated bone marrow or peripheral blood stem cells from HLA-identical sibling donors in patients with first chronic phase chronic myeloid leukemia. *Blood* 2000;101:446–453.
173. Mackinnon S, Papadapoulos EB, Carabasi MH, et al. Adoptive immunotherapy evaluating escalating doses of donor leukocytes for relapse of chronic myeloid leukemia after bone marrow transplantation: Separation of graft-versus-leukemia responses from graft-versus-host disease. *Blood* 1995;86:1261–1268.
174. Dazzi F, Szydlo RM, Craddock C, et al. Comparison of single-dose and escalating-dose regimens of donor lymphocyte infusion for relapse after allografting for chronic myeloid leukemia. *Blood* 2000;95:67–71.
175. Munshi NC, Govindarajan R, Drake R, et al. Thymidine kinase (TK) gene-transduced human lymphocytes can be highly purified, remain fully functional, and are killed efficiently with ganciclovir. *Blood* 1997;89:1334–1340.
176. Alyea EP, Weller E, Schlossman R, et al. T Cell depleted allogeneic bone marrow transplantation followed by donor lymphocyte infusion in patients with multiple myeloma: reduced transplant related toxicity with preservation of graft versus myeloma effect. *Blood* 2001;98:934–939.
177. Soiffer RJ, Murray C, Gonin R, et al. Effect of low-dose interleukin-2 on disease relapse after T-cell-depleted allogeneic bone marrow transplantation. *Blood* 1994;84:964–971.
178. Ruggeri L, Capanni M, Casucci M, et al. Role of natural killer cell alloreactivity in HLA-mismatched hematopoietic stem cell transplantation. *Blood* 1999;94:333–339.
179. Ruggeri L, Capanni M, Urbani E, et al. Effectiveness of donor natural killer cell alloreactivity in mismatched hematopoietic transplants. *Science* 2002;295:2097–2100.

180. Shlomchik WD, Couzens MS, Tang CB, et al. Prevention of graft-versus-host disease by inactivation of host antigen presenting cells. *Science* 1999;285:412–415.
181. Davies SM, Ruggieri L, DeFor T, et al. Evaluation of KIR ligand incompatibility in mismatched unrelated donor hematopoietic transplants. Killer immunoglobulin-like receptor. *Blood* 2002;100:3825–3827.
182. Chen BJ, Cui X, Liu C, et al. Prevention of graft-versus-host disease while preserving graft-versus-leukemia effect after selective depletion of host-reactive T cells by photodynamic cell purging process. *Blood* 2002;99:3083–3089.
183. Koh MB, Prentice HG, Lowdell MW. Selective removal of alloreactive cells from haematopoietic stem cell grafts: graft engineering for GVHD prophylaxis. *Bone Marrow Transplant* 1999;23:1071–1079.
184. Garderet L, Snell V, Przepiorka D, et al. Effective depletion of alloreactive lymphocytes from peripheral blood mononuclear cell preparations. *Transplantation* 1999;67:124–130.
185. Harris DT, Sakiestewa D, Lyons C, et al. Prevention of graft-versus-host disease (GVHD) by elimination of recipient-reactive donor T cells with recombinant toxins that target the interleukin 2 (IL-2) receptor. *Bone Marrow Transplant* 1999;23:137–144.
186. Blazar BR, Taylor PA, Linsley PS, et al. In vivo blockade of CD28/CTLA4 : B7/BB1 interaction with CTLA4-Ig reduces lethal murine graft-versus-host disease across the major histocompatibility complex barrier in mice. *Blood* 1994;83:3815–3825.
187. Blazar BR, Taylor PA, Panoskaltsis-Mortari A, et al. Coblockade of the LFA1 : ICAM and CD28/CTLA4 : B7 pathways is a highly effective means of preventing acute lethal graft-versus-host disease induced by fully major histocompatibility complex-disparate donor grafts. *Blood* 1995;85:2607–2618.
188. Blazar BR, Taylor PA, Panoskaltsis-Mortari A, et al. Blockade of CD40 ligand–CD40 interaction impairs CD4+ T cell-mediated alloreactivity by inhibiting mature donor T cell expansion and function after bone marrow transplantation. *J Immunol* 1997;158:29–39.
189. Guinan EC, Boussiotis VA, Neuberg D, et al. Transplantation of anergic histoincompatible bone marrow allografts [see comments]. *N Engl J Med* 1999;340:1704–1714.
190. Tiberghien P, Ferrand C, Lioure B, et al. Administration of herpes simplex-thymidine kinase-expressing donor T cells with a T-cell-depleted allogeneic marrow graft. *Blood* 2001;97:63–69.
191. Aubin F, Cahn JY, Ferrand C, et al. Extensive vitiligo after ganciclovir treatment of GvHD in a patient who had received donor T cells expressing herpes simplex virus thymidine kinase. *Lancet* 2000;355(9204):626–627.
192. Fowler DH, Gress RE. Th2 and Tc2 cells in the regulation of GVHD, GVL, and graft rejection: considerations for the allogeneic transplantation therapy of leukemia and lymphoma. *Leuk Lymphoma* 2000;38(3–4):221–234.
193. Pan L, Delmonte J Jr, Jalonen CK, et al. Pretreatment of donor mice with granulocyte colony-stimulating factor polarizes donor T lymphocytes toward type-2 cytokine production and reduces severity of experimental graft-versus-host disease. *Blood* 1995;86:4422–4497.
194. Fowler DH, Gress RE. Th2 and Tc2 cells in the regulation of GVHD, GVL, and graft rejection: considerations for the allogeneic transplantation therapy of leukemia and lymphoma. *Leuk Lymphoma* 2000;38:221–234.
195. Hoffmann P, Ermann J, Edinger M, et al. Donor-type CD4(+)CD25(+) regulatory T cells suppress lethal acute graft-versus-host disease after allogeneic bone marrow transplantation. *J Exp Med* 2002;196:389–399.
196. Cohen JL, Trenado A, Vasey D, et al. CD4(+)CD25(+) immunoregulatory T cells: new therapeutics for graft-versus-host disease. *J Exp Med* 2002;196:401–406.
197. Taylor PA, Lees CJ, Blazar BR. The infusion of ex vivo activated and expanded CD4(+)CD25(+) immune regulatory cells inhibits graft-versus-host disease lethality. *Blood* 2002;99:3493–3499.
198. Johnson BD, Konkol MC, Truitt RL. CD25+ immunoregulatory T-cells of donor origin suppress alloreactivity after BMT. *Biol Blood Marrow Transplant* 2002;8:525–535.
199. Teshima T, Mach N, Hill GR, et al. Tumor cell vaccine elicits potent antitumor immunity after allogeneic T-cell-depleted bone marrow transplantation. *Cancer Res* 2001;61:162–167.

Part V

Graft-vs-Tumor Effect

21 Donor Lymphocyte Infusions

Clinical Applications and the Graft-vs-Leukemia Effect

Edwin P. Alyea III, MD

Contents

1. INTRODUCTION

Donor lymphocyte infusions (DLIs) have emerged as an effective strategy to treat patients who have relapsed after allogeneic stem cell transplantation (alloSCT). The success of DLI in the induction of long-lasting remissions in some patients has provided the first direct evidence of the graft-vs-leukemia (GVL) effect. In the decade since the first reports of the use of DLI by Kolb and Slavin, the diseases that respond to DLI have been identified and efforts to further enhance the GVL response have been explored *(1,2)*. The principle toxicity of DLI, graft-vs-host disease (GVHD), is now well recognized and strategies aimed at limiting this toxicity have been investigated. Finally, the demonstration that a profound antitumor effect can be mediated by the donor graft has led to the development of nonmyeloablative transplants, or minitransplants, that depend on the GVL response for success.

The dramatic clinical responses noted after DLI have led to extensive laboratory efforts to identify the effector mechanism of response and potential targets of the GVL reaction. Potential targets include allo-antigens, such as minor histocompatibility antigens, as well as tumor-specific antigens. Responses may be mediated either by direct cytotoxic effects or by indirect effects such as cytokines. In this chapter, we review both the current clinical DLI data and potential future applications of DLI, as well as discuss potential targets of the GVL effect.

From: *Stem Cell Transplantation for Hematologic Malignancies*
Edited by: R. J. Soiffer © Humana Press Inc., Totowa, NJ

2. EXPERIMENTAL MODELS OF GVL

Early preclinical studies of transplantation suggested the presence of a GVL effect. In 1956, Barnes and colleagues observed that radiation alone was not sufficient to eliminate 100% of leukemic cells in murine transplant models and proposed the existence of the GVL effect *(3,4)*. Following this initial observation, numerous investigators using a variety of murine models demonstrated that adoptively transferred lymphocytes given either prior to or following transplant are able to eliminate leukemia cells *(5)*. The effector cell population and the target of the GVL reaction in these models depends not only on the human leukocyte antigen (HLA) relationship between donor and host cells but also on the antigens expressed by the leukemic cells. Despite the increasing recognition of the preclinical GVL effect, there was no direct evidence of a GVL in human transplantation until recently.

Several lines of indirect evidence suggested the existence of a GVL effect in human transplantation. This indirect evidence included the oberservation of a higher relapse rate in recipients of syngeneic transplants compared with allogeneic transplants from sibling donors *(6,7)* and also in recipients of T-cell-depleted (TCD) transplants *(7–10)*. A reduced risk of relapse was also observed in patients who developed GVHD after blood marrow transplantation (BMT) *(11,12)*. Because withdrawal of immune suppression in relapsed transplant patients can induce remission, often in the presence of GVHD *(13–15)*, it appeared that a GVL effect may be induced by immune manipulation and that the GVL effect was tightly linked to GVHD. Direct evidence of the existence of a GVL effect was obtained when DLIs were successfully used to treat patients with chronic myelogenous leukemia (CML) who had relapsed after BMT.

3. DLI: CLINICAL RESULTS

3.1. Chronic Myelogenous Leukemia

Since the initial report by Kolb in 1990, numerous series have confirmed the effectiveness of DLI in the treatment of patients with relapsed CML after allogeneic BMT (alloBMT) *(2,16–20)*. Registry reports from Europe and North America of patients with CML who relapsed after HLA-matched sibling donor transplants demonstrate a complete cytogenetic response rate of greater than 70% in patients with CML when treated in either cytogenetic or hematologic DLI *(22,23)* (*see* Table 1). Unfortunately, patients with CML in more advanced stages of relapse, accelerated or blast crisis, have a much lower response rate following DLI *(16,22)* (*see* Fig. 1).

The time to complete cytogenetic response in patients with CML after DLI is prolonged, often 8–16 wk following the initial infusion of donor cells *(24)*. The time to complete molecular response, defined by elimination of the bcr-abl transcript as detected by polymerase chain reaction (PCR), can be 6 mo or greater after cell infusion (*see* Fig. 2). Several studies have demonstrated that interferon-α (IFN-α) is not required to achieve a response in patients with CML treated with DLI. Both the number of cells infused and the time after transplant when cells are infused appear to be important factors in limiting GVHD.

The responses obtained in patients with CML after DLI appear to be durable. Two studies have reported long-term follow-up of patients who achieved a complete remission following DLI. Five (13%) of 39 patients who achieved complete cytogenetic remission after DLI relapsed with extended follow-up *(25)*. The 3-yr overall survival (OS) for these 39 patients was 70%. The EBMTR has reported on 44 patients with CML who achieved a molecular remission after treatment DLI *(26)*. Four (9%) of 44 patients developed evidence of recurrent disease by PCR with extended follow-up. The 3-yr OS for this group of patients was excellent, 95%.

Table 1
Results of CML Treated With DLI

Stage of disease	*North American*[a]	%	*EBMTR*[b]	%
Early relapse	27/38	71%	126/164	78%
Cytogenetic	3/3	100%	40/50	80%
Hematologic	24/35	74%	88/114	77%
Advanced Phase	5/18	28%	13/36	36%
Accelerated	4/12	33%		
Blast Phase	1/6	17%		

[a] Data from ref. *22*.
[b] Data from ref. *23*.

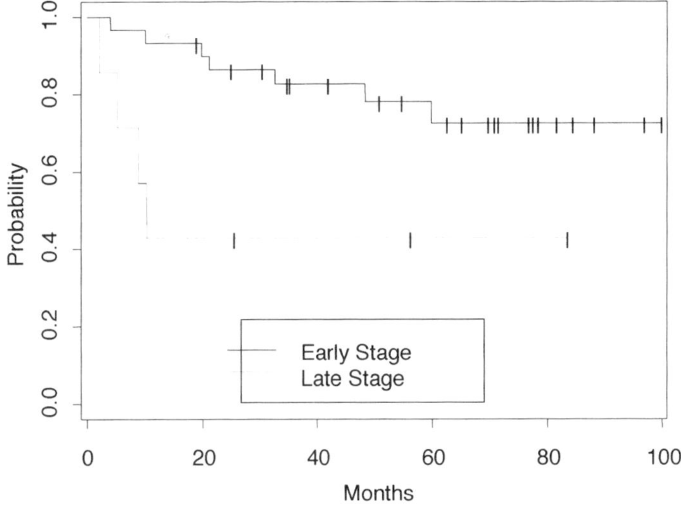

Fig. 1. Response to DLI in patients with CML.

Although these initial results are encouraging, 5- and 10-yr follow-up will be needed to fully assess the impact of this treatment modality.

Donor lymphocyte infusion has also been used in the treatment of patients with CML relapsing after unrelated donor (URD) transplant *(27)*. Eleven (46%) of 24 patients treated with DLI from URDs achieved complete remission (CR). Seven (58%) of 12 patients treated in early phase of relapse obtained remission. Similar to the results of DLI from matched siblings, the response to DLI in advanced-stage CML was poor, with only 4 (31%) of 13 patients achieving remission. All four patients were in the accelerated phase; no responses were noted in patients in blast crisis.

The stage of disease at the time of transplant is the most significant predictor of response in patients with CML. Studies consistently demonstrate that patients receiving DLI in cytogenetic or hematologic relapse have a much higher response rate than patients treated in more advanced phases of the disease. T-cell dose also appears to impact both response rate and risk of development of GHVD. When the impact of cell dose on response was assessed in the large

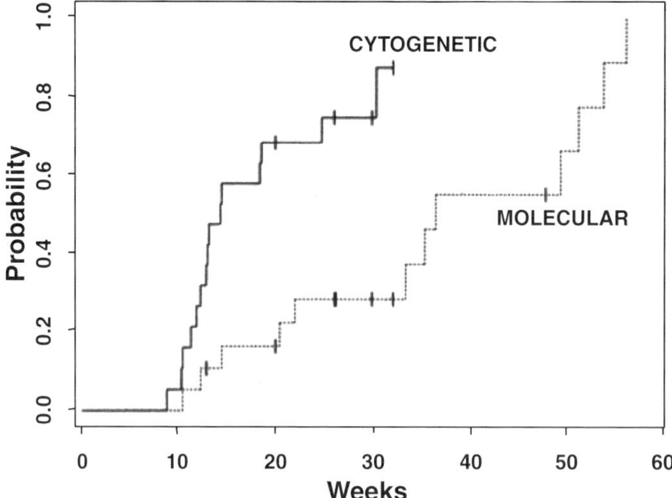

Fig. 2. Time to complete cytogenetic and molecular response in patients with chronic myelogenous leukemia.

registry studies, no clear correlation between cell dose infused and response was noted *(21,22)*. However, the doses of cells infused in the majority of these patients may have been so high that the beneficial effects of low-dose cell infusion were not apparent.

Two prospective trials of unmanipulated DLI have analyzed T-cell number and the impact on response and GVHD. MacKinnon et al. have reported a high response rate and low incidence of GVHD in patients receiving 1×10^7 CD3+ cells/kg *(28)*. Of eight patients receiving this dose, only one patient developed GVHD. Lower doses of cells appear less effective, with no responses seen in patients receiving less than 1×10^7 CD3+ cells/kg. A subsequent trial compared a single-bulk-dose regimen with infusion of escalating doses of T cells *(29)*. Patients receiving a single bulk infusion received a median infusion of 1.5×10^8 T cells/kg, whereas patients receiving the escalating regimen received 1×10^7, 5×10^7, and 1×10^8 T cells/kg if no response or toxicity was observed after each infusion. The incidence of GVHD was significantly lower with the escalating-dose regimen (10%) compared with the single bulk infusion (44%) ($p = 0.011$). There was no difference in the remission rate. In DLI from unrelated donors, no correlation between cell dose and response rate or incidence of acute GVHD was noted.

3.2. Multiple Myeloma

Several studies of allogeneic transplantation in patients with myeloma had suggested the presence of a graft-vs-myeloma (GVM) effect *(30–32)*. DLI studies have have provided direct evidence of the GVM effect with DLI inducing significant responses in patients with multiple myeloma who have relapsed after transplantation (*see* Table 2). The overall response rate to DLI in patient with myeloma approaches 45%, with CRs noted in about 25% of patients. Durable CRs are noted in half of the patients who obtain a CR with follow-up over 7 yr in some patients. Patients who do not obtain a CR eventually develop progressive disease. These patients may benefit from repeat DLIs.

Both the dose of cells infused and timing of DLI after transplantation may influence response rates. The optimal dose of cells to be infused and timing of DLI has yet to be determined. Lokhorst and colleagues reported that patients receiving greater than 1×10^8 CD3+ cells/kg

Table 2
Results of Multiple Myeloma Treated With DLI

	N	*Prior chemotherapy*	*CR (%)*	*PR (%)*	*Overall RR (%)*
Salama et al.*(33)*	25	3	7 (33%)	2 (8%)	9 (36%)
Lokhorst et al. *(34)*	27	13	6 (22%)	8 (29%)	14 (52%)
DFCI	21	0	9 (43%)	6 (29%)	15/21 (71%)

Abbreviations: CR, complete remission; PR, partial remission; RR, relative risk; DFCI, Dana-Farber Cancer Institute.

were associated with an improved response; however, responses have been noted in patients with infusion of doses as low as 1×10^7 CD3+ cells/kg *(34)*. Early administration of DLI after allogeneic transplantation may improve response rates and improve GVM after transplantation. Fourteen patients received prophylactic DLI 6–9 mo after TCD myeloablative allogeneic transplantation in an attempt to augment GVM after transplantation *(35)*. Of the 14 patients receiving DLI, 11 patients had evidence of disease at the time of DLI. Ten of the 11 patients with evidence of disease demonstrated significant GVM responses, with 6 patients obtaining a CR. Although a significant GVM effect could be induced by the addition of prophylactic DLI after allogeneic transplant, only 58% of myeloma patients were able to receive DLI after transplantation because they had developed complications, such as GVHD, which prevent DLI administration.

As with other diseases, GVHD is the main complication associated with DLI in patients with multiple myeloma. The overall incidence of acute and chronic GVHD in the study by Lokhorst were 66% and 56%, respectively *(34)*. As with CML, there appears to be a strong association between GVHD and graft vs malignancy. In the same study, acute and chronic GVHD, developed in 87% and 85% of patients responding, respectively.

3.3. Myelodysplastic Syndrome and Acute Leukemia

Patients with myelodysplasic syndrome (MDS) and large numbers of patients with acute leukemia have been treated with DLI (*see* Table 3). In the North American registry report, CRs were noted in two of five patients with MDS treated with DLI, whereas in the European experience, three of nine patients with MDS achieved a remission *(22,36)*. Response rates in acute myelogenous leukemia (AML) and acute lymphocytic leukemia (ALL) are low and are similar to the response rates noted in patients with advanced-stage CML. The CR rate to DLI in patients with AML is 15–29%, and in ALL, it is 5–18%. The durability of response in patients with acute leukemia is less that that seen in patients with CML. In a study assessing the long-term outcome of patients treated with DLI, 36% of patients with acute leukemia who achieved remission after DLI relapsed, including 4 of 15 with AML and 3 of 4 with ALL *(24)*. The median time to relapse was 10 mo (range: 1–37 mo).

Donor lymphocyte infusion from URDs in patients with acute leukemia is associated with a higher response rate than that seen with DLI from related donors, with 8 of 19 patients (42%) achieving a CR after unrelated DLI *(26)*. Of patients achieving a CR after DLI, 30% died of treatment-related complications and 30% relapsed. The median survival of patients receiving unrelated DLI was short (11 wk).

Table 3
Results of MDS and Acute Leukemia Treated With DLI Alone

Disease	*North American experience*[a]	*European experience*[b]
Myelodysplasia	2/5 (40%)	3/9 (33%)
Acute myeloid leukemia	6/39 (15%)	12/42 (29%)
Acute lymphocytic leukemia	2/15 (13%)	1/22 (5%)

[a]Data from ref. *22*.
[b]Data from ref. *23*.

Many patients with relapsed acute leukemia after allogeneic transplantation have been treated with chemotherapy followed by DLI. In some cases, chemotherapy was administered because of rapidly progressive disease or in an attempt to debulk patients prior to DLI. Although the overall response rate to chemotherapy plus DLI is higher than DLI alone, long-term outcome does not appear significantly improved. A clinical trial that combined chemotherapy and DLI demonstrated an overall CR rate of 47% *(37)*. Unfortunately, the toxicity associated with this approach was high, with a treatment-related mortality of 23% and a disappointing 2-yr OS for all patients of 19%.

3.4. Chronic Lymphocytic Leukemia and Lymphoma

Although there is indirect evidence of the existence of a graft-vs-lymphoma (GVL) effect *(38)*, the DLI experience in patients with chronic lymphocytic lymphoma (CLL) and low-grade lymphoma is limited. Patients with CLL have obtained a CR following DLI. The time to CR may be prolonged, with one patient being followed 12 mo after a single infusion of donor lymphocytes before obtaining a remission *(39,40)*. There are case reports of patients with follicular lymphoma responding to DLI *(38)*. In the report from the North American registry, no responses were noted in patients with non-Hodgkin's lymphoma or in two patients with Hodgkin's disease *(22)*. Future reports of DLI will, no doubt, contain additional information about the response rate in these patients.

3.5. GVHD Following DLI

Graft-vs-host disease is the principle complication of DLI. GVHD occurs in 45–100% of patients with CML who achieve a complete cytogenetic response *(21,22,41)*. GVHD that develops after DLI often has characteristics of chronic GVHD involving the liver and skin; however, GVHD with characteristics of acute GVHD has also been noted. GVHD and complications related to its treatment are the primary reason for the 10–20% treatment-related mortality associated with DLI. The association between response to DLI and the development of GVHD, suggests that GVL and GVHD may be closely related. Importantly, responses are noted in some patients without the development of GVHD, suggesting that GVL may be distinct from GVHD (*see* Fig 3). Efforts to separate GVL and GVHD both experimentally and in the clinic have been explored (*see* Table 4). These efforts include infusion of low doses of cells, defining the proper timing of cell infusion after BMT and selective T-cell infusions.

As previously discussed, infusion of low doses of T cells results in high response rates in patients with CML with minimal GVHD. This has led to a strategy of using escalating doses of lymphocytes, with infusion of higher doses of cells being reserved for patients who do not

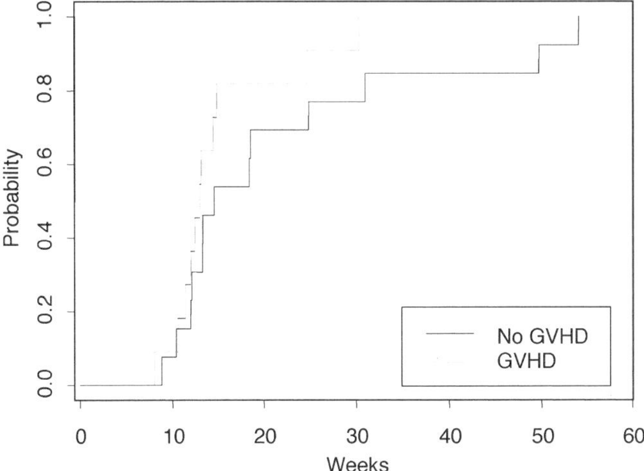

Fig. 3. Impact of GVHD on response in patients with CML.

Table 4
Possible Mechanisms to Limit Toxicity and Enhance Efficacy of Donor Lymphocyte Infusions

Limit Toxicity
Infusion of limited number of cells
CD8 depletion of donor lymphocytes
Infusion of tumor selective cells
Infusion of suicide gene transduced cells
Enhance Efficacy
IL-2
IL-12
Infusion of tumor-specific cells
Vaccination of donor or patient

respond to the initial DLI *(28)*. To minimize toxicity associated with the infusion of a larger number of cells, patients must be followed for prolonged periods because response to DLI may be delayed. Responses have been noted up to 9 mo after a single course of DLI. The relationship among cell dose, response, and toxicity is not well established in other diseases. No relationship between cell dose and response or the development of GVHD was noted in patients receiving DLIs from unrelated donors; however, the number of patients available for evaluation was limited *(26)*.

The administration of DLI very early after transplantation is associated with significant GVHD. In an early study by Sullivan et al., a high incidence of GVHD was noted with DLI given within the first weeks after BMT *(42)*. Examining DLI at a later time-point. Barrett et al. noted an increased risk of GVHD associated with early T-cell infusion at d 30 after BMT compared with infusions at d 45 after TCD alloBMT *(43)*. Larger registry studies of DLI did not demonstrate an increased risk GVHD when DLI was administered either within the first year or beyond 1 yr after transplantation *(21,22)*.

Two strategies using selective T-cell infusion have been explored to limit GVHD while preserving GVL: DLI depleted of CD8+ cells or DLI in which a suicide gene has been transduced into the infused cells. In clinical transplantation, evidence suggests that CD8+ cells play a role in the development of GVHD in humans. This evidence includes the observation that patients with a higher number of circulating CD8+ T cells during the period of early lymphoid reconstitution have an increased risk of developing GVHD *(44)*. In a clinical transplant model, selective TCD of donor marrow with an anti-CD8 monoclonal antibody was found to be capable of reducing the incidence of GVHD without leading to an increased risk of relapse *(45)*.

Two trials of CD8+-cell depletion prior to DLI have been performed *(23,46)*. The incidence of GVHD noted in these trials was low when compared with trials using unmanipulated donor cell infusions. In one study, approx 50% of patients with CML who achieved a complete cytogenetic response did not develop evidence of clinical GVHD (*see* Fig. 2). In addition, no patient receiving CD8-depleted donor lymphocytes developed GVHD in the absence of a response. GVHD has been noted to occur in some patients who have not achieved a response when treated with unmanipulated DLI. These two studies suggest that CD4+ donor cell infusions are capable of inducing a GVL effect while reducing the risk of GVHD. The responses to CD4+ DLI also appear durable *(47)*. A direct comparison of CD4+ DLI with unmanipulated DLI administered 6 mo after TCD DLI has been performed and a significantly lower incidence of GVHD was noted in patients receiving CD4+ DLI. Larger comparative trials will be needed to confirm this finding.

If GVL and GVHD are closely linked, it may be necessary for the effector cells to be tightly controlled. Investigators have designed donor T cells with a suicide gene, thymidine kinase, which may be activated if a patient develops GVHD after DLI *(48–50)*. These transduced cells appear to remain fully functional; however, these cells may be killed by the administration of ganciclovir *(51)*. This strategy may allow for the induction of a GVL response able to be terminated when GVHD begins to develop by the administration of ganciclovir.

4. METHODS TO ENHANCE THE GVL RESPONSE AFTER DLI

Strategies to enhance the GVL effect mediated by DLI have included activation of the infused cells as well as methods to improve potential target antigen presentation. Slavin et al. administered IL-2 to patients following DLI. In addition, some patients received allogeneic cells which had been activated ex-vivo by IL-2 *(1)*. Five of six patients with advanced hematologic malignancies who did not respond to DLI alone achieved remissions with the addition of IL-2 to DLI. In a trial at Dana–Farber, low-dose IL-2 was given for 12 wk following DLI to patients with MDS, acute leukemia, and advanced-phase CML. The IL-2 was well tolerated and no significant additional toxicity was noted. Responses were noted in some patients but were rarely durable.

Several groups have attempted to prime the donor cells prior to infusion. One approach has been to prime donor T cells by immunization of donors with immunoglobulin idiotype, as in multiple myeloma. This approach has been used in patients with myeloma undergoing conventional transplantation *(52)*. A second approach has been to generate in vitro and infuse T-cell clones that have antileukemic activity. Falkenburg et al. have reported the successful treatment of a patient with accelerated-phase CML using this approach *(53)*. A similar approach by Slavin has used in vitro primed donor lymphocytes *(54)*. Cells from the donor are incubated with irradiated lymphocytes obtained from the recipient in an attempt to "immunize" the donor cells. Future efforts to improve the response to DLI may employ methods that increase tumor antigen presentation to DLI. To design strategies that lead to a significant improvement in responses to DLI, identification of the mediators and targets of the GVL effect is needed.

5. MEDIATORS OF THE GVL EFFECT

The majority of evidence suggests that donor T cells mediate the GVL effect in animal models. In murine models, the relative contribution of either CD8+ or CD4+ T-cell subsets in mediating the GVL effect depends on the HLA and minor antigen relationship between donor and host, as well as the target antigens expressed by the malignant cell. CD8+ cells appear to mediate the GVL effect in the majority of models through direct cytotoxicity of the target cell. Demonstrating the importance of CD8+ cells, mice receiving BM depleted of CD8+ cells had an increased risk of leukemia relapse compared with mice receiving marrow depleted of CD4+ cells *(55)*. In contrast, infusion of CD8-depleted marrow with the addition of CD4+ T cells leads to a low incidence of GVHD while preserving GVL in other models *(56)*. The mechanism by which CD4+ cells mediate a GVL response is not clear.

Indirect evidence suggests that T cells mediate GVL in humans. Clinical trials have demonstrated that TCD BMT results in the loss of significant GVL. This loss of GVL is responsible for the increased relapse rate seen in CML patients after TCD BMT, which approaches 40–60% as compared with only 10–20% after non-TCD BMT. In vitro, both CD4+ and CD8+ T-cell subsets that demonstrate antileukemic activity have been generated *(57–69)*. CD4+ T cells with selective cytotoxicity of Philadelphia chromosome-positive (Ph+) clones have been identified in vivo; however, with prolonged culture, specificity appears to wane *(58)*.

Serial phenotypic analysis has not revealed the in vivo expansion of either a population of CD8+ or CD4+ T cells in patients responding to DLI. T-Cell repertoire analysis has been employed as a more sensitive method to assess changes in the T-cell compartment following DLI. In some patients with CML and myeloma who respond to DLI, selective T-cell clonal expansion has been noted at the time of response *(61,62)*.

Natural killer (NK) cells have also been identified as potential mediators of GVL. NK cells appear during hematopoietic recovery after alloBMT and are able to recognize differences in the target's major histocompatibility complex (MHC) class I *(63,64)* and class II molecules *(65)*. Activated NK cells mediate cytotoxicity through MHC unrestricted killing. A correlation between the high number of circulating NK cells and remission status has been noted in patients after BMT *(66)*. Murine models do not support the role of NK cells is the GVL reaction mediated by DLI *(67)*.

6. POTENTIAL TARGETS OF THE GVL EFFECT

Potential targets include both tumor-specific antigens and allo-specific antigens. It is likely that the target of the GVL effect may vary by disease (*see* Table 5). Tumor-specific targets may include unique fusion proteins created by gene translocations specific for certain diseases, such as p210, which is formed by the bcr-abl rearrangement found in patients with CML. Other tumor-specific antigens include immunogloblin idiotype, as in patients with lymphoma or multiple myeloma. Other targets include allo-antigens, which include minor antigens or sex-specific antigens, as in H-Y antigens.

T Cells have been generated in vitro that are capable of recognizing proteins created by the fusion gene product associated that human leukemias *(68–71)* and may serve as potential

Table 5
Potential Target Antigens of the GVL Response

Tumor specific	*Allospecific antigens*
p210 BCR-ABL gene product	unrestricted minor antigens
CML	HA-3, HA-4, HA-6, H-Y
p190 BCR-ABL gene product	tissue-restricted minor antigens
ALL	HA-1, HA-2
	lymphoid and myeloid cells
idiotype	
multiple myeloma, lymphoma,	Proteinase 3
chronic lymphocytic leukemia	AML
abherrently expressed antigens	other antigens
AML, ALL	

targets for T-cell recognition. Four peptides specific for the b3a2 fusion in CML were identified as having high or intermediate binding efficiency to HLA A3, A11 and B8 *(70)*. In contrast, peptides generated from b2a2 and PML-RARα were not found to have high binding affinity in the presence of class I molecules.

Assessment of humoral responses after DLI may also identify potential targets of GVL. Immunophenotyping often demonstrates an expansion of B cells after DLI, suggesting a role for humoral immunity. Using SEREX, 11 potential target antigens have been identified in patients with CML responding to DLI *(72)*. One novel target identified, CML66, has been characterized and is a broadly expressed tumor antigen also found in patients with lung cancer, prostate cancer, and melanoma.

Despite the expression of leukemia-specific antigens, malignant cells may not present proper costimulatory molecules, therefore preventing the generation of an immune response. The engagement of CD28 on T cells by the B7-1/B7-2 (CD80, CD86) on B cells and antigen-presenting cells is needed to elicit an immune response. T-Cell receptor (TCR) signals in the absence of costimulation may lead to anergy. Because not all tumor cells appear to express the proper costimulatory molecules, the immune response may be inhibited.

Many suspect that the GVL response is directed toward allo-antigens. Often, the conversion from mixed chimerism to complete donor hematopoiesis is noted after response to DLI *(16,73)*. A detailed assessment of chimerism and response to DLI demonstrated that patients had a predominance of donor-derived lymphopoiesis at the time of relapse, whereas granulopoiesis and erythropoiesis were mainly recipient derived *(74)*. Following DLI and at the time of response, a significant decrease in recipient cells was noted in all lineages, suggesting that the GVL response is directed toward a broadly expressed allo-specific antigen.

Several candidates for targets of an allo-immune response have been identified. Some of these antigens are ubiquitous, including HA-3, HA-4, HA-6, and H-Y, whereas several minor antigens are specific for certain tissues on lymphoid and myeloid cells, including HA-1 and HA-2. Whether these minor antigens serve as targets is unclear. Leukemic cells of lymphoid origin that expressed mHA with specificities HA-1 to HA-5 and HA-Y were identified; however, the leukemic cells were less susceptible to lysis. The mechanism responsible for the impaired lysis appears to be the low expression of LFA-1 adhesion molecules *(75)*. If minor histocompatibility antigens (mHA) antigens are the target of the GVL effect, this would provide a link between GVL and GVHD.

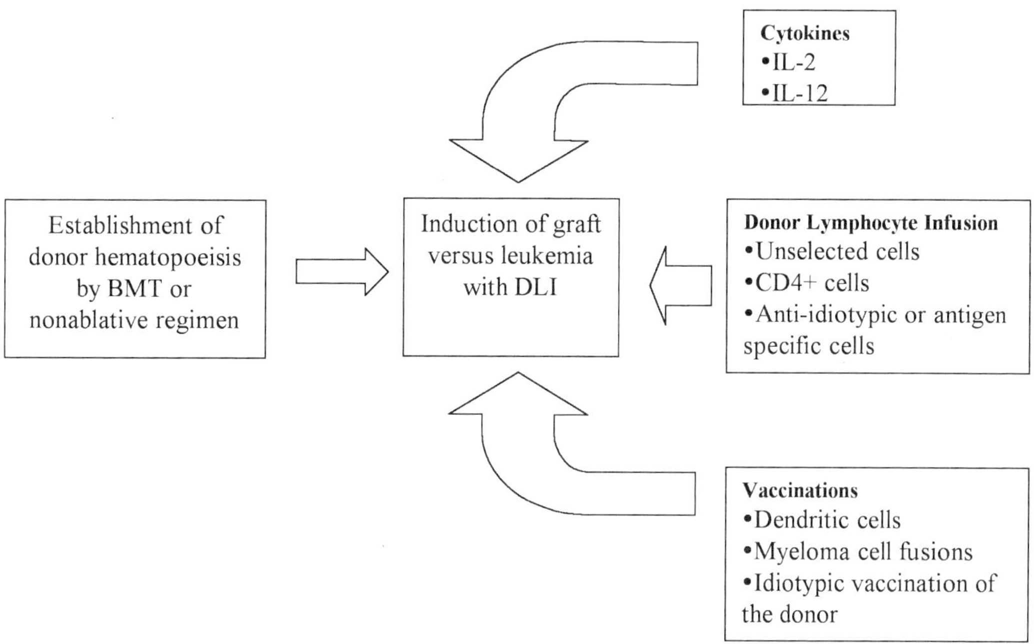

Fig. 4. Strategies to improve response to DLI.

Three pathways by which the GVL effect may eliminate tumor cells have been suggested *(76–78)*. Direct killing of leukemia cells by perforin and granzyme attack mediated by CD4+ or CD8+ cytotoxic lymphocytes or NK cells has been postulated. T-Cells may also mediate killing via cytokines such as tumor necrosis factor (TNF)-α and IFN-γ, which have been shown to inhibit hematopoiesis *(79)*. The involvement of Fas/Fas-ligand interactions and the induction of apoptosis has also been implicated in the GVL effect. Fas/Fas-ligand appears to be an important pathway for T cells to mediate antigen-specific killing. Both chronic and acute leukemias have been shown to express Fas antigen *(80)*. A more through understanding of the mechanisms of the GVL reaction will lead to targeted strategies that enhance the GVL effect as well as limit toxicity (*see* Fig. 4).

7. FUTURE DIRECTIONS

Efforts are focusing on methods to make DLI both more effective and less toxic. Current trials are defining the appropriate timing of DLI as well as the number of cells to be infused. An improved understanding of both the effector cells and targets of the GVL response will allow for more selected therapies to be developed in the future. Ultimately, for DLI to be a viable treatment option and available to a large number of patients, DLI must be separated from conventional stem cell transplantation and its toxicities. Nonmyeloablative transplant strategies, which markedly reduce the treatment-related toxicity, may provide the appropriate platform for DLI.

REFERENCES

1. Slavin S, Naparstek E, Nagler A, et al. Allogeneic cell therapy with donor peripheral blood cells and recombinant human interleukin-2 to treat leukemia relapse after allogeneic bone marrow transplantation. *Blood* 1996;87:2195–2204.

2. Kolb H, Mittermuller J, Clemm C, et al. Donor leukocyte transfusions for treatment of recurrent chronic myelogenous leukemia in marrow transplant patients. *Blood* 1990;76:2462–2465.
3. Barnes DWH, Loutit JF. Immunological and histological response following spleen treatment in irradiated mice. In: Mitchel JS, Holmes BE, SCL, eds. *Progress in Radiobiology*. Edinburgh: Oliver and Boyd, 1956;291.
4. Barnes DWH, Loutit JF. Treatment of murine leukaemia with X-rays and homologous bone marrow: II. *Br J Haematol* 1957;3:241–252.
5. Truitt RL, Johnson BD. Principles of graft-vs-leukemia reactivity. *Biol Blood Marrow Transplant* 1995;1:61–68.
6. Gale RP, Horowitz MM, Ash RC, et al. Identical-twin bone marrow transplants for leukemia. *Ann Intern Med* 1994;120:646–652.
7. Horowitz MM, Gale RP, Sondel PM, et al. Graft-versus-leukemia reactions after bone marrow transplantation. *Blood* 1990;75:555–562.
8. Goldman JM, Gale RP, Horowitz MM, et al. Bone marrow transplantation for chronic myelogenous leukemia in chronic phase. Increased risk for relapse associated with T-cell depletion. *Ann Intern Med* 1988;108:806–814.
9. Apperley JF, Mauro FR, Goldman JM, et al. Bone marrow transplantation for chronic myeloid leukaemia in first chronic phase, Importance of a graft-versus-leukaemia effect. *Br J Haematol* 1988;69:239–245.
10. Marmont A, Horowitz MM, Gale RP, et al. T-Cell depletion of HLA-identical transplants in leukemia. *Blood* 1991;78:2120–2130.
11. Weiden PL, Flournoy N, Thomas ED, et al. Antileukemic effect of graft-versus-host disease in recipients of allogeneic-marrow grafts. *N Engl J Med* 1979;300:1068–1073.
12. Weiden PL, Sullivan K, Flournoy N, et al. Antileukemic effect of chronic graft-versus-host disease. Contribution to improved survival after allogeneic marrow transplantation. *N Engl J Med* 1981;304:1529–1533.
13. Odom LF, August CS, Githens JH, et al. Remission of relapsed leukaemia during a graft-versus-host reaction. A "graft-versus-leukaemia reaction" in man? *Lancet* 1978;2:537–540.
14. Higano CS, Brixey M, Bryant EM, et al. Durable complete remission of acute nonlymphocytic leukemia associated with discontinuation of immunosuppression following relapse after allogeneic bone marrow transplantation. A case report of a probable graft-versus-leukemia effect. *Transfusion* 1990;50:175–177.
15. Collins RH, Rogers ZR, Bennett M, et al. Hematologic relapse of chronic myelogenous leukemia following allogeneic bone marrow transplantation. Apparent graft-versus-leukemia effect following abrupt discontinuation of immunosuppression. *Bone Marrow Transplant* 1992;10:391–395.
16. Porter DL, Roth MS, McGarigle C, et al. Induction of graft-vs-host disease as immunotherapy for relapsed chronic myelogenous leukemia. *N Engl J Med* 1994;330:100–106.
17. Frassoni F, Fagioli F, Sessarego M, et al. The effect of donor leucocyte infusion in patients with leukemia following allogeneic bone marrow transplantation. *Exp Hematol* 1992;20:712.
18. Helg C, Roux E, Beris P, et al. Adoptive immunotherapy for recurrent CML after BMT. *Bone Marrow Transplant* 1993;12:125–129.
19. Drobyski WR, Keever CA, Roth MS, et al. Salvage immunotherapy using donor leukocyte infusions as treatment for relapsed chronic myelogenous leukemia after allogeneic bone marrow transplantation: efficacy and toxicity of a defined T-cell dose. *Blood* 1993;82:2310–2318.
20. Jiang YZ, Kanfer EJ, Macdonald D, et al. Graft-versus-leukaemia following allogeneic bone marrow transplantation: emergence of cytotoxic T lymphocytes reacting to host leukaemia cells. *Bone Marrow Transplant* 1991;8:253–258.
21. Kolb HJ, Schattenberg A, Goldman JM, et al., the European Group for Blood and Marrow Transplantation Working Party Chronic Leukemia. Graft-versus-leukemia effect of donor lymphocyte transfusions in marrow grafted patients. *Blood* 1995;86:2041–2050.
22. Collins R, Shpilberg O, Drobyski W, et al. Donor leukocyte infusions in 140 patients with relapsed malignancy after allogeneic bone marrow transplantation. *J Clin Oncol* 1997;15:433–444.
23. Kolb H. Donor leukocyte transfusions for treatment of leukemic relapse after bone marrow transplantation. *Vox Sang* 1998;74:321–329.
24. Alyea EP, Soiffer RJ, Canning C, et al. Toxicity and efficacy of defined doses of CD4(+) donor lymphocytes for treatment of relapse after allogeneic bone marrow transplant. *Blood* 1998;91:3671–3680.
25. Porter DL, Collins RH Jr, Shpilberg O, et al. Long-term follow-up of patients who achieved complete remission after donor leukocyte infusions. *Biol Blood Marrow Transplant* 1999;5:253–261.
26. Dazzi F, Szydlo RM, Cross NC, et al. Durability of responses following donor lymphocyte infusions for patients who relapse after allogeneic stem cell transplantation for chronic myeloid leukemia. *Blood* 2000;96:2712–2716.

27. Porter DL, Collins RH Jr, Hardy C, et al. Treatment of relapsed leukemia after unrelated donor marrow transplantation with unrelated donor leukocyte infusions. *Blood* 2000;95:1214–1221.
28. Mackinnon S, Papadapoulos EB, Carabasi MH, et al. Adoptive immunotherapy evaluating escalating doses of donor leukocytes for relapse of chronic myeloid leukemia after bone marrow transplantation: separation of graft-versus-leukemia responses from graft-versus-host disease. *Blood* 1995;86:1261–1268.
29. Dazzi F, Szydlo RM, Craddock C, et al. Comparison of single-dose and escalating-dose regimens of donor lymphocyte infusion for relapse after allografting for chronic myeloid leukemia. *Blood* 2000;95:67–71.
30. Bensinger WI, Buckner CD, Anasetti C, et al. Allogeneic marrow transplantation for multiple myeloma: an analysis of risk factors on outcome. *Blood* 1996;88:2787–2793.
31. Bjorkstrand B, Ljungman P, Svensson H, et al. Allogeneic bone marrow transplantation versus autologous stem cell transplantation in multiple myeloma: a retrospective case-matched study from the European Group for Blood and Marrow Transplantation. *Blood* 1996;88:4711–4718.
32. Le Blanc R, Montminy-Metivier S, Belanger R, et al. Allogeneic transplantation for multiple myeloma: further evidence for a GVHD-associated graft-versus-myeloma effect. *Bone Marrow Transplant* 2001;28:841–848.
33. Salama M, Nevill T, Marcellus D, et al. Donor leukocyte infusions for multiple myeloma. *Bone Marrow Transplant* 2000;26:1179–1184.
34. Lokhorst HM, Schattenberg A, Cornelissen JJ, van Oers MH, Fibbe W, Russell I, Donk NW, Verdonck LF. Donor lymphocyte infusions for relapsed multiple myeloma after allogeneic stem-cell transplantation: predictive factors for response and long-term outcome. *J Clin Oncol* 2000;18:3031–3037.
35. Alyea E, Weller E, Schlossman R, et al. T-Cell-depleted allogeneic bone marrow transplantation followed by donor lymphocyte infusion in patients with multiple myeloma: induction of graft-versus-myeloma effect. *Blood* 2001;98:934–939.
36. Kolb HJ. Donor leukocyte transfusions for treatment of leukemic relapse after bone marrow transplantation. EBMT Immunology and Chronic Leukemia Working Parties. *Vox Sang* 1998;74(suppl 2):321–329.
37. Levine JE, Braun T, Penza SL, et al. Prospective trial of chemotherapy and donor leukocyte infusions for relapse of advanced myeloid malignancies after allogeneic stem-cell transplantation. *J Clin Oncol* 2002;20:405–412.
38. Jones RJ, Ambinder RF, Piantadosi S, et al. Evidence of a graft-versus-lymphoma effect associated with allogeneic bone marrow transplantation. *Blood* 1991;77:649–653.
39. Alyea E, Canning C, Houde H, et al. A pilot study of CD8+ cell depletion of donor lymphocyte infusions (DLI) using CD8 monoclonal antibody coated high density microparticles (HDM). *Blood* 1999;94:161a.
40. Mandigers CM, Meijerink JP, Raemaekers JM, et al. Graft-versus-lymphoma effect of donor leucocyte infusion shown by real-time quantitative PCR analysis of t(14;18). *Lancet* 1998;352:1522–1523.
41. Antin JH. Graft-versus-leukemia: no longer an epiphenomenon. *Blood* 1993;82:2273–2277.
42. Sullivan KM, Storb R, Buckner CD, et al. Graft-versus-host disease as adoptive immunotherapy in patients with advanced hematologic neoplasms. *N Engl J Med* 1989;320:828–834.
43. Barrett AJ, Mavroudis D, Tisdale J, et al. T Cell-depleted bone marrow transplantation and delayed T cell addback to control acute GVHD and conserve a graft-versus-leukemia effect. *Bone Marrow Transplant* 1998;21:543–551.
44. Soiffer RJ, Gonin R, Murray C, et al. Prediction of graft-versus-host disease by phenotypic analysis of early immune reconstitution after CD6-depleted allogeneic bone marrow transplantation. *Blood* 1993;82:2216–2223.
45. Nimer SD, Giorgi J, Gajewski JL, et al. Selective depletion of CD8+ cells for prevention of graft-versus-host disease after bone marrow transplantation. A randomized controlled trial. *Transplantation* 1994;57:82–87.
46. Giralt S, Hester J, Huh Y, et al. CD8-depleted donor lymphocyte infusion as treatment for relapsed chronic myelogenous leukemia after allogeneic bone marrow transplantation. *Blood* 1995;86:4337–4343.
47. Shimoni A, Gajewski JA, Donato M, et al. Long-Term follow-up of recipients of CD8-depleted donor lymphocyte infusions for the treatment of chronic myelogenous leukemia relapsing after allogeneic progenitor cell transplantation. *Biol Blood Marrow Transplant* 2001;7:568–575.
48. Bonini C, Verzeletti S, Servida P, et al. Transfer of the HSV-TK gene into donor peripheral blood lymphocytes for in vivo immunomodulation of donor antitumor immunity after ALLO-BMT. *Blood* 1994;84:110a [Abstract].
49. Verzeletti S, Bonini C, Traversari C, et al. Transfer of the HSV-tK gene into donor peripheral blood lymphocytes for in vivo immunomodulation of donor antitumor immunity after allo-BMT. *Gene Ther* 1994;1:S24 [Abstract].
50. Verzeletti S, Bonini C, Traversari C, et al. Retroviral vector gene transfer into donor peripheral blood lymphocytes for in vitro selection and in vivo immunomodulation of donor antitumor immunity after allo-BMT. *J Cell Biochem* 1995;(suppl 21A):356 [Abstract].

51. Glazier A, Tutschka PJ, Farmer ER, et al. Graft versus host disease in cyclosporine treated rats after syngeneic and autologous bone marrow reconstitution. *J Exp Med* 1983;158:1.
52. Kwak LW, Taub DD, Duffey PL, et al. Transfer of myeloma idiotype-specific immunity from an actively immunised marrow donor. *Lancet* 1995;345:1016–1020.
53. Falkenburg JH, Wafelman AR, Joosten P, et al. Complete remission of accelerated phase chronic myeloid leukemia by treatment with leukemia-reactive cytotoxic T lymphocytes. *Blood* 1999;94:1201–1208.
54. Slavin S. Immunotherapy of cancer with alloreactive lymphocytes. *Lancet Oncol* 2001;2:491–498.
55. Truitt RL, Atasoylu AA. Contribution of CD4+ and CD8+ T cells to graft-versus-host disease and graft-versus-leukemia reactivity after transplantation of MHC-compatible bone marrow. *Bone Marrow Transplant* 1991;8:51–58.
56. Korngold R, Sprent J. T Cell subsets and graft versus host disease. *Transplantation* 1987;44:335.
57. Jiang Y, Mavroudis D, Dermime S, et al. Alloreactive CD4+ T lymphocytes can exert cytotoxicity to chronic myeloid leukaemia cells processing and presenting exogenous antigen. *Br J Haematol* 1996;93:606–612.
58. Oettel KR, Wesly OH, Albertini MR, et al. Allogeneic T-cell clones able to selectively destroy Philadelphia chromosome-bearing (Ph1+) leukemia leines can also recognize Ph1– cells from the same patient. *Blood* 1994;83:3390–3402.
59. Faber LM, van Luxemburg-Heijs SAP, Veenhof WFJ, et al. Generation of CD4+ cytotoxic T-lymphocyte clones from a patient with severe graft-versus-host disease after allogeneic bone marrow transplantation: implications for graft-versus-leukemia reactivity. *Blood* 1995;86:2821–2828.
60. van Lochem E, de Gast B, Goulmy E. In vitro separation of host specific graft-versus-host and graft-versus-leukemia cytotoxic T cell activities. *Bone Marrow Transplant* 1992;10:181–183.
61. Claret EJ, Alyea EP, Orsini E, et al. Characterization of T cell repertoire in patients with graft-versus-leukemia after donor lymphocyte infusion. *J Clin Invest* 1997;100:855–866.
62. Orsini E, Alyea EP, Schlossman R, et al. Changes in T cell receptor repertoire associated with graft-versus-tumor effect and graft-versus-host disease in patients with relapsed multiple myeloma after donor lymphocyte infusion. *Bone Marrow Transplant* 2000;25:623–632.
63. Kurago ZB, Smith KD, Lutz CT. NK cell recognition of MHC class I. NK cells are sensitive to peptide-binding groove and surface alpha-helical mutations that affect T cells. *J Immunol* 1995;154:2631–2641.
64. Malnati MS, Peruzzi M, Parker KC, et al. Peptide specificity in the recognition of MHC class I by natural killer cell clones. *Science* 1995;267:1016–1018.
65. Jiang YZ, Couriel D, Mavroudis DA, et al. Interaction of natural killer cells with MHC class II: reversal of HLA-DR1-mediated protection of K562 transfectant from natural killer cell-mediated cytolysis by brefeldin-A. *Immunology* 1996;87:481–486.
66. Jiang YZ, Barrett AJ, Goldman JM, et al. Association of natural killer cell immune recovery with a graft-versus-leukemia effect independent of graft-versus-host disease following allogeneic bone marrow transplantation. *Ann Hematol* 1997;74:1–6.
67. Johnson BD, Dagher N, Stankowski WC, et al. Donor natural killer (NK1.1+) cells do not play a role in the suppression of GVHD or in the mediation of GVL reactions after DLI. *Biol Blood Marrow Transplant* 2001;7:589–595.
68. Cullis J, Barrett A, Goldman J, et al. Binding of BCR/ABL junctional peptides to major histocompatibility complex (MHC) class I molecules: studies in antigen-processing defective cell lines. *Leukemia* 1994;8:165–170.
69. Bocchia M, Wentworth P, Southwood S, et al. Specific binding of leukemia oncogene fusion protein peptides to HLA class I molecules. *Blood* 1995;85:2680–2684.
70. Bocchia M, Korontsvit T, Xu Q, et al. Specific human cellular immunity to bcr-abl oncogene derived peptides. *Blood* 1996;87:3587–3592.
71. Greco G, Fruci D, Accapezzato D, et al. Two brc-abl junction peptides bind HLA-A3 molecules and allow specific induction of human cytotoxic T lymphocytes. *Leukemia* 1996;10:693–699.
72. Wu CJ, Yang XF, McLaughlin S, et al. Detection of a potent humoral response associated with immune-induced remission of chronic myelogenous leukemia. *J Clin Invest* 2000;106:705–714.
73. Porter DL, Roth MS, Lee SJ, et al. Adoptive immunotherapy with donor mononuclear cell infusions to treat relapse of acute leukemia or myelodysplasia after allogeneic bone marrow transplantation. *Bone Marrow Transplant* 1996;18:975–980.
74. Dazzi F, Capelli D, Hasserjian R, et al. The kinetics and extent of engraftment of chronic myelogenous leukemia cells in non-obese diabetic/severe combined immunodeficiency mice reflect the phase of the donor's disease: an in vivo model of chronic myelogenous leukemia biology. *Blood* 1998;92:1390–1396.

75. van Els CA, Bakker A, Zwinderman AH, et al. Effector mechanisms in graft-versus-host disease in response to minor histocompatibility antigens. II. Evidence of a possible involvement of proliferative T cells. *Transplantation* 1990;50:67–71.
76. Grogg D, Hahn S, Erb P. CD4+ T cell-mediated killing of major histocompatibility complex class II-positive antigen-presenting cells (APC). III. CD4+ cytotoxic T cells induce apoptosis of APC. *Eur J Immunol* 1992;22:267–272.
77. Ziegler TR, Young LS, Benfell K, et al. Clinical and metabolic efficacy of glutamine-supplemented parenteral nutrition after bone marrow transplantation. A randomized, double-blind, controlled study. *Ann Intern Med* 1992;116:821–828.
78. Susskind B, Iannotti MR, Shornick MD, et al. Indirect allorecognition of HLA class I peptides by CD4+ cytolytic T lymphocytes. *Hum Immunol* 1996;46:1–9.
79. Zoumbos NC, Djeu JY, Young NS. Interferon is the suppressor of hematopoiesis generated by stimulated lymphocytes in vitro. *J Immunol* 1984;133:769–774.
80. Munker R, Lubbert M, Yonehara S, et al. Expression of the Fas antigen on primary human leukemia cells. *Ann Hematol* 1995;70:15–17.

22 Nonmyeloablative Transplantation

Lyle C. Feinstein, MD *and Brenda M. Sandmaier,* MD

Contents

1. INTRODUCTION

The myeloablative doses of chemotherapy and total-body irradiation (TBI) used in allogeneic hematopoietic stem cell transplant (alloHSCT) can produce considerable morbidity and mortality, particularly in older or medically infirm patients. These toxicities restrict this treatment to patients who are younger than 50 yr of age and in good medical condition *(1)*. Patients older than 50 yr account for only 10% of those followed by the International Bone Marrow Transplant Registry *(2)*. Such a restriction is problematic in that many hematologic malignancies for which alloHSCT may be curable typically are present after age 50 *(3)*.

2. GRAFT-VS-TUMOR EFFECTS

Allogeneic marrow transplants for hematologic malignancies were originally based on the theory that marrow ablative doses of chemotherapy and radiation would overcome the host's immune responses while eradicating the underlying disease *(4)*. The marrow infusion was a supportive measure to restore hematopoiesis. Weiden et al. recognized that the allograft itself conferred an immune-mediated graft-vs-tumor (GVT) effect *(5,6)*. Evidence supporting a GVT effect, known in part to be a T-cell-mediated phenomenon, includes (1) lower relapse rates and improved survival among patients receiving alloHSCT as compared to autologous grafts *(7,8)*, (2) greater incidence of relapse following syngeneic compared to alloHSCT *(9)*,

From: *Stem Cell Transplantation for Hematologic Malignancies*
Edited by: R. J. Soiffer © Humana Press Inc., Totowa, NJ

(3) greater incidence of relapse after T-cell-depleted compared to nondepleted allografts *(10)*, (4) reduced risk of relapse among recipients with acute and chronic graft-vs-host disease (GVHD) compared to those without GVHD *(5,6,10–13)*, and (5) reinduction of remission by donor lymphocyte infusion (DLI) for relapse after allografting *(14–19)*.

3. RATIONALE FOR NONMYELOABLATIVE ALLOGRAFTING

The rationale for nonmyeloablative allografting is that reducing regimen-related toxicities while preserving GVT effects could expand treatment options for patients previously ineligible for conventional allografting because of age or medical infirmity. The reduced toxicity of nonmyeloablative preparative regimens may decrease the incidence of hepatic veno-occlusive disease *(20)* and reduce the incidence and/or duration of cytopenias. Furthermore, a less intense regimen may reduce the risk for severe acute GVHD, as there is less tissue damage and consequent cytokine release *(21,22)*. This approach, however, shifts the burden of tumor eradication to the GVT immune response presumably mediated through T-cell immune responses against minor histocompatibility antigens. Diseases susceptible to GVT killing would be the most obvious to benefit from such an approach.

4. BIOLOGY OF NONMYELOABLATIVE ALLOGRAFTING

Recent strategies to reduce transplant-related toxicities have involved combining nonmyeloablative conditioning regimens with pretransplant and posttransplant immunosuppression to facilitate donor hematopoietic stem cell engraftment. Recipient and donor T cells and dendritic cells locate to the thymus, where both host-reactive and donor-reactive T cells are deleted and a state of mixed chimerism is established *(23,24)*. A peripheral T-cell repertoire tolerant toward both donor and host is created. Stable mixed chimerism allows for adoptive immunotherapy to eradicate the malignancy through either withdrawal of immunosuppression with resultant GVT effect or, less frequently, the administration of DLI.

5. CONDITIONING REGIMENS

Several groups have investigated methods of reducing the regimen-related toxicities of allotransplants while optimizing GVT effects (*see* Table 1) *(25–34)*. Strategies can be categorized as (1) reduced intensity regimens that retain a degree of regimen-related toxicity and (2) minimally myelosuppressive regimens. Reduced intensity regimens rely on the cytotoxic conditioning to suppress the host-vs-graft (HVG) effect. Minimally myelosuppressive regimens use postgrafting immunosuppression to control GVHD and suppress residual HVG effects that would prevent engraftment.

Conditioning regimens typically include two of the following: a nucleoside analog, such as fludarabine, an alkylating agent, or low-dose TBI. Fludarabine is an ideal agent given its relatively low nonhematologic toxicity profile, activity in many hematologic malignancies, and immunosuppressive nature, which likely facilitates engraftment *(35,36)*.

5.1. Reduced-Intensity Regimens

5.1.1. Hematologic Malignancies

Patients at the M.D. Anderson Cancer Center in Houston received purine nucleoside analog-based regimens for treatment of myeloid and lymphoid malignancies. Fifteen patients (median age: 59 yr; range: 27–71 yr) with myeloid malignancies were conditioned with a regimen of

Table 1

Nonmyeloablative Allografting for HSCT From HLA-Matched Donors

Transplant center	*No. of patients studied*	*Conditioning regimen*	*Postgraft immuno-suppression*	*Diagnosis*	*No. of patients achieving 90% donor chimerism*	*No. of patients achieving CR*	*GVHD*		*Outcomes no. of patients*
							Acute Grade II–V	*Chronic*	
M.D. Anderson *(25)*	15	F+I+A F+I+M 2-CDA+A	CSP+MP	AML MDS	6	8	3	0	OS: 6 DFS: 2 Median 100 d
M.D. Anderson *(26)*	15	F+Cy F+C+A	T±MTX	CLL NHL	8	8	4 3 after DLI	2	OS: 7 Median 180 d
Jerusalem *(27)*	26	F+B+ATG	CSP	HM GD	7 2 after DLI	NA	10	9 2 after DLI	OS:22 DFS: 21 Median 240 d
Jerusalem *(28)*	23	F+B+ATG	CSP	L	16	NA	8	4 2 after DLI	DFS: 10 Median 675 d
NIH *(29)*	15	F+Cy	CSP	HM ST	7 3 after stopping CSP	5	10 1 after DLI	4	OS: 8 121–409 d posttransplant
Boston *(30)*	21	Cy+ATG±TI	CSP	HM	NA 7 after DLI	8	12 6 after DLI	NA	OS: 11 DFS: 7 Median 445 d
Freiburg *(31)*	21	F+Ca+M	CSP+MTX	HM ST	16	15	13	14	OS: 13 DFS: 11 Median 354 d
Seattle *(34)*	192	2 Gy TBI±F	MMF+CSP	HM	NA	NA	88	NA	OS: 114 Nonrelapse mortality: 43 Relapse mortality: 35 Median 289 d

Abbreviations: A, ara-C; AML, acute myelogenous leukemia; ATG, antithymocyte globulin; B, busulfan; C, cisplatin; Ca, carmustine; CLL, chronic lymphocytic leukemia; CSP, cyclosporine; Cy, cyclophosphamide; DLI, donor lymphocyte infusion; GD, genetic diseases; HM, hematologic malignancies; I, idarubicin; L, lymphoma; MDS, myelodysplastic syndrome; MP, methylprednisolone; NA, not available; MTX, methotrexate; ST, solid tumors; T, tacrolimus; TBI, total body irradiation; T, thymic irradiation; 2-CDA, 2-chlorodeoxyadenosine; OS, overall survival; DFS, disease-free survival fludarabine with idarubicin and ara-C (*n*=7) or melphalan (*n*=1) or 2-chlorodeoxyadenosine and ara-C (*n*=7) prior to allografting from a human leukocyte antigen (HLA)-identical (*n*=13) or single-antigen mismatch (*n*=2) sibling donor *(25)*. Nine patients were refractory to salvage chemotherapy. GVHD prophylaxis included cyclosporine (CSP) and methylprednisolone. Four patients failed to engraft. The only treatment-related death occurred prior to the stem cell infusion. Eight patients achieved a complete remission (CR) that lasted a median of 60 d (range: 34–170). At a median follow-up of 100 d (range: 34–175), six patients were alive and two were disease-free. Fifteen patients (median: 55 yr; range: 45–71 yr) with lymphoid malignancies received allografts from an HLA-identical sibling after conditioning with fludarabine and cyclophosphamide or cisplatin, fludarabine, and cytarabine *(26)*. Six patients had advanced refractory relapse. GVHD prophylaxis included tacrolimus alone or with methotrexate. Eleven patients engrafted and eight achieved CR. Three nonrelapse deaths occurred. At a median follow-up of 180 d (range: 90–767), five of six patients (83.3%) with chemosensitive disease were alive compared with two of nine patients (22.2%) with refractory or untreated disease.

Investigators at Hadassah University in Israel used a regimen of fludarabine, antithymocyte globulin (ATG), and busulfan to condition 26 patients (median age: 31 yr; range: 1–61 yr) with hematologic malignancies (*n*=22) and genetic diseases (*n*=4) *(27)*. CSP was used as GVHD prophylaxis. All patients achieved complete chimerism or stable partial donor chimerism. Four nonrelapse deaths occurred as a result of acute GVHD. Although no regimen-related deaths were observed, four patients developed moderate to severe hepatic veno-occlusive disease. At a median of 8 mo posttransplant, 22 of 26 patients (85%) were alive and 21 (81%) were disease-free. Using the same regimen, 23 heavily treated, high-risk malignant lymphoma patients (median age: 41 yr; range: 13–63 yr) received allografts from HLA-matched related (*n*=22) or unrelated (*n*=1) donors *(28)*. Resistant disease was present in 12 patients, and 5 had preceding autologous transplants. All patients engrafted. Four nonrelapse and six relapse related deaths occurred. Ten patients were alive a median of 22.5 mo (range: 15–37) after HSCT. Actuarial survival and disease-free survival (DFS) at 37 mo were both 40%.

Researchers at the National Cancer Institute described 15 patients (median age: 50 yr; range: 23–68 yr) with hematologic malignancies (*n*=8) or solid tumors (*n*=7) who received allografts from HLA-identical (*n* =14) or 5/6 HLA antigen-matched (*n*=1) sibling donors after conditioning with cyclophosphamide and fludarabine *(29)*. CSP was used as GVHD prophylaxis. Full chimerism was achieved in seven patients by d 30 and in six further patients by d 200 after CSP withdrawal and DLI. One patient rejected the allograft with recovery of autologous hematopoiesis. Nine patients developed grade II–III acute GVHD, and four developed treatable chronic GVHD. Five patients died of progressive disease and two of transplant-related causes. Ten of 14 (71.4%) patients surviving more than 30 d demonstrated delayed disease regression. Five had a sustained CR, including one with metastatic renal cell carcinoma (RCC). Eight patients survived 121–409 d following transplant. Full donor T-cell chimerism preceded both acute GVHD and disease regression.

The Boston group at the Massachusetts General Hospital evaluated 21 patients conditioned with cyclophosphamide, ATG, and thymic irradiation (among patients without previous mediastinal radiotherapy) who received HLA-matched donor marrow infusions *(30)*. CSP was used for GHVD prophylaxis. Of eight evaluable patients who received prophylactic DLI to improve chimerism, six achieved full donor chimerism. Fourteen of 20 evaluable patients (70%) had responses; eight achieved CR. Five of the nine evaluable patients (56%) who received prophylactic DLI achieved a CR, compared with 3 of 11 patients (27%) who did not receive prophylactic DLI. One regimen-related death occurred, and one patient died from DLI-induced GVHD. At a median follow-up of 445 d (range: 105–548), 11 patients were alive and 7 were free of disease progression.

Investigators in Freiburg, Germany studied 21 patients (median age: 49 yr; range: 36–62 yr) who received peripheral blood stem cells (PBSCs) from HLA-matched related donors after conditioning with fludarabine, carmustine, and melphalan *(31)*. CSP and reduced-dose methotrexate were used as GVHD prophylaxis. Acute GVHD developed among 13 patients (62%) and 9 of 17 (53%) evaluable patients developed extensive chronic GVHD. Eight patients died; seven with relapsed or progressive disease. With a median follow-up of 354 d (range: 258–577), 15 patients (71%) achieved a CR and four patients achieved a partial response (PR). The overall survival (OS) and DFS were 62% and 52%, respectively.

Researchers in London, England treated 44 patients (median age: 41 yr; range: 18–56 yr) with hematologic malignancies with a PBSC allograft from HLA-identical sibling donors (*n*=36) or marrow from matched unrelated donors (*n*=8) after conditioning with Campath-1H, fludarabine, and melphalan *(32)*. GVHD prophylaxis included CSP alone (*n* =38) or CSP and methotrexate (*n*=6). Sustained engraftment occurred among 42 of 43 evaluable patients. No grade III–IV acute GVHD occurred. Four patients died of relapse or progression, and four treatment-related deaths occurred. Among 19 patients, the nonmyeloablative allograft was their second transplant, and only 3 of the 19 (16%) died of transplant-related complications. At a median follow-up of 9 mo (range: 2–9), 36 patients were alive and 22 were in CR. The estimated probabilities of nonrelapse mortality, progression-free survival, and OS at 12 mo were 11%, 71%, and 73%, respectively.

5.1.2. HLA-Mismatched Related and HLA-Matched Unrelated Donor Allografting

Sykes et al. treated five refractory NHL patients (median age: 30 yr; range: 20–51 yr) with a marrow transplant from haploidentical related donors sharing at least one HLA-A, -B, or -DR allele on the mismatched haplotype after conditioning with cyclophosphamide and thymic irradiation, and ATG *(37)*. GVHD prophylaxis included CSP. Four evaluable patients engrafted. All patients developed grade II–III acute GVHD that responded to steroid therapy. Three patients died of systemic aspergillus, pulmonary hemorrhage, and progressive lymphoma, respectively. Two patients without GVHD were in CR and PR at 460 and 103 d posttransplant, respectively.

Chakraverty et al. studied 47 patients (median age: 44 yr; range: 18–62 yr) who received allografts from unrelated donors after nonablative conditioning with Campath-1H, fludarabine, and melphalan *(38)*. Twenty-nine patients had failed prior autografts. Twenty donors were mismatched for HLA class I and/or class II alleles. GVHD prophylaxis was with CSP. Primary graft failure occurred in only 2 of 44 evaluable patients. Only three patients developed grade III–IV acute GVHD, and no chronic extensive GVHD was observed. Estimates of nonrelapse mortality at d 100 and 1 yr were 14.9% and 19.8%, respectively. With a median follow-up of 344 d (range: 79–830), OS and progression-free survivals at 1 yr were 75.5% and 61.5%, respectively.

5.1.3. Solid Tumors

The largest published experience of nonmyeloablative allografting for treatment of a solid tumor has been for RCC. The modest response rates observed with the immunomodulatory agents interleukin-2 (IL-2) and interferon-α (IFN-α) *(39)* in the treatment of metastatic RCC provided the rationale for a trial evaluating the feasibility of a nonmyeloablative HSCT. Childs et al. treated 19 patients (median age: 48 yr; range; 37–65 yr) with refractory metastatic RCC with a regimen of cyclophosphamide and fludarabine followed by PBSC transplant from an HLA-identical (*n*=17) or a single-antigen mismatch (*n*=2) donor *(40)*. Seventeen patients had previous therapy with IL-2, IFN-α, or both. GVHD prophylaxis was with CSP. Eight patients received DLI (median: 2.5 doses; range: 1–3 doses) to facilitate full donor chimerism and/or treat progressive disease. Ten patients died, 8 of progressive disease and 2 of transplant-related complications. Grade II–IV acute GVHD occurred among 10 patients (53%), 1 of whom died. Seven patients had a PR and three were in CR at 27, 25, and 16, mo posttransplant. At a median follow-up of 402 d (range: 287–831) after transplant, nine patients were alive. Responses occurred at a median of 55 d (range: 21–113) after HSCT and only after complete donor chimerism was achieved. Responses were associated with acute GVHD.

5.1.4. Nonmalignant Conditions

Nonmyeloablative HSCT may be useful for the treatment of nonmalignant diseases because there is no tumor burden to overcome and a state of stable mixed chimerism may be sufficient to correct abnormalities or deficiencies in the host.

Amrolia et al. described eight patients with severe immunodeficiency states who received marrow transplants from HLA-matched unrelated (*n*=6) or sibling (*n*=2) donors after conditioning with fludarabine, melphalan, and antilymphocyte globulin *(41)*. All patients engrafted, and none had grade II–IV acute GVHD. One patient died of infectious complications following disease recurrence. At a median follow-up of 12 mo, five of seven evaluable patients achieved normal age-related CD3 counts, and six had normal phytohemagglutinin stimulation indices.

Horwitz et al. reported on 10 patients with chronic granulomatous disease who received TCD PBSC transplants from HLA-identical siblings after conditioning with cyclophosphamide, fludarabine, and ATG *(42)*. Two patients rejected their grafts. Grade II–IV acute GVHD developed among three of four evaluable adults and was not observed among the five pediatric patients. Three recipients died of nonrelapse causes. At a median follow-up of 17 mo (range: 8–26), eight patients had oxidase-positive neutrophils in their blood at levels that would be expected to provide normal host defense (median level: 100% donor neutrophils; range: 33–100%); in six patients, the proportion was 100%.

5.2. Minimally Myelosuppressive Regimens

Although reduced-intensity regimens often have less regimen-related toxicities than conventional alloHSCT, patients still experience cytopenias, may require hospitalization, and may be at risk for developing hepatic veno-occlusive disease. In an attempt to further reduce toxicities and move alloHSCT into the outpatient setting, Storb and colleagues used the canine model to develop a conditioning regimen of only 2 Gy TBI, the dose necessary to maintain engraftment when coupled with the postgrafting immunosuppressive agents CSP and mycophenolate mofetil (MMF) *(43)*.

5.2.1. HLA-Matched Sibling Donors

Preclinical canine studies by Storb et al. prompted multi-institutional trials conducted at the Fred Hutchinson Cancer Research Center, University of Leipzig, Stanford University, City of Hope National Medical Center, Baylor University, University of Torino, and University of Colorado *(34,44)*. One hundred ninety-two patients (median age: 55 yr; range: 18–73 yr) received PBSCTs from HLA-matched sibling donors for hematologic malignancies. Graft rejection occurred among 10 of the first 59 (17%) patients receiving 2 Gy TBI as conditioning. With the addition of fludarabine pretransplant, only 3% of all subsequent patients failed to engraft. All rejections were nonfatal. Relapse mortality and nonrelapse mortality were 18% and 22%, respectively. Grades II, III, and IV acute GVHD occurred among 33%, 11%, and 5% of patients with stable grafts, respectively. With a median follow-up of 289 d (range: 100–1177), 114 patients (59%) were alive. Two-yr estimates of overall and progression-free survival were 50% and 40%, respectively.

5.2.2. HLA-Matched Unrelated Donors

Using a longer duration of postgrafting immunosuppression with MMF and CSP, 63 patients with median age 53 yr (range: 4–69) received HLA-matched unrelated donor grafts after conditioning with fludarabine and 2 Gy TBI *(45)*. The incidence of rejection was 27%. Grades II, III, and IV acute GVHD occurred among 50%, 13%, and 0%, respectively, of patients with stable grafts. Chronic extensive GVHD was present in 50% of patients with stable grafts. Nonrelapse mortality was 14%, and 32% of patients died of relapse. With a median follow-up of 5.5 mo (range: 0.6–15.6), 54% of patients were alive and 37% were in CR.

6. CONSOLIDATIVE ALLOGRAFTS FOLLOWING PLANNED AUTOGRAFTS

As GVT effects may not be sufficient to eradicate large volume disease, a recent strategy has been to follow an autoHSCT with a nonmyeloablative allograft. The rationale of the regimen is that the autotransplant debulks the patient's tumor allowing the subsequent allograft to eliminate residual disease.

Carella et al. evaluated nonmyeloablative allografting following autoHSCT for treatment of refractory Hodgkin's disease (n=10) and non-Hodgkin's lymphoma (n=5) *(33)*. The median age was 34 yr (range: 19–60). The median number of chemotherapy regimens was 2, and 13 of 15 patients had mediastinal and/or retroperitoneal bulky disease. Autotransplant conditioning included carmustine, etoposide, cytarabine, and melphalan. At a median of 61 d after autotransplant, patients were conditioned with fludarabine and cyclophosphamide followed by PBSC infusion from an HLA-matched sibling. GVHD prophylaxis included CSP and methotrexate. Seven patients received DLI for failure to achieve full donor chimerism after CSP withdrawal. Three patients died with progressive disease and two nonrelapse deaths occurred. Nine patients who were in PR after autotransplant achieved a CR after allografting. Five of seven patients receiving DLI achieved a CR. With a median follow-up of 337 d (range: 210–700), 10 patients were alive and 5 maintained a CR a median of 270 d (range: 210–340) after allografting.

The high nonrelapse mortality *(46,47)* and documented GVT effect *(48)* observed with multiple myeloma prompted an evaluation of the feasibility of a tandem approach. Maloney et al. evaluated 32 patients with a median age of 55 yr (range: 39–71), with previously treated stage II–III myeloma (43% refractory or relapsed disease) who received 200 mg/m^2 melphalan followed by autoHSCT *(49)*. Forty to 120 d later, 31 patients received 200 cGy TBI followed by an allograft from an HLA-identical sibling. GVHD prophylaxis was CSP and MMF. All patients engrafted without subsequent rejection. Four nonrelapse deaths occurred and one patient died of disease progression. With a median follow-up of 328 d after allografting, overall survival was 81%, with 53% of patients achieving a CR.

7. NONMYELOABLATIVE ALLOGRAFTING AFTER FAILING A CONVENTIONAL TRANSPLANT

For many patients with hematologic malignancies who fail a conventional allogeneic or autologous transplant because of relapse, rejection, or the development of a new secondary malignancy, salvage allografting is the only option with curative intent. Unfortunately, outcomes with conventional allografting following a failed autologous or allogeneic transplant are typically poor because of high nonrelapse mortality *(50–56)*. Nonmyeloablative allografting offers the potential for curative GVT effects with reduced regimen-related toxicities (*see* Table 2) *(57–60)*.

Nagler et al. evaluated 12 patients (median age: 33 yr; range: 8–63 yr) with hematologic malignancies who received an allograft from HLA-identical sibling donors for relapsed disease or secondary malignancy following an autologous transplant *(57)*. Recipients were conditioned with fludarabine, busulfan, and ATG and received CSP as GVHD prophylaxis. Only one nonrelapse death occurred and six patients were disease-free, with a median follow-up of 23 mo. Actuarial survival and DFS at 34 mo were 56% and 50%, respectively.

Dey et al. described 13 patients with hematologic malignancies who relapsed following an autoHSCT and received an HLA-matched related donor allograft following conditioning with cyclophosphamide and ATG with or without thymic irradiation *(58)*. CSP was used as GVHD prophylaxis, and DLI was administered at 5–6 wk posttransplant to facilitate full donor chimerism and optimize GVT effects. Only one nonrelapse death occurred. Median survival was 10 mo (range: 3–39) with 2-yr estimates of OS and DFS of 45% and 38%, respectively.

Devine et al. studied 11 patients (median age: 41 yr; range: 22–58 yr) with hematologic malignancies who relapsed after an autoHSCT or alloHSCT and received a second transplant from an HLA-identical (*n*=7) or HLA-mismatched related (*n*=4) donor after a reduced intensity regimen of fludarabine and melphalan with or without ATG *(59)*. Tacrolimus and methotrexate were used for GVHD prophylaxis. Although full donor engraftment was achieved in all but 1 patient, 10 of 11 died a median of 140 d (range: 9–996) after transplant: 5 from relapse and 5 from nonrelapse causes. The authors suggested that disease status at the time of nonmyeloablative allografting was significant, as only one of the patients was in a complete remission at the time of transplant.

Feinstein et al. reported on 48 patients (median age: 44 yr; range: 18–69 yr) who failed a conventional autologous (*n*=43), allogeneic (*n*=4), or syngeneic (*n*=1) HSCT and subsequently received an HLA-matched related (*n*=29) or unrelated (*n*=19) donor allograft after conditioning with 2 Gy TBI or 2 Gy TBI and fludarabine *(60)*. Postgrafting immunosuppression was with CSP and MMF. One rejection occurred in a patient receiving an unrelated donor allograft. Day +100 transplantation and overall nonrelapse mortality were 6% and 15%, respectively. With a median follow-up of 8.4 mo (0.6–31.5), 24 patients were alive and 14 were disease-free.

8. UNRESOLVED ISSUES AND FUTURE DIRECTIONS

The optimal regimen may ultimately be defined by the nature of the disease being treated. The disappointing response to DLI observed in acute leukemias of lymphoid (0–18%) or myeloid (15–29%) origin after conventional allografting suggests that cytoreduction may be necessary to permit time for an adequate GVT effect to develop *(17,19,61)*. Furthermore, antigen-presenting host dendritic cells, which play an important role in GVHD *(62)* and possibly the GVT effect, are reduced or absent after myeloablative transplants, but likely persist

Table 2
Nonmyeloablative Allografting Following a Failed Conventional HSCT

Transplant center	*No. of patients studied*	*Conditioning regimen*	*Postgraft immuno suppression*	*No. of patients achieving 90% donor chimerism*	*No. of patients achieving CR*	*GVHD*		*Outcomes no. of patients*
						Acute grade II–IV	*Chronic extensive*	
Jerusalem *(57)*	12	F+B+ATG	CSP	12	6	5	1	OS: 7 DFS: 6 Median 23 mo
Boston *(58)*	13	Cy+ATG±TI	CSP	12 6 afterDLI	7	5 4 after DLI	1	OS: 5 DFS: 5 Median 10 mo
Chicago *(59)*	11	F+M±ATG	T+MTX	10	6/10	2	4/7	OS: 1 DFS: 1 Median 5 mo
Seattle *(60)*	48	F+2 Gy TBI	MMF+CSP	47	NA	NA	NA	OS: 24 DFS: 14 Median 8.4 mo

Abbreviations: ATG, antithymocyte globulin; B, busulfan; CSP, cyclosporine; Cy, cyclophosphamide; DLI, donor lymphocyte infusion; HM, hematologic malignancies; NA, not available; M, melphalan; MTX, methotrexate; T, tacrolimus; TBI, total-body irradiation; TI, thymic irradiation after nonmyeloablative regimens. This may allow for a greater GVT effect with or without DLI in relapsed acute leukemias after nonmyeloablative allografting.

The urgency to achieve full donor chimerism is also likely to be disease-specific. For many nonmalignant diseases, patients need not achieve full donor chimerism. Experience with hemoglobinopathies *(63–67)* supports this strategy. For more aggressive diseases, conversion to full donor chimerism may be necessary to eradicate the malignant process *(29,40)*. Minor histocompatibility antigen-sensitized DLI can facilitate a more rapid conversion to full donor chimerism in the canine model *(68)*.

Although reduced-intensity and minimally myeloablative regimens limit regimen-related toxicity, even low doses of radiation or chemotherapy may entail some risk of secondary malignancy. CTLA4-Ig, a peptide that binds B7 and blocks the T-cell-activating CD28 : B7 pathway and the T-cell-inhibitory B7 : CTLA4 pathway, facilitated both engraftment and a reduction in TBI to 1 Gy for dogs receiving PBSCs from dog leukocyte antigen-identical littermates and posttransplant immunosuppression with CSP and MMF *(69)*. Similarly, only 3 Gy TBI was necessary for engraftment among mice receiving tacrolimus, antilymphocyte globulin, and T-cell depleted bone marrow from major and minor histocompatible antigen-mismatched donors *(70)*. Administration of the α-emitter bismuth-213 conjugated to an anti-CD45 monoclonal antibody obviated the need for TBI as conditioning and facilitated stable mixed hematopoietic chimerism in the canine model *(71)*. Finally, murine studies using only 0.7–1 Gy thymic irradiation and host peripheral blood TCD suggest that, by mass action, high doses of PBSCs can overcome the immunologic "niche" for engraftment that would otherwise be created by TBI *(72)*. Major histocompatibility disparity can also be overcome with high doses of stem cells *(73)*.

Selective blockade of T-cell costimulatory pathways involving B7 : CD28 and CD154 : CD40 facilitates T-cell tolerance and ameliorates GVHD in murine nonmyeloablative HSCT regimens. Targeting of the B7 : CD28 activation signal with anti-CD28 monoclonal antibodies (MAbs) inhibited donor T-cell expansion and prevented lethal GVHD in sublethally irradiated mice more effectively than the less specific CTLA4-Ig, suggesting that it may produce better immunologic tolerance *(74)*. Host CD8 TCD and anti-CD40 ligand permitted the induction of mixed chimerism and donor-specific skin graft tolerance in 3-Gy-irradiated mice receiving fully major histocompatibility complex-mismatched marrow grafts *(75)*. Similarly, a MAb directed to the cellular adhesion molecule CD44 was able to facilitate stable mixed hematopoietic chimerism among haploidentical canine recipients conditioned with low-dose TBI *(76)*.

In the nonmyeloablative setting, the optimal source of stem cells, peripheral blood, or marrow remains unclear. Following myeloablative conditioning, hematologic recovery is faster with a PBSC allograft than with marrow *(77–80)*. However, recovery of counts is usually rapid with nonmyeloablative regimens, regardless of the source of hematopoietic stem cells. A recent abstract by Maris et al. suggests that PBSCs confer superior engraftment, OS, and progression-free survival over marrow for patients receiving HLA-matched unrelated donor allografts after nonmyeloablative conditioning with fludarabine and 2 Gy TBI *(45)*.

Infection remains a barrier to reducing nonrelapse mortality. Mohty et al. reported on 21 patients conditioned with fludarabine, busulfan, and ATG who received CSP as GVHD prophylaxis *(81)*. Early viral infection, especially cytomegalovirus (CMV), occurred at a high rate (65%), and 33% of patients developed late bacterial infections (predominantly Gram-negative organisms) despite not being neutropenic. A matched control study was done to compare 56 patients conditioned with 2 Gy TBI to controls who received conventional allotransplants. It was concluded that CMV disease was significantly delayed in the nonmyeloablative setting; however, the overall 1-yr incidence was similar between the two groups *(82)*.

9. CONCLUSION

Despite relatively short follow-up, preliminary results from studies of nonmyeloablative HSCT are encouraging. A less toxic regimen can be implemented while preserving potent GVT effects. Current challenges include defining the optimal regimen to facilitate full donor engraftment while further minimizing regimen-related toxicities and the incidences of infection and GVHD. Such strategies would expand treatment options for patients who would otherwise be ineligible for potentially curative therapy with alloHSCT.

REFERENCES

1. Molina AJ, Storb RF. Hematopoietic stem cell transplantation in older adults. In: Rowe JM, Lazarus HM, Carella AM, eds. *Handbook of Bone Marrow Transplantation*, 1st ed. London: Martin Dunitz, 2000:111–137.
2. Horowitz MM, Keating A. Report on state of the art in blood and marrow transplantation—the IBMTR/ABMTR summary slides with guide. *IBMTR/ABMTR Newslett* 2000:7:3–10.
3. Jemal A, Thomas A, Murray T, et al. Cancer statistics, 2002. *CA Cancer J Clin* 2002;52:23–47.
4. Thomas ED, Storb R, Clift RA, et al. Bone-marrow transplantation. *N Engl J Med* 1975;292:832–843, 895–902.
5. Weiden PL, Flournoy N, Thomas ED, et al. Antileukemic effect of graft-versus-host disease in human recipients of allogeneic-marrow grafts. *N Engl J Med* 1979;300:1068–1073.
6. Weiden PL, Sullivan KM, Flournoy N, et al. Antileukemic effect of chronic graft-versus-host disease. Contribution to improved survival after allogeneic marrow transplantation. *N Engl J Med* 1981;304:1529–1533.
7. Gorin NC, Labopin M, Fouillard L, et al. Retrospective evaluation of autologous bone marrow transplantation vs allogeneic bone marrow transplantation from an HLA identical related donor in acute myelocytic leukemia. *Bone Marrow Transplant* 1996;18:111–117.
8. Zittoun RA, Mandelli F, Willemze R, et al. Autologous or allogeneic bone marrow transplantation compared with intensive chemotherapy in acute myelogenous leukemia. *N Engl J Med* 1995;332:217–223.
9. Fefer A, Sullivan KM, Weiden P, et al. Graft versus leukemia effect in man: the relapse rate of acute leukemia is lower after allogeneic than after syngeneic marrow transplantation. In: Truitt RL, Gale RP, Bortin MM, eds. *Cellular Immunotherapy of Cancer*. Edited by. New York: Alan R. Liss, 1987:401–408.
10. Horowitz MM, Gale RP, Sondel PM, et al. Graft-versus-leukemia reactions after bone marrow transplantation. *Blood* 1990;75:555–562.
11. Sullivan KM, Fefer A, Witherspoon R, et al. Graft-versus-leukemia in man: relationship of acute and chronic graft-versus-host disease to relapse of acute leukemia following allogeneic bone marrow transplantation. In: Truitt RL, Gale RP, Bortin MM, eds. *Cellular Immunotherapy of Cancer*. New York: Alan R. Liss, 1987:391–399.
12. Sullivan KM, Weiden PL, Storb R, et al. Influence of acute and chronic graft-versus-host disease on relapse and survival after bone marrow transplantation from HLA-identical siblings as treatment of acute and chronic leukemia. *Blood* 1989;73:1720–1728.
13. Ringden O, Horowitz MM. Graft-versus-leukemia reactions in humans. *Transplant Proc* 1989;21:2989–2992.
14. Drobyski WR, Keever CA, Roth MS, et al. Salvage immunotherapy using donor leukocyte infusions as treatment for relapsed chronic myelogenous leukemia after allogeneic bone marrow transplantation: efficacy and toxicity of a defined T-cell dose. *Blood* 1993;82:2310–2318.
15. van Rhee F, Lin F, Cullis JO, et al. Relapse of chronic myeloid leukemia after allogeneic bone marrow transplant: the case for giving donor leukocyte transfusions before the onset of hematologic relapse. *Blood* 1994;83:3377–3383.
16. Porter DL, Roth MS, McGarigle C, et al. Induction of graft-versus-host disease as immunotherapy for relapsed chronic myeloid leukemia. *N Engl J Med* 1994;330:100–106.
17. Kolb HJ, Schattenberg A, Goldman JM, et al. Graft-versus-leukemia effect of donor lymphocyte transfusions in marrow grafted patients. European Group for Blood and Marrow Transplantation Working Party Chronic Leukemia. *Blood* 1995;86:2041–2050.

18. Mackinnon S, Papadopoulos EB, Carabasi MH, et al. Adoptive immunotherapy evaluating escalating doses of donor leukocytes for relapse of chronic myeloid leukemia after bone marrow transplantation: separation of graft-versus-leukemia responses from graft-versus-host disease. *Blood* 1995;86:1261–1268.
19. Collins RH Jr, Shpilberg O, Drobyski WR, et al. Donor leukocyte infusions in 140 patients with relapsed malignancy after allogeneic bone marrow transplantation. *J Clin Oncol* 1997;15:433–444.
20. McDonald GB, Hinds MS, Fisher LD, et al. Veno-occlusive disease of the liver and multiorgan failure after bone marrow transplantation: a cohort study of 355 patients. *Ann Intern Med* 1993;118:255–267.
21. Antin JH, Ferrara JLM. Cytokine dysregulation and acute graft-versus-host disease. *Blood* 1992;80:2964–2968.
22. Hill GR, Crawford JM, Cooke KR, et al. Total body irradiation and acute graft-versus-host disease: the role of gastrointestinal damage and inflammatory cytokines. *Blood* 1997;90:3204–3213.
23. Sykes M, Szot GL, Swenson KA, et al. Induction of high levels of allogeneic hematopoietic reconstitution and donor-specific tolerance without myelosuppressive conditioning. *Nature Med* 1997;3:783–787.
24. Manilay JO, Pearson DA, Sergio JJ, et al. Intrathymic deletion of alloreactive T cells in mixed bone marrow chimeras prepared with a nonmyeloablative conditioning regimen. *Transplantation* 1998;66:96–102.
25. Giralt S, Estey E, Albitar M, et al. Engraftment of allogeneic hematopoietic progenitor cells with purine analog-containing chemotherapy: harnessing graft-versus-leukemia without myeloablative therapy. *Blood* 1997;89:4531–4536.
26. Khouri IF, Keating M, Körbling M, et al. Transplant-lite: induction of graft-versus-malignancy using fludarabine-based nonablative chemotherapy and allogeneic blood progenitor-cell transplantation as treatment for lymphoid malignancies. *J Clin Oncol* 1998;16:2817–2824.
27. Slavin S, Nagler A, Naparstek E, et al. Nonmyeloablative stem cell transplantation and cell therapy as an alternative to conventional bone marrow transplantation with lethal cytoreduction for the treatment of malignant and nonmalignant hematologic diseases. *Blood* 1998;91:756–763.
28. Nagler A, Slavin S, Varadi G, et al. Allogeneic peripheral blood stem cell transplantation using a fludarabine-based low intensity conditioning regimen for malignant lymphoma. *Bone Marrow Transplant* 2000;25:1021–1028.
29. Childs R, Clave E, Contentin N, et al. Engraftment kinetics after nonmyeloablative allogeneic peripheral blood stem cell transplantation: full donor T-cell chimerism precedes alloimmune responses. *Blood* 1999;94:3234–3241.
30. Spitzer TR, McAfee S, Sackstein R, et al. Intentional induction of mixed chimerism and achievement of antitumor responses after nonmyeloablative conditioning therapy and HLA-matched donor bone marrow transplantation for refractory hematologic malignancies. *Biol Blood Marrow Transplant* 2000;6:309–320.
31. Wäsch R, Reisser S, Hahn J, et al. Rapid achievement of complete donor chimerism and low regimen-related toxicity after reduced conditioning with fludarabine, carmustine, melphalan and allogeneic transplantation. *Bone Marrow Transplant* 2000;26:243–250.
32. Kottaridis PD, Milligan DW, Chopra R, et al. In vivo CAMPATH-1H prevents graft-versus-host disease following nonmyeloablative stem cell transplantation. *Blood* 2000;96:2419–2425.
33. Carella AM, Cavaliere M, Lerma E, et al. Autografting followed by nonmyeloablative immunosuppressive chemotherapy and allogeneic peripheral-blood hematopoietic stem-cell transplantation as treatment of resistant Hodgkin's disease and non-Hodgkin's lymphoma. *J Clin Oncol* 2000;18:3918–3924.
34. Sandmaier BM, Maloney DG, Gooley T, et al. Nonmyeloablative hematopoietic stem cell transplants (HSCT) from HLA-matched related donors for patients with hematologic malignancies: clinical results of a TBI-based conditioning regimen. *Blood* 2001;98(Pt 1):742a–743a [Abstract #3093].
35. Chun HG, Leyland-Jones B, Cheson BD. Fludarabine phosphate: a synthetic purine antimetabolite with significant activity against lymphoid malignancies. *J Clin Oncol* 1991;9:175–188.
36. Cheson BD. Infectious and immunosuppressive complications of purine analog therapy [review]. *J Clin Oncol* 1995;13:2431–2448.
37. Sykes M, Preffer F, McAfee S, et al. Mixed lymphohaemopoietic chimerism and graft-versus-lymphoma effects after non-myeloablative therapy and HLA-mismatched bone-marrow transplantation. *Lancet* 1999;353:1755–1759.
38. Chakraverty R, Peggs K, Chopra R, et al. Limiting transplantation-related mortality following unrelated donor stem cell transplantion by using a nonmyeloablative conditioning regimen. *Blood* 2002;99:1071–1078.
39. Negrier S, Escudier B, Lasset C, et al. Recombinant human interleukin-2, recombinant human interferon alfa-2a, or both in metastatic renal-cell carcinoma. Groupe Francais d'Immunotherapie. *N Engl J Med* 1998;338:1272–1278.
40. Childs R, Chernoff A, Contentin N, et al. Regression of metastatic renal-cell carcinoma after nonmyeloablative allogeneic peripheral-blood stem-cell transplantation. *N Engl J Med* 2000;343:750–758.

41. Amrolia P, Gaspar HB, Hassan A, et al. Nonmyeloablative stem cell transplantation for congenital immunodeficiencies. *Blood* 2000;96:1239–1246.
42. Horwitz ME, Barrett AJ, Brown MR, et al. Treatment of chronic granulomatous disease with nonmyeloablative conditioning and a T-cell-depleted hematopoietic allograft. *N Engl J Med* 2001;344:881–888.
43. Storb R, Yu C, Wagner JL, et al. Stable mixed hematopoietic chimerism in DLA-identical littermate dogs given sublethal total body irradiation before and pharmacological immunosuppression after marrow transplantation. *Blood* 1997;89:3048–3054.
44. McSweeney PA, Niederwieser D, Shizuru JA, et al. Hematopoietic cell transplantation in older patients with hematologic malignancies: replacing high-dose cytotoxic therapy with graft-versus-tumor effects. *Blood* 2001;97:3390–3400.
45. Maris M, Niederwieser D, Sandmaier B, et al. HLA-matched unrelated donor hematopoietic cell transplantation after nonmyeloablative conditioning for patients with hematologic malignancies. *Blood* 2003;102:2021–2030.
46. Bensinger WI, Buckner CD, Anasetti C, et al. Allogeneic marrow transplantation for multiple myeloma: an analysis of risk factors on outcome. *Blood* 1996;88:2787–2793.
47. Gahrton G, Tura S, Ljungman P, et al. Prognostic factors in allogeneic bone marrow transplantation for multiple myeloma. *J Clin Oncol* 1995;13:1312–1322.
48. Lokhorst HM, Schattenberg A, Cornelissen JJ, et al. Donor leukocyte infusions are effective in relapsed multiple myeloma after allogeneic bone marrow transplantation. *Blood* 1997;90:4206–4211.
49. Maloney DG, Sahebi F, Stockerl-Goldstein KE, et al. Allografting with non-myeloablative conditioning following cytoreductive autografts for the treatment of patients with multiple myeloma. *Blood*, in press.
50. Radich JP, Gooley T, Sanders JE, et al. Second allogeneic transplantation after failure of first autologous transplantation. *Biol Blood Marrow Transplant* 2000;6:272–279.
51. de Lima M, van Besien KW, Giralt SA, et al. Bone marrow transplantation after failure of autologous transplant for non-Hodgkin's lymphoma. *Bone Marrow Transplant* 1997;19:121–127.
52. Ringdén O, Labopin M, Gorin NC, et al. The dismal outcome in patients with acute leukaemia who relapse after an autograft is improved if a second autograft or a matched allograft is performed. *Bone Marrow Transplant* 2000;25:1053–1058.
53. Mehta J, Tricot G, Jagannath S, et al. Salvage autologous or allogeneic transplantation for multiple myeloma refractory to or relapsing after a first-line autograft? *Bone Marrow Transplant* 1998;21:887–892.
54. Tsai T, Goodman S, Saez R, et al. Allogeneic bone marrow transplantation in patients who relapse after autologous transplantation. *Bone Marrow Transplant* 1997;20:859–863.
55. Ringdén O, Labopin M, Frassoni F, et al. Allogeneic bone marrow transplant or second autograft in patients with acute leukemia who relapse after an autograft. *Bone Marrow Transplant* 1999;24:389–396.
56. Bosi A, Laszlo D, Labopin M, et al. Second allogeneic bone marrow transplantation in acute leukemia: results of a survey by the European Cooperative Group for Blood and Marrow Transplantation. *J Clin Oncol* 2001;19:3675–3684.
57. Nagler A, Or R, Naparstek E, et al. Second allogeneic stem cell transplantation using nonmyeloablative conditioning for patients who relapsed or developed secondary malignancies following autologous transplantation. *Exp Hematol* 2000;28:1096–1104.
58. Dey BR, McAfee S, Sackstein R, et al. Successful allogeneic stem cell transplantation with nonmyeloablative conditioning in patients with relapsed hematologic malignancy following autologus stem cell transplantation. *Biol Blood Marrow Transplant* 2001;7:604–612.
59. Devine SM, Sanborn R, Jessop E, et al. Fludarabine and melphalan-based conditioning for patients with advanced hematological malignancies relapsing after a previous hematopoietic stem cell transplant. *Bone Marrow Transplant* 2001;28:557–562.
60. Feinstein LC, Sandmaier BM, Maloney DG, et al. Allografting after nonmyeloablative conditioning as a treatment after a failed conventional hematopoietic cell transplant. *Biol Blood Marrow Transplant* 2003;9:266–272.
61. Carlens S, Remberger M, Aschan J, et al. The role of disease stage in the response to donor lymphocyte infusions as treatment for leukemic relapse. *Biol Blood Marrow Transplant* 2001;7:31–38.
62. Shlomchik WD, Couzens MS, Tang CB, et al. Prevention of graft versus host disease by inactivation of host antigen-presenting cells. *Science* 1999;285:412–415.
63. Andreani M, Nesci S, Lucarelli G, et al. Long-term survival of ex-thalassemic patients with persistent mixed chimerism after bone marrow transplantation. *Bone Marrow Transplant* 2000;25:401–404.

64. Andreani M, Manna M, Lucarelli G, et al. Persistence of mixed chimerism in patients transplanted for the treatment of thalassemia. *Blood* 1996;87:3494–3499.
65. Walters MC, Patience M, Leisenring W, et al. Collaborative multicenter investigation of marrow transplantation for sickle cell disease: current results and future directions. *Biol Blood Marrow Transplant* 1997;3:310–315.
66. Walters MC, Storb R, Patience M, et al. Impact of bone marrow transplantation for symptomatic sickle cell disease: an interim report. *Blood* 2000;95:1918–1924.
67. Vermylen C, Cornu G, Ferster A, et al. Haematopoietic stem cell transplantation for sickle cell anaemia: the first 50 patients transplanted in Belgium. *Bone Marrow Transplant* 1998;22:1–6.
68. Georges GE, Storb R, Thompson JD, et al. Adoptive immunotherapy in canine mixed chimeras after nonmyeloablative hematopoietic cell transplantation. *Blood* 2000;95:3262–3269.
69. Storb R, Yu C, Zaucha JM, et al. Stable mixed hematopoietic chimerism in dogs given donor antigen, CTLA4Ig, and 100 cGy total body irradiation before and pharmacologic immunosuppression after marrow transplant. *Blood* 1999;94:2523–2529.
70. Li S, Thanikachalam M, Pang M, et al. Combined host-conditioning with CTLA4-Ig, tacrolimus, anti-lymphocyte serum, and low-dose radiation leads to stable mixed hematopoietic chimerism. *Exp Hematol* 2001;29:534–541.
71. Sandmaier BM, Bethge WA, Wilbur DS, et al. Bismuth-213 labeled anti-CD45 radioimmunoconjugate to condition dogs for nonmyeloablative allogeneic marrow grafts. *Blood*, 2002;100:318–326.
72. Fuchimoto Y, Huang CA, Yamada K, et al. Mixed chimerism and tolerance without whole body irradiation in a large animal model. *J Clin Invest* 2000;105:1779–1789.
73. Bachar-Lustig E, Rachamim N, Li HW, et al. Megadose of T cell-depleted bone marrow overcomes MHC barriers in sublethally irradiated mice. *Nature Med* 1995;1:1268–1273.
74. Yu XZ, Bidwell SJ, Martin PJ, et al. CD28-specific antibody prevents graft-versus-host disease in mice. *J Immunol* 2000;164:4564–4568.
75. Ito H, Kurtz J, Shaffer J, et al. CD4 T cell-mediated alloresistance to fully MHC-mismatched allogeneic bone marrow engraftment is dependent on CD40–CD40 ligand interactions, and lasting T cell tolerance is induced by bone marrow transplantation with initial blockade of this pathway. *J Immunol* 2001;166:2970–2981.
76. Sandmaier BM, Yu C, Gooley T, et al. Haploidentical stem cell allografts after nonmyeloablative therapy in a preclinical large animal model. *Blood* 1999;94(suppl 1):318a [Abstract 1424].
77. Bensinger WI, Martin PJ, Storer B, et al. Transplantation of bone marrow as compared with peripheral-blood cells from HLA-identical relatives in patients with hematologic cancers. *N Engl J Med* 2001;344:175–181.
78. Powles R, Mehta J, Kulkarni S, et al. Allogeneic blood and bone-marrow stem-cell transplantation in haematological malignant diseases: a randomised trial. *Lancet* 2000;355:1231–1237.
79. Heldal D, Tjonnfjord GE, Brinch L, et al. A randomised study of allogeneic transplantation with stem cells from blood or bone marrow. *Bone Marrow Transplant* 2000;25:1129–1136.
80. Champlin RE, Schmitz N, Horowitz MM, et al. Blood stem cells compared with bone marrow as a source of hematopoietic cells for allogeneic transplantation. *Blood* 2000;95:3702–3709.
81. Mohty M, Faucher C, Vey N, et al. High rate of secondary viral and bacterial infections in patients undergoing allogeneic bone marrow mini-transplantation. *Bone Marrow Tranplant* 2000;26:251–255.
82. Junghanss C, Boeckh M, Carter RA, et al. Incidence and outcome of cytomegalovirus infections following nonmyeloablative compared with myeloablative allogeneic stem cell transplantation, a matched control study. *Blood* 2002;99:1978–1985.

Index